Principles of
Animal Nutrition and
Feed Technology
Third Edition

Principles of
Animal Nutrition and
Feed Technology
Third Edition

DV Reddy BVSc, MVSc, PhD
Professor and Head
Department of Animal Nutrition
Rajiv Gandhi College of Veterinary and
Animal Sciences, Puducherry

Oxford & IBH Publishing Co. Pvt. Ltd.
New Delhi
(*A Unit of* CBS Publishers & Distributors Pvt Ltd)

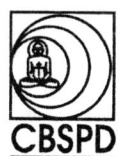

CBSPD

CBS Publishers & Distributors Pvt Ltd

New Delhi • Bengaluru • Chennai • Kochi • Kolkata • Lucknow • Mumbai
Hyderabad • Jharkhand • Nagpur • Patna • Pune • Uttarakhand

Principles of
Animal Nutrition and
Feed Technology
Third Edition

ISBN-13: 978-81-204-1796-0
ISBN-10: 81-204-1796-8

OXFORD & IBH
New Delhi
(A Unit of CBS Publishers & Distributors Pvt Ltd)

Published by **Satish Kumar Jain** and produced by **Varun Jain** for

CBS Publishers & Distributors Pvt Ltd
4819/XI Prahlad Street, 24 Ansari Road, Daryaganj, New Delhi 110 002, India.
Ph: 011-23289259, 23266861
Fax: 011-23243014
Website: www.cbspd.com
e-mail: delhi@cbspd.com

Corporate Office: 204 FIE, Industrial Area, Patparganj, Delhi 110 092
Ph: 011-4934 4934
Fax: 011-4934 4935
e-mail: publishing@cbspd.com; publicity@cbspd.com

Branches

- **Bengaluru:** Seema House 2975, 17th Cross, KR Road, Banasankari 2nd Stage, Bengaluru 560 070, Karnataka, India
  Ph: +91-80-26771678/79   Fax: +91-80-26771680   e-mail: bangalore@cbspd.com
- **Chennai:** 7, Subbaraya Street, Shenoy Nagar, Chennai 600 030, Tamil Nadu, India
  Ph: +91-44-26680620, 26681266   Fax: +91-44-42032115   e-mail: chennai@cbspd.com
- **Kochi:** 42/1325, 1326, Power House Road, Opp KSEB, Power House, Ernakulum Kochi 682 018, Kerala, India
  Ph: +91-484-4059061-65,67   Fax: +91-484-4059065   e-mail: kochi@cbspd.com
- **Kolkata:** 147, Hind Ceramics Compound, 1st Floor, Nilgunj Road, Belghoria, Kolkata-700056, West Bengal, India
  Ph: +033-25633055, 033-25633056   e-mail: kolkata@cbspd.com
- **Lucknow:** Basement, Khushnuma Complex, 7 Meerabai Marg (Behind Jawahar Bhawan),Lucknow-226001, UP, India
  Ph: +0522-4000032   e-mail: tiwari.lucknow@cbspd.com
- **Mumbai:** PWD Shed, Gala no 25/26, Ramchandra Bhatt Marg, Next to JJ Hospital Gate no. 2, Opp. Union Bank of India, Noorbaug, Mumbai-400009, Maharashtra, India
  Ph: 022-66661880/89   e-mail: mumbai@cbspd.com

Representatives

• Hyderabad	0-9885175004	• Jharkhand	0-9811541605	• Nagpur	0-9421945513
• Patna	0-9334159340	• Pune	0-9923910676	• Uttarakhand	0-9716462459

Printed at Chaman Enterprises, Daryaganj, New Delhi, India

Preface to the Third Edition

The science of animal nutrition continues to advance. The third edition consists of 21 chapters with addition of new chapter 7 "Digestion, Absorption and Postabsorptive nutrient utilization". This new edition of the text has been extensively revised by way of adding several new flow charts and illustrations. Diagrams that integrate all key aspects of a metabolic pathway: the enzymes, intermediates and the mechanisms that guide and regulate metabolic flow help the student a quick grasp and better comprehension.

New information has been added in several chapters to make the textbook more meaningful; notably in chapter four: basics of biochemistry of carbohydrates, fats and proteins are described and illustrated in a user-friendly manner; in chapter six: gastrointestinal tract (GIT), its functions, control systems, gastric secretion and motility patterns of GIT are described and illustrated; carbohydrate metabolism and control of glucose metabolism are delineated with flow charts and illustrations in chapter eight; similarly lipid metabolism and fatty acid synthesis and oxidation are explained in chapter 10. **All these efforts have been made to meet the objective: "Complete information in a comprehensible way".**

Suggestions from students and colleagues from several veterinary colleges have been most helpful in the formulation of this edition. I am indebted to my students: to my undergraduates who have shared in my experiments with nutrition syllabuses and my postgraduates who motivated me to deliver on contemporary thoughts on the subject. For the same reasons I am indebted to my colleague teachers / researchers / extension workers in several institutions spread over the Indian Union. I give my heartfelt thanks to all.

I extend my sincere appreciation to Thiru V.Srinivasan, Librarian and Thiru B.Kumaran, Computer Assistant for their helpful attitude. I am thankful to the publishers for meticulous planning and publication of the textbook. Above all, I thank God for His guidance and inspiration.

January2016   **Duvvuru Venka Reddy**

Preface to the Second Edition

Eminent nutrition teachers and scientists gave rave reviews. My esteemed colleague teachers find them very useful. My beloved students follow them avidly.

The overwhelming response was visible.....demonstrated during my visits to some of the colleges. The enthusiastic response was expressed and gratitude was felt when students visited our department during their study tours.

Several of my colleagues in teaching and research institutes expressed 'Job is well done'. With all these expressions, I have the gratification of knowing that I have done my duty as mentioned in the Veterinarian's oath.

I 'thank you very much'. I request your feedback about my books corrections needed and suggestions to improve the text. I promise to take care all due things with acknowledgement.

I wish to make my book more effective as a teaching resource and as a comprehensive resource.

Yours sincerely

D.V. REDDY

Response to Feedback Request and Action Taken

Response to my request letters for feedback by post as well as by email had been quite substantial and satisfying, from all Veterinary Colleges and majority Animal and Veterinary Research Institutes of India. I am extremely grateful to all those of my colleagues and students who have offered numerous helpful suggestions.

Nutritional science is dynamic. Information on micronutrients and feed additives to further the nutrient utilization in precision animal nutrition mode, for a profitable enterprise, animal well-being and consumer food safety is rapidly changing. Accordingly, new useful information has been added in several of those related chapters to update them; chapter 18: conservation of fodders has been thoroughly revised; new useful information has been provided in Appendix II in an effort to make the textbook a more complete text on Principles of Animal Nutrition and Feed Technology.

I take this opportunity to express my thanks to Messrs Oxford & IBH Publishing Co. Pvt. Ltd., New Delhi for meticulous planning and intelligent publishing of the book.

June 2010

Duvvuru Venka Reddy

Preface to the First Edition

There are several textbooks on Animal Nutrition and Feeding written by eminent teachers and scientists. But no single textbook caters the needs of undergraduate students of Veterinary Science by providing all the needed information comprehensively on Animal Nutrition subject at a single source. As per the Veterinary Council of India (Minimum Standards of Veterinary Education Degree Course-BVSC and AH) Regulations, 1993, Animal Nutrition courses encompass principles of animal nutrition, evaluation of feedstuffs and feed technology and applied nutrition covering feeding of livestock, poultry, human beings, pet, rabbit and laboratory animals. The examination system comprises an internal assessment (50%) at the end of each semester and an external assessment (50%) conducted by an annual board appointed by the university at the end of the academic year. The new syllabus and the examination system make the student and the teacher as well, to run to different sources for procuring the needed information for each of the four Animal Nutrition courses (ANN 211, ANN 212, ANN 221 and ANN 222). Being in the teaching line since 1981 and specifically teaching Animal Nutrition as per the new syllabus since its introduction from 1995, I have prepared the manuscript. It will be published as two books: 1. Principles of Animal Nutrition and Feed Technology and 2. Applied Nutrition (Livestock, Poultry, Human, Pet, Rabbit and Laboratory Animal Nutrition).

Each textbook consists of two sections (Part I and II) and thus the four sections correspond to the four courses. Each section provides a structured approach to learning by covering all the topics in a uniform, systematic format. This (section – or) course-wise topic-led organization is a distinct advantage of these books since they meet the needs of the students for each course of Animal Nutrition Semester-wise. Some of the topics have been detailed beyond the syllabus level to enlarge the knowledge of the readers because of their importance in applied feeding practice, for example feed additives. These books are designed to give students rapid, easy access to all the material in a course wise format which benefits them prepare for the internal examinations and external examinations economically and ensure exploit their potential to a greater extent. The topics are detailed in a straightforward and hopefully lucid manner. "Complete information in a comprehensible way" is the watchword of the books.

These textbooks are also useful to teachers and scientists of department of Animal Nutrition, personnel of feed industry involved in feed manufacturing and marketing, postgraduate students of Animal Sciences i.e. Animal Nutrition, Avian Production and Management, Livestock Production and Management and Animal Husbandry Extension. Further, they are useful to field veterinarians, extension workers of departments of Animal Husbandry and Dairying and Rural Development, Progressive Animal farmers and Animal lovers. I appreciate the contribution of my wife, Prasuna and children, Amar and Vamsee for providing me cheerful environment and allowing me to spend many hours with drafts of manuscripts rather than with them.

January 2001   *Duvvuru Venka Reddy*

Suggested Reference Books

1. **ANIMAL NUTRITION**
   by L.A. Maynard, J.K. Loosli, H.F. Hintz and R.G. Warner, 7th edition, 1979.

2. **ANIMAL NUTRITION**
   by P McDonald, R A Edwards, J F D Greenhalgh, C A Morgan, L A Sinclair and R G Wilkinson, 7th edition, Pearson Education Limited, United Kingdom, 2011, 7th Revised edition.

3. **FEEDS AND PRINCIPLES OF ANIMAL NUTRITION**
   (Revised edition of Animal Nutrition) by G.C. Banerjee, 1st edition, 1988. Reprint 1998, 1999.

4. **VITAMINS IN ANIMAL NUTRITION** (Comparative Aspects to Human Nutrition) by L.R. McDowell, 1st edition, 1989.

5. **MINERALS IN ANIMAL AND HUMAN NUTRITION**
   by L.R. McDowell, 1st edition, 1992.

6. **ANIMAL NUTRITION**
   by J.W. Lassiter and H.M. Edwards, Jr. 1st edition, 1982.

7. **TRACE ELEMENTS IN HUMAN AND ANIMAL NUTRITION**
   by E.J. Underwood, 4th edition 1977, 5th edition by Walter Mertz, 1987.

8. **THE MINERAL NUTRITION OF LIVESTOCK**
   by E.J. Underwood and N.F. Suttle, 3rd edition, 1999.

9. **THE RUMEN AND ITS MICROBES**
   by R.E. Hungate, Ist edition, 1966.

10. **ADVANCED ANIMAL NUTRITION FOR DEVELOPING COUNTRIES**
    edited by U.B. Singh, 1st edition, 1987.

11. **ADVANCES IN DAIRY ANIMAL PRODUCTION**
    by V. D. Mudgal , K.K. Singhal and D.D. Sharma, 1st edition, 1995.

12. **COMMERCIAL POULTRY NUTRITION**
    by S. Leeson and J.D. Summers, 1st Indian reprint, 1993.

13. **APPLIED ANIMAL NUTRITION**
    by E.W. Crampton and L.E. Harris, 2nd edition, 1968.

14. **LIVESTOCK FEEDING**
    by S.N. Ray; 1st edition, 1978.

15. **ANIMAL NUTRITION IN THE TROPICS**
    by S.K. Ranjhan, 4th edition, 1997.

16. **AGROINDUSTRIAL BYPRODUCTS AND NONCONVEN-TIONAL FEEDS FOR LIVESTOCK FEEDING**
    by S.K. Ranjhan, 1st edition, 1990.

17. **CHEMICAL COMPOSITION AND NUTRITIVE VALUE OF INDIAN FEEDS AND FEEDING OF FARM ANIMALS**
    by S.K. Ranjhan, 1st edition, 1991.

18. **NUTRITIVE VALUE OF INDIAN CATTLE FEEDS AND FEEDING OF ANIMALS**
    by K.C. Sen, S.N. Ray and S.K. Ranjhan, 6th edition, 1978.

19. **TEXTBOOK OF FEED PROCESSING TECHNOLOGY**
    by N.N. Pathak, 1st edition, 1997.

20. **NUTRIENT REQUIREMENTS OF LIVESTOCK AND POULTRY**
    by S.K. Ranjhan, 2nd revised edition, 1998.

21. **FEEDING OF POULTRY**
    by B. Panda, V.R. Reddy, V.R. Sadagopan and A.K. Shrivastav, 1st edition, 1984.

22. **DICTIONARY OF ANIMAL NUTRITION AND FEED TECHNOLOGY**
    by K.K. Singhal, 1st edition, 1992.

23. **CLINICAL NUTRITION OF THE DOG AND CAT**
    by J.W. Simpson, R.S. Anderson and P.J. Markwell, 1st edition, 1993.

24. **THE WALTHAM BOOK OF CLINICAL NUTRITION OF THE DOG AND CAT**
    by J.M. Wills and K.W. Simpson, 1st edition, 1994.

25. **NUTRITIVE VALUE OF INDIAN FOODS**
    by National Institute of Nutrition, Indian Council of Medical Research, 1989.

26. **CUNNINGHAM'S TEXTBOOK OF VETERINARY PHYSIOLOGY**
    by Bradley G. Klein, 5th edition, 2013 Published by Elsevier Saunders, USA; section IV: Physiology of the Gastrointestinal tract by Thomas H. Herdt and Ayman I. Sayegh, pp263-358.

27. **ANTHONY'S TEXTBOOK OF ANATOMY & PHYSIOLOGY**
    20th edition, 2013.

28. **ESSENTIALS OF ANATOMY AND PHYSIOLOGY**
    by K.T.Patton et al., 2012.

29. **PHYSIOLOGY OF DOMESTIC ANIMALS**
    by Oystein V.Sjaastad, Knut Hove and Olav Sand, 1st edition 2003 Scandinavian Veterinary Press, Oslo (Norwy), first Indian reprint 2005 by International Book Distributing Co, Lucknow, pp 489-579.

30. **HARPER'S ILLUSTRATED BIOCHEMISTRY**
    by Robert K. Murray, Daryl K. Granner and Victor W. Rodwell 27th International Edition, 2006 Published by The McGraw-Hill Companies, Inc.

31. **PRINCIPLES OF BIOCHEMISTRY, INTERNATIONAL STUDENT VERSION**
    4th edition, Wiley Plus; 2013.

Contents

Part I
Principles of Animal Nutrition

What is nutrition? antoine lavoisier, father of the science of nutrition, the origin of life–biological molecules arose from inorganic materials, living organisms, prokaryotes and Eukaryotes, molecular data reveal three evolutionary domains of organisms, objective of nutrition, babcock single plant experiments, role of laboratory animals in discovery of nutrients, role of specialists in expansion of nutritional knowledge, importance of nutrients in animal health and production, essentiality of nutrients in animal health and production, soil-plant-animal relationship, precision animal nutrition concept.

Dief of animals, factors that affect the chemical composition of the forage, composition of animal body, composition of plants and animal products, main reasons.

Proximate composition, importance of proximate analysis, digestion and metabolism, proximate principles, significance of moisture content of feeds, detergent method of forage analysis—main features, chemical constituents of weende and van soest schemes for feed analysis, modern analytical methods, non-structural carbohydrates (NSC) and non-starch polysaccharides (NSP), methods for measurement of NSP fall into two categories, contribution of NSP, resistant starch (RS), the cornell net carbohydrate and protein system (CNCPS), spectroscopy and chromatography, near-infrared reflectance spectroscopy (NIRS), nuclear magnetic resonance spectroscopy (NMRS), classification of carbohydrates, monosaccharides and their derivatives, glycosides, oligosaccharides, polysaccharides, glucosaminans, heteroglycans, pectic substances, hemicellulose, exudate gums and acid mucilages, hyaluronic acid and chondroitin, classification of carbohydrates by dietary form, fibre carbohydrates and non-fibre carbohydrates, physically effective fibre (peNDF), proteins, amino acids, amino acids found in natural proteins, essential amino acids, dispensable and indispensable amino acids, amino acid requirements for several species, critical and limiting amino acids, forms of amino acids, their utilisation and interconversion, classification of proteins, nucleic acids, nucleoside and nucleotide, amines, amides, lipids, the noncaloric functions of fat, essential fatty acids (EFAs), nomenclature, omega-3 and 6 fatty acids or n-3 and n-6 fatty acids, conjugated linoleic acid (CLA), properties of fats of nutritional significance, auto-oxidation of methylene-interrupted unsaturated fatty acid, eicosanoids, functions of essential fatty acids, sources of EFA, deficiency symptoms of EFA, toxicity of EFA, glycolipids, galactolipids, glycosphingolipids, phospholipids, phosphoglycerides or glycerophospholipids, lecithins, cephalin, plasmalogens, sphingomyelins or sphingopho-spholipids, waxes, steroids, sterols, 7-dehydrocholesterol, ergosterol, steroid hormones, terpenes, amphipathic lipids.

5. **The Role and Requirement of Water**   81–86
Role of water, properties and functions of water, sources of water, metabolic or oxidation water, factors governing the water requirements of livestock and poultry, effect of excess of water, effect of lack of water, effects of water deprivation, water economy among animals, nature of nitrogenous end product, mammals, birds, nutrients and toxic elements in water.

hindgut, the rate of fermentation and VFA production in the equine colon is similar to that in the rumen, postabsorptive nutrient utilization, regulation of energy-supplying nutrients, fuel metabolism, general scheme of metabolism during the absorptive phase, the conversion of glucose to fatty acids is an irreversible process, transport of fatty acids out of the liver is through chylomicron-like particles known as VLDLs, amino acids are extensively modified during absorption, general scheme of metabolism during the postabsorptive phase, hepatic metabolism switches to glucose production during the postabsorptive phase, the reaction of adipose tissue during the postabsorptive phase is to mobilize fatty acids, general scheme of metabolism during prolonged catabolic periods, a large portion of the fatty acids released from adipose tissue is taken up directly by the liver, fatty acids cannot be used for glucose synthesis, hepatic VLDLs may be synthesized from adipose-derived fatty acid as well as from newly synthesized fatty acid, hormonal conditions direct the distribution of VLDL fatty acids in the body, special fuel considerations of ruminants, ruminants exist in a perpetual state of gluconeogenesis because of their unique digestive process, efficient conservation of glucose in ruminants, lactational ketosis in dairy cows and pregnancy toxemia in ewes and does control of glucose metabolism, glucose is always required by the central nervous system and erythrocytes, homeostasis of blood glucose concentration.

and oxidation of fat, glycerol metabolism, β-oxidation of fatty acids occurs in mitochondria, importance of carnitine in fatty acid oxidation, oxidation of unsaturated fatty acids, peroxisomal β oxidation, oxidation of unsaturated fatty acids, comparison of fatty acid synthesis and oxidation, conversion of fat into glucose, interrelations among fats, proteins and carbohydrates.

toxicity, chromium toxicity in humans, nickel (Ni), symptoms of deficiency, effects of lead poisoning and symptoms, organic minerals, chelation, balanced trace element nutrition helps to neutralize oxidative stress.

animal feeds, absorbable and nonabsorbable antibiotics, ban on the antibiotic growth promoters, the effects of these in-feed antibiotics, potential consequences of a ban on growth-promoting antibiotics, sulfa drugs, arsenicals, copper supplements, hormones, anabolic hormones; catabolic hormones; exogenous hormones and their effect, exogenous bovine somatotropin (bST) injections, milk production, meat production, porcine somatotropin (pST), equine somatotropin (eST), thyroprotein and goitrogens, β-adrenergic agonists (β-agonists), clenbuterol, cimaterol, ractopamine, immunomodulators, growth promoters for fattening ruminants, coccidiostats, use of hormones in animal production and food safety, phytoestrogens, feed enzyme additives, commercial feed enzymes, probiotics, yeast culture and acidifiers, characteristics of a good probiotic, pigs and probiotics, poultry and probiotics, yeast culture, yeast cultures vs yeast blends, live yeast culture as a feed additive, examples of commercial preparations, mannan oligosaccharides (MOS), fructo oligosaccharides (FOS), prebiotics, silver nanoparticles, nanoparticles, direct-fed microbials (DFM), direct-fed microbials (DFM) for calves, acidifiers, organic acids, antioxidants, sequestrants, mycotoxin binders, commercial preparations, anticaking agents, humectants, firming and crisping agents, preservatives, antifungal agents, deodourising agents, flavouring agents, flavour in poultry feed, food colours, pigments, pellet binders, buffers, magnesium oxide, sodium bentonite, sodium bicarbonate for poultry, pigs, methane inhibitors, roughage substitutes, propionate production promoters, defaunating agents, ketosis controlling agents, bloat controlling compounds, microbial growth factors (for ruminants), surfactants, sweetening agents, tranquilizers, emulsifiers, stabilizer, bile acid, nutraceuticals, essential oils, methyl donors, feed odditives for transition cows, feed additive sweeteners, amino acids, commercial preparations, carnitine, β-carotene, niacin, encapsulated nutrients, meat and bone meal (MBM), dicalcium phosphate, chromium supplement.

Part II
Evaluation of Feedstuffs and Feed Technology

monogastric animals, weight gain methods, nitrogen balance experiments, calculation of BV of a protein, body nitrogen retention method, estimation of protein quality from amino acid composition, amino acid availability, estimation of the availability of amino acids, ileal digestibility of protein, ileal digestibility and faecal digestibility, measures of protein quality used in practice in the feeding of pigs and poultry, ideal protein concept, measures of protein quality for ruminants, protein rationing, characterization of proteins in feeds, cornell net carbohydrate and protein system (CNCPS), methods for estimating RUP digestibility.

roughages, ammoniation through urea hydrolysis, effect of ammonia treatment on feeding value of wheat straw, biological treatments, indo-dutch project on bioconversion of crop residues, complete feed manufacturing machine, densified feed blocks, expander-extruder processing of complete feeds.

Part I
Principles of Animal Nutrition

Chapter 1

Contribution of Scientists of the Past Years to the Science of Animal Nutrition

An appreciation of the history of earlier discoveries can stimulate future progress.

A person can't appreciate the present or contemplate the future without an awareness of the past!

Santario Sanctorius (1561-1636) of Italy weighed himself on a balance before and after eating food, to find out what happened to the food. His weight increased by the amount of food he consumed which came to original after a time. But what happened to the food he could not answer. This is the first experiment on human metabolism.

Antoine Laurent de Lavoisier (1743-1794) of France introduced the balance and thermometer into nutrition studies. He discovered that combustion was an oxidation and he showed that respiration in the body involved the combination of carbon and hydrogen with oxygen from inspired air and that the quantities of oxygen absorbed and carbon dioxide given off dependent on the food intake and the work done. With Laplace (1749-1827), he designed a (animal) calorimeter by means of which it was demonstrated that respiration is the essential source of body heat. He stated that life is a chemical process. He is acknowledged as the 'Founder of the science of nutrition'/'Father of Nutrition' 'Father of Modern chemistry'. The science of nutrition was undoubtedly set back many years when Lavoisier's career was ended by the guillotine.

Lazaro Spallanzani (1729-1799) of Italy swallowed linen bags containing meat and bread and retrieved by strings attached to them periodically and found some chemical changes that took place.

G.J. Mulder (Netherlands) gave the name 'Protein' to nitrogenous food. The term protein means 'to take first place'.

Francois Magendie (1783-1855) the great French Physiologist, is recognized as the 'founder' of the modern experimental method in animal-feeding experiments. He employed diets of pure carbohydrates and fats to prove that food nitrogen is essential. In 1816, he stated that N present in the body had its origin in N compounds present in food. He published 'gelatin report' in 1841 which conclusively stated that all proteins were not of equal value. Later Escher and Kauffmann reported that gelatin was deficient in tyrosine and cystine.

Justus von Liebig (1803-1873) was the foremost organic chemist of his time and is frequently spoken of as the 'founder of agricultural chemistry'. He was the father of the modern methods of organic analysis. He postulated that nitrogenous compounds, which comprised the complex chemical group of proteins in feeds, were utilized by the animal for body building and the nonprotein materials were oxidized to produce heat.

Agricultural Science owes a tremendous debt to John B. Lawes (1814-1900) and Joseph H. Gilbert (1817-1901) for their pioneer work in the fields of agronomy and animal nutrition, begun in 1843 and continued for over half a century. The famous English Scientists performed the pioneer and laborious task of analyzing the entire bodies of farm animals.

Stephen M. Babcock (1843-1931) is most widely known for his invention, the Babcock test. He made many pioneer contributions in the fields of dairy chemistry and animal nutrition. Following six years at the New York Experiment Station, he served for twenty five years as chemist and Assistant Director at the Wisconsin Experiment Station.

He conceived the idea of trying out rations made up entirely from a single plant. He carried out feeding experiments with cows, heifer calves on rations made entirely from the corn, wheat, oat plants. This experiment made it clear that there were marked differences in nutrition values which could not be detected by any chemical means available at that time. The experiment, more importantly, led to the conviction that simplified diets must be used for the solution of nutritional problems.

It stimulated the use of the purified-diet method, which resulted in the discovery of the first Vitamin in 1913. This purified-diet method has been so largely responsible for the newer knowledge of nutrition.

Nathan Zuntz (1847-1920) was a pioneer in the field of basal metabolism and in respiration studies with farm animals. He developed the first portable respiration apparatus. Trained as a physician, he preferred to become a teacher and investigator in physiology, first at Bonn and later at Berlin. He devoted himself particularly to work with farm animals and to basic problems related to their nutrition. His publications, numbering over 400, deal with a wide variety of physiological problems. He was the first to formulate clearly the "fermentation" hypothesis to explain the mechanism of forage utilization by ruminants in 1879. That asparagine could support weight gain and a positive nitrogen balance in sheep (Weiske et al., 1879) led to **Zuntz's hypothesis** (1891) that microorganisms of the rumen might synthesize their cell protein from simple nitrogenous components and so effect a saving of the dietary protein. The research on synthesis of protein by ruminants was thus based on the feeding on NPN substrates such as urea, amide, ammonium salts, etc., as there could be an economic advantage in such practice.

Wilbur Olin Atwater (1844-1907) served for thirty five years as Professor of Chemistry at Wesleyan University, Middle town, Conn.

In 1892, with the assistance of E.B. Rosa, Professor of Physics at Wesleyan, Atwater began the construction of the first human-respiration calorimeter which he later employed in his pioneer studies of heat production in man, of energy requirements for various body functions and of the nutritive value of foods.

Oscar Kellner (1851-1911), following short periods of service in the agricultural experiment stations at Proskau and Hohenhein and an extended period as professor of agricultural chemistry at the University of Tokyo, became director of the experiment station at Mockern, Germany in 1893. Here he served until his death. His many accurately conducted respiration studies with farm animals made a large contribution to the fundamental knowledge of nutritional physiology and found practical application in his feeding standards, starch equivalent system of energy evaluation.

Henry Prentiss Armsby (1851-1921), following periods of service at the New Jersey, Connecticut, and Wisconsin Experiment Stations, became director of the newly established Pennsylvania Experiment Station at State College in 1887. In 1907 the Institute of Animal Nutrition was established at this Institution with Armsby as Director, and here he served until his death, winning lasting fame for himself and his institute.

He constructed a respiration calorimeter for farm animals and studied heat production in cattle. These epoch-making studies, led to the development of the net energy system of evaluating feeds.

Thomas B. Osborne (1859-1929), Lafayette B. Mendel (1872-1935) collaborated in nutrition research for over twenty years. They had outstanding discoveries particularly in the fields of proteins and vitamins. Osborne and Mendel published their work on classic purified diet studies. In 1909 Osborne and Mendel began their classic purified diet studies with rats using pure proteins and supplemented with various amino acids and found that nutritional quality of certain proteins could be maintained by the addition of missing amino acids. Osborne became the leading authority of the world on the vegetable proteins while Mendel made many important contributions on various aspects of nutritional physiology.

Max Rubner (1854-1932), served for over 40 years at the University of Berlin, first as Professor of hygiene and later of physiology. He made many pioneer contributions to the science of nutrition, particularly in the field of energy metabolism. He showed that carbohydrate and fat were interchangeable in metabolism on the basis of energy equivalents.

H.H. Mitchell (1886-1966) received his bachelor's degree and doctorate in chemistry at the Illinois State University, USA, where he rose to Professor and Head of the division of Animal Nutrition. He was an outstanding teacher and investigator. He published his two-volume work, 'Comparative Nutrition of Man and Domestic Animals', Academic Press, New York in 1963.

F.B. Morrison (1887-1958), worked at the University of Wisconsin and Cornell University. He wrote 'Feeds and Feeding' which was first published in 1936.

Leonard Amby Maynard (1887-1972), a doctorate in chemistry, worked in different capacities at Cornell University, USA. Many students were attracted to Cornell University because of his ability in teaching and inspiring students in nutrition research. As chairman of the NRC committee on Animal Nutrition in 1942, he was responsible to prepare Recommended Nutrient Allowances for various farm animals. His research included studies on the requirements of minerals, amino acids and vitamins; the development of purified diets; utilization and metabolism of protein, minerals and lipids in feed supplies especially for lactating animals. He authored a book on Animal Nutrition, first published in 1937 which is a very popular textbook.

Max Kleiber (1893-1976): Studied in Switzerland in agricultural chemistry and energy metabolism. He constructed a respiration apparatus at the University of California, Davis for energy metabolism studies with large animals. He developed the use of weight to the 0.75 power instead of surface area to describe energy metabolism.

R.W. Swift (1895-1975): Devoted much of his career to studies on energy metabolism with the Armsby calorimeter.

In 1884 Tappeiner in Germany showed that large quantities of VFA, notably acetic acid, were produced from the *in vitro* fermentation of cellulose by bacteria from the rumen of the ox. Quantitative knowledge of this rumen activity and of its role in nutrition has developed particularly through the use of the permanent rumen fistula technique described in 1886 by the French Physiologist Colin.

Pioneering studies on ruminant digestive physiology were carried out by Barcroft and coworkers at Cambridge during 1940s. Knowledge of quantitative digestion and metabolism in ruminants was developed most rapidly when isotope dilution techniques become easy to apply, facilitated by improved instrumentation and mathematical approaches. Annisan and Lindsay contributed substantially to our knowledge of cellular metabolism and quantitative nutrition of ruminants with the help of isotope dilution techniques linked to arteriovenous difference measurements and blood flow data. The opportunity arose for the first time to examine ketone body metabolism in the whole animal (Leng and Annison, 1964) when radioactivity labelled β-hydroxy butyrate was first prepared by incubating C^{14}-butyrate with sheep liver slices *in vitro*.

Leng and Nolan using the isotope dilution and also the stable isotope of $N(N^{15})$ provided detailed information on VFA production and N transactions in the reticulo rumen.

Kurt Nehring a German agricultural chemist, strongly promoted the development of agricultural chemistry and soil science in Rostock and in particular the development of animal nutrition and science of evaluating feedstuff. He was instrumental in getting the "Oscar Kellner-Institute for Animal Nutrition" established in Rostock. He had worked out the Rostock system of feed evaluation with the association of Schiemann, L. Hoffmann, Jentsch and Chudy. He legitimately considered himself as the systems spiritual father and initiator.

Burch H. Schneider (1901-1973), an American animal nutritionist, worked as Professor at Allahabad Agricultural Institute, India during 1933-1938 and at Lahore, Pakistan for ten years. He was associated with University of Georgia in the USA. He wrote a highly respected book on animal nutrition, "Feeds of the World· Their digestibility and composition". His life long study of the "Evaluation of feeds through digestibility experiments" was completed and edited by William P. Flatt.

Tony Joseph Cunha is a distinguished scientist and has made outstanding scientific discoveries, especially in the area of swine nutrition. In 1950 Cunha and coworkers were the first to reveal the growth-promoting effect of aureomycin in pigs, which was the beginning of the antibiotic era in swine feeding. He was appointed Chairman of NRC committee on the Nutrient Requirements of Swine in 1965 to which he was a member since 1951. He has been the author, co-author, or contributor to 10 textbooks, and has written many practical nutritional articles on beef cattle, horses and swine. He is the author of a textbook on "Swine Feeding and Nutrition".

G.P. Lofgreen is known for the use of net energy system in the evaluation of feedstuffs and in determining the energy requirements of livestock.

W.N. Garrett published a bulletin "Net energy tables for use in feeding beef cattle" in 1968. This represents the fruits of 15 year's work beginning with his significant Ph.D. thesis.

Erle Bartley born of British parents in Bangalore, India, studied abroad and joined the Kansas State University faculty in 1949. His research on bloat led him to the development of poloxalene, Antizymotic (**Bloat Guard** is the trade name), the most effective bloat preventative drug. He and his colleagues demonstrated that the probable cause of the sudden death syndrome is endotoxin produced by rumen bacteria during high grain feeding. Dr. Bartley and his colleagues have worked on feed processing treatments that improve microbial protein synthesis in the rumen, improve urea utilization, reduce ammonia toxicity and improve the palatability of urea. e.g. Starea.

J.P. Fontenot a ruminant nutritionist, studied the magnesium requirements of cattle and sheep and its metabolism. This information is essential for the proper control of hypomagnesemia. He was the first to publish the nutritive value of broiler litter for ruminants. The finding that litter nitrogen could supply up to half of total nitrogen needs of the ruminant is important in the economy of meeting the dietary protein needs of livestock.

E.J. Underwood (1905-1980) was born in London but reared in Australia and worked in the University of Western Australia. A doctorate in Animal Nutrition from the University of Cambridge in 1931, he studied at the University of Wisconsin in the Department of Biochemistry from 1936 to 1938 with Professors E.B. Hart and C.A. Elvehjem. His field of scientific research was trace element nutrition and physiology. He contributed more to the development of this field more than any other person through his own research, which laid the foundation for our understanding of the physiological role of cobalt, through his numerous national and international consulting activities, and through his book "Trace Elements in Human and Animal Nutrition", which he authored in four editions. He also wrote "The mineral nutrition of livestock".

Asok Nath Bhattacharya an Indian, went abroad for higher studies and received Ph.D. in Biochemistry and Nutrition in 1964 from Virginia Polytechnic Institute (VPI). He worked in Cornell University, USA and American University of Beirut, Lebanon. Latter he became a consultant for the World Bank Projects in livestock Development in Turkey in 1975. At VPI, he was one of the early workers to conduct controlled investigations to study the subject of recycling poultry waste as a feedstuff. Later while in the Middle East he made significant contributions to reduce the cost of feeding by supplementing dried beet pulp, or citrus pulp as a grain replacement for beef, sheep and dairy cattle.

Peter J. Van Soest is well remembered for his pioneering work on developing procedures to estimate fibre in feedstuffs. Working as research chemist at the ARS, Beltsville, Maryland he developed the detergent system of fractionation of forage carbohydrates and new methods for lignin. He discovered the Maillard reaction and provided a simple assay for protein availability. He became Professor of Animal Nutrition at Cornell University in 1968. At Cornell his research interests have diversified into human nutrition as well. He studied the digestion capacities of more than 47 species of herbivores including man. He is a member of the AOAC. He published an advanced book on ruminant nutrition 'Nutritional Ecology of the Ruminant' and he was the Chief Editor of Animal Feed Science and Technology Journal.

Indian Scientists

Animal Nutrition research was started in the Indian subcontinent with the establishment of the laboratory of Physiological Chemist at Imperial Agricultural Research Institute, Pusa, Bihar in 1921 which was later shifted to Imperial Institute of Animal Husbandry and Dairying at Bangalore in 1923 and later to Mukteswar in 1935 and finally to its present location in Indian Veterinary Research Institute, Izatnagar in 1939. Till 1952 Division of Animal Nutrition at IVRI was the only principal centre of research in the field of animal nutrition in India. Later around the same period National Dairy Research Institute at Karnal was established with a Division on Dairy Cattle Nutrition.

The evaluation of feeds and fodders was the beginning of the animal nutrition research in India which led to the publication of "Nutritive value of Indian cattle feeds and feeding of Farm animals" by K.C. Sen, the first Head of the Division of Animal Nutrition at IVRI, Izatnagar, in 1954. This was later revised by S.N. Ray and S.K. Ranjhan in 1978 and finally by S.K. Ranjhan in 1991.

Nutritive value of non-conventional feeds (agroindustrial byproducts, tree leaves, etc.) was initiated at IVRI, under the leadership of N.D. Kehar. Work on nutrient requirement of Indian cattle was also initiated by N.D. Kehar. Enrichment of straws using wet alkali treatment was started by N.D. Kehar in late forties and early fifties. The Government of India established the Postgraduade College of Animal Sciences at IVRI in 1958. Dr. N.D. Kehar took over as the first Principal cum Joint Director of the college. Dr. N.D. Kehar is an architect of vast network of Animal Nutrition research in India.

It has been acknowledged that Dr. K.C. Sen, Dr. N.D. Kehar and Dr. S.N. Ray laid the solid foundation for animal nutrition research in India with their vision, zeal and perseverance.

Highly sophisticated area of research was started in early seventies on rumen digestion and metabolism using radioisotopes by Dr. U.B. Singh and coworkers at IVRI and Drs. S.P. Arora, V.D. Mudgal, B.N. Gupta and coworkers at NDRI. Radioisotopes have also been used to predict the body composition of live sheep and pigs by Dr. M.Y. Khan and coworkers from IVRI and Dr. D. Anjaneya Prasad and Dr. D. Venka Reddy from College of Veterinary Science, Tirupati. Respiration chamber (open circuit) was established in early eighties at IVRI, Izatnagar to undertake studies on energy metabolism.

Dr. S.K. Talapatra conducted lot of work on assessing grasses for their nutritive value at Veterinary college, Mathura. He is remembered for the development of methods to estimate minerals in feeds and fodders.

The work on protein degradability of feedstuffs as proposed by E.R. Orskov was initiated by D. Anjaneya Prasad, N. Krishna, Z. Prabhakara Rao and coworkers at Tirupati.

Chapter 2

History of Animal Nutrition, Importance of Nutrients in Animal Health and Production

The primary objective of raising livestock and poultry is to produce good quality animal products in the form of milk, meat and eggs to the consumers as a profitable enterprise with least contribution to climate change. Towards meeting this, livestock and poultry need to be fed with wholesome feed and thus nutrition plays a major role.

What is Nutrition?

Nutrition involves various chemical reactions and physiological processes which transform foods into body tissues and activities. It involves the ingestion, digestion, and absorption of the various nutrients, their transport to all body cells, and the removal of unusable elements and waste products of metabolism.

Nutrition had its beginning as an art, and remained an art until the chemist became interested in the nature of foods and give analytical methods for their analysis. The physiologists and biochemists contributed a great deal for the advancement of nutrition.

Antoine Lavoisier, Father of the Science of Nutrition

The great French chemist Antoine Lavoisier (1743-1794) is frequently referred to as the founder of the science of nutrition. He established the chemical basis of nutrition in his famous respiration experiments carried out before the French Revolution. Antoine Lavoisier for the first time demonstrated that respiration was a process of oxidation in which food was burnt to produce necessary heat in the body to maintain life. His studies led him to state, "Life is a chemical process". Thereafter chemistry became an important tool in nutrition studies.

A. Lavoisier introduced the balance and thermometer into nutrition studies. He discovered that combustion was an oxidation and he showed that respiration in the body involved the combination of carbon and hydrogen with oxygen from inspired air and that the quantities of oxygen absorbed and carbon dioxide given off depended on the food intake and the work done. With Laplace, he designed a (animal) calorimeter by means of which it was demonstrated that respiration is the essential source of body heat.

Through application of chemistry in physiological studies the old idea that the nutritive value of food resided in a single "aliment" was proved wrong in the first quarter of the nineteenth century, i.e. by 1825.

The need for protein, fat, and carbohydrates became recognized during 1826 to 1900. For the remainder of the century, nutritional science and practice were concerned primarily with these nutrients and a few mineral elements Ca, Cl, F, Fe, Mg, K, Na, S were known and considered to be important in the body although critical research proving their essentiality was meagre or lacking. The large expansion in the nutrition field has occurred from around 1910 onwards with the discovery of the vitamins, of the role of amino acids, and of several more essential mineral elements. By late 1970's we knew that the body needs over forty different nutrients, in contrast to the three recognized a century ago.

The origin of life–biological molecules arose from inorganic materials

Although it is impossible to describe exactly how life first arose, paleontological and laboratory studies have provided some insights about the origin of life. Living matter consists of a relatively small number of elements (Table 1). For example, C, H, O, N, P, Ca and S account for about 97 % of the dry weight of the human body. Living organisms may also contain trace amounts of many other elements. The earliest known fossil evidence of life is about 3.5 billion years old. The preceding prebiotic era, which began with the formation of the earth about 4.6 billion years ago, left no direct record, but scientists can experimentally duplicate the sorts of chemical reactions that might have given rise to living organisms during that billion-year period.

Table 1   Most abundant elements in the human body

Element	Dry weight, %
C	61.7
N	11.0
O	9.3
H	5.7
Ca	5.0
P	3.3
K	1.3
S	1.0
Cl	0.7
Na	0.7
Mg	0.3

The atmosphere of the early earth probably consisted of small, simple compounds such as H_2O, N_2, CO_2, and smaller amounts of CH_4 and NH_3. In the 1920s, Alexander Oparin and J.B.S. Haldane independently suggested that ultraviolet radiation from the sun or lightning discharges caused the molecules of the primordial atmosphere to react to form simple organic (carbon-containing) compounds. This process was replicated in 1953 by Stanley Miller and Harold Urey, who subjected a mixture of H_2O, CH_4, NH_3, and H_2 to an electric discharge for about a week. The resulting solution contained water-soluble organic compounds, including several amino acids and other biochemically significant compounds. It was contested by other scientists. Whatever their actual origin, the early organic molecules became the precursors of an enormous variety of biological molecules.

Later, complex self-replicating systems were evolved from simple molecules: For example, proteins from amino acids, nucleic acids from nucleotides and polysaccharides from monosaccharides with the help of functional groups and linkages (see the table in the Appendix II). Obviously, combining different monomers and their various functional groups into a single large molecule increases the chemical versatility of that molecule, allowing it to perform chemical feats beyond the reach of simpler molecules. (This principle of emergent properties can be expressed as "the whole is greater than the sum of its parts.")

Living organisms

Living organisms thrive virtually everywhere on the earth's surface. These hot springs host a variety of microbial species, including some that provide commercially useful products that function optimally at high temperatures.

Prokaryotes and Eukaryotes

All modern organisms are based on the same morphological unit, the cell. There are two major classifications of cells: the eukaryotes and the prokaryotes. **Prokaryotes** range in size from 1 to 10 µm and have one of the three basic shapes: spheroidal (cocci), rodlike (bacilli) and helically coiled (spirilla). Except for an outer cell membrane, which in most cases is surrounded by a protective cell wall, nearly all prokaryotes lack cellular membranes. The best characterized prokaryote is *Escharichia coli*, a 2 µm by 1 µm rodlike bacterium that inhabits the mammalian colon.

Eukaryotic cells are generally 10 to 100 µm in diameter. It is not size, however, but a profusion of membrane-enclosed organelles that best characterizes eukaryotic cells. Membrane-bounded organelles include the nucleus, endoplasmic reticulum, lysosome, peroxisome, mitochondrion, vacuole and Golgi apparatus. The nucleus contains chromatin (a complex of DNA and protein) and the nucleolus (the site of ribosome synthesis). The rough endoplasmic reticulum is studded with ribosomes, while the smooth endoplasmic reticulum is not. The cytosol (the cytoplasm minus its membrane-bounded organelles) is organized by the cytoskeleton, an extensive array of filaments that also gives the cell its shape and the ability to move (see the figure 1).

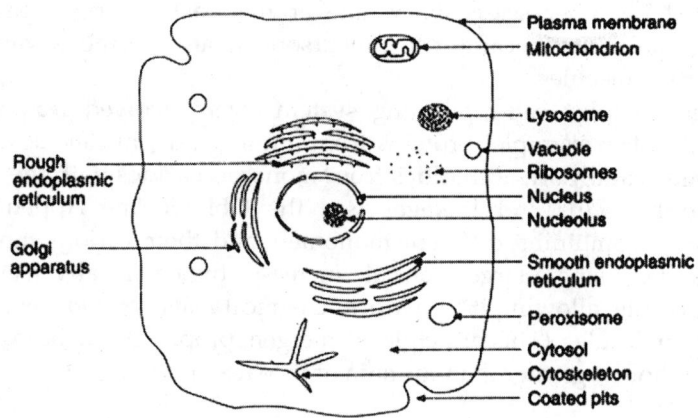

Figure 1   Diagrammatic representation of a rat liver cell

Molecular data reveal three evolutionary domains of organisms

Traditional taxonomic schemes that are based on gross morphology have proved inadequate to describe the actual relationships between organisms as revealed by their evolutionary history (phylogeny). Phylogenetic relationships are best deduced by comparing polymeric molecules - RNA, DNA, or protein - from different organisms. For example, analysis of RNA led Carl Woese in 1992 to group all organisms into **three domains: bacteria, archaea and eukarya** (Figure 2). The **archaea** (also known as archaebacteria) are a group of prokaryotes that are as distantly related to other prokaryotes (the bacteria, sometimes called eubacteria) as both groups are to eukaryotes (eukarya). The archaea include some unusual organisms: the methanogens (which produce methane), the halobacteria (which thrive in concentrated brine solutions) and certain thermophiles (which inhabit hot springs). The three-domain scheme also shows that animals, plants and fungi constitute only a small portion of life-forms.

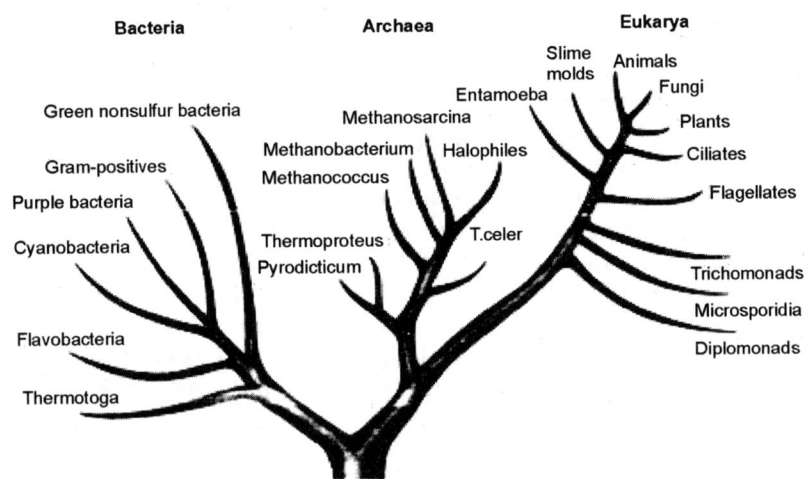

Figure 2   Phylogenetic tree showing three domains of organisms: the branches indicate the pattern of divergence from a common ancestor. The archaea are prokaryotes, like bacteria, but share some features with eukaryotes. [Wheelis, M.L.,Kandler, O., and Woese, C.R., Proc. Natl. Acad. Sci. 89, 2931 (1992)]

Objective of Nutrition

The objective of nutrition is to provide all essential nutrients in adequate amounts and in optimum proportions.

Babcock Single Plant Experiments

Grain and forage from either corn or wheat plant were combined and fed to 5-month old heifer calves (along with salt) through till they calved. Though weight gain was similar, large differences became evident during reproduction. Wheat plant-fed cows delivered bad or dead calves and milk production was also less. This was before the vitamins had been identified and very little was known about mineral requirements. This feeding experiment planned by M. Babcock (1843-1931; the inventor of Babcock Test for butterfat) at Wisconsin Experiment Station with single plants revealed that simplified diets must be used for the solution of nutrition problems. It stimulated the use of the purified diet method which resulted in the discovery of the first vitamin in 1913. Vitamin A was discovered by two independent teams of scientists—McCollum and Davis and Osborne and Mendel.

Role of Laboratory Animals in Discovery of Nutrients

The modern discoveries in nutrition have resulted from studies with a wide variety of species. The contributions of the laboratory rat to our knowledge of vitamins, amino acids and minerals have been enormous. The discovery of insulin and of the role of nicotinic acid in the prevention and cure of pellagra exemplifies the debt that we owe to the dog. Guinea pig experiments showed us the specific cause of scurvy and how to prevent it. Chick helped the discovery of thiamin and has continued to help solve many puzzles in the field of vitamins.

The chicken has played a prominent role as an experimental animal throughout the history of the discovery, isolation and identification of all the vitamins. Hart and associates of Wisconsin used chicks in their classic studies of vitamin A & D. Norris and Heuser used chicks in the studies which led to discoveries and development of information concerning pantothenic acid, B_2, folic acid, and vit. B_{12}. Henrik Dam in Copenhagen and Almquist in California used chicks in their studies on Vit. K.

Monkey, mice and hamsters all have contributions to their credit. Even the lower forms, particularly bacteria, have played a large role in the discovery of growth factors, in the assay of our foods for various nutrients, and in explaining how these nutrients function in metabolism.

Today the nutritional scientist realizes that basic, or pilot, experiments with one of these various species, selected in accordance with the objective of the study, provide the best approach for the solution of many of the problems in the nutrition of man and farm animals, although the final answers must be obtained with the animal species concerned.

Role of Specialists in Expansion of Nutritional Knowledge

The expanding developments in the field of nutrition have resulted from the application of the knowledge and techniques of many different sciences. Physiologists and biochemists have long worked as a team in studying the body's need for food and how this food is metabolized.

Then organic chemists isolated and synthesized the various vitamins. Thanks to their efforts, commercial sources of many of them have become available both for further experimental work and also for use in feeding practice. Physicists have given radiographs, the spectrograph, isotopes, chromatography, etc. and have shown us how they can be used for the advancement of nutrition. e.g. Nuclear magnetic resonance (NMR), Near Infrared Spectroscopy (NIRS). X-ray crystallography has joined with computers to enable molecular biochemists to unravel the structure of certain proteins and thus help explain their functions.

Geneticists have discovered breed differences in nutritive requirements and in the efficiency of food utilization. They have even developed new strains of certain lower forms that will detect specific vitamin and amino acid deficiencies in our foods. e.g. *Tetrahymena pyriformis, Streptococcus zymogenes.*

Microbiologists have assisted greatly in the discoveries of the nutritional roles that bacteria play in the rumen of ruminants and in the intestine of other species. R.E. Hungate discovered rumen bacteria, while M.P. Bryant did considerable work on them, Gruby and Delafond discovered rumen protozoa in 1843 while C.G. Orpin (1975) and T. Bauchop (1979) discovered the presence of rumen fungi. R.E. Hungate published a book 'The Rumen and its Microbes' in 1966. Some of the rumen fungi (zoospores of phycomycete fungi) are *Neocallimastix frontalis, Piromyces* (*Piromonas*) *communis, Caecomyces* (*Sphaeromonas*) *communis.* Microbiological and chemical methods have greatly speeded up the development of our knowledge regarding the vitamin and amino acid content of foods.

Food/Feed Technology has made large contributions in developing special feed ingredients and additives and in processing animal products to improve their usefulness in human nutrition.

Importance of Nutrients in Animal Health and Production

The efficiency of animal production depends on genetic makeup and nutritional status of the animal and management practices.

Nutrition plays a pivotal role because of the following factors: Balanced feeding only can bring out the genetic potential of the animal; cost of feeding of animals accounts for 70-75% of total animal production cost; it minimizes the competition between human and animal for food by introducing nonconventional feeds in animal feed formulation; it manipulates feed ingredients for effective utilization of nutrients.

Essentiality of Nutrients in Animal Health and Production

Several essential nutrients are needed in trace amounts only. About 0.1 mg of cobalt or selenium per day makes the difference between life and death in sheep. A lack of that minute amount was responsible for tremendous livestock losses in certain parts of the world before their specific cause was discovered. We express protein and energy requirements in kilos or grams, but a few milligrams or micrograms in case of certain other nutrients e.g. vitamins, minerals. But they are just as important for health and production as energy and protein. Soil may contribute toxic elements as well as essential elements through the plants to the livestock. Some of the vitamins as well as the minerals that are essential in small amounts may prove harmful at higher intakes. Poor nutrition can result from too much as well as too little. A suitable balance between certain nutrients is important.

Soil-Plant-Animal Relationship

Studies on some of the "trace" mineral elements have shown that the character of the soil on which we grow our food crops plays an important role in determining their nutritive value. Varieties of the same crop differ in nutritional quality and various cultural factors have an influence on nutritional quality. Thus, animal and human nutrition ties back into agriculture and to the soil, stressing the importance of yields of nutrients as distinguished from yields of a crop per unit of land.

The recent developments have served to stress the interrelationships between human and animal nutrition. The foods of both human and animals are products of the soil from captured solar energy and contain the same essential nutrients. Plants make use of the carbon dioxide, water, nitrate, and other mineral salts to form carbohydrates, fats and proteins which the animals must have to build their bodies and which are broken down in life processes. Thus plants store energy and animals dissipate energy.

The metabolic processes which absorbed nutrients undergo for the support of various body functions are largely identical, whatever the species. While animals concentrate the nutrients of food crops into more nutritious and palatable forms for the human diet, they waste basic food resources in the process if they are fed cereals and other foods which humans can eat.

Precision Animal Nutrition Concept

With the objective of raising animals to produce quality animal products for human beings in an environment-friendly way and profitably, an earnest attempt has been made to define 'precision animal nutrition' and to identify the tools needed to realize it. The Abstract has been published in the Proceedings of the International Animal Nutrition Conference (Reddy 2007) held at National Dairy Research Institute, Karnal (Haryana), India.

Precision animal nutrition (PAN) is defined as providing the animal with the feed that precisely meet its nutritional requirements for optimum productive efficiency to produce better quality animal products (milk, meat and eggs) and to contribute cleaner environment and thereby ensure profitability. Cleaner environment means reducing the enteric emission of methane, excretion of nitrogen (ammonia), phosphorus and other compounds into the environment. It is aimed at supplying the nutrients to the animals matching their requirements to improve not only the animal physiology and health but also the enrichment of their products for the well being of the consumer (Reddy and Krishna, 2009).

Chapter 3

Composition of Animal Body and Plants—Comparison between Plants and Animals

Diet of Animals

The diet of farm animals consists of primarily, plants and plant products though animal products such as fish meal, etc. are used in limited amounts in young ruminants, swine, poultry and may be in high yielding adult ruminants. Animals depend upon plants for their existence and consequently a study of animal nutrition must necessarily begin with the plant itself.

Factors that Affect the Chemical Composition of the Forage

1. *Soil Composition:* Soils deficient in zinc, copper, iodine, etc. have shown that the fodders are also deficient in the same minerals. Excess of toxic minerals like selenium and fluorine present in the soil is reflected in the pastures grown on such soils.

2. *Application of manures and fertilizers:* Application of nitrogenous fertilizers, superphosphate increase the nitrogen and phosphorus content of the plants, respectively; other nutrients are also increased.

3. *Irrigation:* With higher level of irrigation the absorption of mineral matter, specially the calcium increases.

4. *Stage of growth and frequency of cutting:* The nutritive value of the fodder is higher just before flowering and goes down at bloom and seed setting stage (see Table 1). Cutting the fodder at frequent intervals provide good quality fodder.

5. *Variety and Strains:* There is a marked difference in the chemical composition between the different varieties of the same species of forage.

TABLE 1   The Chemical Composition (%) of Ryegrass Cut at Different Stages of Growth

	Stage of growth			
	Young leafy	Late leafy	Head emergence	Seed setting
Ether Extract	9.1	7.6	6.5	4.7
Crude protein	18.5	15.2	13.8	9.6
Cellulose	21.3	22.1	23.9	26.7
Hemicellulose*	15.8	18.9	19.4	25.7
Lignin	2.7	3.6	4.3	7.3
Total Ash	8.1	8.5	7.8	5.7
Nitrogen free extract	20.4	18.8	18.1	15.7
Total	95.9	94.7	93.8	95.4

* Xylan, Araban, Glucan, Galactan, etc.

As the plant ages, the concentration of protein decreases and that of cellulose and hemicellulose (structural carbohydrates) and lignin increase. There is therefore a reciprocal relationship between the CP and CF contents in a given species under uniform application of nitrogenous fertilizers. The total ash content decreases as the plant matures and the content of silica increases.

The two major plant families that form bulk of forages and browses are Graminae and Fabaceae (legumes). Forage legumes are miniaturized trees, with unlignified leaves at the end of lignified stems (Figure 1). Legume leaves do not decline in digestibility with age, but the lignifying stems do. In contrast, greater part of lignified tissue is in the midrib portions of the leaves in the grasses, while stems can be more digestible if the pith is a storage site for reserves. Only the stem cortex is lignified (Figure 2). A resulting feature in both grasses and legumes is a varied digestibility of parts within a standing plant.

6. *Environmental temperatures:* Higher environmental temperatures promote lignification. Temperate plants grown at low temperature are less lignified and more digestible, while tropical forages and C4 grasses can be very much lower in quality. The lignin concentration of plants increases with age and ambient temperature. Thus young, cool-season plants are more digestible than mature plants grown in hot weather.

The main components of foods, plants and animals are moisture, organic matter (carbohydrates, proteins, fats, vitamins, etc.) and inorganic matter. The composition of selected feeds is presented in Table 2 and perusal of the

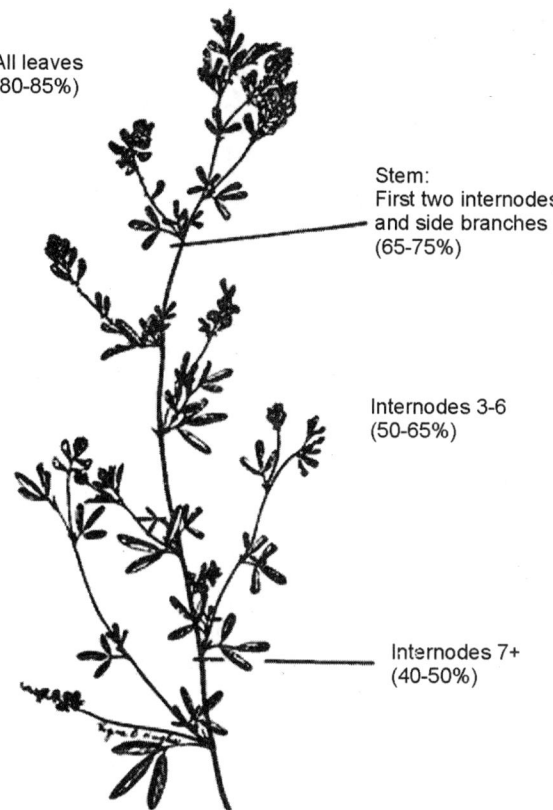

All leaves
(80-85%)

Stem:
First two internodes
and side branches
(65-75%)

Internodes 3-6
(50-65%)

Internodes 7+
(40-50%)

Figure 1   Morphology of alfalfa or lucerne as an example of a typical forage legume, showing the variation in digestibility of plant parts (Van Soest, 1994).

data reveal the following.

TABLE 2. Percentage Composition of Selected Feeds.

	Water	Protein	Fat	CHO	Ash	Ca	P
Maize plant (Mature, but before seed formation)	66.4	2.6	0.9	28.7	1.4	0.09	0.08
Maize grain	14.6	8.9	3.9	71.3	1.3	0.02	0.27
Maize stover	15.6	5.7	1.1	71.4	6.2	0.50	0.08
Soybean seed	9.1	37.9	17.4	30.7	4.9	0.24	0.58
Lucerne plant	74.1	5.7	1.1	16.8	2.4	0.44	0.07
Lucerne leaves	10.6	22.5	2.4	55.6	8.9	2.22	0.24
Lucerne stems	10.9	9.7	1.1	74.6	3.7	0.82	0.17

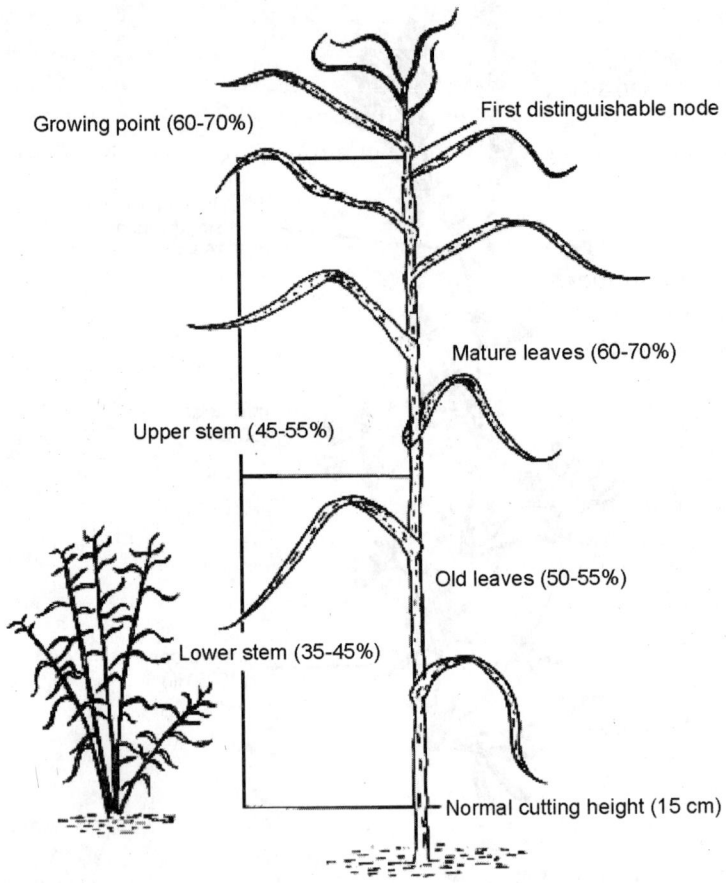

Figure 2 The variation in digestibility of portions of the stems and leaves of tropical grasses (McDowell, 1972).

- The water content of plant decreases as the seed matures.
- Leaves are richer in protein than are stems. Legumes are rich in protein compared to grasses and cereals.
- As the plant matures there is a movement of protein from the vegetative parts to the seed.
- Fat is also higher in leaves than in stems and is generally highest in seeds.
- Legumes are rich in calcium. Calcium is associated with the vegetative portion of the plant.
- Seeds are low in calcium but rich in phosphorus.
- Cereal grains are low in calcium and sodium.

Composition of Animal Body

J.B. Lawes and J.H. Gilbert performed the pioneer and laborious task of analyzing the entire bodies of farm animals and published it in 1859. Based on literature survey involving data from mammals, birds and fish over a wide age range, it is reported that water, protein and ash content of the fat-free body is in a ratio of about 19:5:1 (74-76% water, 20-22% protein and 3-5% ash) while J.T. Reid and associates published it as 72.9% water, 21.6% protein and 5.3% ash. The two major variables in animal body composition are the concentrations of water and fat, and that these two components vary inversely.

The percentage of fat normally increases with age (Table 3), but it is highly variable, depending upon the level of food intake. Its variation affects the percentages of the other constituents, and this is particularly true for water. Very fat animals may have as little as 40% of water. Very small amount of carbohydrate, as much less than 1% at any given moment is present in the body. It is constantly being formed and broken down in metabolism and thus performs a multitude of vital functions.

Body composition on fat-free and moisture-free basis is practically constant, which averages 80% and 20%, protein and ash, respectively. However, higher protein percentages are observed in case of pig, rat and hen and this reflects relatively smaller size of skeleton.

TABLE 3. Percentage Composition of the Animal Body (less contents of digestive tract).

Species	Water	Protein	Fat	Ash
Sheep, thin	74	16	5	4.4
Sheep, fat	40	11	46	2.8
Pig, 8 kg	73	17	6	3.4
Pig, 30 kg	60	13	24	2.5
Pig, 100 kg	49	12	36	2.6
Human	60	18	18	4.3

Percentage of the principal mineral constitutents of the body of steers on empty body weight (EBW) are Ca-1.33, P-0.74, Na-0.16, K=0.19, Cl-0 11, Mg-0.041 and S-0.15.

Composition of Plants and Animal Products

Plants contain the same substances that are found in the animal body, but the relative amounts present are very different. Plants also show larger differences in composition among species than do animals as shown in tables 1, 2 and 3.

The main component of the dry matter (DM) of plant is carbohydrate. Oil seeds such as groundnuts contain large amounts of protein and lipid material in the form of oil. In contrast the carbohydrate content of the animal body is very low.

Main Reasons

1. Cell walls of plants consist of carbohydrate material, mainly cellulose while the walls of animal cells are composed almost entirely of lipid and protein.
2. In the plant, cellulose chains are formed in an ordered manner to produce compact aggregates (microfibrils), which are held together by both inter- and intramolecular hydrogen bonding. In the plant cell wall, cellulose is closely associated, physically and chemically, with other components, especially hemicelluloses and lignin. The cell-wall structure of plants can be roughly compared to the connective tissue structure of animals. In animals collagen may be compared to cellulose, while hyaluronic acid and chondroitin sulfate (see later page no 52) do in animal connective tissue as what hemicellulose, pectin and lignin do in cementing themselves with cellulose. With the exception of lignin, all these cell-wall molecules are carbohydrates.
3. Plants store energy in the form of carbohydrates such as starch and fructans, whereas animal's main energy store is in the form of lipid.

The lipid content of animal body is variable and is related to age. The lipid content of living plants is relatively low (4 to 5%).

In both plants and animals, proteins are the major nitrogen containing compound.

In plants most of the protein is present as enzymes, the concentration is high in the young growing plant and falls as the plant matures. In animals, muscle, skin, hair, feathers, wool and nails consist mainly of protein. Like proteins, nucleic acids are also nitrogen containing compounds and they play a basic role in the synthesis of proteins in all living organisms. They also carry the genetic information of the living cell.

The organic acids which occur in plants and animals include citric, malic, fumaric, succinic and pyruvic acids. They are present in small quantities and play an important role as intermediates in the general metabolism of the cell. Other organic acids occur as fermentation products in the rumen, or in silage. These include acetic, propionic, butyric and lactic acids.

Vitamins are present in plants and animals in minute amount and many of them are important as components of enzyme systems. Plants can synthesize all the vitamins they require for metabolism. Animals can't, or have very limited powers of synthesis and are dependent upon an external supply. A ruminant animal synthesize vitamin C in its tissues, vitamin B-complex group and vitamin K in its rumen while monogastrics have limited/negligible capacity to synthesize. The inorganic matter contain all those elements present in plants and animals other than carbon, hydrogen, oxygen and nitrogen. Calcium and phosphorus are the major inorganic components of animals (70% of body ash) and potassium and silicon are the main inorganic elements in plants.

Chapter 4

Nutritional Terms, Proximate Composition and Chemical Composition

Food/Feed is the source of energy and tissue building constituents. Carbohydrates, fats and proteins yield energy. Water, protein and mineral matter form body tissue.

Proximate Composition

Wilhelm Henneberg and Friedrich Stohmann devised a method called Proximate analysis in 1865 at Weende, a village near the University of Goettingen in Germany. Hence it is called Weende analysis. According to this method, the nutrients present in a sample of feed are analysed and expressed in terms of 6 broad fundamental groups or principles (empirical categories) called the Proximate Principles. They are 1. Water 2. Ether Extract (EE) 3. Crude Fibre (CF) 4. Crude Protein (CP) 5. Total Ash (TA) 6. Nitrogen Free Extract (NFE). None of the Proximate Principles is a chemical compound.

Importance of Proximate Analysis

1. It is the basis for the description of feeds.
2. It is a common basis for feed purchasing and for ration formulation.
3. It is the starting point for more detailed analysis.

Proximate analysis is a system for approximating the nutritive value of a feedstuff without actually using it in a feeding trial. It is simple and yet descriptive method for evaluating the nutritive value of feeds. That is why, though this method was discovered more than 100 years ago, it is being followed all over the world. The Weende's system of proximate analysis is described in Fig. 1. Of the six proximate principles, only five are actually analysed and the 6th principle, NFE is calculated by difference. The proximate principles are expressed on percentage by weight basis,

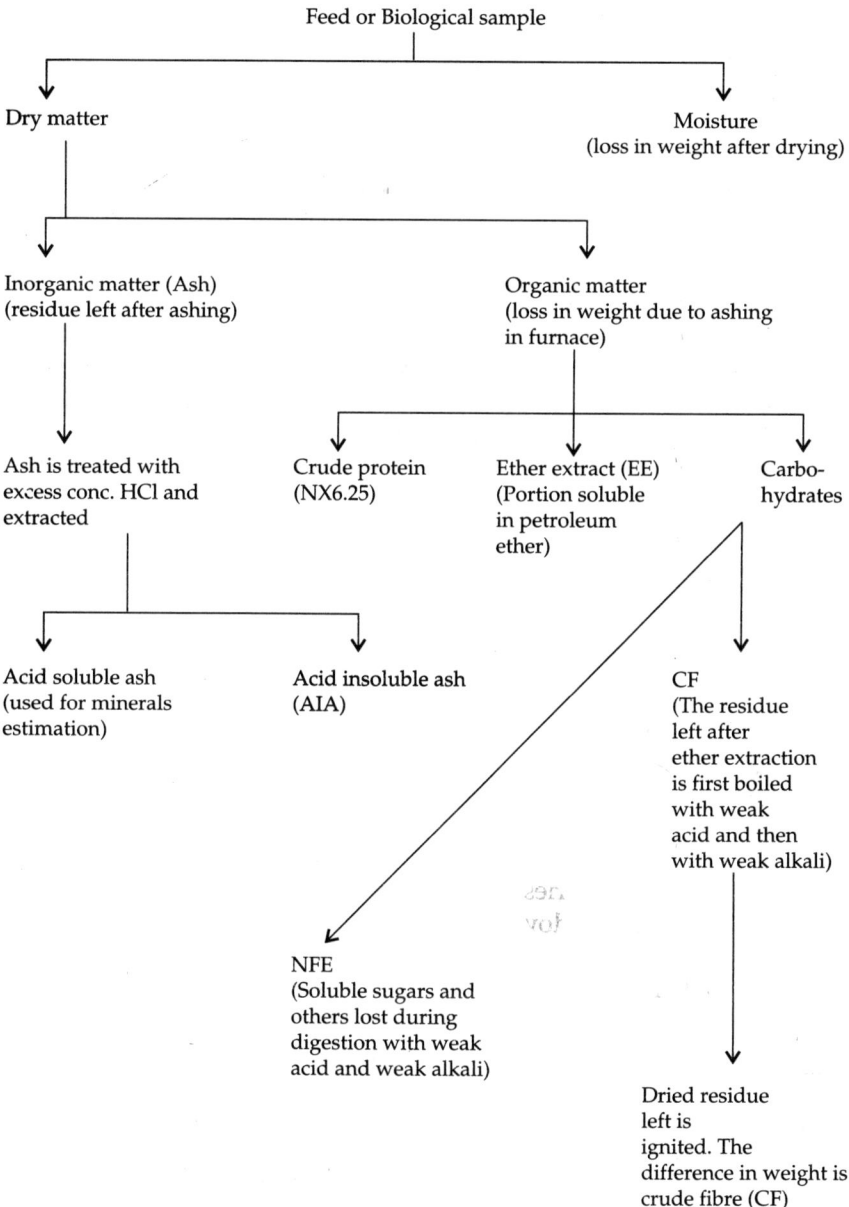

Figure 1 Weende's System of Proximate Analysis.

and more commonly on dry matter basis (see Appendix II). See figure 1 for more details.

Weight of NFE = Weight of sample–Weight of moisture + CP+EE+CF+Ash on DMB, NFE% = 100—(CP% + EE% + CF% + Ash%)

New analytical techniques have been introduced in recent times, and the information about feed/food composition is rapidly expanding. However, the proximate analysis system still forms the basis for the statutory declaration of the feed/food composition.

Chemical composition: To know the chemical composition of the food/feed, it has to be analysed for all the individual chemical compounds that may be present as glucose, starch, fat, protein, amino acids, Vitamin A, riboflavin, calcium, phosphorus, acid insoluble ash (AIA), etc. Such a method of analysis to determine all the individual chemical compounds present in a feed is laborious, expensive and time consuming.

Nutrient: A nutrient is defined (by F.B. Morrison) as any food constituent or group of food constituents of the same general chemical composition that aids in the support of animal life. In the order of priority for nutrients ranking is as follows: water, energy, protein, minerals and vitamins.

In terms of survivability, water is the single most important nutrient for the body. With the exception of water, energy is the most critical component that must be considered in a diet.

Digestion and Metabolism

Digestion involves a series of processes in the gastrointestinal tract by which feeds are broken down in particle size and finally rendered soluble so that absorption of nutrients is possible.

Metabolism is the name given to the sequence, or succession, of chemical processes that take place in the animal. Some of the processes involve the degradation of complex compounds to simpler materials and are designated by the general term catabolism. Anabolism describes those metabolic processes in which complex compounds are synthesized from simpler substances.

Proximate Principles

1. *Water:*   Water is an important constituent of all plant and animal tissues. It is determined by drying a feed sample in a hot air oven at 100°C for a specified length of time. The loss of weight is the moisture content of

the sample. (Dry matter is the residue that is left after the removal of moisture).

Moisture content in feeds: All leafy succulent roughages contain about 80% water, green grasses about 75%, thick-stemmed crops like maize and sorghum about 70%, hays about 12-14%, straws about 10% and concentrates like grains, brans, oil cakes, etc. about 10% water. Feeds containing about 10% water are also known as air-dry feeds.

Significance of Moisture Content of Feeds

1. As the moisture content of a feed varies, its proximate composition will also vary and consequently its nutritive value. Hence while expressing the proximate composition of a feed, its moisture content should always be specified or the composition should be reported in terms of the total dry matter present.
2. Moisture content of feeds is also significant in calculating the cost per unit weight of feeds. As the moisture level increases dry matter level decreases. Therefore while purchasing feed, the dry matter content of the feed should be considered rather than the gross weight of the feed.
3. Useful in the classification of feeds into succulent and non-succulent feeds.
4. Moisture content is significant in the storage of feeds. In general feeds with more than 11% moisture get mouldy and spoiled.
5. Moisture levels determine the keeping quality of hay and losses in silage making.

Total carbohydrates: According to the Weende method of analysis the total carbohydrates in a feed are expressed as crude fibre and NFE.

Crude fibre: Crude fibre composed of cellulose, hemicellulose and lignin. Cellulose is a linear polymer of β-1, 4-linked d-glucose units in trans position. Hemicellulose includes pentosans and hexosans and is also a polysaccharide. Hemicelluloses is widely distributed in forage crops and in certain other feeds. Lignin is not a true carbohydrate as it contains 1 to 5% of nitrogen and 5 to 15% of methoxy groups (OCH_3). Yet lignin is grouped together with cellulose and hemicellulose, as all the three are closely associated in their occurrence in the walls of plant cells. Therefore they are collectively known as "Crude Fibre". The crude fibre is determined by subjecting the fat-free residual feed to successive refluxing treatments with 1.25% solutions of sulphuric acid and sodium hydroxide; the organic residue remained after ignition of the dry matter is the crude fibre.

Crude fibre content forms an useful basis for the classification of feeds into roughages and concentrates. All feeds with 18% or more crude fibre on DMB are classified under roughages and those with less than 18% under concentrates.

Cellulose, hemicellulose and lignin are not acted upon by any digestive enzyme secreted by the mammals.

Lignin which occurs in the woody parts of the plant like the stem, husk, stalks and seed coats has absolutely no feeding value in any species as it is not only indigestible but will also depress the digestibility of the cellulose and other complex carbohydrates.

Lignins are the only non-saccharadic polymer of the cell wall. They originate from three derivatives of phenylpropane: coumaryl alcohol, coniferyl alcohol and sinapyl alcohol. The lignin molecule is made up of many phenylpropanoid units associated in a complex cross-linked structure:

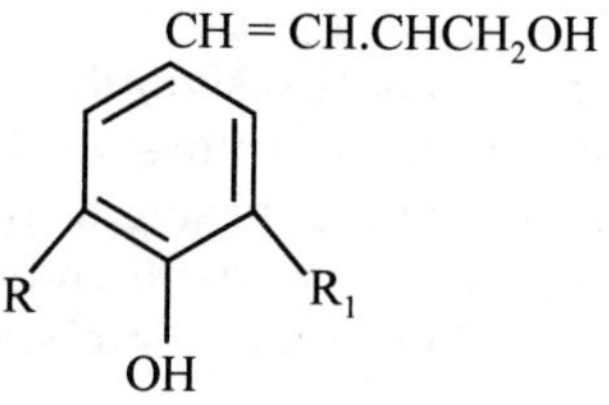

$$CH = CH.CHCH_2OH$$

(1) Coumaryl alcohol, where $R = R_1 = H$.

(2) Coniferyl alcohol, where $R = H$, $R_1 = OCH_3$.

(3) Sinapyl alcohol, where $R = R_1 = OCH_3$.

Lignin

Lignin is of particular interest in animal nutrition because of its high resistance to chemical degradation. Physical incrustation of plant fibres by lignin renders them inaccessible to enzymes that would normally digest them. There is evidence that strong chemical bonds exist between lignin and many plant polysaccharides and cell wall proteins that render these compounds unavailable during digestion. Wood products, mature hays and straws are rich in lignin and consequently are poorly digested unless treated chemically to break the bonds between lignin and other carbohydrates.

Nitrogen free extract: A variable proportion of the cell wall material, depending upon the species and stage of growth of the plant material, is dissolved during the crude fibre extraction and thus is contained in the nitrogen-free extract. This leads to an underestimation of the fibre and an overestimation of the starch and sugars. Thus the nitrogen-free extract fraction is a heterogenous mixture of components, which includes starch, sugars, fructans, pectins, organic acids and pigments. The simple sugars are readily absorbed from the digestive tract. The starches and dextrins undergo hydrolysis by the action of digestive enzymes into glucose and then absorbed. This process of utilization of soluble carbohydrates to yield energy is common to all animals though in the ruminants soluble carbohydrates are wastefully decomposed in the rumen due to the activity of microorganisms.

Ether extract: The fat content in a feed is determined by extracting a feed sample in a soxhlet apparatus for 8-16 hours. Such an extract contains not only true fats namely, the glycerides of fatty acids which are saponifiable, but also other ether soluble substances, pseudofats like free fatty acids, cholesterol, lecithin, chlorophyll, alkali substances, volatile oils and resins. Due to the presence of these substances together with true fats in the extract obtained from the soxhlet apparatus, the whole extract is called crude fat or ether extract.

Crude protein: It includes true protein and non-protein nitrogen. It is estimated indirectly by determining the nitrogen content of the feed and multiplying it with 6.25 (See Page No. 448 also). True protein in a feed is estimated by precipitating the true proteins by stutzer's reagent (alkaline $CuSO_4$) and estimating the N content of the precipitate which is multiplied by 6.25 to arrive at the true protein content. True proteins are made up of amino acids which are the end products of protein digestion.

Total ash and AIA: When a sample of feed is burnt in a muffle furnace at 600°C for 2 hours, only the inorganic/mineral matter is left behind. This is the total ash or mineral content of the feed. The most important reason to determine total ash is to calculate the NFE by difference. Though it gives an apparent idea about the quantity of minerals, its analysis is of little value either for expressing mineral requirements or for indicating the useful mineral content of feeds (because of AIA content), for two basic reasons: body requirements are specific for certain inorganic elements; ash may not be a measure of total inorganic matter present, since some organic carbon may be bound as carbonate, and some inorganic elements such as S, Se, I, F, and even Na and Cl may be lost during combustion.

When hydrochloric acid is added to the ash some substance remains insoluble. This insoluble portion is known as acid insoluble ash (AIA). This indicates the content of silica (mature plant byproducts such as straw, husk, hulls, shells are rich in silica) and sand that is found in the feed due to faulty handling or as an adulterant. The soluble portion of the total ash is soluble ash which contains all macro and micro minerals. The AIA is estimated to know the quality of the feed.

Detergent Method of Forage Analysis—Main Features

Partition of carbohydrates of forage by Weende System of proximate analysis into nitrogen free extract and crude fibre is not realistic either chemically or nutritionally. To overcome the limitations, a rapid method of partitioning of feed carbohydrates into fractions based on nutritional availability was developed by Van Soest and his associates (Fig. 2) in 1960's while working at the U.S.D.A.'s ARS research laboratory in Beltsville, Maryland. Dry matter of forages is divided into cell contents or Neutral detergent solubles and cell wall constituents or Neutral detergent fibre.

Cell contents: sugars, soluble carbohydrates, starch, pectin, non-protein nitrogen, proteins, lipids and other solubles. These are soluble and digestible by the enzymes secreted in the digestive tract of all animals.

Cell wall constituents: cellulose, hemicellulose, lignin, silica, fibre-bound protein, lignified nitrogen compounds, heat-damaged proteins, etc. These are insoluble and are digested by only microorganisms in the gastrointestinal tract.

(A) Neutral detergent fibre: The method utilizes detergents which complex with protein to render it soluble and utilizes a chelating agent (EDTA) to remove heavy metal and alkaline earth contamination. This procedure involves the separation of feed dry matter into two fractions-one of high digestibility and the other of low digestibility—by boiling a 0.5-1.0 gm sample of the feed in a neutral detergent solution (3% sodium lauryl sulfate buffered to a pH of 7.0) for one hour and filtering.

NDF as determined by the Van Soest procedure is considerably higher than the conventional crude fibre values for some feeds since all of the lignin and hemicellulose are included in the NDF fraction. Crude protein content of NDF is neutral detergent insoluble CP (NDICP).

NDF can be equated with the cell wall content of grasses and cereals. If preceded by a starch extraction, it can be equated with the cell wall content of many other feed ingredients. It underestimates the cell wall content of legumes. Legumes and other non-grass species contain relatively high concentrations of pectic polysaccharides that are extracted by neutral detergent and not included in their NDF fraction. Hence NDF and cell wall are not synonyms.

(B) Acid detergent fibre: This procedure is used for the purpose of determining the lignin in a forage sample. In this method the acid detergent fibre procedure is used as a preparatory step. This involves the boiling of a 1.0 gm sample of feed in an acid detergent solution (49.04 g of

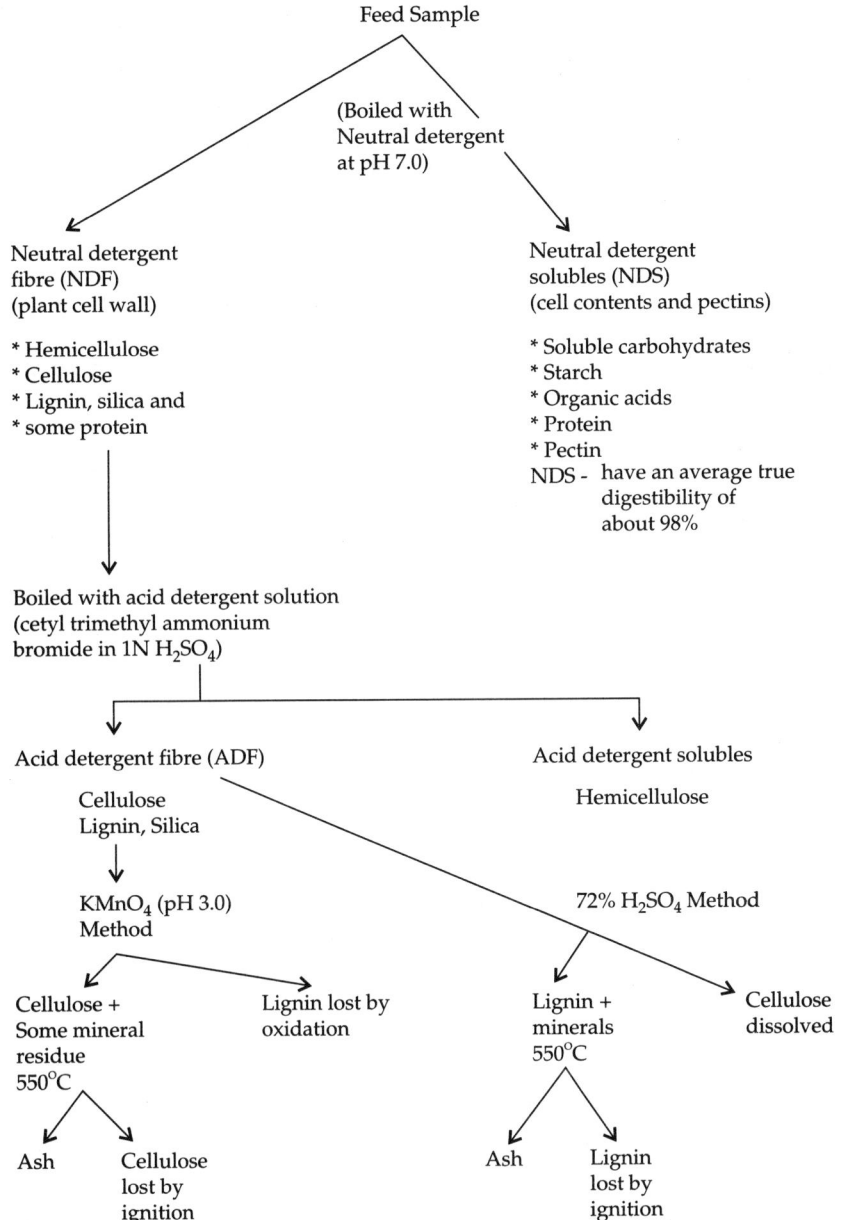

Figure 2. Van Soest Method of Partitioning Fibre in Feeds.

sulfuric acid and 20 gms of cetyl trimethyl ammonium bromide per litre) for one hour and filtering. The insolubles or residue makes up A.D.F.

N.D.F. - A.D.F. = hemicellulose (+ limited amount of protein)

In the UK the ADF method has been modified slightly, the duration of boiling and acid strength being increased. The term 'modified acid-detergent fibre' (MADF) is used to describe this determination.

(C) Acid detergent lignin and permanganate lignin: In order to determine the amount of lignin present, the ADF is then digested in 72% H_2SO_4 at 15°C for 3 hrs and filtered. The residue remaining after washing and drying is weighed and ashed. The ash remaining approximates the silica present, while the loss in weight during ashing approximates the lignin and is referred to as acid detergent lignin (ADL) or more specifically as acid insoluble lignin.

An alternative method for determining lignin which has advantages for certain materials involves the oxidation of the lignin of ADF with an excess of acetic acid-buffered potassium permanganate solution. Lignin so determined is referred to as permanganate lignin. A variation of this method may be used to allow for the cutin present in many seed hulls, which otherwise would be measured as lignin.

(D) Acid detergent insoluble nitrogen: Forage processing temperatures of over 50°C tend to increase the lignin yields with either of the above methods largely by the production of artifact lignin via the nonenzymic browning reaction. The nitrogen content of the ADF is considered to be a sensitive measure of the extent of such damage and serves as a basis for estimating artifact lignin. This is called acid detergent insoluble nitrogen (ADIN). CP of ADF is acid detergent insoluble CP (ADICP).

The analytical method for determining NDF was originally devised for forages, but it can also be used for starch-containing foods provided that an alpha-amylase treatment is included in the procedure (Van Soest et al., 1991). The NDF is expressed exclusive of residual ash (referred henceforth as NDFom) and ADF is corrected by the ash content of the ADL residue (ADFom), as recommended by Van Soest (2006), because of varying soil contamination in forages and feeds. For other details in detergent analysis of feeds, readers may refer Appendix in Advanced Animal Nutrition by D.V.REDDY.

A hormonised global standardization method for the determination of "Acid detergent fibre and lignin (H_2SO_4) in animal feed" has been published by the AOAC (Official Method 973.18) and jointly by the International Organisation for Standardisation (ISO) and the European Committee for Standardisation (CEN) (EN ISO 13906: 2008 method). A globally accepted standard for amylase treated NDF has already been issued - ISO 16472:2006 and AOAC 2002.04. These standards describe the use of a manual refluxing apparatus and give the FOSS Fibertec system (Autoanalyser) as a suitable option. Similar autoanalyser methods are available for determination of nitrogen and fat extraction.

Chemical constituents of Weende and Van Soest schemes for feed analysis

Cellulose has a flat, straight structure. This allows cellulose molecules to align tightly together in straight, parallel rows to provide structural rigidity. Cellulose interacts with other cell wall components such as hemicellulose, lignin, pectin, cutin and minerals to various extents. The extent and nature of the interactions alter the nutritional characteristics of the cellulose.

Hemicellulose is more heterogenous than cellulose. Generally, the base polymer is xylose linked by β1-4 glycosidic bonds. The interactions of hemicellulose and lignin are numerous and varied. Cellulose and hemicellulose are occasionally grouped as holocellulose.

Pectin is a water-soluble linear polymer composed primarily of D-galacturonic acid linked by α1-4 glycosidic bonds. The α1-4 bond is similar in character to a β1-4 glucosidic bond. Pectin is present in soft tissues such as the peel of citrus fruits, (citrus pulp), pulp from sugar beet. Pectins are found in relatively high level in leguminous plant and in cell wall of fruits.

Pectins are readily digested by symbiotic bacteria and protozoa. For animals without significant gastrointestinal fermentation, pectin is termed **soluble fibre** as it adds bulk to the faeces even though it is soluble.

Basically, the plant cell wall is composed of microfibrils of cellulose forming a strong framework that gives rigidity to the plant. These microfibrils are embedded in a matrix composed of a lignin network which cements other matrix polysaccharides, such as hemicellulose and pectins. These polymers have different proportions according to the structure of the cell wall (Figure 3). For instance, as the plant is ageing the lignin network is enlarging from secondary to primary wall, and is laid down encrusting the microfibrills leading to a lower accessibility for cell wall polysaccharides to be hydrolysed by bacterial enzymes.

Various gums are found in the cell wall of the seeds of many plants. The gums are polymers of various sugars linked by β1-4 with β1-3 branch points. The branching prevents these molecules from packing together, rendering them as open structures that are soluble in water or form viscous gels in water. The gum are indigestible by mammalian enzymes but are fermented readily by enteric microorganisms.

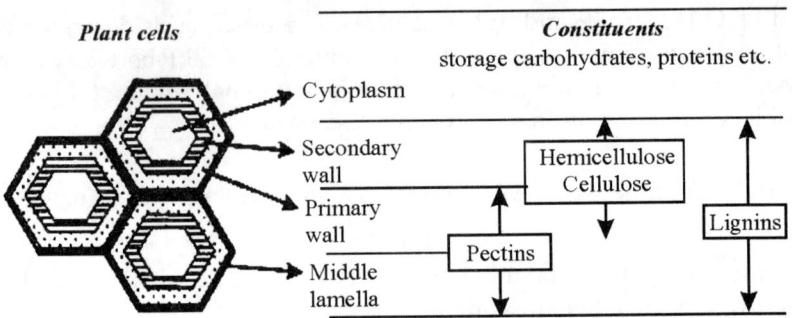

Figure 3   Schematic representations of plant cell walls and their main constituents
(T.Gidenne, 2003).

Table 2   Weende and Van Soest schemes for analysis of feeds and
corresponding chemical constituents

Weende analysis	Chemical constituents			Van Soest analysis	
Moisture	Water				
Crude protein	Dry matter	Organic matter	Protein	Neutral detergent soluble	
			Non-protein N		
Crude fat			Lipids		
			Pigments		
			Starch		
Nitrogen free Extract			Sugars		
			Organic acids		
			Pectins		
			Hemicellulose		NDF
			Cellulose	ADF	
Crude fibre			Lignin		
			Fibre-bound N		
Crude ash		Inorganic matter	Insoluble ash	Silica	
			Soluble ash		

Source: FAO 2011. Quality assurance for animal feed analysis laboratories FAO Animal
Production and Health Manual No. 14, Rome, pp 83

Analytical methods in a nutshell: The international standard method for
the analysis of protein is that which was first introduced by Johann
Kjeldahl in Copenhagen in 1883. The method involves digestion of the
sample in H_2SO_4 to convert all the N to ammonium sulphate. Ammonia is
then liberated by alkaline distillation and quantified titrimetrically with
standard acid solution.

Dumas method of CP determination: Now Dumas method is also used for determination of nitrogen and CP. The equipment used for this method is Dumas apparatus, which is expensive. However, this method is rapid and does not rely on hazardous chemicals. Nitrogen is determined by total combustion of the sample (0.22 g for solids; 0.2–0.5 g for liquids depending on expected N concentration) at 950° C in the presence of oxygen where the nitrogen is converted to NO_x gas. The NO_x is reduced to N_2 which is measured in a thermal conductivity cell.

Calculation: % CP = % N x F, where F = 6.25 for all forages, feeds and mixed feeds; 5.70 for wheat grains and 6.38 for milk and milk products.

Table 3   Proximate principles-equipment required for their analysis.

S.No.	Proximate principle	Equipment required	Scientists developed	Type of the sample needed
1.	Moisture	Hot air oven at 100° C for 8 hours	---	Sample as received
2.	Crude protein	Macro-Kjeldahl apparatus, Micro-Kjeldahl apparatus and Kjeltek; Dumas apparatus	Johann Kjeldahl in Copenhagen, in 1883	1. Ground sample: Air-dry sample; 2. Green fodder / silage 'as it is'
3.	Ether extract	Soxhlet extraction apparatus	Franz von Soxhlet, a German chemist in 1879	Ground sample: Dried sample
4.	Crude fibre	Refluxing apparatus: Spoutless beaker and round bottom flask	Wilhelm Henneberg and Friedrich Stohmann (German Scientists) in 1860	Ground sample: Dried and fat-free sample
5.	Total ash	Muffle furnace at 600° C for 2 hours	-----	Ground sample: Air-dry sample/ dried sample
6.	Nitrogen free extract	By calculation	-----	-------

The traditional method for the analysis of fat is that developed by the German Chemist Franz von Soxhlet in 1879.

Fibre has a very long tradition which can be traced back to 1672, when Nahemiah Drew introduced his method for plant fibre. However in 1860, Henneberg and Stohmann at Weende, Germany, introduced a technique involving acid and alkaline hydrolysis followed by washing, filtration and ashing to gravimetrically evaluate "crude fibre". This method received AOAC approval in 1886.

AOAC: The procedures for analysis of nutrients are described in the book 'Official Methods of Analysis', published by Association of Official

Analytical Chemists (AOAC), formerly (prior to 1965) known as Association of Official Agricultural Chemists. In 1991, it was renamed as Association Of Analytical Communities. This was founded in Philadelphia (USA) on September 9, 1884 by Agricultural chemists with the cooperation of federal and commercial chemists. From 1920, it started publishing "Official Methods of Analysis". This is published once in every five years. In 1995 16th edition had been published and it consists of two volumes containing analytical methods in the areas of consumer protection and public health.

Modern analytical methods

The proximate analysis procedure has been severely criticised by many nutritionists as being archaic and imprecise, and in the majority of laboratories it has been partially replaced by other analytical procedures.

Non-structural carbohydrates (NSC) and non-starch polysaccharides (NSP)

Inadequacies in the nitrogen-free extract fraction have been addressed by the development of methods to quantify the non-structural carbohydrates, which are mainly starches and sugars. The term 'non-structural carbohydrate' (NSC) is sometimes used for the fraction obtained by subtracting the sum of the amounts of CP, EE, ash and NDF from 100. See later 'fibre carbohydrates and non-fibre carbohydrates' in the same chapter (page no. 53).

In monogastric nutrition and particularly human nutrition, the term 'dietary fibre' is often used and attention has been focused on its importance in relation to health. Dietary fibre (DF) may be defined as lignin plus those polysaccharides that cannot be digested by monogastric endogenous enzymes but may be fermented in the large intestine and promote beneficial physiological effects. By virtue of its definition, DF is difficult to determine in the laboratory. The non-starch polysaccharides (NSP) in most foods, along with lignin, are considered to represent the major components of cell walls. The NSP is a fraction of carbohydrate in feed and it does not include starch and free sugars. The NSP include pectins, galactans and beta-glucans. Total NSP consists of soluble NSP and insoluble NSP. Cell wall polymers are water insoluble cell wall and water soluble NSP (Figure 4).

Methods for measurement of NSP fall into two categories

Enzymic-gravimetric methods and Enzymic-chromatographic methods. The enzymic-chromatographic methods identify the individual

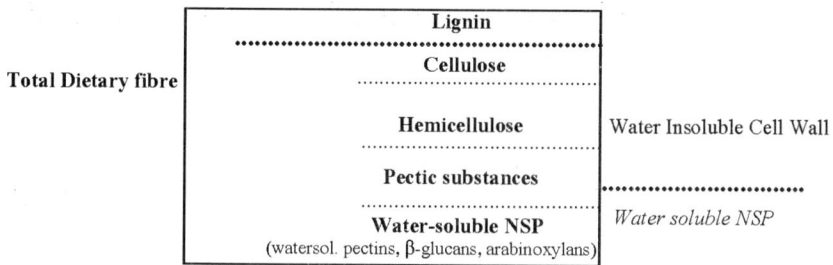

Figure 4 Global classification of dietary fibre (T.Gidenne, 2003; Livestock Production Science, 81, 105-117)

carbohydrates in the dietary NSP. The Englyst method can be used to determine total, soluble and insoluble dietary fibre. Total NSP and insoluble NSP are determined directly by analysis of separate subsamples and the soluble NSP are calculated by difference. The major constituents of NSP are rhamnose, arabinose, xylose, glucose, galactose, mannose and glucuronic and galacturonic acids. (Also see Applied Nutrition 3rd edition 2015 for values in certain feeds). Cellulose is the major source of glucose, and hemicellulose provides xylose, mannans and galactose. The degradation of pectins releases arabinose, galactose and uronic acids. Following the adoption of methods to determine NSP, it became apparent that *non-digestible oligosaccharides* and *resistant starch* also contributed to DF based on their physiological behaviour. In recognition of this, enzymic procedures have been developed to determine these components.

Contribution of NSP

Water-soluble NSP is known to lower serum cholesterol, and insoluble NSP increases faecal bulk and promotes peristalsis of the intestines, accelerates colonic transit and thus prevents constipation. The soluble NSP (gel-forming NSPs such as beta-glucan) increase viscosity of the intestinal contents and depress the digestibility in pigs and poultry, and thereby reduce the absorption of other nutrients from the small intestine.

The soluble / highly fermentable NSP of foods may be degraded in the gut of monogastrics by microbial fermentation yielding nutrients (volatile fatty acids, etc) for the colon flora, which in turn contribute to stabilization of colon bacterial flora and reduce the risk of bacterial translocation. Butyric acid (volatile fatty acid) is an important source of energy for the growth of colonocytes and thus promotes development of the cells and enhances absorption. The extent of degradation depends on the conformation of the polymers and their structural association with non-carbohydrate components, such as lignin. In addition, the physical properties of the NSP, such as water-holding capacity and ion exchange properties, can influence the extent of fermentation.

Resistant Starch (RS)

The concept of resistant starch has gained increasing attention in pig nutrition, as for human beings (G.Giuberti et al., 2015, Animal Feed Science and Technology, 201: 1-13). Resistant starch is defined as a fraction of dietary starch that can escape digestion in the upper gastrointestinal tract therefore passing into the large bowel where can act as fermentative substrate. Nutritionally RS, along with other NSP and non-digestible oligosaccharides, is regarded as *non-digestible carbohydrate. Resistant starch may act as a potential prebiotic source* favouring butyrate production. Its fermentation could reduce the nitrogen emission from pig farms.

The Cornell Net Carbohydrate and Protein System (CNCPS)

The Cornell Net Carbohydrate and Protein System (CNCPS) is a mathematical model to evaluate diet and animal performance. It was developed from basic principles of rumen function, microbial growth, feed digestion and passage and animal physiology. See Table 4 for the several fractions of protein and carbohydrates based on their rumen availability. For more details, readers may refer Appendix in Advanced Animal Nutrition by D.V. REDDY.

Table 4   Protein and Carbohydrate fractionation relative to ruminal availability

Fraction	Protein	Carbohydrate	Rumen availability
A	Ammonia N, soluble amino acids, proteins; instantly degraded in the rumen	Sugars, some starch, fructans, organic acids; highly degradable	Soluble (generally highly available, 4% per min to 2% per hour)
B1	Rapidly degrading proteins in the rumen (10% per hour)	Fast degrading starch, pectin, oligosaccharides; intermediate in solubility	Insoluble potentially digestible (1-30% per hour)
B2	Fast degrading protein	Available plant cell wall and is slowly degradable; this fraction is particularly large in forages.	....
B3	Slowly degrading proteins in the rumen (0.1 - 1.5% per hour)	....	....
C	ADF bound proteins	Lignin	Nondigestible (0% per hour)

Spectroscopy and chromatography

Spectroscopy

A simple total ash determination provides very little information about the exact mineral profile of the feed/food. Analytical techniques involving spectroscopy are generally used to obtain the macro- and micro - mineral contents except the phosphorus. Atomic absorption spectroscopy (AAS) and flame emission spectroscopy had been used. Atomic absorption and flame emission spectrometry are being replaced by inductively coupled plasma emission spectroscopy, as this has a greater sensitivity for the relatively inert elements and can be used to determine several elements simultaneously or sequentially. Just as with other nutrients, a measure of the concentration of the element alone is not sufficient to describe its usefulness to the animal. Accordingly availability of minerals is to be assessed.

Chromatography

Knowledge of the crude protein content of a feed/food is not a sufficient measure of its usefulness for non-ruminants. Similarly, the total ether extract content does not give sufficient information on this fraction since it is important to know its fatty acid composition. In nonruminants, this has large effects on the composition of body fat and, if soft fat is to be avoided, the level of unsaturated fatty acids in the diet must be controlled. In ruminants, a high proportion of unsaturated fatty acids will depress fibre digestion in the rumen.

Techniques involving chromatographic separation can be used for detailed information on amino acid composition of protein, fatty acid composition of fat or individual sugars in NSP. Gas-liquid chromatography (GLC) and high-performance liquid chromatography (HPLC) are used for the purpose. They can also be used for determination of vitamins (e.g. A, E, B_6, K).

Near-infrared reflectance spectroscopy (NIRS)

Currently, rapid methods of feed analysis are needed to comply with the rules under Hazard Analysis of Critical Control Points (HACCP), Good Manufacturing Practice (GMP) and International Organization for Standardization (ISO). It is now common for laboratories to use near-infrared reflectance spectroscopy (NIRS) to estimate the composition of foods. NIRS is an ideal method for the testing, quantification and qualification of large numbers of samples from raw materials to the final compound feeds. Within a minute it gives simultaneous data on constituents like protein, fat, moisture, fibre and starch of various products. The basis of this methodology lies in the absorption of infrared rays by hydrogen-containing functional groups (C–H, O–H, N-H and S–H) and C=O groups in organic compounds present in the food. Therefore, absorption of infrared rays gives a unique spectrum for each of the chemicals, and therefore helps us to understand the chemical property and content (protein, moisture, fibre, fat and starch). NIRS has difficulty in measuring minerals because minerals do not absorb light in the near-infra red region.

Calibration: NIRS is not a stand-alone technology. Being a secondary method the performance of the reference laboratory limits the reliability of the NIRS calibrations. Its accuracy is dependent upon the accuracy of the reference method. Separate calibrations are required for each constituent or parameter. A portion of unknown samples must routinely be analysed by the reference method to ensure that calibrations remain reliable.

The equipment: These equipments are of different types working with a limited number of fixed frequencies (filter instruments, light-emitting diodes) and scanning instruments. Scanning instruments can be divided into monochromators (grating, diode-array, acousto-optical tunable filter (AOTF) and those working with Fourier Transform infrared (FTIR) Spectroscopy involving the use of interferometers. The highest spectral resolution (<0.1cm-1.0) can be obtained with Fourier transform Michelson interferometer instrumentation.

NIRS offers unique advantages over conventional methods of nutrient analysis and prediction. It can be used to determine the composition and nutritive values of ingredients. With small amounts (4-5 g) of sample, numerous constituents are simultaneously analysed precisely. It gives instantaneous results and is non-destructive of the sample. It is particularly useful in the compound feed industry where rapid analysis of raw materials and finished product is required for efficient mixing and quality control standards. The technique has been extended to the analysis of fresh silage samples, eliminating the need to drying and grinding the sample. FTIR spectroscopy is being considered as a low-cost alternative to the in situ technique to predict the nutritional value of a wide range of feeds for ruminants (A.Belanche et al., 2014, Journal of Dairy Science 97: 2361-2375).

Nuclear magnetic resonance spectroscopy (NMRS)

NMRS makes use of the fact that some compounds contain certain atomic nuclei which can be identified from a nuclear magnetic resonance spectrum, which measures variations in frequency of electromagnetic radiation absorbed. It provides more specific and detailed information of the conformational structure of compounds than, for example, NIRS. But is more costly and requires more time and skill on the part of the operator. Hence it is more suited to research work and for cases in which the results from simpler spectroscopy techniques require further investigation. Nuclear magnetic resonance spectroscopy has been useful in the investigation of the soluble and structural components of forages. NMRS is a research technique for determining the chemical structure of food components.

Classification of Carbohydrates

Carbohydrates are compounds containing carbon, hydrogen and oxygen, with the last two elements present in the same proportions as in water, and are found especially in plant foods.

The carbohydrates may be divided broadly into sugars and nonsugars according to their chemical nature, the term 'sugar' being restricted to those containing less than ten monosaccharide residues. Nonsugars include polysaccharides and complex carbohydrates. The term 'oligosaccharide' is used to include all sugars others than the monosaccharides.

Monosaccharides and their derivatives

The monosaccharides have an active aldehyde or ketone group and can take the mirror image, stereoisomeric forms, dextro and laevo (D- or L-formation; see below), depending upon the orientation of the hydroxyl group at carbon atom 5. Biologically the D-forms are more important. Sugars containing aldehyde (CHO) are grouped under aldoses. Naturally occurring aldoses are D-glucose, D-galactose and D-mannose. Sugars containing ketone are grouped under ketoses. The most important naturally occurring ketohexose is D-fructose.

Under physiological conditions the monosaccharides exist mainly in cyclic forms, which can be alpha - or beta - isomers, depending upon the configuration of carbon atom 1. Glucose forms a pyranose ring and fructose most commonly forms a furanose ring. Starch and glycogen are both polymers of the alpha-form, while cellulose is a polymer of the beta-glucose.

The phosphate derivatives of D-xylulose and D-ribulose occur as intermediates in the pentose phosphate metabolic pathway. D-Sedoheptulose (a monosaccharide containing seven carbon atoms) phosphate is also an intermediate in the pentose phosphate metabolic pathway

Phosphoric acid esters: The phosphoric acid esters of sugars play an important role in a wide variety of metabolic reactions in living organisms.

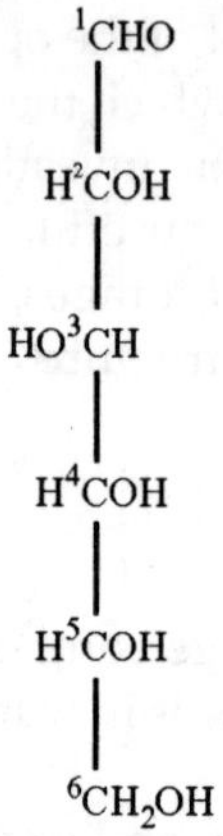

^{1}CHO H^{2}COH HO^{3}CH H^{4}COH H^{5}COH ^{6}CH$_2$OH

D-Glucose

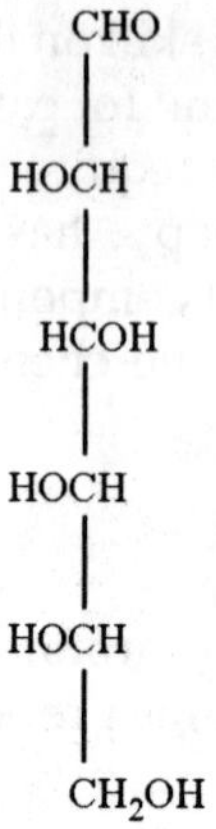

CHO HOCH HCOH HOCH HOCH CH$_2$OH

L-Glucose

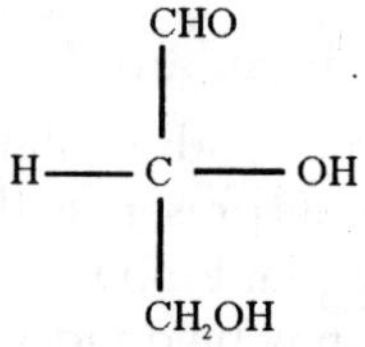

CHO — C — OH, H — , CH$_2$OH

D-Glyceraldehyde

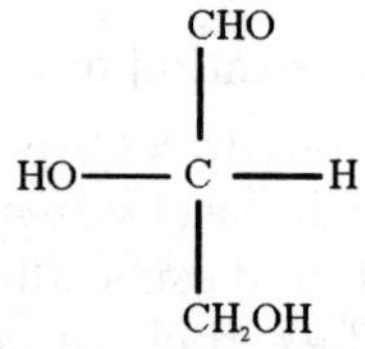

CHO — C — H, HO — , CH$_2$OH

L-Glyceraldehyde

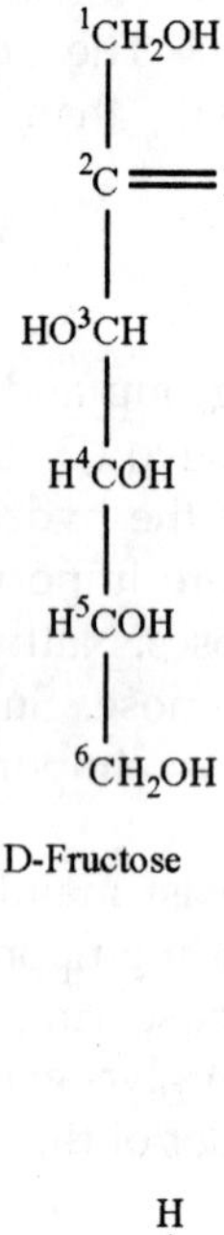

^{1}CH$_2$OH ^{2}C = H HO^{3}CH H^{4}COH H^{5}COH ^{6}CH$_2$OH

D-Fructose

CH$_2$OH ^{2}C = H HO^{3}CH H^{4}COH H^{5}COH ^{6}CH$_2$OH

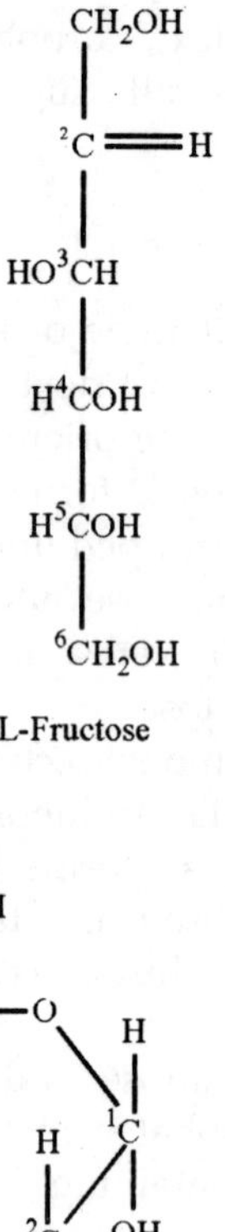

L-Fructose

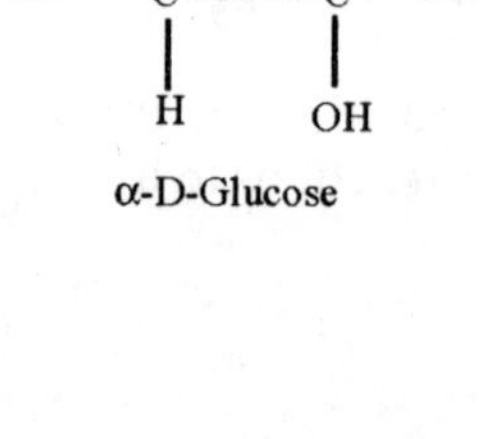

α-D-Glucose

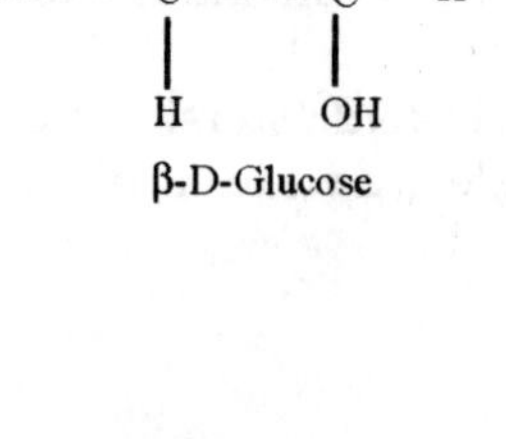

β-D-Glucose

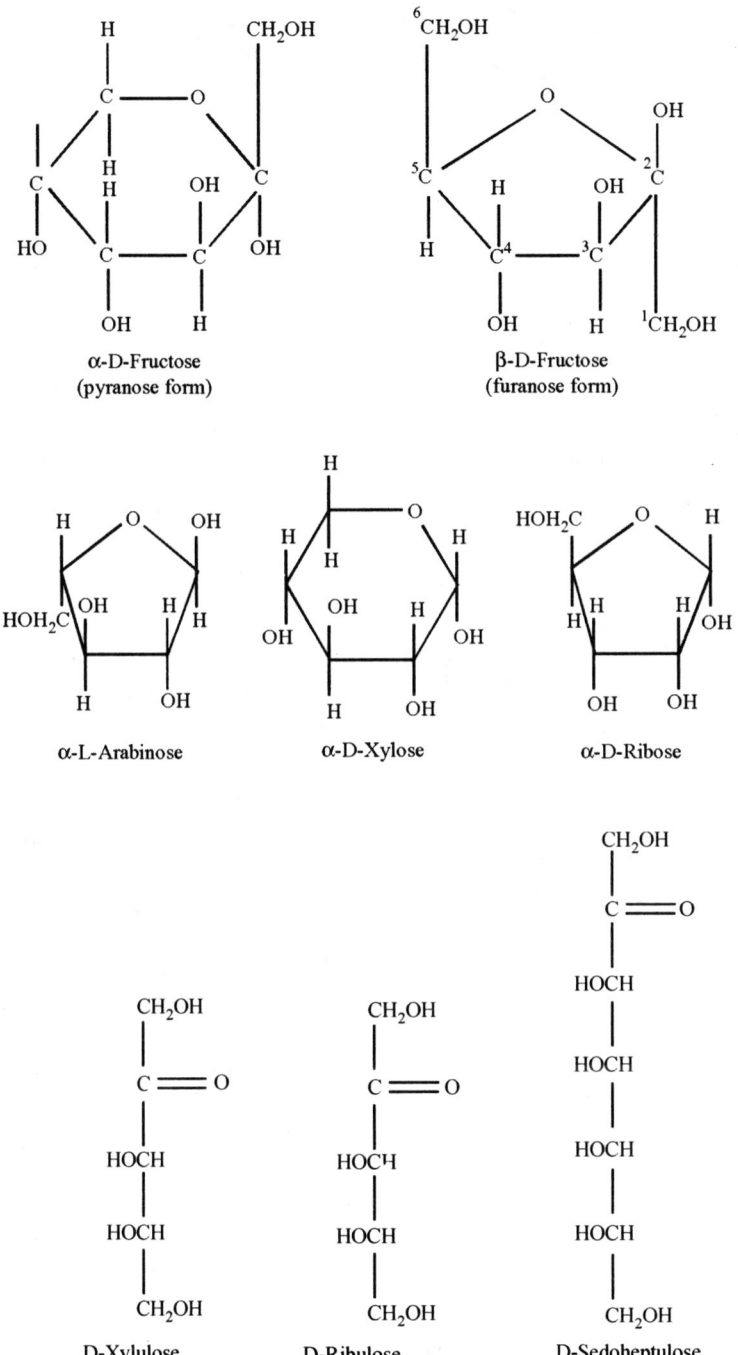

α-D-Fructose
(pyranose form)

β-D-Fructose
(furanose form)

α-L-Arabinose

α-D-Xylose

α-D-Ribose

D-Xylulose

D-Ribulose

D-Sedoheptulose

The most commonly occurring derivatives are those formed from glucose, the esterification occurring at either carbon atoms 1 or 6 or both (see below).

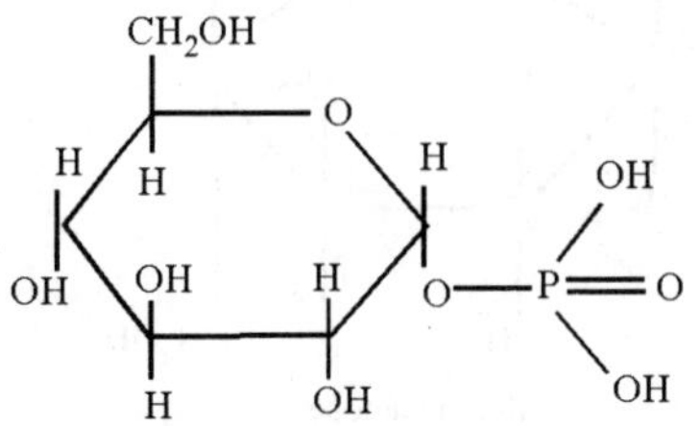

α-D-Glucose 1-phosphate 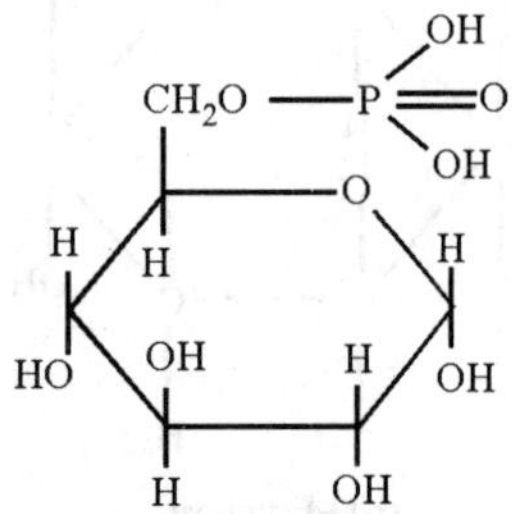   α-D-Glucose 6-phosphate

Amino sugars: If the hydroxyl group on carbon 2 of an aldohexose is replaced by an amino group (-NH2), the resulting compound is an amino sugar. Chitin has D-glucosamine, while cartilage has D-galactosamine (see below).

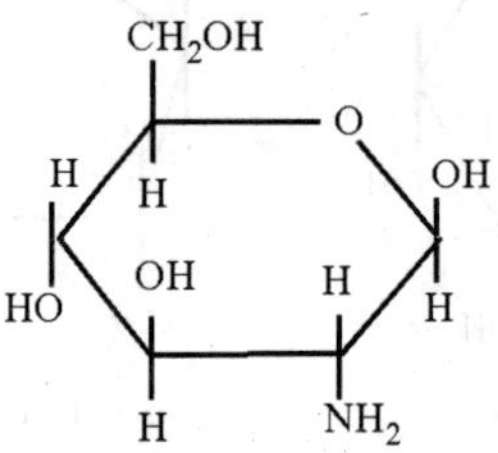

β-D-Glucosamine 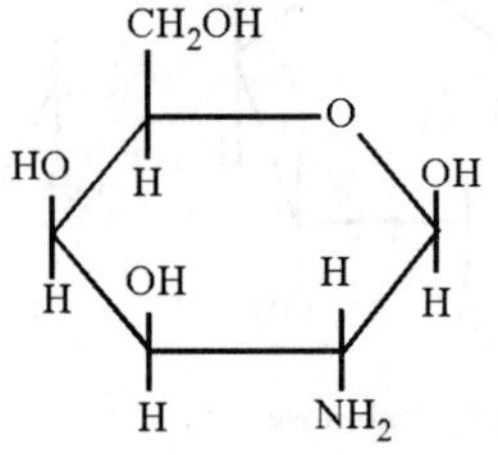   β-D-Galactosamine

Deoxy sugars: Replacement of a hydroxyl group by hydrogen yields a deoxy sugar. The derivative of ribose, deoxy ribose (see below), is a component of deoxyribonucleic acid (DNA).

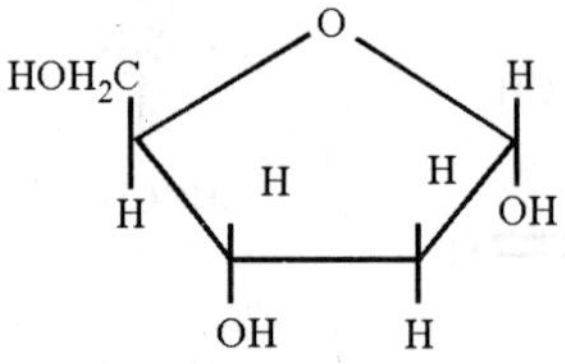

α-D-Deoxyribose 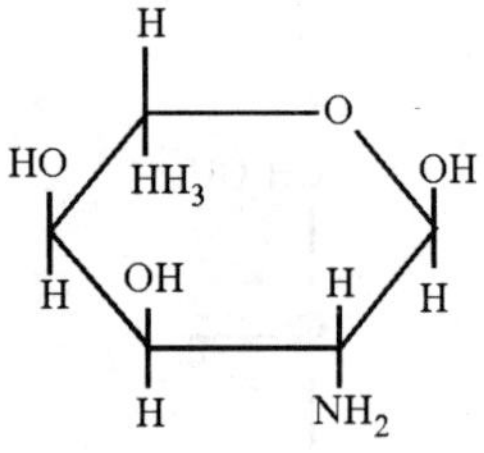   α-L-Rhamnose

Sugar acids: The aldoses are oxidized to produce a number of acids. The most important acids for glucose are gluconic, glucaric and glucuronic acids. Glucuronic and galacturonic acids are important components of a number of heteropolysaccharides.

COOH   COOH   CHO

| | | |

$(CHOH)_n$ $(CHOH)_n$ $(CHOH)_n$

CH_2OH COOH   COOH

Aldonic acids   Aldaric acids   Uronic acids

Sugar alcohols: Simple sugars can be reduced to polyhydric alcohols. For example, glucose yields sorbitol, galactose yields dulcitol while both mannose and fructose yield mannitol.

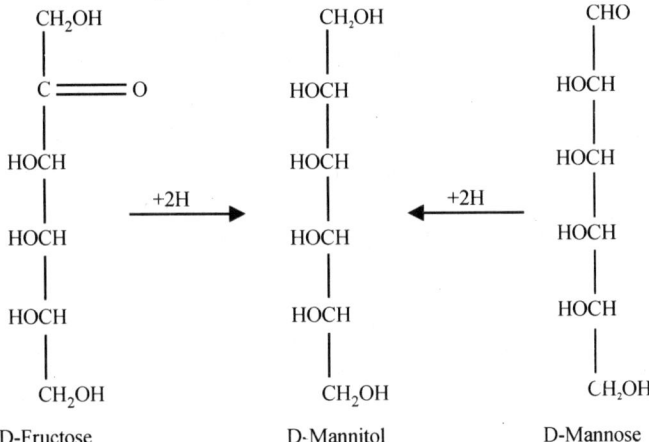

D-Fructose   D-Mannitol   D-Mannose

Glycosides

If the hydrogen of the hydroxyl group attached to the carbon 1 atom of glucose is replaced by esterification, or by condensation, with an alcohol (including a sugar molecule) or a phenol, the derivative so produced is termed a glucoside. Similarly galactose forms galactosides and fructose forms fructosides. The general term glycoside is used collectively to describe these derivatives and the linkage is described as a glycosidic bond.

Oligosaccharides and polysaccharides are classed as glycosides, and these compounds yield sugars or sugar derivatives on hydrolysis. Certain naturally occurring glycosides contain non-sugar residues. For example, the nucleosides contain a sugar combined with a heterocyclic nitrogenous base.

Some important naturally occurring cyanogenetic glycosides are linamarin in linseed, cassava and java beans and dhurrin in leaves of sorghum (see page no 546).

1. Monosaccharides

- Trioses $(C_3H_6O_3)$, tetroses $(C_4H_8O_4)$, heptoses $(C_7H_{14}O_7)$ occur as intermediates in the metabolism of carbohydrates.
- Pentoses $(C_5H_{10}O_5)$: ribose, xylose, arabinose are some examples.
- Hexoses $(C_6H_{12}O_6)$: glucose (dextrose/grape sugar), galactose, fructose (levulose/fruit sugar), mannose are some examples. Amino sugars (D-glucosamine and D-galactosamine), deoxy sugars (deoxyribose), sugar alcohol (mannitol), glycosides (glucoside, galactoside, fructoside) are derivaties of the monosaccharides.

2. Disaccharides $(C_{12}H_{22}O_{11})$: lactose [galactose and glucose, $\beta(1\text{-}4)$ linkage], milk sugar; maltose [glucose and glucose, $\alpha(1\text{-}4)$ linkage], malt sugar; sucrose [glucose and fructose, $\alpha(1\text{-}4)$ linkage], table sugar/non-reducing sugar; cellobiose [glucose and glucose, $\beta(1\text{-}4)$ linkage] are some examples.

Sucrose (see below) consists of one molecule of alpha-D-glucose and one molecule of beta-D-fructose joined together through an oxygen bridge between their respective carbon atoms (1,2). Hence, sucrose has no active reducing group, in contrast to lactose, maltose and cellobiose (see below).

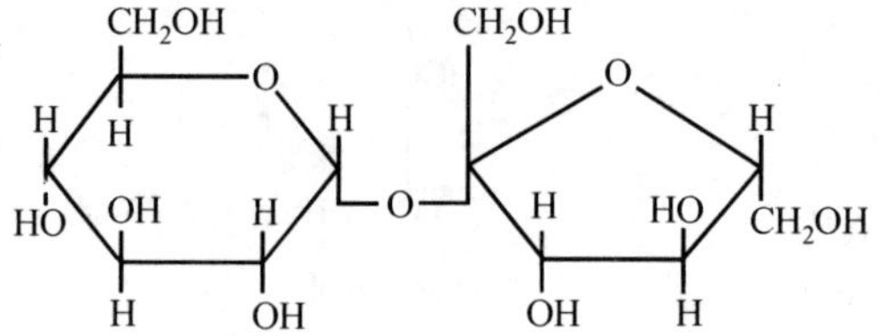

Sucrose

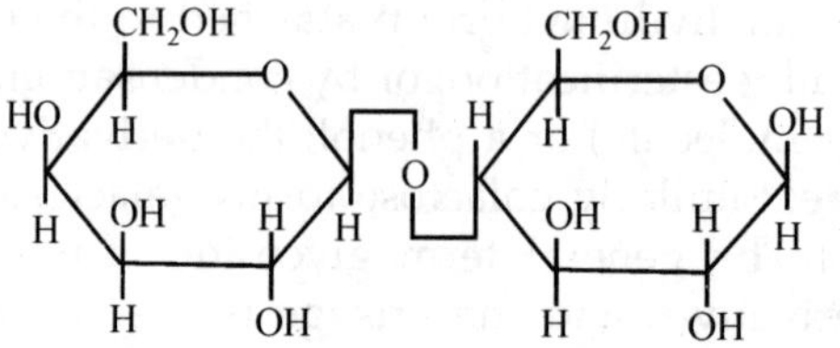

Lactose

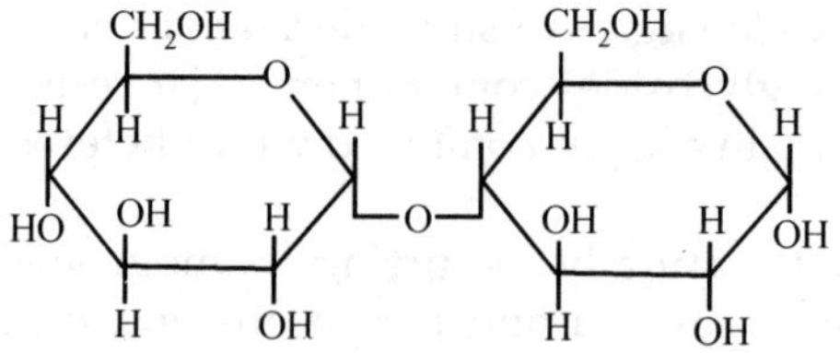

Maltose

CH$_2$OH

HO

H

H

OH

H

OH

H

O

O

H

OH

H

H

H

H

OH

OH

CH$_2$OH

O

Cellobiose

3. Trisaccharides ($C_{18}H_{32}O_{16}$): raffinose (fructose, glucose and galactose) and melezitose (glucose, fructose and glucose) are some examples.

4. Tetrasaccharides ($C_{24}H_{42}O_{21}$): stachyose (galactose, galactose, glucose and fructose; non-reducing sugar) is an example.

5. Polysaccharides/glycans

Polysaccharides

Polysaccharides / glycans are polymers of monosaccharide units. They are classified into two groups, the homoglycans, which contain only a single type of monosaccharide unit, and the heteroglycans, which on hydrolysis yield mixtures of monosaccharides and derived products. Homoglycans are arabinans, xylans, glucans, fructans, galactans, mannans, glucosamines. Heteroglycans include hyaluronic acid, chondroitin, acidic mucilages, pectic substances.

- Pentosans ($C_5H_8O_4$)x: are found in hay, corn cobs, oat hulls, gums. Xylan (xylose) and araban/arabinan (arabinose) are examples.
- Hexosans
    (i)   Glycogen or animal starch: [glucose, α(1-4) + α(1-6) linkages]. It is a glucan analogous to amylopectin in structure.
    (ii) Starch: [amylose, glucose, α(1-4); amylopecin, glucose, α(1-4) + α(1-6) linkages]. Amylose is mainly linear in structure while amylopectin has a bush-like structure.
    (iii) Cellulose: [glucose, β(1-4) linkage]
    (iv) Dextrin: [glucose, α(1-4) + α(1-6) linkages]. Dextrins are intermediate products of the hydrolysis of starch and glycogen.
    (v)   Inulin: [fructose, β(2-1) linkage]. It is a fructan.

    Galactans are polymers of galactose while mannans are polymers of mannose. These occurs in the cell walls of plants.
- Mixed polysaccharides are hemicellulose, chitin, pectins, mucilages.

6. Complex carbohydrates are glycolipids and glycoproteins.

The principal structural carbohydrates of terrestrial plants are cellulose (beta-1,4 linkage), hemicellulose (a common core of xylose chain with a beta-1,4 linkage) and pectins (primarily of alpha-1,4 linked galacturonic acid chain), while chitin is the one in animals. Chitin (polymer of beta-1,4-linked N-acetyl-D-glucosamine) is present in the cell walls of bacteria and fungi and in the exoskeleton of insects and many marine invertebrates. See below for their chemical structures (Figure 5).

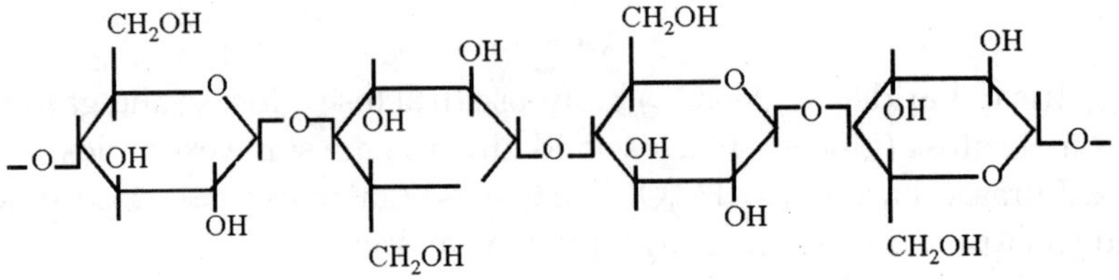

Cellulose

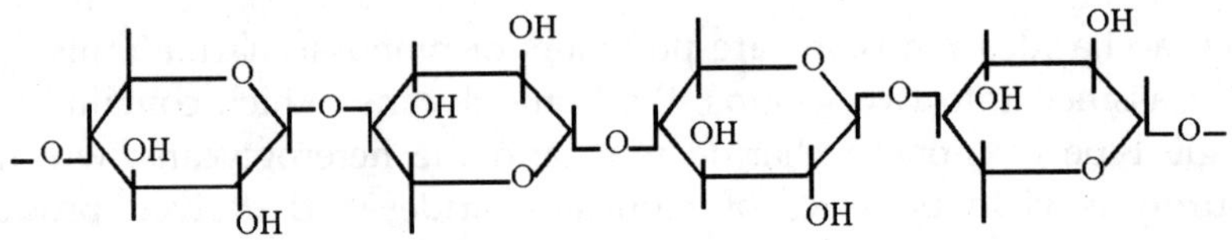

Xylan (Hemicellulose)

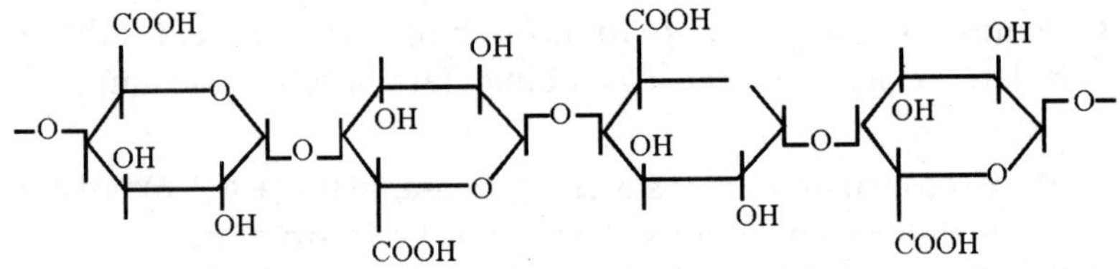

Polygalacturonic acid (Pectin)

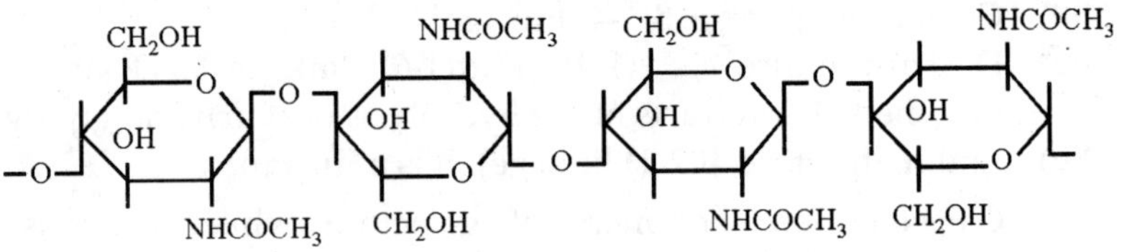

Chitin

Figure 5   Haworth projections of cellulose, xylan, pectin (Van Soest 1994) and chitin (Fruton and Simmonds 1958)

Callose is a collective term for a group of polysaccharides consisting of β-(1,3)-and frequently β-(1,4)-linked glucose residues. These β-glucans occur in higher plants as components of special walls appearing at particular stages of development. A large part of the endosperm cell wall of cereal grains is composed of β-glucans of this type. They are also deposited by higher plants in response to wound healing and infection.

Fructans occur as reserve material in roots, stems, leaves and seeds of a variety of plants, but particularly in the Compositae and Gramineae. All known fructans contain β-D-fructose residues joined by 2,6 or 2,1 linkages. Most fructans on hydrolysis yield, in addition to D-fructose, a small amount of D-glucose, which is derived from the terminal sucrose unit in the fructan molecule.

Glucosaminans

Chitin (Figure 5) is the only known example of a homoglycan containing glucosamine, being a linear polymer of acetyl-D-glucosamine. Chitin is of widespread occurrence in lower animals and is particularly abundant in Crustacea, in fungi and in some green algae. After cellulose, it is probably the most abundant polysaccharide of nature.

Heteroglycans

Pectic substances

Pectic substances are a group of closely associated polysaccharides. They occur as constituents of primary cell walls and intercellular regions of higher plants. They are particularly abundant in soft tissues such as the peel of citrus fruits and sugar beet pulp. Pectin (Figure 5) consists of a linear chain of D-galacturonic acid units in which varying proportions of the acid groups are present as methyl esters. The chains are interrupted at intervals by the insertion of L-rhamnose residues, while other sugars such as D-galactose, L-arabinose and D-xylose are attached as side chains. Pectic acid is another member of this class of compounds. It is similar in structure to pectin except that it is devoid of ester groups. Pectic substances possess considerable gelling properties and are used commercially in jam making.

Hemicellulose

The name hemicellulose is misleading and implies erroneously that the material is destined for conversion to cellulose. Structurally, hemicellulose consists mainly of D-glucose, D-galactose, D-mannose, D-xylose and L-arabinose units joined together in different combinations and by various glycosidic linkages. It may also contain uronic acids. Hemicellulose from grasses contain a main chain of xylan made up of β-(1-4)- linked D-xylose units with side chains containing methylglucuronic acid and frequently glucose, galactose and arabinose.

Exudate gums and acid mucilages

Exudate gums are often produced from wounds in plants, although they may arise as natural exudations from bark and leaves. Gum arabic (the familiar acacia gum), on hydrolysis, yields arabinose, galactose, rhamnose and glucuronic acid. The gums occur naturally as calcium and magnesium salts and sometimes a proportion of their hydroxyl groups are esterified as acetates.

Acidic mucilages are obtained from the bark, roots, leaves and seeds of a variety of plants. Linseed mucilage is a well-known example that produces arabinose, galactose, rhamnose and galacturonic acid on hydrolysis.

Hyaluronic acid and chondroitin

These two polysaccharides have a repeating unit consisting of an amino sugar and D-glucuronic acid. Hyaluronic acid contains acetyl-D-glucosamine. It is present in the skin, the synovial fluid and the umbilical cord. Solutions of this acid are viscous and play an important part in the lubrication of joints. Chondroitin is similar to hyaluronic acid but contains galactosamine in place of glucosamine. Sulphate esters of chondroitin are major structural components of cartilage, tendons and bones.

Classification of Carbohydrates by Dietary Form

P.J. Van Soest classified carbohydrates into four major categories based on dietary form as free, intracellular, cell wall carbohydrates and chitin. Free and intracellular carbohydrates can be considered together as non-structural carbohydrates.

I. Free: Not associated with the cellular structure of food
   - Lactose—milk
   - Fructose—honey

II. Intracellular: Inside the cell
   A. Soluble: Dissolved in the cytosol of cell
   B. Storage polysaccharide
   - Starches
     1. Amylose, α1-4 glucose polymer
     2. Amylopectin, α1-4 and α1-6 glucose polymer
     3. Glycogen, α1-4 and α1-6 glucose polymer

- Fructans
    1. Levans, β2-6 fructose polymer
    2. Inulins, β2-1 fructose polymer

III. Cell wall
1. Cellulose, β1-4 glucose polymer
2. Hemicellulose, β1-4 xylose polymer
3. Pectin, α1-4 galacturonic acid
4. Gums, β1-4 and β1-3 polymers of various sugars
5. Lignin, phenylpropenoid polymers (not carbohydrate)

IV. Chitin, β1-4 N-acetylglucosamine polymer
1. Exoskeleton
2. Cell wall

Fibre Carbohydrates and Non-fibre Carbohydrates

Carbohydrates can also be divided into fibre carbohydrates (equal to NDF) and non-fibre carbohydrates (NFC). Cellulose, hemicellulose and pectin are structural carbohydrates. Non-structural carbohydrates (NSC) (generally speaking comprise those carbohydrates not included in the cell wall matrix and are not recovered in NDF) are mainly starches and soluble sugars, but also include fructans, galactans, pectins, β-glucans. NSC, NFC or neutral detergent soluble carbohydrates (NDSC) are calculated by difference. But they are distinct fractions (NRC, 2001). NDSC include some fibre carbohydrates such as pectins, β-glucans and fructans.

Non-fibre carbohydrates can be calculated by the following formulae.
NFC = 100 – (% CP + % NDF + % EE + % total ash)
NFC = 100 – [% CP + (% NDF – % NDICP) + % EE + % total ash]

Fibre has come to be recognized as a required dietary ingredient for many herbivorous animal species and is necessary for normal rumen function in ruminants. Quality of fibre varies according to fermentability, particle size, and buffering capacity. Only coarse insoluble fibre is adequate for promoting rumen function. This corresponds to the NDF from forages, and NDF is the preferred measure for ruminant feeds and dietary balancing programmes.

Physically Effective Fibre (peNDF)

The concept of physically effective fibre was created to amalgamate the chemical characteristics and particle size of forages, and to quantify its value to rumen function. The physically effective fibre is a good indicator of the rumination potential of the feed. The physically effective fibre (peNDF) of a feed is the product of its physical effectiveness factor (pef) and NDF concentration. Physically effective fibre (peNDF) could be measured either as a proportion of DM retained by the 19- and 8- mm Penn State Particle Separator screens multiplied by dietary NDF content or as the proportion of DM retained by a 1.18-mm screen multiplied by dietary NDF using a dry sieving technique. The NRC (2001) did not give requirements for peNDF due to lack of a standardized, validated method for measuring effective fibre in feeds and to establish requirements for effective fibre.

Proteins

Proteins are complex organic compounds of high molecular weight. In common with carbohydrates and fats, proteins contain carbon, hydrogen and oxygen, and also nitrogen and generally sulphur.

Amino Acids

Amino acids are produced when proteins are hydrolysed by enzymes, acids or alkalis. Although over 200 amino acids have been isolated from biological materials, only 20 of these are commonly found as components of proteins.

Amino Acids Found in Natural Proteins

1. **Aliphatic amino acids**
   a) **Monoamino-monocarboxylic (Neutral)**
      1. Glycine ⎞   5. Leucine   -tasteless
      2. Alanine ⎟ Sweet   6. Isoleucine
      3. Serine   ⎠   7. Threonine
      4. Valine
   b) **Monoamino-dicarboxylic (acidic)**
      8. Aspartic acid   9. Glutamic acid
   c) **Diamino-monocarboxylic (basic)**
      10. Lysine   12. Arginine (bitter)
      11. Hydroxylysine
   d) **Sulphur containing**
      13. Methionine   15. Cystine
      14. Cysteine
2. **Aromatic amino acids**
      16. Phenylalanine
      17. Tyrosine
3. **Heterocyclic**
      18. Proline (imino acid)
      19. Hydroxyproline (imino acid)
      20. Tryptophan
      21. Histidine

The chemical structures of the 20 amino acids commonly found in natural proteins are shown in Table 5.

1. *Monoamino-monocarboxylic acids*

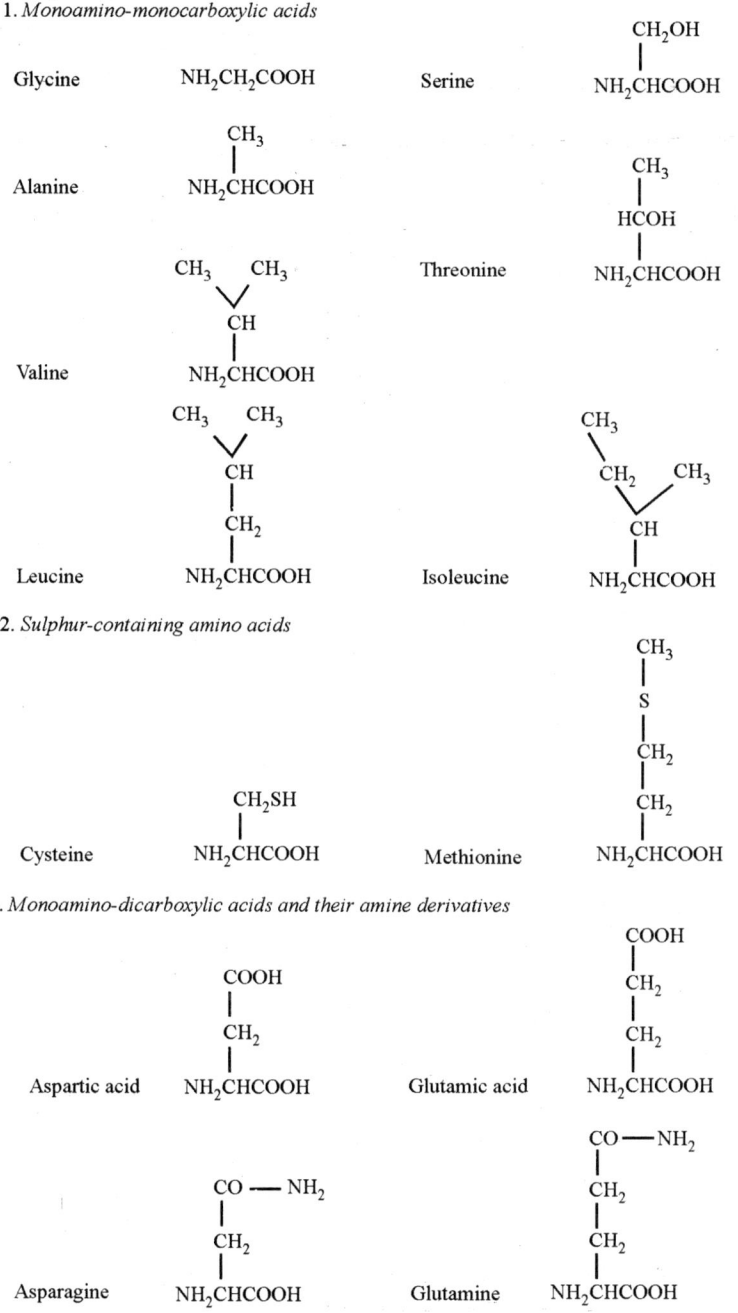

Glycine	NH_2CH_2COOH

Serine

$$CH_2OH$$
$$|$$
$$NH_2CHCOOH$$

Alanine

$$CH_3$$
$$|$$
$$NH_2CHCOOH$$

Threonine

$$CH_3$$
$$|$$
$$HCOH$$
$$|$$
$$NH_2CHCOOH$$

Valine

$$CH_3\ \ CH_3$$
$$\diagdown\diagup$$
$$CH$$
$$|$$
$$NH_2CHCOOH$$

Leucine

$$CH_3\ \ CH_3$$
$$\diagdown\diagup$$
$$CH$$
$$|$$
$$CH_2$$
$$|$$
$$NH_2CHCOOH$$

Isoleucine

$$CH_3$$
$$\diagdown$$
$$CH_2\ \ CH_3$$
$$\diagdown\diagup$$
$$CH$$
$$|$$
$$NH_2CHCOOH$$

2. *Sulphur-containing amino acids*

Cysteine

$$CH_2SH$$
$$|$$
$$NH_2CHCOOH$$

Methionine

$$CH_3$$
$$|$$
$$S$$
$$|$$
$$CH_2$$
$$|$$
$$CH_2$$
$$|$$
$$NH_2CHCOOH$$

3. *Monoamino-dicarboxylic acids and their amine derivatives*

Aspartic acid

$$COOH$$
$$|$$
$$CH_2$$
$$|$$
$$NH_2CHCOOH$$

Glutamic acid

$$COOH$$
$$|$$
$$CH_2$$
$$|$$
$$CH_2$$
$$|$$
$$NH_2CHCOOH$$

Asparagine

$$CO - NH_2$$
$$|$$
$$CH_2$$
$$|$$
$$NH_2CHCOOH$$

Glutamine

$$CO - NH_2$$
$$|$$
$$CH_2$$
$$|$$
$$CH_2$$
$$|$$
$$NH_2CHCOOH$$

4. *Basic amino acids*

Lysine

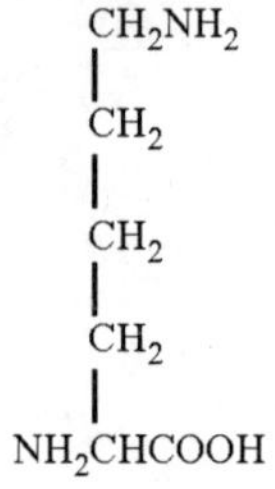

CH_2NH_2
$|$
CH_2
$|$
CH_2
$|$
CH_2
$|$
$NH_2CHCOOH$

Histidine

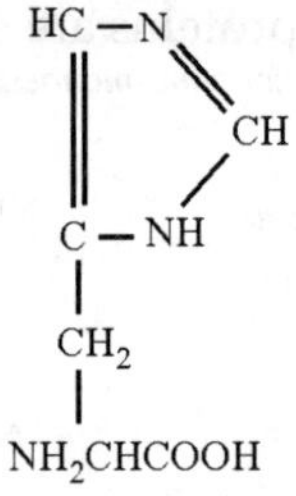

Arginine

NH_2
$|$
$N = NH$
$|$
NH
$|$
$(CH_2)_3$
$|$
$NH_2CHCOOH$

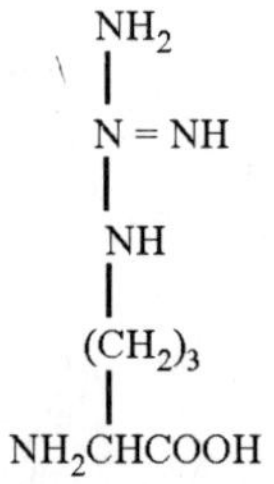

5. Aromatic and heterocyclic amino acids

Phenylalanine $NH_2CHCOOH$

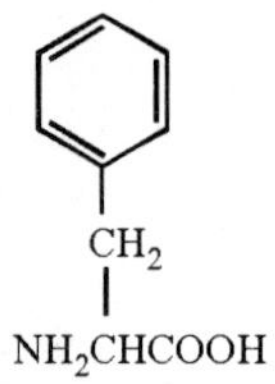

Tyrosine $NH_2CHCOOH$

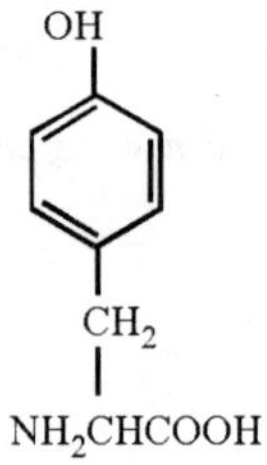

Tryptophan

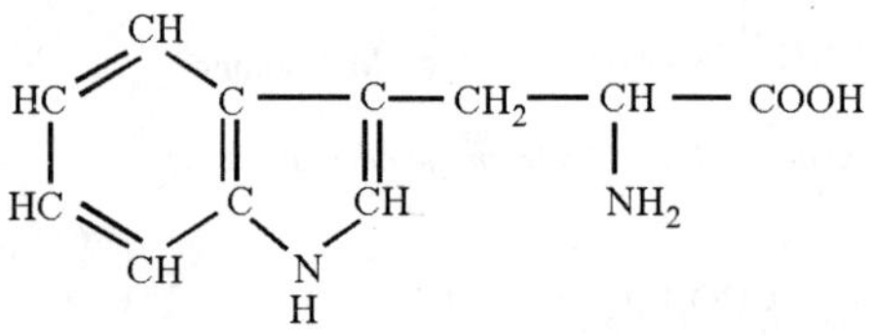

Proline

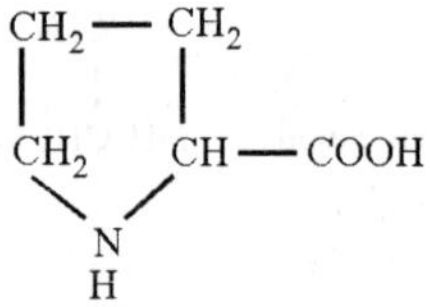

Amino acids are amphoteric since they have both an amino group and a carboxyl group. So in acidic pH, the amino acid is a cation, in basic pH it is an anion and the pH at which it is electrically neutral, it is dipolar. This pH is termed as the *isoelectric point* for that amino acid.

$$
\begin{array}{c}
NH_2 \\
| \\
R\!-\!C\!-\!H \\
| \\
COOH
\end{array}
\qquad\qquad
\begin{array}{c}
NH_4^+ \\
| \\
R\!-\!C\!-\!H \\
| \\
COOH^-
\end{array}
$$

General formula of amino acid　　**Dipolar ion**

The exception is proline, which has an imino (–NH) instead of an amino group. The nature of the R group, which is referred to as the side chain, varies in different amino acids. It may simply be a hydrogen atom, as in glycine, or it may be a more complex radical containing, for example, a phenyl group.

Amino acids in aqueous solution exist as dipolar ions or zwitter ions (from the German Zwitter, a hermaphrodite). Because of their amphoteric nature amino acids act as buffers, resisting changes in pH. All the alpha-amino acids except glycine are optically active. As with the carbohydrates, amino acids can take two mirror image forms, D- and L- (see below).

$$
\begin{array}{c}
COOH \\
| \\
H\!-\!C\!-\!NH_2 \\
| \\
R
\end{array}
\qquad\qquad
\begin{array}{c}
COOH \\
| \\
NH_2\!-\!C\!-\!H \\
| \\
R
\end{array}
$$

D-Amino acid　　　　　L-Amino acid

Essential Amino Acids

W.C. Rose of the University of Illinois (USA) began a brilliant series of studies using semipurified diets and crystalline amino acids. W.C. Rose (1930) classified ten amino acids as essential and others as non-essential amino acids. He defined essential amino acid (EAA) as the one which cannot be synthesized in the body at a rate required for normal growth.

Dispensable and Indispensable Amino Acids

Harper (1974) has taken exception to the concept of nonessentiality and suggested that amino acids that can be "synthesized in the body from whatever precursor" be described by the term dispensable. These are synthesized by the cell using non-specific sources of amino nitrogen (glutamic acid, diammonium citrate, alanine, EAAs, etc.). However, this non-specific nitrogen is clearly "essential" to the animal, since a diet composed solely of essential amino acids is improved by adding mixtures of non-specific nitrogen sources.

Amino Acid Requirements for Several Species

1. There is a marked species difference not only on the protein requirement but also in the qualitative and quantitative amino acid requirements. The very high protein need of the fish is probably a reflection of its basically carnivorous diet and relative inability to utilize carbohydrate.
2. There is a marked reduction in the requirements between the growing infant and the adult.

Ten essential amino acids are required for rats, pigs, and dogs. These may be remembered with ease with their first letters as *PHILLVMATT* for phenylalanine, histidine, isoleucine, leucine, lysine, valine, methionine, arginine, threonine and tryptophan. Rats and pigs require arginine for growth only. Arginine is a product of urea cycle and this meets the requirement for maintenance but not for growth. Adult human beings do not require arginine and histidine.

Chick requires higher level of arginine since they do not have urea cycle and feathers are very high in arginine. Chicken also require high level of glycine because 1. glycine is involved in creatine, porphyrin, uric acid and glutathione synthesis and one-carbon metabolism; 2. excretion of the equivalent of a molecule of glycine with each molecule of uric acid. Hence the required glycine may not be met by synthesis during the early rapid growth period.

Critical and Limiting Amino Acids

Among the essential amino acids, certain amino acids are likely to be low in practical diets and these are known as *critical amino acids*, e.g., lysine, methionine, tryptophan, threonine, arginine, isoleucine. Among the critical amino acids, lysine and methionine are the most deficient amino acids and are known as limiting amino acids. The amino acid in a feed that is most deficient relative to a bird's requirement is referred to as the first limiting amino acid. The next most deficient amino acid is referred to as the second limiting amino acid, etc.

Forms of Amino Acids, their Utilisation and Interconversion

Amino acids requirements refer to the L-isomer, the form in which most amino acids occur in plant and animal proteins. When crystalline A.A. supplements are provided, DL-methionine can replace the L-form. However except for methionine the D-form is used less effectively than the L-form by very young pigs, and other species. In humans, even D methionine is poorly utilized. D-tryptophan has a biological activity of 60 to 70% of that of L-tryptophan for the growing pig. Thus 0.15% DL-tryptophan = 0.12-0.13% L-tryptophan. D-Lysine and D-threonine are not used by any animal species in which they have been tested.

Swine can synthesize arginine at a rate sufficient to meet their needs for postpubertal growth and pregnancy. But the synthesis is not sufficient during the early stages of growth.

Cystine can satisfy at least 50% of the need for total sulphur amino acids (met + cystine). Cystine can be synthesized from methionine but methionine can't be synthesized from cystine. Therefore, methionine can meet the total need for sulphur amino acids in the absence of cystine.

Phenylalanine can meet the total requirement for phenylalanine and tyrosine because it can be converted to tyrosine. Tyrosine can satisfy at least 50% of the total need for these two amino acids. This is because it can't be converted to phenylalanine.

The amino acids requirements of growing-finishing swine, expressed in terms of dietary concentration, increase as the energy density of the diet increases.

Amino acids are also used to synthesize other compounds: For example, tryptophan is used to synthesize niacin; tyrosine is used to synthesize thyroxine, adrenalin and melanin pigment; methionine, a methylating agent can replace some of the dietary choline.

Classification of proteins

Proteins may be classified into two main groups: simple proteins and conjugated proteins.

Simple proteins: These proteins produce only amino acids on hydrolysis. They are subdivided into two groups, fibrous and globular proteins, according to shape, solubility and chemical composition. Fibrous proteins perform structural roles in animal cells and tissues, are insoluble and are very resistant to animal digestive enzymes. They are composed of elongated filamentous chains joined together by cross-linkages. The group includes collagens, elastin and keratins. Globular proteins are so called because their polypeptide chains are folded into compact structures. The group includes all the enzymes, antigens and those hormones that are proteins.

Conjugated proteins: Conjugated proteins contain, in addition to amino acids, a non-protein moiety termed a prosthetic group. Some important examples of conjugated proteins are glycoproteins, lipoproteins, phosphoproteins and chromoproteins.

Nucleic acids

Nucleic acids are polynucleotides that play a fundamental role in living organisms as a store of genetic information. They are the means by which this information is utilised in the synthesis of proteins. Nucleic acids yield, on hydrolysis, a mixture of basic nitrogenous compounds (purines and pyrimidines), a pentose (ribose or deoxyribose) and phosphoric acid. The main pyrimidines found in nucleic acids are cytosine, thymine and uracil (see below). Adenine and guanine are the principal purine bases present in nucleic acids.

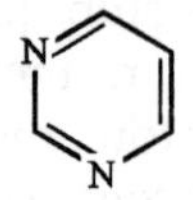

Pyrimidine

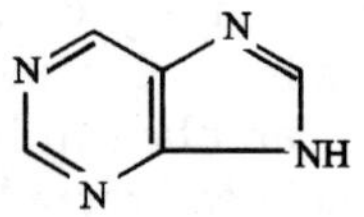

Purine

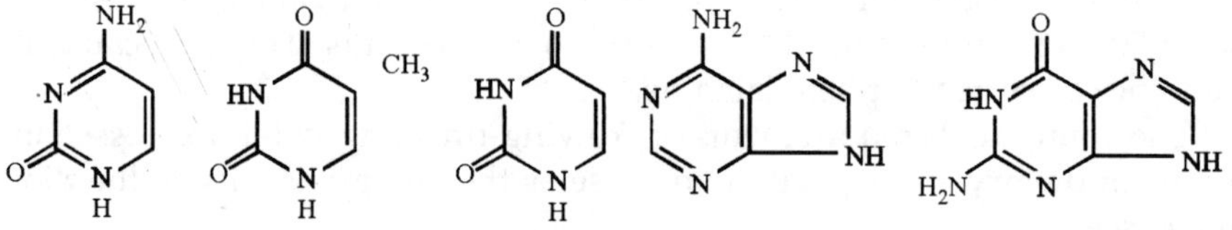

| Cytosine | Thymine | Uracil | Adenine | Guanine |

Nucleoside and nucleotide

The compound formed by linking one of the above nitrogenous compounds to a pentose is termed a nucleoside (see below; adenine + D-Ribose = adenosine). If nucleosides such as adenosine are esterified with

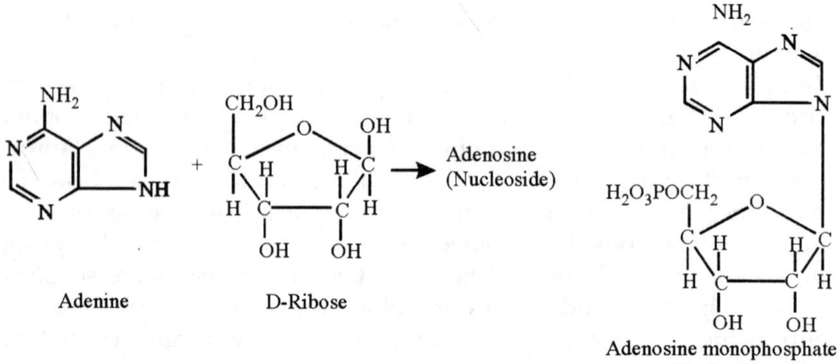

Adenine   D-Ribose

Adenosine (Nucleoside)

Adenosine monophosphate (Nucleotide)

phosphoric acid they form nucleotides, e.g. adenosine monophosphate (AMP) (see below). A nucleotide containing ribose is termed as ribonucleic acid (RNA), while the one that contains deoxyribose is referred to as deoxyribonucleic acid (DNA). AMP upon successive additions of phosphate residues gives adenosine diphosphate (ADP) and then the triphosphate (ATP). ATP plays a pivotal role in energy transformation.

Other nitrogenous compounds: Other important compounds include amines, amides, nitrates and alkaloids.

Amines

Amines are basic compounds present in small amounts in most plant and animal tissues. A number of microorganisms are capable of producing amines by decarboxylation of amino acids (see below). Many occur as decomposition products in decaying organic matter and have toxic properties.

Amino acid	Amine
Arginine	Putrescine
Histidine	Histamine
Lysine	Cadaverine
Phenylalanine	Phenylethylamine
Tyrosine	Tyramine
Tryptophan	Tryptamine

Amides

Asparagine and glutamine are important amide derivatives of the amino acids aspartic acid and glutamic acid. Urea is an amide that is the main end product of nitrogen metabolism in mammals. In humans and other primates, uric acid is the end product of purine metabolism and is found in the urine. In subprimate mammals the uric acid is oxidised to allantoin before being excreted. In birds, uric acid is the principal end product of nitrogen metabolism and thus corresponds, in its function, to urea in mammals.

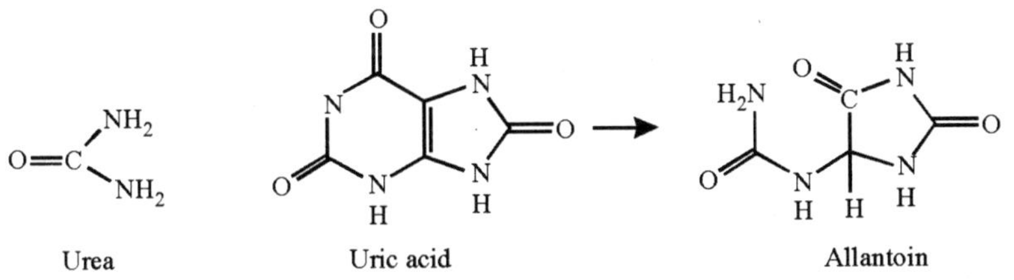

Urea   Uric acid   Allantoin

Lipids

In the proximate analysis of foods they are included in the ether extract fraction. They may be classified as shown in Figure 6. Simple lipids are esters of fatty acids with glycerol. Waxes are esters of fatty acids with alcohol (not glycerol). Compound lipids are esters of fatty acids with glycerol and these contain additional elements like phosphorus, nitrogen and carbohydrate molecule. Phospholipids and glycolipids are examples (page 74).

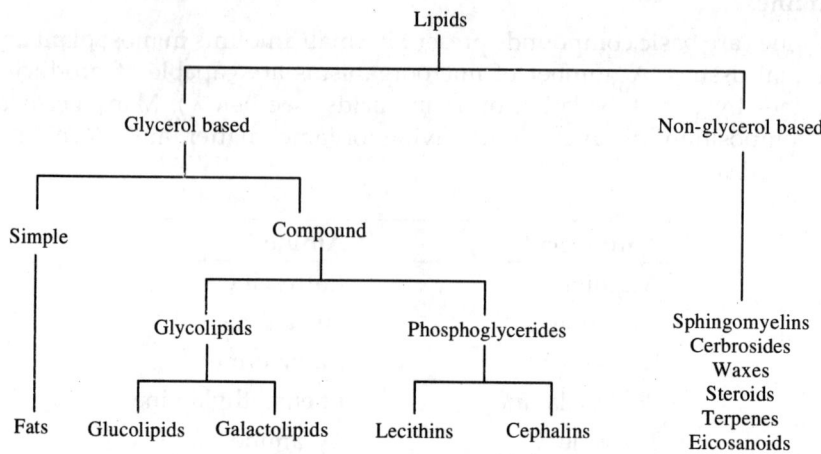

Figure 6   Classification of lipids

In animals, lipids are the major form of energy storage, mainly as fat, which may constitute up to 97 per cent of the adipose tissue of obese animals. Further, stored fat is almost anhydrous. Phospholipids are the structural lipids of animal tissues. Fats are esters of fatty acids with the trihydric alcohol glycerol, and are also referred to as glycerides or acylglycerols (see below). When all three alcohol groups are esterified with fatty acids the compound is a triacylglycerol (triglyceride).

$$^{sn-1}CH_2OH$$
$$^{sn-2}CH_2OH \quad + \quad 3R.COOH \quad \longrightarrow \quad ^{sn-2}CH.O.CO.R \quad + \quad 3H_2O$$
$$^{sn-3}CH_2OH$$

| **Gycerol** | **Fatty acid** | **Triacylglycerol** |

$$^{sn-1}CH_2.O.CO.R$$
$$^{sn-3}CH_2.O.CO.R$$

It is important to appreciate that, in stereochemical terms, the positions occupied by the acid chains are not identical. Under the stereospecific numbering system the positions are designated sn-1, sn-2 and sn-3, as shown. They are readily distinguished by enzymes and this may lead to preferential reactivity at one or more of the positions. Phosphorylation, for example, always takes place at carbon atom sn-3 rather than at carbon atom sn-1. Although triacylglycerols are predominant, mono- and diacylglycerols do occur naturally, but in much smaller amounts. In case of mixed triacylglicerols, R_1, R_2 and R_3 represent the chains of different fatty acids. Naturally occurring fats and oils are mixtures of such mixed triacylglycerols.

Most of the naturally occurring fatty acids have an even number of carbon atoms, which is to be expected in view of their mode of formation. The majority contain a single carboxyl group and an unbranched carbon chain, which may be saturated or unsaturated. The unsaturated acids contain one (monoenoic), two (dienoic), three (trienoic) or many (polyenoic) double bonds. Fatty acids with more than one double bond are frequently referred to as polyunsaturated fatty acids (PUFA) (see Table 6). The unsaturated fatty acids possess different physical and chemical properties compared to the saturated acids; they have lower melting points and are more chemically reactive.

Fats: Fats and oils are constituents of both plants and animals, and are important sources of stored energy. Both have the same general structure and chemical properties but have different physical characteristics. The oils are liquid at ordinary room temperature. The term fat is frequently used in a general sense to include both groups. Fats and oils are primarily composed of various combinations of fatty acids bonded to a glycerine backbone. The common fatty acids of natural fats are presented in Table 6.

The presence of a double bond in a fatty acid molecule means that the acid can exist in two forms, depending upon the spatial arrangement of the hydrogen atoms attached to the carbon atoms of the double bond. When the hydrogen atoms lie on the same side of the double bond, the acid is said to be in the cis form, whereas it is said to be in the trans form when the atoms lie on opposite sides, as shown below. Most naturally occurring fatty acids have the cis configuration.

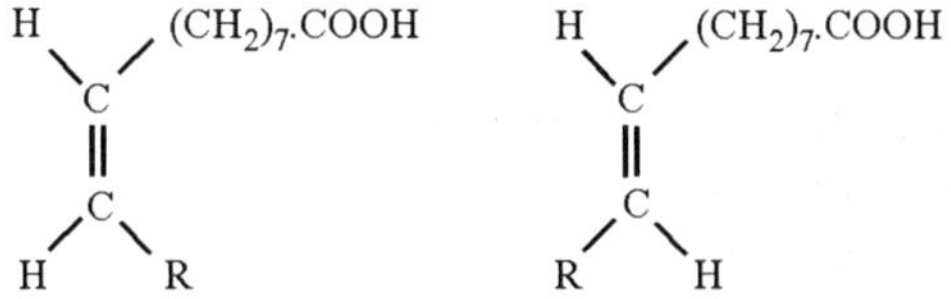

Cis   Trans

Ruminant milk fats are characterised by their high content of low-molecular weight fatty acids, these sometimes forming as much as 20 per cent of the total acids present. As a result they are softer than the depot fats of the respective animals (but not as soft as fats of vegetable and marine origin), being semi-solid at ordinary temperatures. Milk fats of non-ruminants resemble the depot fat of the particular animal.

TABLE 6. Common Fatty Acids of Natural Fats.

Fatty acid	Formula
1. Saturated fatty acids	
Butyric (butanoic)	$C_3H_7.COOH$
Caproic (hexanoic)	$C_5H_{11}.COOH$
Caprylic (octanoic)	$C_7H_{15}.COOH$
Capric (decanoic)	$C_9H_{19}.COOH$
Lauric (dodecanoic)	$C_{11}H_{23}.COOH$
Myristic (tetradecanoic)	$C_{13}H_{27}.COOH$
Palmitic (hexadecanoic)	$C_{15}H_{31}.COOH$
Stearic (octadecanoic)	$C_{17}H_{35}.COOH$
Arachidic (eicosanoic)	$C_{19}H_{39}.COOH$
2. Unsaturated fatty acids	
Palmitoleic (16:1 Δ 9 or n-7-16:1)	$C_{15}H_{29}.COOH$
Oleic (18:1 Δ 9 or n-9-18:1)	$C_{17}H_{33}.COOH$
Linoleic (18:2 Δ 9,12 or n-6, 9-18:2)	$C_{17}H_{31}.COOH$
α-Linolenic (18:3 Δ 9, 12,15 or n-3, 6, 9-18:3)	$C_{17}H_{29}.COOH$
Arachidonic (20:4 Δ 5,8,11,14 or n-6,9,12,15-20:4)	$C_{19}H_{31}.COOH$

Complete formula of Arachidonic acid
$CH_3\text{-}(CH_2)_4\text{-}CH = CH\text{-}CH_2\text{-}CH = CH\text{-}CH_2\text{-}CH = CH\text{-}CH_2\text{-}CH = CH\text{-}(CH_2)_3\text{-}COOH$

Functions of fats: Food fats have two sets of functions—caloric function and noncaloric functions. Fats yield 2.25 times more energy than carbohydrates and proteins.

The Noncaloric Functions of Fat

1. The fat gives shape to the body.
2. It protects the internal organs from shock or injury.
3. Subcutaneous fat serves as an insulation material.
4. Fat helps in the absorption of carotene and the fat soluble vitamins.
5. Fat reduces the heat increment and increases feed efficiency.
6. Fat is a source of metabolic water.

Essential Fatty Acids (EFAs)

The name 'EFAs' was coined to describe the unsaturated fatty acids that cannot be synthesized in the body. A variety of unsaturated fatty acids can be synthesized by combinations of elongation and desaturation reactions. In animals, double bonds are never inserted at positions beyond C9. This precludes the formation of the Δ^{12} double bond of linoleic acid ($\Delta^{9,12}$-octadecadienoic acid), a required precursor of prostaglandins and other eicosanoids. Linoleic acid and alpha linolenic acid must consequently be obtained in the diet (ultimately from plants that have Δ^{12}- and Δ^{15}-desaturases) and are therefore essential fatty acids. Indeed, animals maintained on a fat-free diet develop an ultimately fatal condition that is initially characterized by poor growth, poor wound healing, and dermatitis.

Unlike other mammals, cats have a limited $\Delta6$ desaturase activity. The limited $\Delta6$ desaturase activity can be sufficient for maintenance and conception in adult cats, but for gestation, lactation and growth a dietary supply of arachidonic acid is required. Hence, cats need three EFAs.

Dr. R.T. Holman has contributed more to the knowledge of EFAs. He is responsible for the delineation of metabolic conversions of polyunsaturated fatty acids, and determining quantitative requirements for linoleic and linolenic acids for animals and humans. The omega system was originated by R.T. Holman. The exact structure of an unsaturated fatty acid is given by three numbers:
i)   the number of carbon atoms in the chain
ii) the number of double bonds and
iii) the omega (ω) number, which indicates the number of carbon atoms from the terminal methyl group to the carbon atom of the first double bond.

Nomenclature

Omega-3 and 6 fatty acids or n-3 and n-6 fatty acids

Fatty acid carbon atoms are numbered starting at the carboxyl terminus.

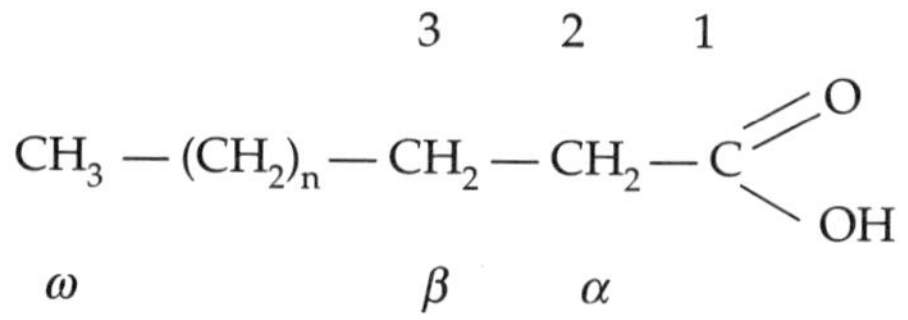

$$CH_3 - (CH_2)_n - \underset{\beta}{CH_2} - \underset{\alpha}{CH_2} - C \overset{\displaystyle O}{\underset{\displaystyle OH}{}}$$

The methyl carbon atom at the distal end of the chain is called the ω (Omega) carbon

$$CH_3 - (CH_2) - C = C - CH_2 - R - COO^-$$

$$\begin{array}{cc} \mid & \mid \\ H & H \end{array}$$

ω — carbon ω — 3 double
atom   bond

That is if the first double bond is on the 3rd carbon atom from the methyl end, it is called n-3 fatty acid e.g. alpha linolenic acid (18:3 n-3). It is also called octadecatrienoic acid. Similarly if the first double bond is on the 6th carbon atom it is called n-6 fatty acid e.g. linoleic acid (18:2 n-6). It is also called octadecadienoic acid.

The Omega-9 (Oleic acid) and Omega-7 (Palmitoleic) series can be derived from endogenously synthesized oleic acid and palmitoleic acid, respectively. The Omega-6 series is derived from linoleic acid e.g. gamma linolenic acid, arachidonic acid. The Omega-3 series is derived from alpha linolenic acid e.g. eicosapentaenoic acid (EPA, 20:5), docosahexaenoic acid (DHA, 22:6) (Fig. 7).

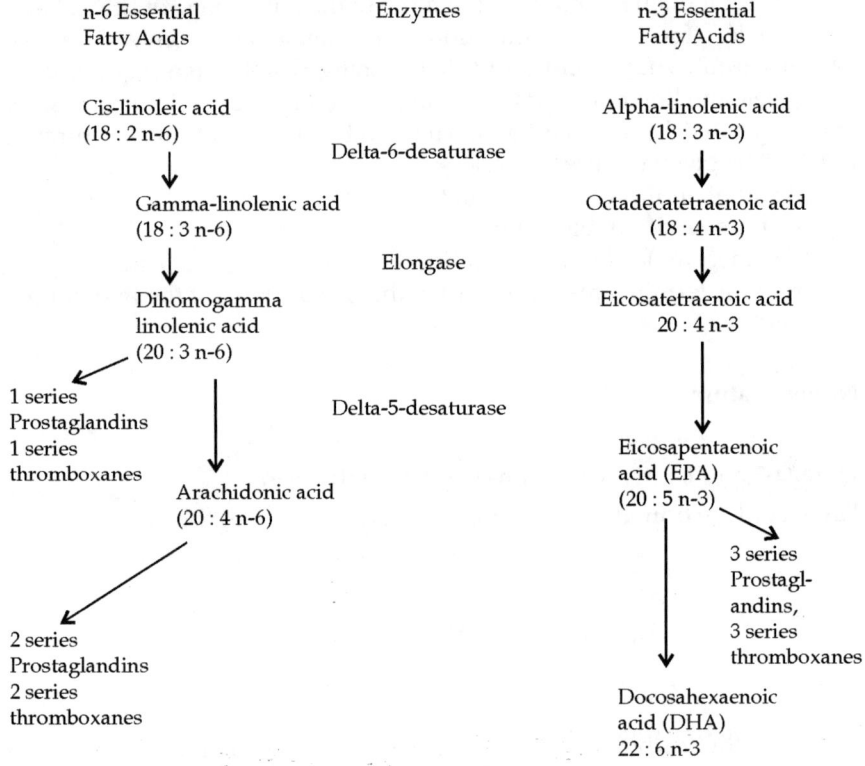

Figure 7. Synthesis of Arachidonic Acid, EPA and DHA.

No conversion from one omega family to another occurs in mammals. Members of the omega-6 and omega-3 families are considered EFAs for mammals because of their inability to introduce double bonds between the ninth carbon atom and the terminal methyl group of the fatty acid chain.

Functions of Essential Fatty Acids

1. Like other polyunsaturated acids, EFA form part of various membranes and play a part in lipid transport and certain lipoprotein enzymes.
2. Linoleic acid is an important constituent of epidermal sphingolipids that function as the skin's water permeability barrier: Animals deprived of linoleic acid must drink far more water than those with an adequate diet.
3. They are the source material for the synthesis of eicosanoids. These include the prostaglandins, thromboxanes and leukotrienes, hormone-like substances that regulate many functions, including blood clotting, blood pressure, smooth muscle contraction and the immune response. (Fig. 8)

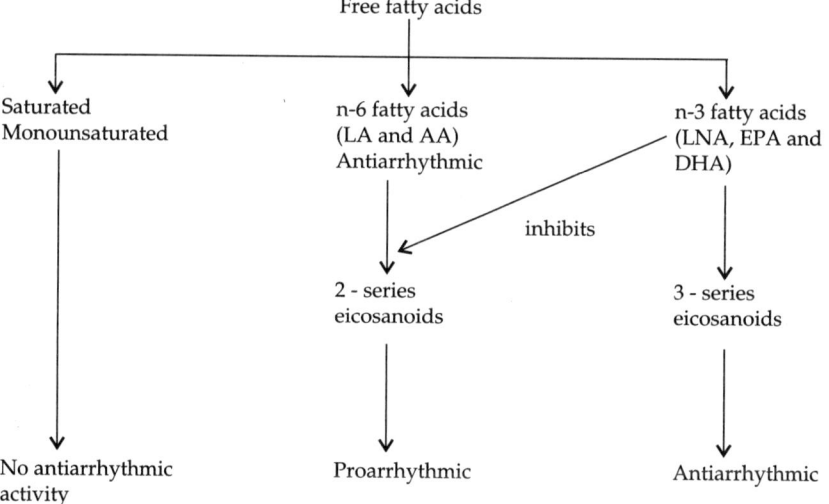

Figure 8. Cardiac Arrhythmia and Fatty Acids.

They are also the source of other important C20 acids in the form of eicosapentaenoic (EPA), hydroxy-eicosatrienoic (HETrR) and docosahexaenoic (DHA) acids.

4. EFA and eicosanoids are involved in maintaining the fluidity of mammalian cell membranes.
5. EPA is the precursor of the 3-series of prostaglandins and thromboxanes and the 5-series of leukotrienes.

6. DHA is thought to play an important role in brain and retinal function, and EPA and HETrR have a modulating effect on the production of eicosanoids from arachidonic acid.

Sources of EFA

Vegetable oils are excellent sources of linoleic acid. Safflower oil contains 80 per cent, Sunflower oil 59 per cent, Soybean oil 46 per cent, Groundnut oil 40 per cent. Linoleic and gamma-linolenic acids are found in abundance in plants while more unsaturated omega-6 fatty acids are found principally in animals. However, as an exception arachidonic and other higher members occur in primitive plants.

Alpha-linolenic acid is a plant version of omega-3 acid and flax or linseed is a concentrated source. Mustard oil is a good source of alpha-linolenic acid (12 per cent). Marine vertebrates accumulate linolenic acid because it is synthesized by phytoplankton, the base of the marine food chain. Seafoods of all kinds, especially seafish-menhaden oil and flax seed are best sources of omega-3 fatty acids.

Deficiency Symptoms of EFAs

Natural diets, even poor ones, usually contain adequate amounts of EFA, and therefore the deficiency is far rarer than deficiencies of protein, vitamins or minerals. Nevertheless, EFA deficiency does occur when animals or human receive insufficient dietary fat.

Anatomical signs of EFA deficiency vary from species to species but biochemical aberrations associated with deficiency are found to be same in all species.

* The chief alterations in various tissues are decreased levels of omega-6 fatty acids (linoleic, arachidonic, docosapentaenoic acids) and increased levels of omega-9 fatty acids (eicosatrienoic and docosatrienoic acids). Accumulation of eicosatrienoic acid (C20 : 3 w-9) in tissues is an important indication of EFA deficiency.

* In EFA deficiency the PUFAs present in phospholipids (the building unit of biomembranes) are replaced by this eicosatrienoic acid with known concomitant deleterious effects on biomembrane function and integrity (less stable biomembranes).

* This altered membrane structure may cause a disruption in spatial arrangements in mitochondria which results in less efficient oxidative phosphorylation in mitochondria.

* The major feature of the deficiency, in all the animals and birds studied, is an impairment of the exterior covering of the animal. Mammals exhibit a dermatitis while chickens show a faulty feathering reflecting the consequences of faulty membrane formation in all cells.

* Deficiency of EFA produces abnormal keratinization resulting in orthokeratotic hyperkeratosis and epidermal hyperplasia. Skin looks dull and dry.

* The symptoms include reduced growth rate, parakeratosis, increased water permeability of the skin, increased susceptibility to bacterial infections, male and female sterility, decreased prostaglandin biosynthesis, decreased visual acuity, reduced myocardial contractility, abnormal thrombocyte aggregation.

Under typical conditions, EFA deficiency would not be expected for humans except for infants not receiving mother's milk. Deficiency of EFA is believed to lead to a skin condition known as 'phrynoderma' (toad skin) in humans in which skin becomes rough, and thick horny papules of the size of a pin head erupt in certain areas of the body, notably thighs, buttocks, anus and trunk. However, recent studies reveal that these conditions respond more effectively to vitamin E and B vitamins than to EFA treatment.

Toxicity of EFA

There are nutritional disadvantages from excessive intakes of EFA. These polyunsaturated fatty acids get readily oxidized and increase the requirement for vitamin E, which is a biological antioxidant in the body. High levels of PUFAs may have undesirable effects due to formation of excess free radicals and consequent tissue damage.

Conjugated Linoleic Acid (CLA)

The term refers to a group of positional and geometric isomers of linoleic acid (18:2) in which the double bonds are separated by a single carbon-carbon bond instead of a methylene group. Important are 18:2 cis-9, trans-11 isomer, the most abundant CLA and trans-10, cis-12 isomer. CLA has received considerable attention due to its powerful anti-carcinogenic activity, and showed anti-obesity and anti-atherogenic activities. It is an effective antioxidant. Trans-10 cis-12 CLA also decreases the concentration of fat in milk of cows and ewes.

Ruminant products are rich sources of CLA. Ruminants produce CLA in two known manners. Dietary polyunsaturated fatty acids (PUFA; linoleic and alpha-linolenic acids), which undergo incomplete ruminal biohydrogenation, are one source of cis-9, trans-11 CLA in milk fat. Another source is endogenous synthesis in the mammary gland or adipose tissue from vaccenic acid (C18:1 trans-11), an intermediate that also escapes complete biohydrogenation in the rumen.

Properties of Fats of Nutritional Significance

Acid value: When fats and oils become rancid, individual fatty acids are "freed" and make the material slightly acidic. These are called free fatty acids (FFA). The presence of high concentrations of free fatty acids in feed-grade fat may mean that the fat is rancid. Acid value indicates the presence of free fatty acids in a fat which cause rancidity of the fat. Rice bran, oil cakes turn rancid when stored for long periods due to the liberation of free fatty acids. Quality of such feeds can be judged by estimating the acid value of ether extract of such feeds. The acid value/number is defined as the number of milligrams of KOH required to neutralize the free organic acids in 1g of fat.

Saponification number: It is defined as the number of milligrams of KOH required to neutralize the free fatty acids and saponify the esterified fatty acids in 1g of fat. The saponification number is a measure of the molecular weight (length of chain) of the fatty acids in the fat.

Iodine number: Iodine will unite with double bonds of the unsaturated fatty acids in fats, each double bond taking up two atoms of iodine. The iodine number thus is a measure of the total amount of unsaturation of the fatty acids in a fat. It is defined as the number of grams of iodine absorbed by 100 g of fat. Iodine value reflects the degree of unsaturation of the fatty acids in a fat or oil. Food fats with high iodine value (e.g. soybean oil, 130) give rise to low grade carcasses. Butter fat has a iodine value of 30 (Table 7).

TABLE 7   Oils and their melting points and iodine value

Oil	Melting point °C	Iodine Value
Coconut oil	25	10
Palm kernel oil	24	37
Mutton tallow	42	40
Palm oil	35	54
Olive oil	−6	81
Castor oil	−18	85
Peanut oil	3	93
Rapeseed oil	−10	98
Cotton seed oil	−1	105
Sunflower oil	−17	125
Soybean oil	−16	130
Linseed oil	−24	178

High grade carcasses have an iodine value of less than 65. Feeds like maize, soybean meal, groundnut cake give rise to body fat with high iodine number in pigs resulting in 'soft pork'. In milch animals, milk fat is softer on rations with higher levels of groundnut cake, linseed. Cotton seed feeding to milch animals gives rise to hard butter fat. Cod liver oil feeding reduce the rumen acetic acid level and eventually result in a fall in milk fat content.

Reichert-Meissl (RM) value: Reichert-Meissl (RM) value is defined as the number of ml of decinormal alkali required to neutralize the steam-volatile, water-soluble fatty acids from 5 g of fat. The RM value is used to assess the quality of butter (Butter has a RM value of 20.37); adulteration of butter with vegetable oils can be detected.

Rancidity of dietary fat: Oils are said to become rancid when they undergo a degradation process known as oxidation. A variety of chemical compounds such as peroxides, aldehydes and free fatty acids are created as oil oxidizes.

TBA rancidity monitors certain types of aldehydes that form when a fat or oil oxidizes. These aldehydes react with 2-Thiobarbituric acid (TBA) in the laboratory to form a complex that is easily measured.

The unpleasant odour and taste that fats may develop on ageing are due to hydrolysis of the glycerides into free fatty acids and glycerol or to oxidation of unsaturated fatty acids in oils.

Hydrolytic rancidity occurs when fats containing short chain fatty acids, such as butyric or caproic, are hydrolysed, releasing these malodourous fatty acids. The edible fat may frequently be rendered completely unacceptable to the consumer. The enzymes, lipases are mostly derived from bacteria and moulds.

Oxidative rancidity is the more important form of rancidity. The unsaturated fatty acids readily undergo oxidation. The products of oxidation include shorter chain fatty acids, fatty acid polymers, aldehydes, ketones, epoxides and hydrocarbons. The acids and aldehydes are major contributors to the smells and flavours associated with oxidized fat and significantly reduce its palatability. This autocatalytic reaction process is explained under lipid peroxidation.

Oxidation of saturated fatty acids results in the development of sweet, heavy taste and smell due to the formation of methlyketones, as in the production of various cheeses. This is known as ketonic rancidity.

Highly refined fats begin to absorb oxygen immediately upon exposure to it. Natural fats, however, may vary considerably in this induction period before oxidation begins. Certain unsaturated fats are quite resistant. This resistance is due to the presence of antioxidants such as phenols, quinones, tocopherols, gallic acid and gallates. Many vegetable oils have these natural antioxidants, whereas, ordinarily animal fats do not.

The prevention or delay of oxidative rancidity is one reason for the great popularity of hydrogenated oils in various commercial products. e.g., peanut butter, margarine, shortenings. Rancid fats deplete the body's vitamin E, vitamin C, and beta-carotene.

Lipid peroxidation: Lipophillic molecules, like polyunsaturated fatty acids (PUFA), are very liable to oxidation by superoxide radicals to form the corresponding peroxides in a process called lipid peroxidation.

Peroxidation is a non-enzymatic process initiated by free radicals which are formed in the course of normal metabolism in the presence of trace metals (e.g. iron, copper) or by ionising radiation. That is why they are prooxidants. Free radicals are molecules that have lost an electron and try to replace it by reacting with other molecules. They can cause damage to the cells, impairing the immune system and leading to various diseases. Unsaturated bonds in lipid molecules are the prime targets of free radicals. Once initiated by free radicals, lipid peroxidation is autocatalytic. These prooxidants are produced during the processing of a fat and the presence of optimum heat, light and moisture greatly accelerate the oxidative process.

Prolonged or repeated heating of PUFAs also produce peroxides, free radicals, etc. PUFA are of the methylene-interrupted type, i.e., a CH_2 group exists between the two double bonds.

$$-CH_2 - CH = CH - CH_2 - CH = CH$$

$$\downarrow \quad H^\bullet \text{ Free radical}$$

$$-CH_2 - CH = CH - \overset{\bullet}{CH} - CH = CH$$

$$\downarrow$$

$$-\overset{\bullet}{C} \quad - CH = CH - CH = CH \quad \text{Conjugated form of}$$
$$\downarrow \quad O_2 + H^\bullet \qquad \text{double bond}$$
$$- CH - CH = CH - CH = CH$$
$$|$$
$$\text{OOH (Hydroperoxide)}$$

Auto-oxidation of Methylene-interrupted Unsaturated Fatty Acid

Any of the free radicals like the peroxy, alkoxy or hydroxyl, radical can propagate the reaction either by abstracting H from methylene carbon or by reacting with oxygen to produce more radicals. The double bond shifts to the conjugated form and the free radical can then unite with oxygen to a form a peroxide and then with hydrogen to form a hydroperoxide.

The hydroperoxides can polymerize with other hydroperoxides to form a film as in the drying of linseed oil paint. It can also break down into aldehydes and ketones which are odourous.

Fatty acid peroxides are very unstable. They disintegrate rapidly into fragments, leading to loss of fatty acids from membrane lipids and damage the biological membrane. Free radical damage may denature the proteins. In addition, certain degradation products of PUFA peroxides can react with biomolecules.

Lipid peroxidation causes extensive damage to biomembranes. Lipid peroxidation in mitochondria would lead to uncoupling of oxidative phosphorylation since enzymes involved in the energy production are associated with mitochondrial membrane.

The reaction (lipid peroxidation) can be stopped if antioxidants are present which promptly replace the H once it has been abstracted.

Eicosanoids

Prostaglandins, and the structurally related molecules prostacyclins, thromboxanes and leukotrienes, are called eicosanoids because they contain 20 carbon atoms (greek eikosi=20; Fig. 9). These hormones are relatively shortlived and hence act locally near to their site of synthesis in the body. They are derived from dihomogamma linolenic acid, arachidonic acid and EPA.

See fig. 7, 8, 9. The 1- and 3-series prostaglandins are anti-inflammatory and inhibit platelet aggregation, whereas the 2-series are pro-

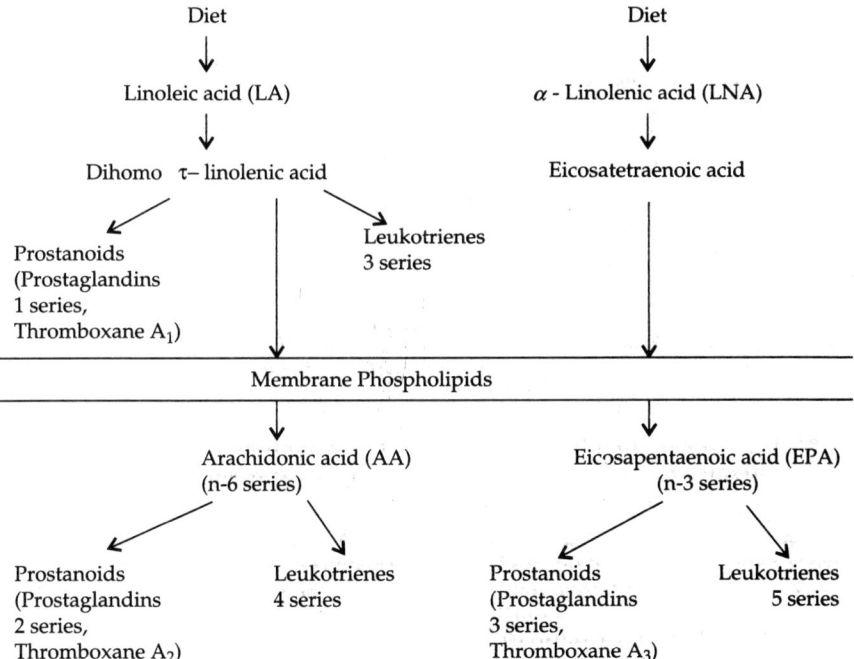

Figure 9. Biosynthesis of Eicosanoids.

inflammatory and pro-aggregatory. The 1- and 3-series thromboxanes mildly stimulate platelet aggregation and stimulate the contraction of respiratory, intestinal and vascular smooth muscle, as do the leukotrienes. The 2-series thromboxanes have a much more powerful action in this respect. Thus eicosanoids have a wide variety of functions, including a major role in the induction and modulation of inflammation.

Glycolipids

In these compounds two of the alcohol groups of the glycerol are esterified by fatty acids and the other is linked to a sugar residue. The lipids of grasses and clovers, which form the major part of the dietary fat of ruminants, are predominantly (about 60 per cent) galactolipids (see the figure). Here the sugar is galactose.

Galactolipids

The galactolipids of grasses are mainly of the monogalactosyl type illustrated here, but smaller quantities of the digalactosyl compounds are also present. In animal tissues, glycolipids are present mainly in the brain and nerve fibres.

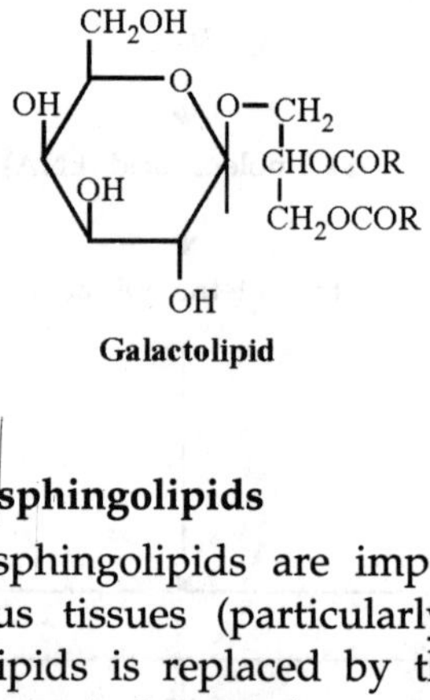

Galactolipid 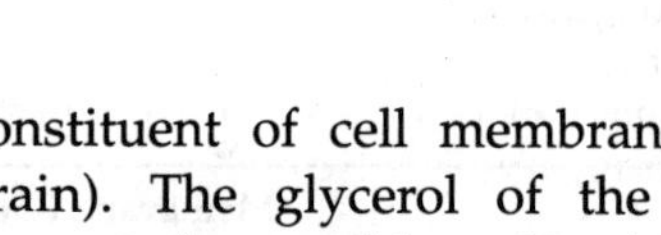   Sphingosine

Glycosphingolipids

Glycosphingolipids are important constituent of cell membrane and nervous tissues (particularly the brain). The glycerol of the plant glycolipids is replaced by the nitrogenous base sphingosine (see the illustration). In simple words, sphingosine bound to fatty acid is a **ceramide;** ceramide bound to monosaccharide is a **cerebroside.**

In their simplest form, the cerebrosides may be described as follows: the glycosphingolipid with the amino group of the sphingosine linked to the carboxyl group of a long-chain fatty acid and the terminal alcohol group to a sugar residue (usually galactose). **The typical structure of galactocerebroside is illustrated here in two ways.** Galactocerebroside is a major component of membrane lipids in the nervous tissue (high in myelin sheath). Glucocerebroside is an intermediate in the synthesis and degradation of complex glycosphingolipids.

1.

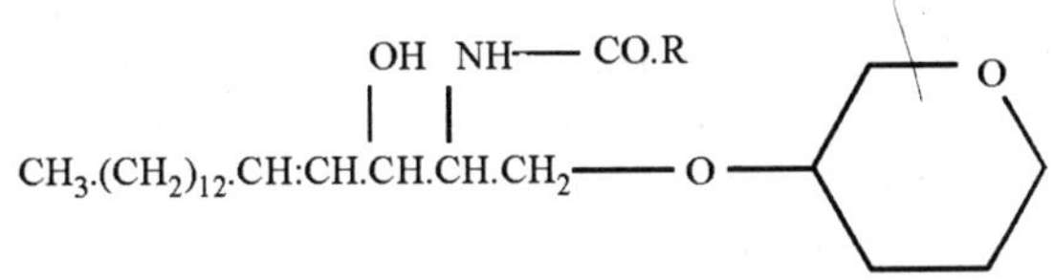

$$CH_3.(CH_2)_{12}.CH:CH.CH.CH.CH_2 — O —$$

with OH, NH—CO.R groups shown above

Sphingosine + (R represents) fatty acid + Galactose = Galactocerebroside

2.

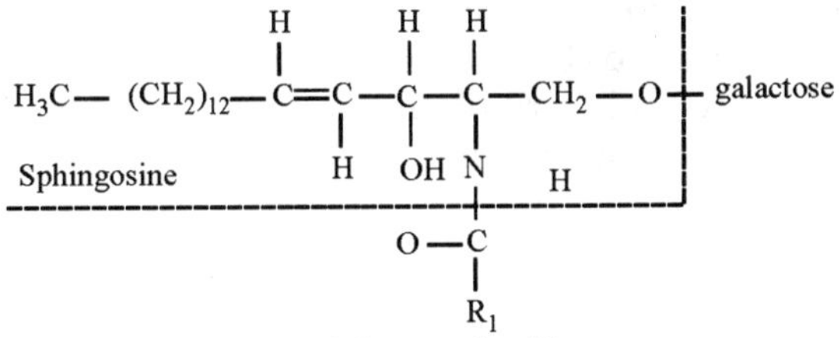

$$H_3C— (CH_2)_{12}—C{=}C—C—C—CH_2—O—galactose$$

Sphingosine   H   OH   N   H

$$O—C$$
$$|$$
$$R_1$$

Galactocerebroside

Gangliosides are predominantly found in ganglions and are the most complex form of glycosphingolipids. They are the derivatives of cerebrosides and contain one or more molecules of N-acetylneuroaminic acid (NANA). NANA is the most important sialic acid.

Phospholipids

Phospholipids contain phosphoric acid, fatty acid, nitrogen base and alcohol. The role of the phospholipids is primarily as constituents of the lipoprotein complexes of biological membranes. Phospholipids are of **two classes: (1) Glycerophospholipids** (or phosphoglycerides) with glycerol as the alcohol and (2) **Sphingophospholipids** (or sphingomyelins) with sphingosine as the alcohol.

Phosphoglycerides or Glycerophospholipids

These are esters of glycerol in which only two of the alcohol groups are esterified by fatty acids (R_1, R_2); with the third esterified by phosphoric

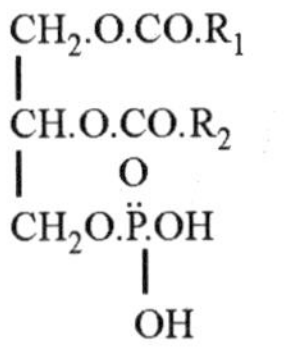

$$CH_2.O.CO.R_1$$
$$|$$
$$CH.O.CO.R_2$$
$$|\quad O$$
$$CH_2O.\overset{..}{P}.OH$$
$$|$$
$$OH$$

Phosphatidic acid

$$R_1{-}\overset{O}{\overset{\|}{C}}{-}O{-}CH_2$$
$$R_2{-}\underset{O}{\overset{\|}{C}}{-}O{-}CH \qquad O$$
$$H_2C{-}O{-}\overset{\|}{P}{-}O^-$$
$$\qquad\qquad O^-$$

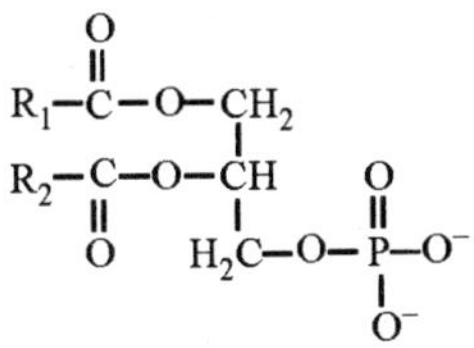

Phosphatidate

acid. The parent compound of the phosphoglycerides is, thus, phosphatidic acid or phosphatidate (diacylglycerol 3-phosphate).

Phosphoglycerides are commonly referred to as **phosphatides.** In the major biologically important compounds, the phosphate group is esterified by one of several alcohols, the commonest of which are serine, choline, glycerol, inositol and ethanolamine. The chief fatty acids present are the 16-carbon saturated and the 18-carbon saturated and monoenoic, although others with 14-24 carbon atoms do occur. The most commonly occurring phosphoglycerides in higher plants and animals are the lecithins and the cephalins. Phosphatidic acid with myoinositol is **phosphatidyl inositol. Phosphatidyl serine** has serine (amino acid). Diphosphatidylglycerol (cardiolipin) is found in the inner mitochondrial membrane (see the illustration).

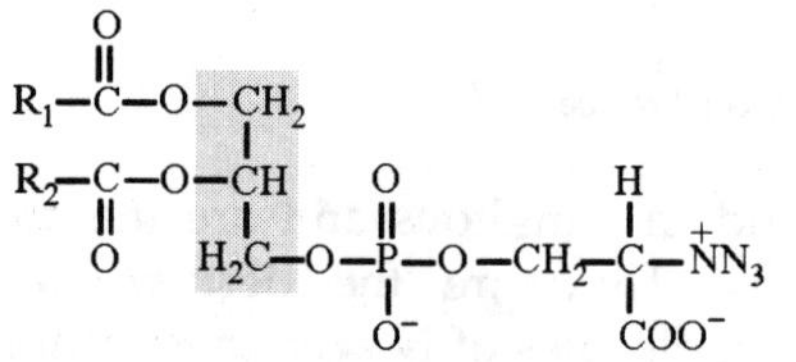

Phosphatidylserine

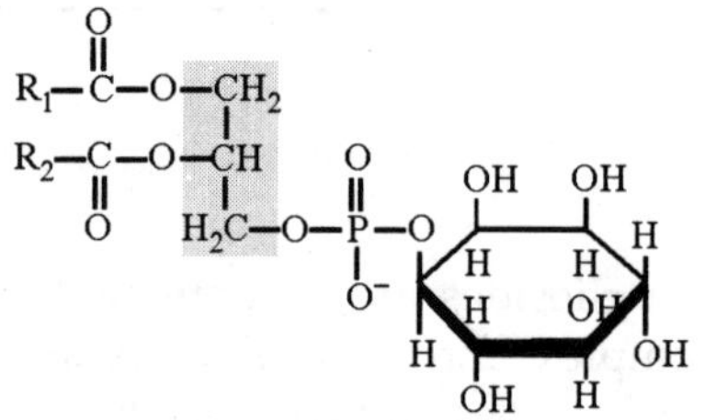

Phosphatidylinositol

Lecithins

Lecithins have the phosphoric acid esterified by the nitrogenous base choline and are more correctly termed **phosphatidyl choline**. A typical example would have the formula:

$$CH_2.O.CO.C_{15}H_{31}$$
$$CH.O.CO.C_{17}H_{33}$$
$$CH_2.O.PO_3.CH_2.CH_2.N+(CH_3)_3$$

OR

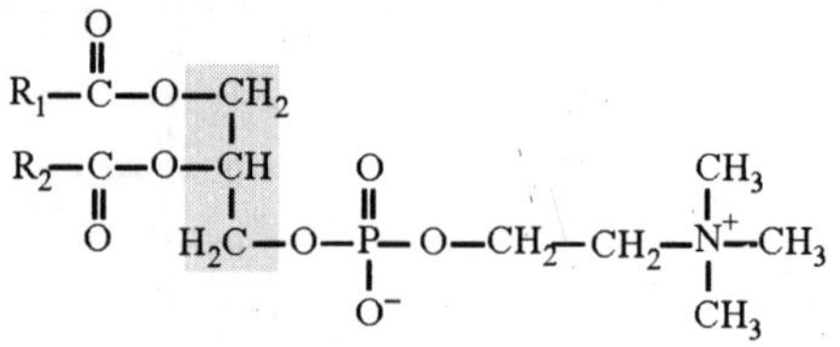

Phosphatidylcholine

$$R_1-\overset{\overset{\displaystyle O}{\|}}{C}-O-CH_2$$

$$R_2-\overset{\overset{\displaystyle}{|}}{\underset{\underset{\displaystyle O}{\|}}{C}}-O-\overset{\overset{\displaystyle}{|}}{\underset{\displaystyle}{CH}}$$

$$H_2C-O-\overset{\overset{\displaystyle O}{\|}}{\underset{\underset{\displaystyle O^-}{|}}{P}}-O-CH_2-\overset{\overset{\displaystyle OH}{|}}{\underset{\underset{\displaystyle H}{|}}{C}}-CH_2OH$$

Phosphatidylglycerol

$$R_1-\overset{\overset{\displaystyle O}{\|}}{C}-O-CH_2$$
$$R_2-C-O-CH \qquad H \qquad H_2C-O-\overset{\overset{\displaystyle O}{\|}}{C}-R_3$$
$$HC-O-C-R_4$$
$$H_2C-O-\overset{\overset{\displaystyle O}{\|}}{\underset{\underset{\displaystyle O^-}{|}}{P}}-O-CH_2-\overset{\overset{\displaystyle}{|}}{\underset{\underset{\displaystyle OH}{|}}{C}}-CH_2-O-\overset{\overset{\displaystyle O}{\|}}{\underset{\underset{\displaystyle O^-}{|}}{P}}-O-CH_2 \qquad O$$

Diphosphatidylglycerol

Cephalin

Cephalins differ from the lecithins in having ethanolamine instead of choline and are correctly termed **phosphatidyl ethanolamines**. See the ethanolamine formula sideby.

$$R_1-\overset{\overset{\displaystyle O}{\|}}{C}-O-CH_2$$
$$R_2-C-O-CH$$
$$H_2C-O-\overset{\overset{\displaystyle O}{\|}}{\underset{\underset{\displaystyle O^-}{|}}{P}}-O-CH_2-CH_2-\overset{+}{N}H_3$$

$$\overset{\overset{\displaystyle NH_2}{|}}{CH_2.CH_2OH}$$

Phosphatidylethanolamine

Plasmalogens

When a fatty acid is attached by an ether linkage (CH=CH) (in place of ester linkage) at C_1 of glycerol in the phosphoglycerides, the resultant compound is plasmalogen. Cephalin or phosphatidyl ethanolamine has ester linkage. Phosphatidal ethanolamine is a plasmalogen (see the figure). Choline, inositol and serine may substitute ethanolamine to give plasmalogens.

$$CH_2-O-CH=CH-R1$$
$$CH-O-\overset{\overset{\displaystyle O}{\|}}{C}-R2$$
$$CH_2-O-\overset{\overset{\displaystyle O}{\|}}{\underset{\underset{\displaystyle O^-}{|}}{P}}-O-CH_2-CH_2-NH_2$$

Phosphatidal ethanolamine

Sphingomyelins or Sphingophospholipids

Sphingomyelins belong to a large group, which have sphingosine instead of glycerol as the parent material. They differ from the cerebrosides in having the terminal hydroxyl group linked to phosphoric acid instead of a sugar residue. The phosphoric acid is esterified by either choline or ethanolamine. The sphingomyelins also have the amino group linked to the carboxyl group of a long-chain fatty acid by means of a peptide linkage:[7]

Sphingosine   Phosphoryl choline

$$CH_3.(CH_2)_{12}CH{:}CH.CHOH.CH.CH_2O.PO_3^-.CH_2.N^+(CH_3)_3$$
$$|$$
$$NH.CO.R$$

Sphingomyelin (sphingosine + fatty acid [ceramide] + phosphoric acid + choline)

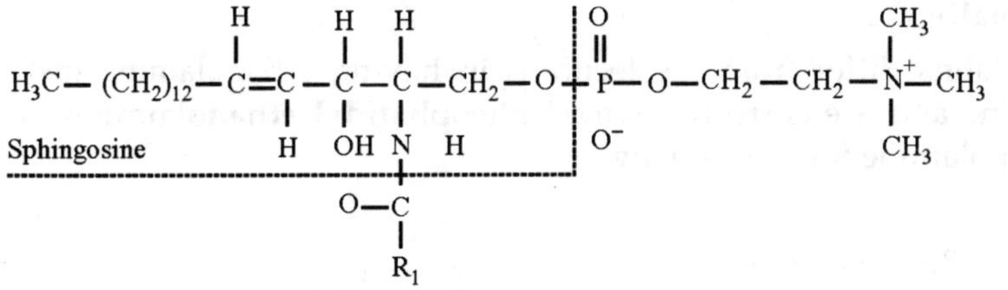

Sphingomyelin

Waxes

Waxes are simple, relatively non-polar lipids consisting of a long-chain fatty acid combined with a monohydric alcohol of high molecular weight. They are usually solid at ordinary temperatures. Cetyl alcohol is the most commonly found in waxes. Natural waxes (beeswax) are usually mixtures of a number of esters.

Waxes are widely distributed in plants and animals, where they often have a protective function. The hydrophobic nature of the wax coating provides wool and feathers with waterproofing in animals. Among the better-known animal waxes are lanolin, obtained from wool, and spermaceti, a product of marine animals.

In plants, waxes are usually included in the cuticular fraction, where they form a matrix in which cutin and suberin are embedded. Phenolic constituents such as p-coumaric acid, paracoumaric and ferulic acids are usually present. Both cutin and suberin are highly resistant to breakdown and are not of any significant nutritional value. The waxes, too, are resistant to breakdown and are poorly utilised by animals. Their presence in foods in large amounts leads to high ether extract figures and may result in the nutritive value being overestimated.

Alkanes (from C21 to C37) make up a large proportion of the whole, with odd-chain compounds predominating. Branched-chain hydrocarbons, aldehydes, free fatty acids (from C12 to C36) and various ketols are commonly occurring though minor constituents. Free alcohols are usually of minor importance but may form up to half of some waxes.

Steroids

The steroids include such biologically important compounds as the sterols, the bile acids, the adrenal hormones and the sex hormones. They have a common structural unit of a phenanthrene nucleus linked to a cyclopentane ring. The individual compounds differ in the number and positions of their double bonds and in the nature of the side chain at carbon atom 17.

Phenanthrene nucleus   Cyclopentane ring   Cholesterol

Basic steroid structural unit

Sterols

These have eight to ten carbon atoms in the side chain, an alcohol group at carbon atom 3, but no carbonyl or carboxyl groups. They may be classified into: the phytosterols of plant origin; the mycosterols of fungal origin; the zoosterols of animal origin. The phytosterols and the mycosterols are not absorbed from the gut and are not found in animal tissues. Cholesterol is a zoosterol that is present in all animal cells.

7-Dehydrocholesterol

This substance is derived from cholesterol and is important as the precursor of vitamin D_3. It is produced when the sterol is exposed to ultraviolet light (see the chemical formula).

Ergosterol

This phytosterol is widely distributed in brown algae, bacteria and higher plants. Upon ultraviolet irradiation, it is converted to ergocalciferol or vitamin D_2.

Steroid hormones

These include the female sex hormones (oestrogens), the male sex hormones (androgens) and progesterone, as well as cortisol, aldosterone and corticosterone, which are produced in the adrenal cortex. The adrenal hormones have an important role in the control of glucose and fat metabolism.

7-Dehydrocholesterol   Cholecalciferol
                              (vitamin D_3)

Formation of vitamin D_3

Terpenes

Terpenes are made up of a number of isoprene units linked together to form chains or cyclic structures. Isoprene is a five-carbon compound. Many terpenes found in plants have strong characteristic odours and flavours and are components of essential oils such as lemon or camphor oil. The word 'essential' is used to indicate the occurrence of the oils in essences and not to imply that they are required by animals. Among the more important plant terpenes are the phytol moiety of chlorophyll, the carotenoid pigments, plant hormones such as giberellic acid and vitamins A, E and K. In animals, some of the coenzymes, including those of the coenzyme Q group, are terpenes.

Amphipathic lipids

Lipids are insoluble (hydrophobic) in water. This is primarily due to the predominant presence of hydrocarbon groups. However, some of the lipids possess polar or hydrophilic groups which tend to be soluble in water. Molecules which contain both hydrophobic and hydrophilic groups are known as amphipathic. Amphipathic lipid has 'polar' head and 'non-polar' tail. Examples include phospholipids, bile salts, sphingolipids.

Chapter 5

The Role and Requirement
of Water

Role of Water

The vital role of water in the body is indicated by Max Rubner (1854-1932). He observed that the body can lose practically all of its fat and over half of its protein and yet live, while a loss of one-tenth of its water results in death. E.F. Adolph (1933) pointed out that water ranks far above every other substance in the body as regards rate of turnover.

W.B. Cannon (1932) stated that the heat produced in maximal muscular effort continued for 20 minutes would be so great that if it were not promptly dissipated it would cause albuminous substances of the body to become stiff like a hard boiled egg.

Water is also a nutrient and is probably the most extraordinary substance in nutrition, being far more complex than its simple chemical formula suggests.

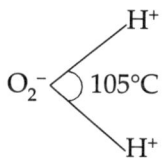 The positive hydrogen of one molecule attracts the negative oxygen of another, and this hydrogen bond has the strength to hold molecules together for the multitude of functions that water performs, hydrogen bonding literally makes the phenomenon of life possible.

Properties and Functions of Water

1. Water is the ideal dispersing medium because of its solvent and ionizing powers which facilitate cell reactions.
2. It has high specific heat. This enables it to absorb the heat of cell reactions with a minimum rise in temperature.
3. The latent heat of vaporization of water also plays an important role in regulating body temperature.
4. Other properties of large significance in physiology are the high surface tension, the tendency to form hydrates and the high dielectric constant of water.
5. It is concerned in digestion, absorption and transport of nutrients and excretion of waste products.

6. Water plays many special roles. As synovial fluid, it lubricates the joints. It acts as a water cushion for the nervous system as cerebrospinal fluid. In the ear, it transports sounds. In the eye, it is concerned with sight. Thus water is necessary for the formation of blood, tissue fluid, synovial fluid, aqueous humour, etc.
7. Water softens coarse feeds and makes them palatable.

Sources of Water

1. Feed
2. Drinking water
3. Metabolic water or oxidation water

Moisture content in feeds and significance of moisture content of feeds has already been described in the earlier chapter.

Metabolic or oxidation water: When the carbohydrate glucose is oxidized to furnish energy for body processes, carbon dioxide and water result:

$$C_6 H_{12} O_6 + 6 O_2 \rightarrow 6 CO_2 + 6 H_2O$$

Metabolism of glucose yields 60% of its weight as water and protein produces approximately 40% of its weight as water, while in the case of fat the figure is over 100%. More specifically 1g each of starch, protein and fat produce 0.56, 0.4 and 1.07 g of metabolic water. Metabolic water is also produced by the dehydration synthesis of body proteins, fats and carbohydrates. Under certain physiological conditions, metabolic water plays an important role in the animal economy. It suffices to meet the needs of hibernating animals. These animals metabolize their reserves of carbohydrate and fat to provide energy for their vital processes. This metabolism produces enough water to balance that lost by respiration and evaporation.

The situation is quite different in the very dry atmosphere of desert regions. Relatively dry air is inhaled to supply O_2 for fat oxidation; Expired air is saturated. The following furnishes the oxygen requirement. Starch requires less oxygen per gram of metabolic water formed than fat and much less than protein.

Nutrient	O_2 needed to oxidize	Metabolic Water formed
1 gram starch	0.83 L	0.56 g
1 g protein	0.97 L	0.40 g
1 g fat	2.02 L	1.07 g

Nutrient	Loss of water by respiration and evaporation
1 g starch	1.49 g
1 g protein	2.44 g
1 g fat	1.88 g

Increased respiration needed to oxidize body fat and protein would result in an increased loss of water by evaporation. Camel, therefore, eats mostly carbohydrates during desert travel.

Clothes moths contain 50% of water in their bodies. Live throughout their cycle on food containing 10% or less of water. They excrete uric acid. The small amount of water obtained from food and metabolic water suffice. Metabolic water comprises only 5 to 10% of total water intake of domestic animals and varied only with the metabolic rate.

Factors Governing the Water Requirements of Livestock and Poultry

Water requirements are equivalent to water consumed *ad libitum* plus water intake through the feeds. The requirements are influenced by the following factors :

I   Biological factors
II   Environmental factors
III Nature of the feed

I Biological factors: 1. Class 2. Species 3. Age 4. Breed 5. Sex 6. Body weight 7. Productivity.

Birds require less water compared to mammals because uric acid is the end product of protein metabolism. Higher evaporative water loss in birds is partially balanced by their reduced urinary water excretion relative to mammals. Among mammals, cats, goats and camels require less water because of their capacity to conserve water. Camel needs only one-seventh as much water per unit body weight as man in the summer. Young animals have higher water needs per unit of body size than do mature ones. Milch animals require more water. A dairy cow needs 1.5 L of water for each litre of milk produced.

II Environmental factors: Temperature and relative humidity.

III Nature of the feed: Water requirements are highly related to dry matter intake (DMI) of the animals.

1. High crude fibre level: Diets of high fibre content involve excretion of faeces of greater water content than when the food is less in fibre. Similarly water losses are more in faeces with the intakes of other feeds which have laxative properties.

2. Diets with high fat level, high protein level and high salt intake increase the water intake.

Species	Water requirement/day	DMI : Water consumption
Adult Cattle	30 L	1 : 3 to 3.5
Calves		1 : 6 to 7
Sheep and Goats	4-6 L	1 : 4
Swine	6-8 L	1 : 3
Poultry	250 ml	1 : 2
Adult buffaloes	40 L	1 : 5 to 5.5
Water 90 ml/kg BW for maintenance		
2.0 to 2.5 litre/kg milk produced		

Effect of excess of water: Dry matter consumption is reduced to too low a level.

Effect of lack of water: Water restriction results in rapid decrease in feed intake, especially in hot environment which accelerate body water loss.
1. Increase the pulse rate, and rectal temperature.
2. Increase the concentration of blood and the reduction in blood volume makes blood circulation difficult.
3. Tingling and numbness of fingers and feet.

Effects of water deprivation: When man is deprived of drinking water in a hot, dry environment, he soon exhibits thirst. When the water deficit approaches 4 to 5 % of BW, there is discomfort and anorexia.

As the water loss increases from 6 to 10% there is headache, his movements lack coordination, speech becomes indistinct, and dyspnea and cyanosis are noted. At a deficit of 12 to 14% the eyes become sunken, the skin becomes shriveled, there is inability to swallow and delirium occurs.

As water is lost from the blood, its viscosity and the resistance to flow increases. When increasing heart rate is no longer able to circulate the blood fast enough to dissipate the heat from the deeper body parts, a fatal increase in body temperature occurs. In a hot environment dehydration of about 12% is fatal to man.

Some desert animals such as camel and gerbil can tolerate a more severe water dehydration than man or dog without suffering an explosive heat rise. A camel can lose water 20% of its body weight before any decrease in appetite was noted.

A camel was exposed to 40°C or more temperature for 7 days without water. It losts 27% of its BW. When water was offered, camel was able to drink enough water within a few minutes to restore its body weight loss with no apparent ill effects.

Water Economy Among Animals

Body water is distributed within the cells (intracellular fluid), outside the cells (extracellular fluid) and interstitial fluid. Water sources to the animal are through feed, drinking water and metabolic water. Water is lost from the body constantly in the respired air, evaporation from the skin and periodically through the faeces and urine.

The water losses through the gastrointestinal tract vary with the nature of the diet i.e. its digestibility and laxative nature. It also depends on the species. Losses are increased with the level of roughage intake and with the intake of other feeds which have laxative nature. In general, the lesser the digestibility the larger the proportion of undigested material, the greater the loss of water in faeces. In cattle and buffaloes, the faecal material contains about 80% water. The faeces are much drier in the case of sheep and goats. In all species and under all normal conditions, the losses through the gut are very small compared with the very large amount of water secreted into the tract in the digestive juices. Almost all the water thus secreted is reabsorbed except in diarrhoea.

The amount of water excreted in the urine is highly variable. The kidneys regulate the volume and composition of body fluids. The kidneys can reduce this loss to a minimum, through its powers of filtration and then of concentration of the filtrate by the reabsorption of water. There are large differences in animals in ability to conserve urinary water losses. Camel and Kangaroo rat have much higher concentrations of electrolytes in their urine compared to humans. Camel eats mostly carbohydrates during desert travel. This minimizes water used for excretion of waste products.

Nature of Nitrogenous End Product

Mammals: Urea is the principal end product of protein catabolism. It is soluble in water and toxic to the tissues in concentrated solution. Much water is required to dilute it to a harmless concentration, remove it from the tissues and excrete it. Urea excretion in mammals requires 20-40 times more water than is required to excrete a similar amount of uric acid in birds.

Birds: Uric acid is the principal nitrogenous end product. It is excreted in nearly solid form with minimum loss of water. Further the breakdown of protein to uric acid provides more metabolic water than does its catabolism to urea. That is why, birds have a lower requirements of water than mammals. Birds are much less sensitive to the temporary deprivation of water.

Mammals will live longer without food than without water. Consumption of food, especially protein food, without water hastens death as the result of the accumulation of toxic end products. Birds, snakes and insects survive much longer under these conditions.

Nutrients and Toxic Elements in Water

Water may carry many of the essential elements as well as toxic materials because of its properties as a solvent. Total dissolved solids (TDS) or salinity is a measure of the usefulness of water for animals or for crop irrigation.

Description	TDS, mg/litre (L)	
Slightly saline	1,000 - 3,000	All species can tolerate
Moderately saline	3,000 - 10,000	
Very saline	10,000 - 35,000	
Brine	> 35,000	

There may be mild temporary diarrhoea when animals are changed suddenly from salt free water to slightly saline water. Water containing 3000 to 5000 mg/L is unsatisfactory for poultry. Ruminants and horses refused at first water containing 5000-7000 mg/L. But after adaptation animals gave satisfactory performance. Sheep are more tolerant than cattle. Cattle are more tolerant than pigs. The most abundant salt in saline water is sodium with calcium and magnesium in lower concentrations occuring as carbonates, bicarbonates, chlorides and sulfates. Sulfates are more harmful than chlorides. Magnesium chloride is more injurious than the Ca or Na salt due to osmotic effect.

National Academy of Sciences (Washington, D.C., 1974) recommended upper limits of some toxic substances in drinking water.

Substance	Safe Upper limit, mg/litre (L)
Arsenic	0.2
Cadmium	0.05
Chromium	1.0
Cobalt	1.0
Copper	0.5
Fluoride	2.0
Lead	0.1
Mercury	0.01
Nickel	1.0
Nitrate	100
Nitrite	10
Vanadium	0.1
Zinc	25.0

Chapter 6

Digestive Process in Different Species

Digestive system - Gastrointestinal tract

The digestive system consists of two parts, the gastrointestinal (GI) tract and the major digestive accessory glands, which include liver and pancreas. The GI tract, also known as the gut, is a tube-like structure that extends from the mouth to the anus. This tube consists of four main layers, histologically: (1) the mucosa comprising epithelial cells (enterocytes, endocrine cells, etc), the lamina propria and the muscularis mucosae; (2) the submucosa; (3) two muscular layers, an inner thick circular layer and an outer thin longitudinal layer and (4) a serosal layer.

Functions of the GI tract

Functionally, the GI tract supplies the body, including the gut itself, with nutrients, electrolytes and water. To supply the body with these substances, the gut performs five functions: motility, secretion, digestion, absorption and storage. The GI tract controls these five functions through intrinsic and extrinsic control systems. The intrinsic control system elements are located between the different layers of the gut, whereas the extrinsic control system resides outside the wall of the GI tract. Each of these systems consists of two components, namely, nerves and endocrine secretions (Figure 1). **The intrinsic control system** has two components: the enteric nervous system (ENS) and gut hormones that include gastrin, gastric inhibitory peptide, cholecystokinin, secretin and motilin. **The extrinsic control system** elements that regulate gut functions consist of the vagus and the splanchnic nerves and the hormone aldosterone. The ENS is a component of the autonomic nervous system (ANS). The other two ANS components are the sympathetic and parasympathetic systems. The ENS controls the majority of the GI functions independent from the central nervous system.

The secretions of the intrinsic and extrinsic control systems of the gut are regulatory in nature but not of digestive type. They regulate the activity of the cells and tissues of the GI tract. They are not secreted into the gut lumen but reach their target tissues by *four different routes*. Endocrine secretions reach by the blood, paracrine secretions reach by diffusion through the interstitial space, whereas autocrine secretions of the paracrine cell modify the function of the same cell. The enteric neurons secrete contents via vesicles located on axon branches of these neurons, namely, from varicosities. The varicosities contain neurotransmitter / neuromodulator (regulatory peptides), which are collectively known as neurocrines.

The **enteric neurons** consist of sensory (afferent) neurons, interneurons and motor (efferent) neurons. Remember that the gut tube has four layers. Sensory / afferent input comes from mechanoreceptors (located within the muscular layers) and chemoreceptors (within the mucosa). Mechanoreceptors monitor distension of the gut wall, whereas chemoreceptors monitor chemical conditions in the gut lumen. Enteric motor nerves supply vascular muscle, gut muscle and glands within the gut wall. Efferent neurons of the ENS may be stimulatory or inhibitory. The action is largely determined by the type of substance they secrete and the receptors activated (Table 1). On the basis of chemical contents, *enteric neurons may be cholinergic neurons* (contain acetyl choline) or *adrenergic neurons* (contain adrenaline or epinephrine). Cholinergic neurons are stimulatory to gut activities while adrenergic neurons are inhibitory to gut activities.

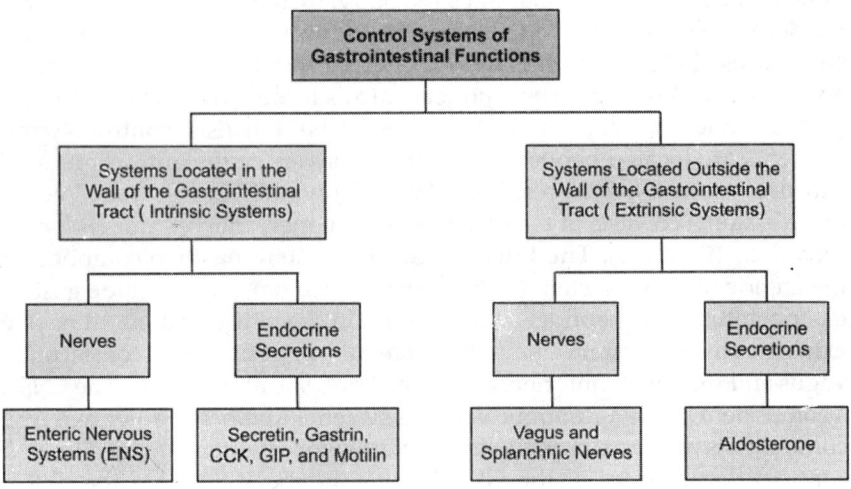

Figure 1 A diagram summarizing the various systems that control the different functions of the GI tract

Gastrointestinal hormones and aldosterone The GI tract contains millions of **epithelial cells**, which are referred to as enterocytes, enterochromaffin cells and endocrine cells. The enterocytes have an absorptive function, whereas the enterochromaffin cells are secretory in nature. These enterochromaffin cells secrete peptides or hormones that help regulate gut motility, food digestion and nutrient absorption. The 'gut peptide' that fulfils certain criteria is termed as a 'gut hormone'. Therefore, all gut hormones are also considered gut peptides, whereas not all gut peptides are gut hormones.

The intrinsic hormonal control system of the gut consists of five hormones including secretin, gastrin, cholecystokinin (CCK), gastric inhibitory polypeptide (GIP) or glucose-dependent insulinotropic peptide (because its secretion is stimulated by the presence of glucose in the duodenum) or enterogastrone (because of its ability to reduce the rate of stomach emptying) and motilin. In addition, the candidate hormones (that do not completely fulfill the criteria) are pancreatic polypeptide, peptide YY and enteroglucagon. The extrinsic hormonal control system of the gut is limited to one hormone: aldosterone; this is the only hormone that is secreted outside the GI tract but still participates in controlling some of the functions of the GI tract (see Table 1 for other details). The secretions of the intrinsic and extrinsic control systems of the gut are regulatory and not digestive in nature.

Digestion

Digestion involves a series of processes in the gastrointestinal (G.I.) tract by which feeds are broken down in particle size and finally rendered soluble so that absorption is possible. This is accompanied by a combination of mechanical and enzymatic processes. Microorganisms provide important enzymes not secreted by mammalian species. The primary enzymes of the GI tract are presented in Table 2. Readers may refer luminal-phase and membranous-phase of digestion in the new chapter 7.

Organs of Digestion

I Mouth (teeth, tongue, cheeks and salivary glands): Its function is to bring in feed, mechanically break it up, and mix it with saliva which acts as a lubricant to facilitate swallowing. Principal organs of prehension are lips, tongue and pointed lower lip, respectively, in horses, ruminants and pigs. Dogs and cats hold food with their forelimbs; the movement of the head and jaws brings the food into the mouth.

Poultry have no teeth and swallow the food as it is. Any grinding done by the action of the grit is in its gizzard. In their natural rearing birds pick

Table 1 Gastrointestinal hormones and aldosterone*

Hormone	Production site	Action	Release stimulus
Secretin	S-cells of the Duodenum and upper jejunum	Stimulates bicarbonate secretion and inhibits acid secretion	In response to fat, protein, gastric acid and bile acids
Gastrin (little gastrin and big gastrin)	G cells of the gastric pylorus, antrum and duodenum	Stimulates acid secretion and growth of stomach epithelium	In response to the presence of protein and gastric distension
Cholecystokinin (CCK)	Endocrine I cells and the enteric neurons of the duodenum and jejunum	CCK controls many GI-related functions. For example, CCK causes gallbladder and smooth muscle contraction while increasing pancreatic secretion and it inhibits gastric emptying and food intake.	In response to fat and protein
Gastric inhibitory polypeptide (GIP) or enterogastrone	K cells of duodenum and jejunum	Inhibits gastric acid secretion and stimulates insulin secretion	In response to fat and glucose
Motilin	M (or Mo) cells of the duodenum and, to a lesser extent, jejunum	Motilin works on both muscles and nerves to regulate the 'migrating motor complex' to push undigested material out of the small intestine to colon; stimulates gastric emptying during the between-meal period and secretion of pepsinogen	Acetylcholine
Aldosterone (steroid hormone – mineralocorticoid)	Outer zona glomerulosa section of the adrenal cortex	Primarily, it acts on the distal convoluted tubules and collecting ducts of the kidney causing secretion of potassium and reabsorption of sodium and water. In GI tract, it stimulates sodium and water reabsorption from the gut and salivary glands in exchange with potassium ions. Promotes increased absorption of water and sodium in the proximal colon and decreased absorption in the distal colon, although it is species-dependent.	Low-salt (low sodium) diet, angiotensin, adrenocorticotropic hormone, or high potassium levels

*Adapted from Cunningham's textbook of Veterinary Physiology** by Bradley G. Klein, 5th edition, 2013 section IV: Physiology of the Gastrointestinal tract pp263-358.

small stones called grit to support the grinding of whole grains, etc. in the gizzard. But birds reared in cages or otherwise with mash feed the effect of grit supply seems to be doubtful.

TABLE 2. Primary Enzymes of the Gastrointestinal Tract.

Food source (Substrate)	Enzyme	Origin	Products of digestion
Carbohydrates			
Starch, glycogen, dextrin	Amylase ″	Saliva, Pancreas	Maltose, glucose
Maltose	Maltase	S. intestine	Glucose
Lactose	Lactase	″	Glu, galactose
Sucrose	Sucrase	″	Glu, fructose
Fats and Oils			
Lipids	Lipase ″	Gastric mucosa, Pancreas	Monoglycerides, Glycerol, fatty acids
Proteins			
Milk proteins	chymosin	Gastric mucosa of young calf	Coagulates milk Proteins
	Endoenzymes		
Proteins	Pepsin	Gastric mucosa	Polypeptides
Protein breakdown products	Trypsin Chymotrypsin	Pancreas ″	Peptides, Proteoses
	Exoenzymes Carboxy- peptidase	″	Pepides, Amino acids
	Amino- peptidase	S. intestine	Peptides, Amino acids
	Dipeptidase	″	Amino acids
Nucleoproteins	Nucleotidase	″	Nucleotides, nucleosides
	Nucleosidase	″	Purines, Phosphoric acid

Principal salivary glands are parotid, mandibular (submaxillary) and sublingual and smaller glands are buccal glands (in cheeks) and labial glands (in lips). In addition to its lubricating function, saliva may have antibacterial, digestive and evaporative cooling functions, depending on the species. Saliva is 99% water, with mucin, inorganic salts and enzymes α-amylase and lysozyme present in the remaining 1%. The antibacterial activity of saliva results from antibodies and antimicrobial enzyme lysozyme. The evaporation of 1 L of water into water vapour requires 580 kcal heat. Evaporative heat loss is the only form of heat loss available when ambient temperature exceeds body temperature; the animal begins to pant and increases its salivation (example, dogs); some animals smear themselves with saliva (example, small rodents).

The quantity of saliva secreted varies from species to species. In large ruminants it is up to 130 to 180 litres per day. In man, pig and rat saliva contains ptyalin (α-amylase) which splits α 1:4 glucosidic linkages. It is inactivated by the acid in the gastric juice. The activity of enzyme is low in pigs. Horse, lacks salivary amylase. Some birds have salivary amylase that is active in the environment of the crop. This enzyme is usually absent from the saliva of carnivorous animals such as cats. The saliva of some species (calves on milk diet) also contains a fat-digesting enzyme known as lingual lipase (pregastric esterase, page no 229).

II Esophagus: It provides passage to the food from the mouth to the stomach or forestomach. In contrast to most species, the horse seldom vomits.

III Stomach: See 'Gastric Secretion' for a description of monogastric-stomach. Ruminants have four compartments in their stomach as rumen, reticulum, omasum and abomasum, the last one being the true stomach. Of these the rumen and reticulum have about 50% of the total capacity of the digestive tract. This large capacity is essential to allow feed retention so that microorganisms can breakdown cellulose and other complex carbohydrates, which mammalian enzymes cannot hydrolyze. Ruminants swallow feed with little mastication. Later they regurgitate the ingesta from reticulorumen, remasticate the solids and reswallow it. This phenomenon of 'chewing the cud' or rechewing rumen content ingested earlier is one of the features characteristic of ruminant animals.

Milk and other liquid drinks reach the omasum and/or abomasum directly through oesophageal groove. Some nonruminants such as kangaroo, hippopotamus, etc. have a voluminous sacculated stomach that serves as the primary site of microbial activity.

In chickens and turkeys, esophagus empties directly into the crop where food is stored and soaked. The food then passes through the proventriculus (glandular stomach), where digestive juices are copiously secreted and mixed with food, to the gizzard (ventriculus) (muscular stomach), where hard seeds and grains are ground before moving into the small intestine.

See figure 2 'avian digestive system'. The gizzard wall produces koilin, a protein-polysaccharide complex similar in its amino acid composition to keratin, which hardens in the presence of hydrochloric acid (Proventriculus produces hydrochloric acid and pepsinogen). Proteolysis occurs in the lumen of the gizzard in addition to grinding action due to the presence of grit. The pancreatic juice of fowls contains the same enzymes as the mammalian secretions. The intestinal mucosa produces mucin, α-amylase, maltase, sucrase and proteolytic enzymes. Unlike young pigs, chicks have maltase and sucrase activities in their small intestine and, it can be assumed that they possess satisfactory amylase activity, because they perform well on uncooked cereal diets.

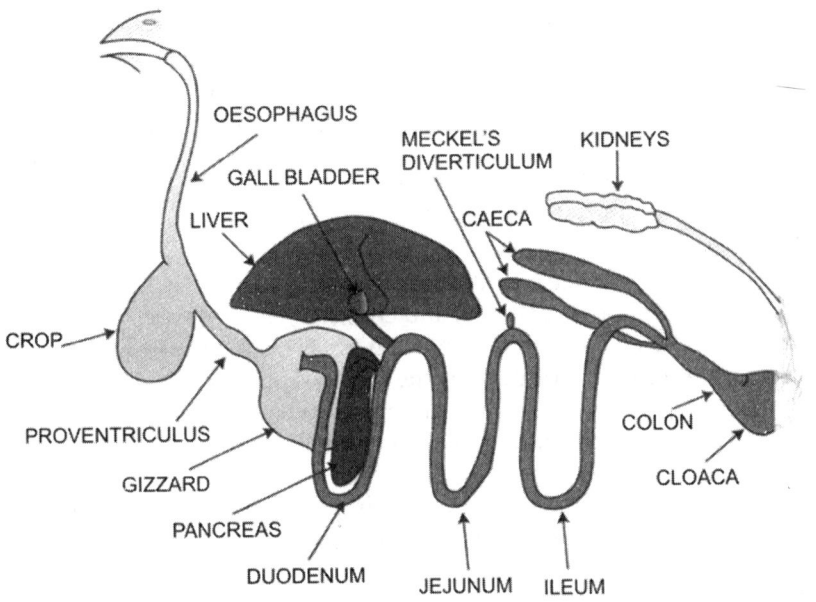

Figure 2 Avian digestive system

Gastric secretion

Most of the domestic monogastric animals have only glandular mucosa in the stomach. Horses and rats, however, have an area in the proximal portion of their stomachs that is covered by nonglandular, stratified squamous epithelium. This area is visibly different from the glandular area. The nonglandular area may serve as a place where a small amount of fermentative digestion could occur. As it is studied in motility section, there is little mixing activity in the proximal stomach. That is how the fermentation activity in the nonglandular area could proceed without impediment from the acid secretions killing the bacteria.

The glandular area of the stomach is divided into three regions: cardiac mucosa, parietal mucosa and pyloric mucosa. These areas contain glands of similar structure but with different types of secretions. The glandular mucosa of the stomach has frequent invaginations or pores known as **gastric pits**. The major surface areas of the stomach, as well as the lining of the pits, are covered with **'surface mucous cells'**. These cells produce 'thick, tenacious mucus' that is important for protecting the stomach epithelium from the acid conditions and grinding activity present in the lumen. When the mucous cells are injured, stomach ulcers result.

The cardiac glands secrete only mucus, which is alkaline in nature and may protect the adjacent esophageal mucosa from the acid secretions of the stomach. Within the parietal area, the glands contain **'parietal cells' (oxyntic cells)**. These cells produce HCl. In this region gastric glands secrete a glycoprotein and fucolipid mucus. This region also produces pepsinogen. The pyloric glands have no parietal cells but contain the gastrin-producing G cells. Pyloric glands do secrete pepsinogen. Thus, gastric juice consists of water, pepsinogen, inorganic salts, mucus, hydrochloric acid and the intrinsic factor important for the efficient absorption of vitamin B_{12}.

When the gastric glands are stimulated, the HCl solution is secreted into the lumen. Both the hydrogen (H^+) and chloride (Cl^-) ions are secreted by the parietal cells. H^+ is secreted through an H^+,K^+–ATPase (adenosine triphosphatase) enzyme located on the luminal surface of the cell. This enzyme is also referred to as a proton pump, exchanges H^+ for potassium ions (K^+), pumping one K^+ into the cell for each H^+ secreted into the lumen. In the exchange process, one molecule of ATP is expended. The K^+ cations that accumulate within the cells are released back into the lumen in combination with Cl^- anions. This allows the recycling of K^+ ions as they are pumped back into the cells in exchange for H^+, resulting in the net secretion of H^+ and Cl^-, with little net movement of K^+.

Hydrogen ions for secretion come from the dissociation of intracellular carbonic acid (H_2CO_3), leaving a bicarbonate ion (HCO_3^-) in the cell for each H^+ secreted into the lumen (Figure 3). Carbonic acid originates from water and carbon dioxide through the action of *carbonic anhydrase*, an enzyme found in high concentration in the gastric mucosa.

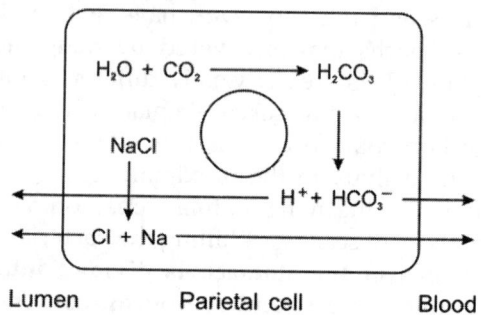

Figure 3   Electrolyte movements during gastric acid secretion

As hydrogen cations (H^+) are secreted, bicarbonate anions (HCO_3^-) accumulate in the cell. To counterbalance this accumulation, bicarbonate anions are exchanged for chloride anions (Cl^-) at the cell's nonluminal surface. Thus additional chloride is made available to the cell for secretion into the glandular lumen, and bicarbonate is secreted into the blood. During periods of intense secretion by the gastric glands, large amounts of bicarbonates are released into the blood. This transient and mild alkalization of the blood during digestion is normally reversed when bicarbonate in the blood is consumed indirectly during the neutralization of gastric secretions as they enter the intestine. On a total-body basis, therefore, gastric acid production results in only small and transient changes in blood pH.

The extent of digestive action in the stomach varies with species. In all the species gastric mucosa secretes hydrochloric acid and pepsin. These help break down protein into polypeptides. In the young lamb, calf, kid and piglet gastric mucosa secretes rennin which coagulates milk proteins. Gastric juice of carnivores contains gastric lipase in low concentration.

IV Small intestine: It is the principal site of absorption of amino acids, vitamins, minerals and lipids and soluble carbohydrates; the duodenal area is the site for mixing digesta and secretions and the jejunal area is the site of absorption. The duodenal (Brunner's) glands produce an alkaline secretion. This secretion acts as a lubricant and also protects the duodenal wall from the hydrochloric acid entering from the stomach.

Certain individuals do not secrete effective amounts of lactase and therefore cannot tolerate significant amounts of lactose in the diet. Mature animals in most species have a lower lactose tolerance than the young. Ruminants do not secrete significant amounts of sucrase.

The duodenum receives bile from the gall bladder and pancreatic secretions from the pancreas. In all farm animals except the horse, bile is stored in the gall bladder until required. Bile consists largely of bile acids and bile pigments with small amounts of cholesterol, lecithin, electrolytes and protein. The secretions of the pancreas include the proteolytic enzymes, a lipase, an alpha amylase.

The endoenzymes break large molecules into smaller ones by acting within the peptide chain, while the exoenzymes attack terminal amino acids and produce free amino acids. The endoenzymes do not cleave at random but are specific for certain peptide bonds; for example, pepsin breaks bonds adjacent to an aromatic amino acid.

V Large intestine: In the pig and other omnivores there is an enlargement of the caecum and the colon. Some herbivorous animals show great extension of the size of the caecum and colon as compared with other parts of the tract. For instance, in the horse and rabbit about 60% of the capacity of the G.I. tract is in the caecum and colon. See Table 3 for comparative figures and figure 4 'The digestive system of a horse'. The equine gut contains a diverse array of microbes, including bacteria, protozoa, anaerobic fungi, archaea and bacteriophages, all of which work together to aid feed and fibre digestion for their host.

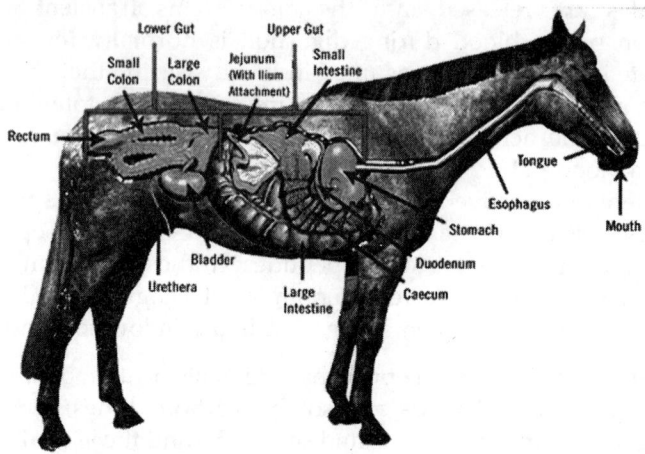

Figure 4   The digestive system of a horse.

TABLE 3. Approximate Capacity of the G.I. Tract (litres) of Various Animals *.

Part of the G.I Tract/	Human	Dog	Pig	Horse	Sheep	Cattle
BW, Kg	75	18	190	450	80	575
Reticulorumen	-	-	-	-	17	125
Omasum	-	-	-	-	1	20
Abomasum	1	0.40	8	8	2	15
Total Stomach	1	0.4	8	8	20	160
S. intestine	4	0.15	9	27	6	65
Caecum	0	0.01	1	14	1	10
L. intestine	1	0.10	9	41	3	25
Gastrointestinal tract	6	0.66	27	90	30	260
%BW	8	3.7	14.2	20	37.5	45.2

* *Note :* The volume of the stomach and intestines increases when animal consumes a bulky diet and the volume decreases when a concentrate, high-energy diet is fed because less food is needed to satisfy appetite.

The colon has multiple functions, including absorption of water and electrolytes, storage of faeces and fermentation of organic matter that escapes digestion and absorption in the small intestine. The relative importance of these functions varies with the species. Accordingly, the size and shape of the colon is variable (see figure 5). The major determinant of colon size is the importance of colonic fermentation to the energy needs of the animal. Horses and rabbits make extensive use of fermentation

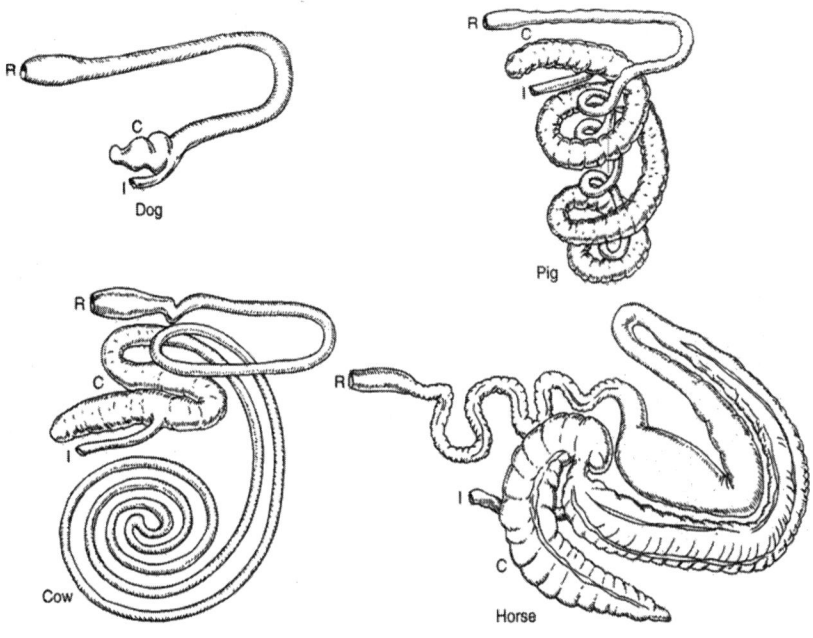

Figure 5   Variations of colon anatomy of four mammals dog, pig, horse and cow; C, caecum; I, ileum; R, rectum.

products for nutritional needs and have large and complex colons. Dogs and cats do not rely on fermentation products and have relatively simple colons. In animals such as pigs and cattle, importance of colonic fermentation to digestive needs is intermediate between horse and dog and this intermediate position is noted in their colon development.

In birds, chicken and turkey have two caeca whereas ostrich has two large caeca with significant bacterial population. Poultry droppings have a characteristic appearance of a brownish and/or black mash with whitish material covering, originating from the uric acid of the urine because of excretion of urine and faeces together.

It has been reported that digestion in the large intestine of the ruminant accounts for between 4 to 26% of the digestible energy (Ulyatt *et al.* 1975). Microbial digestion of fibre is extensive in the horse, guinea pig, rabbit, pig, elephant, and many other *nonruminant* herbivores though it is not as efficient as in the rumen. In mature swine 80 to 90% of the crude fibre is digested here to VFA. There is relatively little fibre digestion in the large intestine of many *nonruminants* such as the dog, chicken, cat and human. Large amounts of bacterial protein and vitamins are synthesized in the large intestine, but the extent of their absorption is negligible except in the animals where caecotrophy is practiced. Volatile fatty acids, amino nitrogen, electrolytes and water are absorbed in ruminants.

Motility patterns of the gastrointestinal tract

Movement of the gut wall is referred to as motility and motility may be of a propulsive, retentive or mixing nature. The time it takes for the material to travel from one portion of the gut to another is referred to as the **transit time.**

The walls of the gastrointestinal tract are muscular and capable of movement. The movements of the GI muscles have direct actions on ingesta in the gut lumen and serve several functions. (1) Propel the ingesta from one location to the next in the GI tract, (2) retain the ingesta at a given site for digestion, absorption or storage, (3) break up the food material physically and mix it with digestive secretions and (4) circulate ingesta so that all portions come into contact with absorptive surfaces.

Before the food is directed into the GI tract, quadruped animals must first grasp it with the lips, teeth or tongue. The exact method of food prehension varies greatly among different species. In all domestic animals, however, prehension is a highly coordinated process involving direct control by the central nervous system (CNS). Mastication or chewing is the first act of digestion. Deglutition or swallowing involves voluntary and involuntary stages and occurs after the food has been well masticated. In the voluntary phase of swallowing, food is made into a bolus by the tongue and pushed back into the pharynx.

The pharynx is the common opening of both the respiratory and the digestive tract. The major physiological function of the pharynx is to ensure that 'only air' enters the respiratory tract and that 'only food and water' enters the digestive tract. When food enters the pharynx, involuntary part of the swallow reflex is initiated and food is directed into the digestive system, which involves series of highly coordinated actions. When all the openings to the pharynx are closed, food bolus is pushed toward the opening of the esophagus with a wave of muscular constriction over the walls of the pharynx.

As food reaches the esophagus, the upper esophageal sphincter relaxes (as the pharynx constricts) to accept the material. This is what happens during the deglutition. Food is pushed into the upper portion of the esophageal body by propulsive movements (known as peristalsis) toward the stomach. As the food bolus reaches the distal end of the esophagus, the lower sphincter relaxes and the ingested matter enters the stomach. If esophagus is not cleared of food material by the primary wave of peristalsis, secondary peristaltic waves are generated.

When deglutition is not taking place, the body of the esophagus is relaxed, but the upper and lower sphincters remain constantly constricted. If the two esophageal sphincters are not tightly closed, inspiration would cause aspiration of air from the pharynx and reflux of ingesta from the stomach into the body of the esophagus. Stomach contents would be drawn into the esophagus because inspiratory pressures in the thorax are lower than intraabdominal pressure. More so the lower esophageal sphincter should remain closed, lest movement of stomach contents into the esophagus would cause damage to the esophageal mucosa.

Dog and cat have simple stomachs while pig, horse and rats have more complex stomachs among the monogastrics. The motility patterns described here are more related to dogs and cats. The complex motility patterns of the ruminant stomach are detailed in chapter 7; Page No. 133. The stomach is divided into two physiological regions, each of which has a different impact on gastric function. The proximal region adjacent to the esophagus retains the food and thus serves a storage function. The distal region serves a grinding and sieving function, breaking solid pieces of food to particles small enough for small-intestinal digestion.

As food enters the proximal stomach, the muscular reflex exhibits adaptive relaxation and thus it can dilate to accept large quantities of food without an increase in intraluminal pressure. Because of a weak, continuous-contraction nature of the muscular activity, little mixing occurs and the ingesta is pushed towards the distal stomach. In the distal stomach (antrum), there is intense slow-wave activity and strong waves of peristalsis move the material towards the pylorus (sphincterlike junction between stomach and duodenum). The pylorus constricts and allows particles of less than 2 mm in diameter only to pass into the duodenum. Some types of ingested materials such as bones and indigestible foreign objects cannot be reduced to particles less than 2 mm in diameter. To clear such indigestible debris, a particular type of motility (migrating motility complex) occurs between the meals.

During the digestive period, the ingesta are subjected to propulsive and nonpropulsive motility patterns. Thus, ingesta are pushed down the gut for a short distance (propulsive) and then subjected to segmentation (localized contraction of circular muscle) (nonpropulsive) - Portions of small intestine (3 to 4 cm long) contract tightly dividing the gut into segments of constricted and dilated lumen. These actions within the small intestine mix the ingesta with digestive juices and circulate them over the absorptive mucosal surfaces. The interaction of segmentation and peristaltic motility that occurs during the digestive-phase may be described as "two steps forward, one step backward".

During the interdigestive period, waves (migrating motility complex, MMC) of powerful peristaltic contractions sweep over a large length of small intestine. The MMC begins in the duodenum and may travel the entire length of the small intestine probably serving to push the undigested material out of the small intestine. It is also important in controlling the bacterial population in the upper gut. Normally the duodenum harbours a relatively small population of bacteria, and the population increases distally into the ileum, while colon is heavily colonized. The MMC may help to impede the migration of bacteria from the ileum to the duodenum.

During the periods of peristaltic activity in the ileum, the ileocaecal sphincter relaxes allowing the material to enter into the colon. The ileocaecal sphincter is at the junction of the small and large intestine and prevents the retrograde movement of colon contents into the ileum.

Mixing activity is prominent in the colons of all species and is achieved by segmentation contractions along with other types of motility. Colonic segmentation is pronounced in horses and pigs and in some areas sacculations (haustra) are formed. A particular characteristic of colonic motility is retropulsion or antiperistalsis. Retrograde or reverse peristalsis in the proximal portions of the colon causes ingesta to be retained there to promote the storage and absorptive functions of the colon.

The colon of the dog and cat is a relatively simple organ consisting of a short caecum, an ascending part, a transverse part and a descending part. During the resting phase, there is a colonic pacemaker (not anatomical structures; rather, areas defined by activities of the ENS) at about the junction of the transverse and descending colons. This gives rise to antiperistaltic activity in the proximal colon, with resultant accumulation of ingesta in the caecum and ascending colon areas. Moderate peristaltic activity usually occurs in the descending colon, whereas the distal colon and rectum are usually constricted and empty. Material entering the carnivore colon is of a fluid consistency. It is thoroughly mixed in the ascending and transverse colons, and much of the water and many of the electrolytes are absorbed. By the time it reaches the descending colon, it is semisolid and becoming faeces.

Despite large anatomical differences, there are important similarities in motility among various species. Equine caecum is large and separated into haustra. It is unique among caeca of most species because a distinct, sphincterlike orifice joins it to the colon. The longitudinal muscles of the caecum and colon form discrete bands or teniae that course along the longitudinal axis of the gut. The teniae divide the haustra longitudinally that give the equine caecum and large colon a sacculated appearance. Motility in the equine caecum consists of active segmentation and mixing that appear to transfer majority of ingesta to the colon. Motility in the colon consists of segmentation, antiperistalsis and peristalsis. A colonic pacemaker appears to exist at the pelvic flexure. The characteristic ball-shaped form of equine faeces probably represents intense segmentation-type motility in the small colon, where the faeces are formed.

In ruminants and pigs, the hindgut consists of a caecum of intermediate complexity, a spiral colon, and a straight colon. Pacemaker may be located in the central point of spiral colon and it generates antiperistaltic motility.

The anal opening is constricted by two sphincters: an internal sphincter of smooth muscle, which is a direct extension of the circular muscle layer of the rectum and an external sphincter of striated muscle. The entry of faeces into the rectum is accompanied by the reflex relaxation of the internal anal sphincter, followed by peristaltic contraction of the rectum. This is known as the rectosphincteric reflex and is an important part of the act of defecation. The reflex normally results in defecation, but in trained animals its effects can be blocked by voluntary constriction of the external anal sphincter.

Microbial Digestion of Carbohydrates

Mammals do not possess enzymes to digest the plant cell walls (structural carbohydrates). They digest them by fermentative digestion with the help of microorganisms. Herbivorous animals are of two types: 1. Pregastric fermentors (e.g. ruminants) and 2. Postgastric fermentors (e.g. swine, horse, guinea pig, rabbit).

Rumen microorganisms

For any microorganism present in the rumen to be called as rumen microorganism, it should be present in as a million of the particular species per gram of rumen ingesta. The life span of amylolytic bacteria, cellulolytic bacteria, protozoa and fungi, respectively, is 20-30 min, 18 h, 6-36 h and 24 h. The contribution of them to the total microbial mass is 50-90% in case of bacteria, 10-50% for protozoa and 5-10% for fungi.

In young calves of less than 3 weeks old the bacteria are mostly of the lactate fermenting type, aerobes and coliforms. By 3 months of age rumen bacteria characteristic of the adult animal, which are anaerobic get themselves established. Rumen protozoa get established in young calves when they are about 3 to 4 months old. They are of two types: ciliates and flagellates.

Microorganisms are continuously removed from the reticulo-rumen by the onward flow of digesta to the omasum. To maintain a stable population in the reticulo-rumen, the microbes that are removed must be replaced. To become established, each type of microorganism must have a retention time in the reticulo-rumen exceeding its lifespan. Microbes possessing a lifespan greater than 8-16 h must thus attach to the rumen wall or to fibre-containing material.

Rumen Bacteria

Population of rumen bacteria· 10^{10} cells per ml of rumen contents. Rumen bacteria are anaerobic. A few bacteria are capable of growing under aerobic conditions and are called as facultative. R.E. Hungate did pioneering work on rumen bacteria and is considered as father of Rumen Microbiology. M.P. Bryant continued work on rumen bacteria.

1. Cellulose digesters (cellulolytic bacteria)

Rod shaped

Bacteroides succinogenes or *Fibrobactor succinogenes*
Butyrivibrio fibrisolvens
Clostridium lochheadii
Clostridium longisporium
Cillobacterium cellulosolvens
Acetigenic rod

Cellulolytic cocci

Ruminicoccus albus
Ruminicoccus flavefaciens

2. Starch digesters (amylolytic bacteria)

Cellulolytic and amylolytic

Bacteroides succinogenes or *Fibrobactor succinogenes*
Butyrivibrio fibrisolvens
Clostridium lochheadii

Non-cellulolytic and amylolytic

Streptococcus bovis
Bacteroides amylophilus or *ruminobacter amylophilus*
Bacteroides ruminicola or *Prevotella ruminicola*
Succinomonas amylolytica
Selenomonas ruminantium

3. Hemicellulose digesters (Hemicellulolytic bacteria)

Eubacterium ruminantium
Bacteroides ruminicola or *Prevotella ruminicola*
Bacteroides amylogenes
Butyrivibrio fibrisolvens
Ruminococcus albus
Ruminococcus flavefaciens

4. Pectin digesters (Pectinolytic bacteria)

Bacteroides ruminicola
Butyrivibrio fibrisolvens
Lachnospira multiparus
Treponema bryantii
Succinovibrio dextrinosolvens
Streptococcus bovis

5. Sugar fermenters or sugar-utilizing

In the young calves, number of species of Lactobacillus are found in their stomach.

Lactobacillus casei, L. plantarum, L. lactis, L. bifidus, L. fermentii, L. vitulinus, L. ruminus, Treponema bryantii

6. Acid utilizing bacteria (lactate utilisers)

Megasphera elsdenii
Selenomonas ruminantium

Formate utilizer

Vibrio succinogenes

Oxalate utilizer

Euryoxic bacterium
Oxalobacter formigenes

7. Methanogenic bacteria

Methanobacterium ruminantium or *Methanobrevibacter ruminantium*
Methanobacterium formicicum
Methanomicrobium mobile

8. Proteolytic bacteria

Bacteroides amylophilus
Bacteroides ruminicola
Butyrivibrio fibrisolvens

9. Lipolytic bacteria

Veillonella alcalescens
Anaerovibrio lipolytica

10. Ureolytic bacteria

Succinivibrio dextrinosovens
Bacteroides ruminicola
Ruminococcus bromii
Selenomonas spp.
Butyrivibrio spp.
Treponema spp.

11. Ammonia-producing

Bacteroides ruminicola
Megasphera elsdenii
Selenomonas ruminantium

Succinic acid producing bacteria

Bacteroides succinogenes
Ruminococcus flavefaciens
Bacteroides amylophilus
Bacteroides ruminicola or *Prevotella ruminicola*
Succinomonas amylolytica
Succinovibrio dextrinosolvens

Strains that are killed by exposure to oxygen

Butyrivibrio fibrisolvens
Clostridium lochheadii
Cellulolytic cocci
Methanobacterium ruminantium

Rumen Protozoa

The rumen protozoa were first observed by Gruby and Delafond in 1843. Protozoal population is up to 10^6 per ml. All the protozoa (2% of the weight of rumen contents) are strictly anaerobic. Flagellates are less; cilates are predominating. The rumen ciliates are of two types:

Holotrichs and entodiniomorphs

- **Holotrichs** use soluble carbohydrates
    1. *Isotricha intestinalis*
    2. *Dasytricha ruminantium*
    3. *Charon equii*
    4. *Blepharoprosthium pierum*

- **Entodiniomorphs** (oligotriphs) use particulate material like starch
  1. *Entodinium bursa*
  2. *Diplodinium cristagalli*
  3. *Diploplastron affine*
  4. *Ostracodinium gracile*
  5. *Epidinium caudatum*
  6. *Ophryoscolex purkynei*
  7. *Eudiplodinium maggaii*
  8. *Metadinium medium*
  9. *Polyplastron multivesiculatum*

G.S. Coleman in 1975 indicated that presence of protozoa in the rumen could be detrimental to ruminant nutrition by lowering net microbial growth efficiency. Now let us see their role in the rumen.

Role of Protozoa in the Rumen

- Protozoa engulf starch and remove it from the rumen liquor; thus it is not available for attack by bacteria. In the absence of protozoa, the production of lactic acid by rumen bacterial attack on the free starch produces a disastrous drop in rumen pH and a loss of fermentative capacity.
- **Digestion of cellulose by the larger entodiniomorphid protozoa:** Rumen protozoa are responsible for 30-40% of total rumen microbial fibre digestion.
- **Breakdown of plant protein and turnover of bacterial nitrogen and carbon:** Protozoa engulf protein, bacteria and small protozoa and digest them. This turnover is probably relatively unimportant in well-fed animals where the small amounts of bacterial nitrogen lost as ammonia are insignificant. However, in animals fed poor quality hay or straw and where supply of nitrogen is insufficient, the loss of nitrogen and carbon due to protozoa is considerable.

Rumen Fungi

Orpin in 1975 isolated certain zoospores of obligate fungi in the rumen. Bauchop in 1979 identified the role of rumen fungi in cellulolytic activities. The anaerobic fungi constitute 8% microbial mass as measured by chitin, when diets are rich in fibre. They are strictly anaerobic, and their lifecycle includes a mobile phase (as a zoospore) and a vegetative phase (sporangium). During the latter phase they become attached to food particles by rhizoids, which can penetrate cell walls. The organisms have been shown to be important for initiation and continuation of rumen fermentation.

Five Genera

1. *Neocallimastix frontalis, N.patriciarum*
2. *Piromyces* (formerly *Piromonas*) *rhizinflata, P. communis*
3. *Caecomyces* (formerly *Sphaeromonas*) *equi, C. communis*
    All these three are *monocentric thalli*.
4. *Orpinomyces joyonii, O. bovis*
5. *Anaeromyces* (*synonymous Ruminomyces*) *mucronatus*
    These two are polycentric thalli.

Symbiotic Bacteria

This comes under interrelationship between bacteria and protozoa. All entodiniomorphid protozoa (tested under experiment) engulf bacteria. Some engulfed bacteria are not killed and digested but survive, live and divide in vesicles in the protozoal endoplasm on the available nutrients. Most of the engulfed bacteria are killed and digested and the resultant amino acids and nucleotides are used for the synthesis of protozoal protein and nucleic acid, respectively. From the experimental results available with *Entodinium caudatum*, the number of 'engulfed' bacteria present is a balance between the rate at which they can grow and synthesize a protective covering, and the rate at which the protozoa can digest them.

Rumen Microorganisms and their Fermentation Characteristics

In ruminants, microorganisms breakdown the higher carbohydrates, cellulose, pentosans and starch (protein as well) to monosaccharides and then fermented to (steam) volatile fatty acids (VFA) and methane. Further, microorganisms synthesize essential nutrients such as B-vitamins, amino acids. Host animals provide space (rumen, large intestine) and other factors most favourable for microbes' activity. This symbiotic relationship is developed to the highest degree in ruminants. Even insects such as termites have significant microbial activity. Important rumen microorganisms and their fermentation characteristics are furnished in Table 4.

The reticulo-rumen provides a continuous culture system for anaerobic bacteria, protozoa and fungi. The rumen microorganisms can be envisaged as operating together as so called consortia to attack and breakdown feeds. Rumen microbes (see figure 6) ferment carbohydrates to VFA and generate significant amounts of reducing equivalents [$FADH_2$ and NADH] and H_2 as end products. Methanogens, both free living and endosymbionts inside protozoa, converts H_2 to CH_4. A small amount of reducing equivalents is utilized in lipid synthesis and fatty acid biohydrogenation. Synthesis of amino acids can result in production or utilization of reducing equivalents, but the net amount is small. Protein synthesis utilizes reducing

TABLE 4. Rumen Microorganisms and their Fermentation Characteristics.

Organism	Substrate	Products of fermentation VFAs and other acids only
Bacteria		
Bacteroides succinogenes or *Fibrobacter succinogenes*	Cellulose, xylan	Acetate, succinate, formate
Ruminococcus flavefaciens	"	Acetate, succinate, formate
R. albus	"	Acetate, formate
Butirivibrio fibrisolvens	"	Acetate, butyrate, formate
Clostridium polysaccharolyticum	Cellulose	Accetate, butyrate, formate
C. lochheadii	"	Acetate, butyrate, formate
Bacteroides ruminicola or *Prevotella ruminicola*	Xylan and soluble carbohydrates	Acetate, succinate, propionate, formate
Selenomonas ruminantium	Soluble carbohydrates (starch, glucose)	Acetate, Propionate "
(Bacteroides) Ruminobacter amylophilus	"	Acetate, succinate, formate
Megasphaera elsdenii	"	Acetate, propionate, butyrate valerate, caproate
Succinovibrio dextrinosolvens	"	Acetate, succinate, formate
Succinomonas amylolytica	"	Acetate, succinate
Streptococcus bovis	"	Lactate, acetate, formate
Lactobacillus vitulinus	"	Lactate
Ciliate Protozoa	Cellulose, starch	Acetate, propionate, butyrate
Rumen fungi	Initiate fibre fermentation	

equivalents. Microbial mass synthesized in the rumen provides about 20% of the nutrients absorbed by the host animal. Bacterial DM contains 100g N/kg, 80% of which is in the form of amino acids while the remaining 20% as nucleic acid N. Moreover, some of the amino acids are contained in the peptidoglycan of the cell wall membrane and are not digested by the host animal. Microbial fermentation of carbohydrates and proteins yield volatile and short chain fatty acids which provide 60-80% of the ME of ruminants on most diets.

Microbial digestion of fibre is extensive in the large intestine in the horse, guinea pig, elephant, pig, rabbit and other nonruminant herbivore though it is not as efficient as in the rumen. About 25 to 30% of the total dry matter consumed by a ruminant may be made up of crude fibre. Ruminants are able to digest more than 50% of the crude fibre consumed in their rations for the following reasons:

Great size of the rumen (10-20% of their live weight) to allow feed to accumulate and ensure sufficient time for breakdown of cellulose.

Movements of the reticulo-rumen and the act of rumination play a role in breaking up the feed and exposing it to attack by microorganisms.

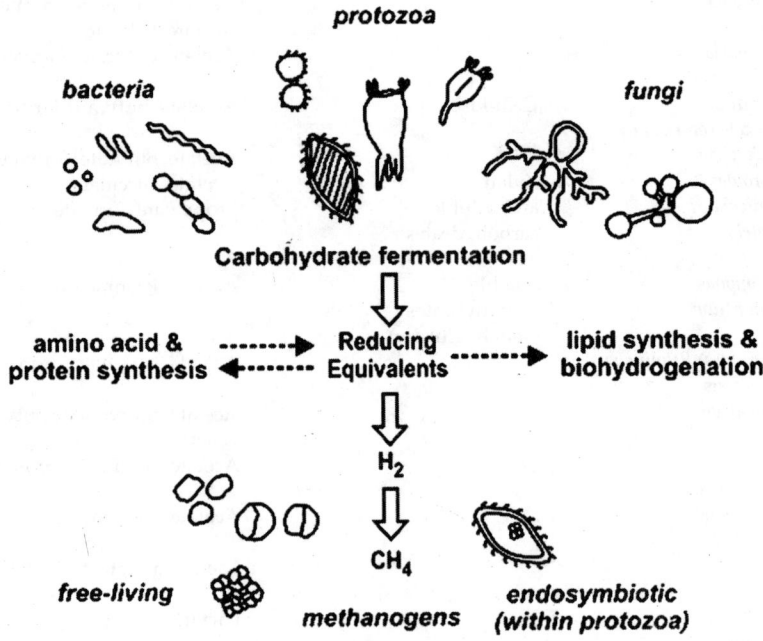

Figure 6 Rumen microorganisms (organisms are not drawn to scale [after Czerkawski, 1986])

Factors that Affect Microbial Digestion of Fibre

1. Character of the feed: It influences the kind and number of the microorganisms present. For example, addition of easily digestible carbohydrates, such as molasses, starch to the ration reduces the digestibility of fibre because the rumen bacteria prefer to attack the simpler carbohydrates.

2. Character of the roughage: Irrespective of its fibre content, roughage has an influence on the nature of the bacterial flora and on their activity. Replacement of a straw with a hay stimulate microbial activity because hay supply the critical nutrients for microbial growth.

3. *Chemical and physical nature of the fibre:* The complex polysaccharides of mature plants are less well digested than they are in young, growing plants. Mature plants have higher lignin content and this encrusts the cellulose and hemicellulose and thus carbohydrates are not accessible for bacterial attack. That is how lignin is not only indigestible itself in the animal but it also lowers the digestibility of cell walls. The reduced digestibility may also be due to increased rate of passage from the rumen.

4. *Rumen environment:* The following conditions must be satisfied for the digestion of crude fibre in the rumen.

(a) The feed consumed should remain in the rumen for sufficient length of time.
(b) The ingesta should be sufficiently moist for the microorganisms to thrive and for their enzymes to act.
(c) An optimum rumen temperature of 38-40°C.
(d) An optimum rumen pH. It should not be less than 6.2 for optimum cellulolytic activity.
(e) The internal rumen environment should be anaerobic.
(f) A negative oxidation-reduction potential must be maintained (– 250 to –450 mV).
(g) Ionic strength (osmolality) of the rumen fluid must be kept within an optimal range (near 300 mOsm).
(h) Regular supply of nutrients through feed should be maintained to serve as substrate for microorganisms.
(i) End products of microbial fermentative digestion should not accumulate in the rumen.

Metabolism of toxins in the rumen

The rumen microbes have a high capacity for degrading toxic organic compounds, including many plant alkaloids. Ruminants can therefore consume fungi and many plants that cannot be tolerated by other animals. Microorganisms in the rumen also detoxify bioactive amines such as histamine, formed by degradation of plant proteins during silage fermentation. However, microbes in the reticulorumen lack enzymes to detoxify several commonly occurring noxious compounds, such as aflatoxins from fungi of the Aspergillus genus, which cause liver damage, photosensitivity and renal impairment.

Bulk

There are two constituents which contribute bulk or volume to a feed. They are water and crude fibre. Highly succulent feeds like green legumes, roots, tubers are bulky because of their high water content. Coarse feeds are bulky because crude fibre contributes to the major portion of the dry matter of such feeds. They are light and occupy a greater volume than concentrates. The weight per unit volume of feeds is their **bulk density**. Look for more information on bulk density in chapter 17. Straws are bulky roughages and brans are bulky concentrates.

Importance of Bulk

1. Bulk satisfies the appetite of an animal.
2. Digestive tract functions more efficiently due to distension and peristalsis. Distension is particularly accomplished by the fibre.
3. Bulk has the property of breaking up the concentrates thereby presenting a larger surface area for the digestive enzymes to act on the concentrate feeds.
4. Bulk has a laxative effect in the animal. This is due to the water absorbing capacity of crude fibre especially the hemicellulose. A fibre which readily absorbs water and swells has more laxative effect.

   A nonfibrous feed which absorbs a large amount of water is less effective, because it is largely digested and thus do not reach the portion of the G.I. tract occupied primarily by feed residues. Of course, bulk is not the sole cause of laxative effect. Many feeds are laxative because of specific chemical substances contained in them which promote peristalsis.
5. Bulk is promoted by ability to absorb water. Some fibrous materials, such as agar, absorb large quantities of water while others, such as regenerated cellulose, do not. Linseed oil meal, which is much lower in fibre than wheat bran, absorbs three times as much water and thus, in this sense, is a more bulky feed in the digestive tract.

Effect of too much bulk: Feeding a ration of very low bulk density lowers digestibility of the feed and productivity of the animal due to consumption of less digestible nutrients. Such ration may cause atony and digestive disturbances like impaction.

Effect of too less bulk: Rations with very less fibre decreases rumen activity and animals develop a craving for food initially. Later the animal loses its appetite gradually. Too less bulk reduces the water absorbing capacity of the ration. There is a decrease in the milk yield and fat per cent due to decreased acetic acid and enhanced propionic acid in the rumen liquor.

Lambs grow normally on low fibre purified diets when sodium and potassium bicarbonates were included to serve as buffers. All concentrate rations consisting of rolled barley or ground maize supplemented with protein, minerals and vitamins gave satisfactory rates and efficiency of gain in finishing beef cattle. However, injury to the rumen epithelium (parakeratosis) and liver abscesses occur in some animals. Adding long hay prevents these pathological changes. Gastric ulcers are observed in swine on feeding finely ground (less than 600 μ particle size) feeds.

Lactating dairy cows tend to produce milk with a lower fat content as the crude fibre in the ration falls below about 17% (35% NDF) of the DM. In humans low fibre diets are associated with appendicitis, cancers of colon and rectum, gallbladder disorders and ischemic heart disease. A human diet should have 8-10% fibre and humans need 40 grams of fibre a day. Thus the indigestible materials also influence health.

Digestibility of Crude Fibre by Various Species

Species	Site of digestion	Percent of contained crude fibre digested
Ruminants	Rumen	50-90
Horse	Caecum	13-40
Pig	Caecum	3-25
Rabbit	Caecum	65-78
Rat	Caecum	34-46
Dog	Caecum	10-30
Man	Small and large intestine	25-62
Poultry	Caecum	20-30

This data do not mean that unlimited quantities of fibre can be digested to the extent shown but do show their capacity to digest crude fibre.

Benefits and costs of ruminant mode of digestion

Benefits of ruminant mode of digestion

1. The ecological success of ruminants is due to the benefits of a pregastric fermentation vat, the forestomach. Because of this, ruminants are able to digest fibrous carbohydrate sources not digested by monogastric species. Ruminants are able to break down cellulose and related compounds, thus not only releasing the enclosed cell contents but more importantly, utilizing the cellulose itself, which is the most abundant carbohydrate of the plants.

2. Ruminants are able to synthesize high biological value microbial protein (rich in essential amino acids) from low biological value plant proteins (lacking in essential amino acids), from dietary nonprotein nitrogen (NPN) such as urea, uric acid, etc. and from recycled urea.

3. Ruminants upgrade lignocellulosic crop residues and poultry droppings and urea to higher-quality microbial protein and energy for their nutrition and provide valuable animal products for well being of human population.
4. Ruminants are able to synthesize B-complex group of vitamins (provided that adequate cobalt is available in the case of vitamin B_{12}), vitamin K and conjugated linoleic acid (CLA).

Cost of ruminant mode of digestion

1. Fermentation of readily digestible feeds: Loss of metabolizable energy as heat and methane. Methane loss is inevitable at 6 to 9% of gross energy due to fermentative digestion.
2. Fermentation of protein means loss of protein as source of essential amino acids. Protein fermentation is inefficient as a source of ATP for microbial growth. Ruminants downgrade high quality protein and waste nitrogen when protein is fed in excess of microbial needs. Nitrogen for microbial growth can be supplied through urea or poultry droppings.
3. Hydrogenation of unsaturated fatty acids into saturated fatty acids is usual occurrence in the rumen due to the presence of excess hydrogen. This results in higher levels of saturated fatty acids in the ruminant meat.

Protected nutrients

Many denatured proteins escape rumen fermentation/degradation. Commercially this principle has been exploited by subjecting protein supplements to denaturation by formaldehyde (formalin) to protect them from rumen degradation. This process prevents the microbial degradation of high-quality proteins so that their essential amino acids are directly available to the host animal in the small intestine.

In a similar way lipids are protected (see p. 239 for details) from rumen degradation. Lipids can be encapsulated in a coating of protected protein. Protection of lipids prevents the saturation of unsaturated fatty acids in the rumen and allows higher levels of lipids to be fed without their adverse effect of depressing rumen fermentation and motility in the forestomach and gastrointestinal tract, and appetite.

Chapter 7

Digestion, Absorption and Postabsorptive Nutrient Utilization

Digestion and Absorption: The Nonfermentative Processes

Digestion is the process of breaking down complex nutrients into simple molecules and absorption is the process of transporting those simple molecules across the intestinal epithelium. Both the processes are necessary for the assimilation of nutrients into the body.

Structural characteristics of the small-intestinal epithelium

Contact between the small-intestinal mucosa and the luminal contents is facilitated by an extensive intestinal surface area. Large folds of mucosa add to the intestinal surface area in some animals. But in all species of animals, mucosal surface is covered with fingerlike epithelial projections called **villi**. The greater villi length provides greater digestive and absorptive capacity as demanded by greater energy need during physiological conditions such as lactation. Villi themselves are covered with a brushlike surface membrane known as the **brush border**. At the base of the villi are glandlike structures known as **Crypts of Lieberkuhn**. The villi and crypts are covered with a continuous layer of cellular epithelium. The epithelial cells covering the villi and crypts are called **enterocytes**.

Division and replication of enterocytes occur in the crypts only. Crypt enterocytes are highly mitotic and regenerate rapidly. In fact, the intestinal crypt cells are among the most rapidly regenerating cells of the body. As crypt cells multiply, they migrate upward onto the villi, and get changed to highly specialized absorptive cells on the villi. As the cells reach the tips of the villi they are lost because of age and exposure to gut contents. On an average, the turnover time (the time taken for an enterocyte to migrate from its site of origin in the crypt to the tip of a villus) of enterocytes is 4 to 7 days.

The cell surface (of enterocyte) facing the lumen is covered by the **apical membrane**. Attached to the apical membrane has many glycoproteins.

These glycoproteins are enzymes and transport molecules responsible for the digestive and absorptive functions of the intestinal epithelium. This rich area of glycoproteins on the surface of the apical membranes is given the name **'glycocalyx'**. Goblet cells are liberally interspersed among the enterocytes. They secrete a rich layer of **'mucus'** that covers the mucosa. In addition to the mucus and glycocalyx layers, there is an area near the intestinal surface known as the **'unstirred water layer'**. The unstirred water layer, mucus, and glycocalyx form an important diffusion barrier through which nutrients must pass before entering the enterocytes.

Tight junctions

Each enterocyte has two distinct types of cell membranes: The cell surface facing the lumen is called apex and is covered by the apical membrane (It contains microvilli. Under the light microscope, the microvilli give the cell surface its 'brushlike' appearance, which is synonymous with apical membrane); the part not facing the gut lumen is called the basolateral membrane (nutrients that are absorbed into the enterocytes through the apical membrane must exit the cell through the basolateral membrane before gaining access to the bloodstream).

   The attachments between adjacent enterocytes are called tight junctions. These connections serve a special function in the process of digestion and absorption. The tight junctions form a narrow band of attachment between adjacent enterocytes. The junctions may be called "tight," but from a molecular standpoint, they are rather loose. This is especially true in the duodenum and jejunum, where the tight junctions are loose enough to allow the free passage of water and small electrolytes. However, the tight junctions are never permeable enough to permit the passage of organic molecules. Understanding the anatomical relationships of the enterocytes, tight junctions, apical membrane, basolateral membrane and lateral spaces is critical to appreciate the physiology of intestinal absorption. Please see the figure 1.

Free flow of water and electrolytes among the intestinal lumen, ECF and blood

Majority of the basolateral membranes of adjacent enterocytes are unattached. This arrangement creates a potential space between enterocytes. This **area between the lateral surfaces of the enterocytes is called the lateral space**. The lateral spaces are normally distended and filled with extracellular fluid (ECF). At the end of the lateral spaces nearest the apical membrane, ECF is separated from the fluid of the intestinal lumen only by the tight junctions. At the opposite end of the lateral spaces,

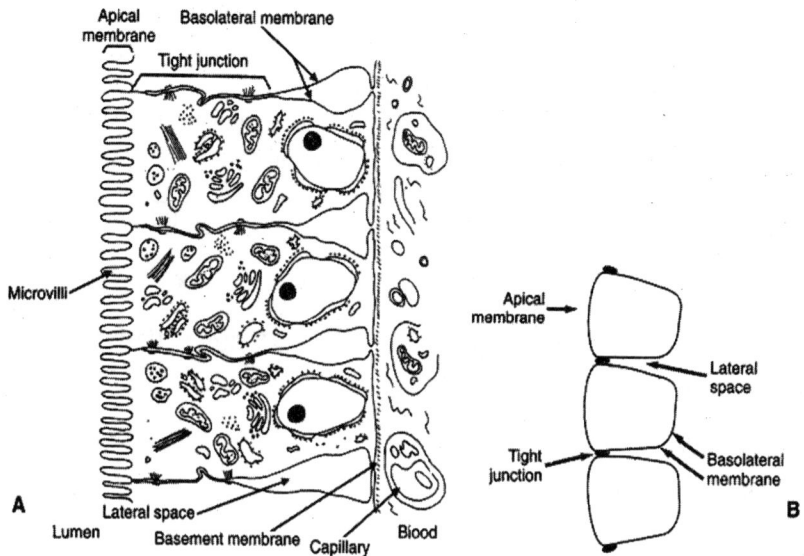

Figure 1   A. Anatomic illustration of intestinal epithelium; B. Line sketch of the epithelium, including an intestinal capillary.

the ECF is separated from the blood only by the **basement membrane** of the intestinal capillaries. Both the **tight junctions** and the capillary endothelium are permeable barriers that allow the free passage of water and small molecules. Thus, there is relatively free flow of water and most electrolytes among the fluid in the lumen of the intestine, the ECF in the lateral spaces, and the blood.

Digestion of Carbohydrates and Proteins

The overall process of digestion is the physical and chemical breakdown of food particles into subunits suitable for absorption. Physical reduction of food particle size begins with mastication (chewing) but is completed by the grinding action of the distal stomach. In the distal stomach the physical action of grinding is aided by the chemical actions of pepsin and hydrochloric acid.

Chemical digestion of each major nutrient is accomplished by the process of hydrolysis, the splitting of a chemical bond by the insertion of a water molecule. Glycosidic linkages in carbohydrates, peptide bonds in proteins, ester bonds in fats, and phosphodiester bonds in nucleic acids are all cleaved by hydrolysis during digestion (Figure 2). The reader may see Appendix to view these chemical bonds among the polymers.

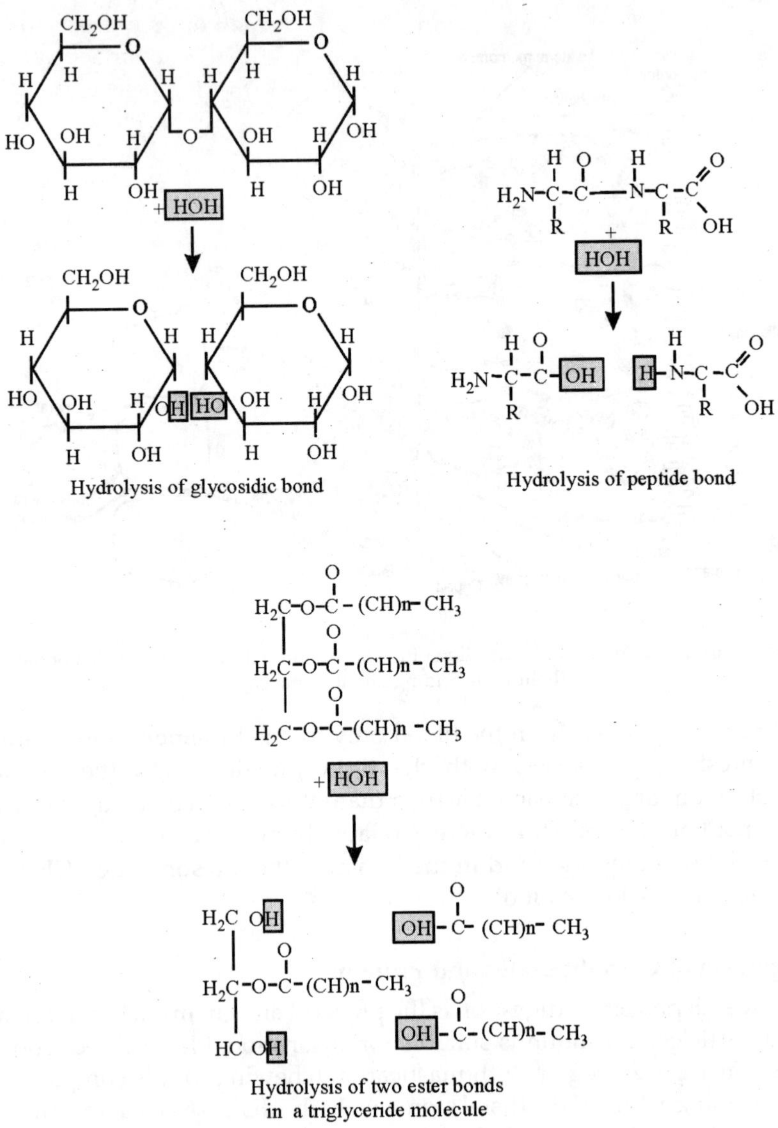

Hydrolysis of glycosidic bond

Hydrolysis of peptide bond

Hydrolysis of two ester bonds
in a triglyceride molecule

Figure 2 Hydrolytic cleavage of macromolecules.

Luminal-phase and membranous-phase of digestion

Hydrolysis in the digestive tract is catalysed by the action of enzymes. **There are two types of enzymes**: those who act within the lumen of the gut and those that act at the membrane surface of the epithelium. Major gastrointestinal glands such as salivary glands, gastric glands, pancreas secrete the corresponding enzymes into the lumen of their associated gut segments where they get mixed with ingesta and exert their actions. Thus the actions they catalyze are referred to as the **luminal phase of digestion**. Here original macromolecules are hydrolysed to short-chain polymers leading to incomplete hydrolysis of nutrients. The hydrolytic process is completed by enzymes that are present at the small intestinal epithelial membrane surface. These enzymes break the short-chain polymers of luminal-phase digestion into monomers, which can be absorbed across the epithelium. This final phase is referred to as the **membranous-phase of digestion**.

The difference between the two phases is that membranous-phase enzymes are chemically bound to the surface membrane of the small intestine. They constitute a large and important portion of the glycocalyx. The substrates for these enzymes must diffuse into the glycocalyx before hydrolysis can occur. These enzymes are synthesized within the enterocytes and subsequently transported to the luminal surface of the apical membrane. The membranous-phase enzymes of carbohydrate digestion include maltase, isomaltase, sucrase and lactase. The enzymes for digestion of peptides are peptidases. The extracellular enzymes responsible for luminal phage of carbohydrate digestion and intestinal mucosal enzymes are presented in Table 1.

TABLE 1   Carbohydrates and endogenous enzymes of vertebrates
[Source: Modified from Stevens (1977)].

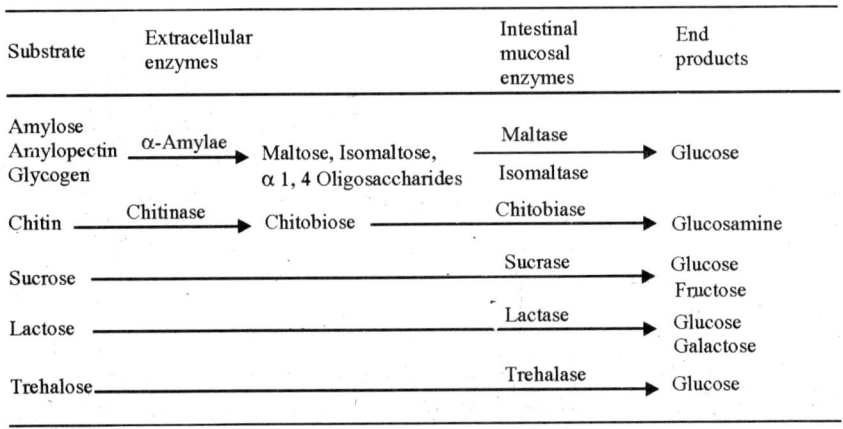

Substrate	Extracellular enzymes		Intestinal mucosal enzymes	End products
Amylose Amylopectin Glycogen	α-Amylae →	Maltose, Isomaltose, α 1, 4 Oligosaccharides	Maltase ————→ Isomaltase	Glucose
Chitin	Chitinase →	Chitobiose —————	Chitobiase ————→	Glucosamine
Sucrose	————————————		Sucrase ————→	Glucose Fructose
Lactose	————————————		Lactase ————→	Glucose Galactose
Trehalose	————————————		Trehalase ————→	Glucose

Luminal phase of digestion

Carbohydrates: Dietary carbohydrates are primarily from the plants and are fibres, sugars and starches. Plant (cell wall) fibres are not digested by hydrolytic digestion but by microbial digestion, while sugars and starches are digested by hydrolytic digestion with the help of mammalian enzymes. Dietary starch consists of amylose and amylopectin. Amylose is composed of repeating glucose units joined by α[1-4] linkages. Amylopectin is a similar molecule, except that it has branch points formed by α[1-6] linkages. That is why, luminal-phase carbohydrate digestion results in the production of various short-chain polysaccharides (maltose, maltotriose, isomaltose and limit dextrins). These disaccharides, trisaccharides and oligosaccharides are digested in the membranous-phase (see the figure 3 below).

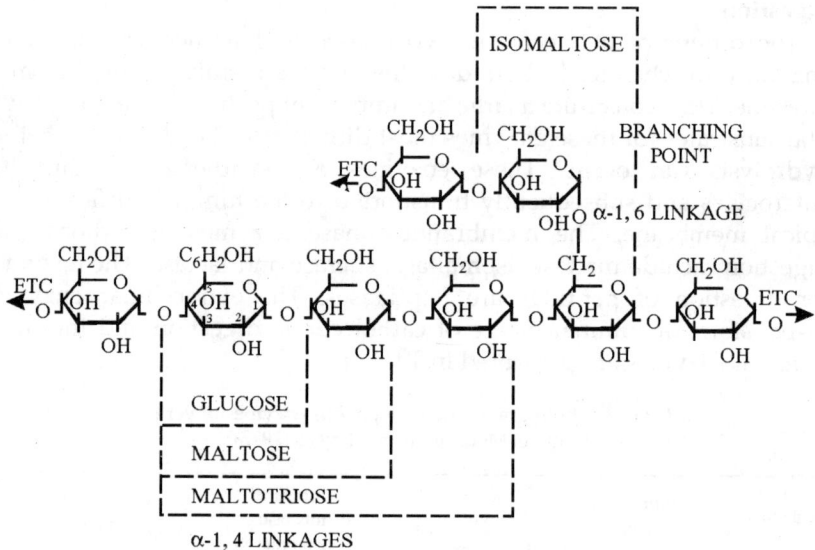

Figure 3   The structure of starch and its hydrolytic products. [Pancreatic amylase cleaves the starch at the α-1, 4-linkage, but not at the α-1, 6-linkages. Further hydrolysis is catalyzed by the maltase and isomaltase of the brush border of intestinal epithelial cells (Davenport 1982)].

Proteins: Starch molecules are made up of only one type of monomer (glucose), while protein molecules are made up of a variety of amino acids. Hence various proteolytic enzymes (Table 2) are necessary for digestion of proteins. Proteins are digested by a variety of luminal-phase enzymes. The proteolytic enzymes are secreted from the stomach glands or pancreas in the form of **inactive zymogens**, which are activated in the stomach or intestinal lumen, respectively. These enzymes must be secreted in an inactive form, otherwise the active enzymes would digest the cells in which they are synthesized. Duodenal mucosal cells elaborate **enterokinase enzyme** and this activates the trypsinogen and the active trypsin enzyme serves as an autocatalytic agent to activate additional trypsinogen as well as the other pancreatic protein-digesting enzymes.

TABLE 2   Luminal - Phase Enzymes of Protein Digestion

Enzyme	Source	Precursor	Activator
Pepsin	Gastric glands	Pepsinogen	Hydrochoric acid, pepsin
Chymosin (rennin)	Gastric glands	Chymosinogen	?
Trypsin	Pancreas	Trypsinogen	Enterokinase, trypsin
Chymotrypsin	Pancreas	Chymotrypsinogen	Trypsin
Elastase	Pancreas	Proelastase	Trypsin
Carboxypeptidase A	Pancreas	Procarboxypeptidase A	Trypsin
Carboxypeptidase B	Pancreas	Procarboxypeptidase B	Trypsin

Luminal-phase protein digestion begins in the stomach. Gastric digestion of protein is facilitated by pepsin and HCl. The acid environment of the stomach is suited to the action of pepsin, which has its optimal activity at pH 1 to 3. Gastric hydrolysis of protein is probably important to the physical as well as the chemical digestion of protein, because (1) most connective tissue of animal origin is protein and (2) digestion of connective tissue aids in breaking food down into particles small enough to pass the pylorus. Animals without stomachs can digest proteins, provided they have a functional pancreas and are fed small, frequent meals of soft, moist food. Luminal-phase of protein digestion is completed in the small intestine by the action of pancreatic enzymes (see table 2).

Most proteolytic enzymes are endopeptidases, which break proteins at internal points along the amino acid chains; complex proteins are hydrolysed to short chain peptides. Endopeptidases produce essentially no free amino acids. The two exopeptidases (carboxypeptidase A and carboxypeptidase B) release individual amino acids from ends of peptide chains and are active in luminal-phase digestion (see Tables 2 and 3).

Membranous-phase of digestion

Membranous-phase digestion occurs within the microenvironment of the unstirred water layer, intestinal mucus and glycocalyx. Peptides and polysaccharides in the intestinal lumen must diffuse into the surface layer before membranous-phase digestion can take place. Most of the products of digestion are absorbed, soon after formation, into the underlying epithelial cells. This arrangement is efficient because it ensures that the final products of carbohydrate and protein digestion are formed near their site of absorption, avoiding the need for long diffusion distances (Figure 4). All polysaccharides are digested to monosaccharides before absorption. However in case of proteins, a large portion of dietary amino acids is absorbed directly in the form of dipeptides and tripeptides, though peptidases hydrolyse the peptides into free amino acids.

Dipeptides and tripeptides that are absorbed intact are subsequently hydrolysed by the action of intracellular peptidases; the resulting free amino acids are then available for passage into the blood.

TABLE 3   Protein and endogenous enzymes of vertebrates
[Source: Modified from Stevens (1977)].

Substrate	Extracellular enzymes	Intestinal mucosal enzymes	End products

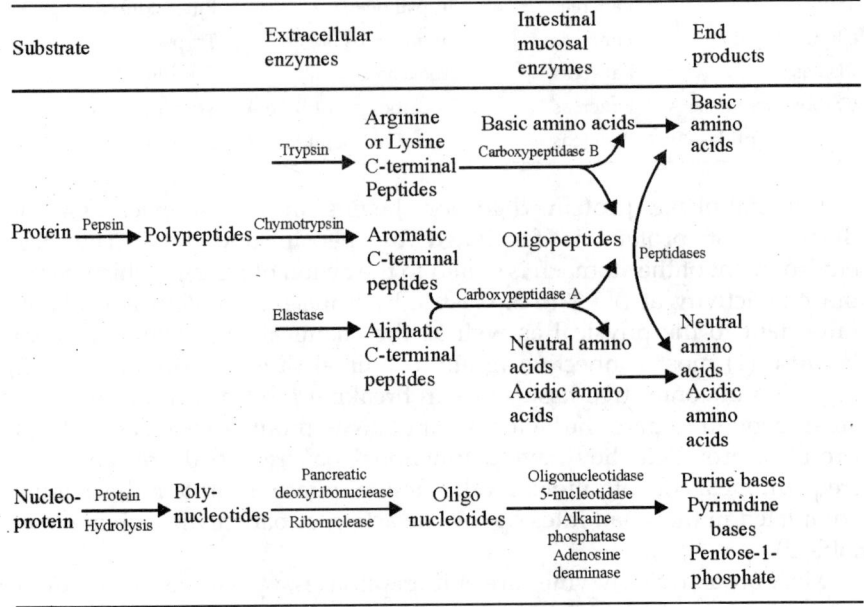

| Nucleo-protein | Protein Hydrolysis → Poly-nucleotides | Pancreatic deoxyribonuciease → Ribonuclease → Oligo nucleotides | Oligonucleotidase 5-nucleotidase Alkaine phosphatase Adenosine deaminase → Purine bases Pyrimidine bases Pentose-1-phosphate |

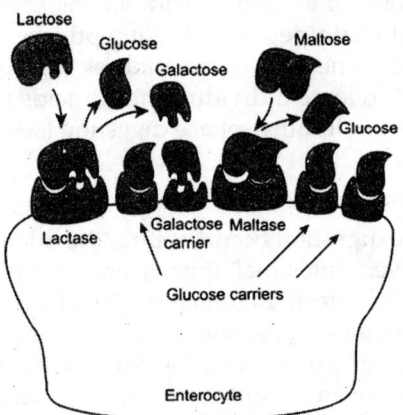

Figure 4 Relationship of membranous-phase digestion to absorption. [The enzymes responsible for digestion and the carrier molecules responsible for absorption are both part of the apical membrane. The products of digestion are thus formed in the immediate vicinity of the carrier proteins, avoiding long diffusion distances. Specific enzymes and carrier molecules are present for the various substrates]. Source: Cunningham's textbook of Veterinary Physiology by Bradley G. Klein, 5th edition, 2013, pp 303

Intestinal absorption of organic and inorganic nutrients

Absorption refers to the movement of the products of digestion across the intestinal mucosa and into the vascular system for distribution. When molecules can freely penetrate a membrane, their movement across it is completely determined by the laws of diffusion and differences in chemical and electrical gradients. Molecules flow to areas of lower concentration and charged particles move to areas of opposite charge. However, charged ions (especially cations) and most organic nutrient molecules do not freely penetrate the gastrointestinal epithelium. Therefore, a mechanism is needed to facilitate their transport across membranes.

Specialized transport mechanisms: Specialized transport mechanisms exist in the apical and basolateral membranes. Specialized transport mechanisms are needed for the movement of molecules across membranes in the intestinal epithelium. **The transport mechanism can be classified as active transport, secondary active transport, tertiary active transport, and passive transport.**

Active transport involves the direct consumption of metabolic energy. During active transport, energy stored as ATP is expended to move ions or molecules across membranes against an electrical or chemical gradient. In the large and small intestine, the active transport pathway of greatest importance is the sodium-potassium (Na^+, K^+) - adenosine triphosphatase (ATPase) pump.

Secondary and tertiary active transport mechanisms utilize the transcellular (through the cells) sodium ion electrochemical gradient as their source of energy. **Sodium co-transport process** can provide the energy to "pull" the co-transported molecule, such as glucose, from an area of lower concentration to one of higher concentration. Although the movement of a molecule against its concentration gradient represents expenditure of energy, there is no direct expenditure of metabolic energy by the sodium co-transport process. The energy expenditure is indirect and result from the direct expenditure of energy by the Na^+, K^+- ATPase pump in creating and maintaining the sodium electrochemical gradient. This is the definition of secondary active transport, with glucose transport being secondary to the active transport of sodium. Many organic nutrients, including glucose, amino acids, several vitamins, and bile acids, are absorbed by sodium co-transport processes.

Passive transport occurs either through specialized channels in cell membranes or directly through the tight junctions. Ions move through the channels in a completely passive manner, responding only to electrochemical gradients. No metabolic energy is directly required to effect ion movement. A second form of passive molecular movement through the intestinal epithelium is through the tight junctions. The "tight junctions" are not so tight especially in the duodenum and upper jejunum and are freely permeable to water and small inorganic ions. Thus, water and ions move across the tight junctions in response to osmotic pressure and electrochemical gradients. Movement of materials through the tight junctions is called **paracellular (around the cells) absorption**, in contrast to absorption through to apical membrane, which is called transcellular (through the cells) absorption. Transcellular absorption and paracellular absorption work in a complementary manner to produce an efficient absorptive process.

The **products of membranous-phase digestion are absorbed by sodium co-transport**. Sodium co-transport proteins for glucose and galactose are located in the apical membrane, in proximity to the membranous-phase digestive enzymes. Sodium co-transport systems exist for free amino acids and might also exist for dipeptides and tripeptides.

Absorption of water and electrolytes

Conservation of the body's supply of water and electrolytes, primarily sodium, potassium, chloride, and bicarbonate, is a high priority for sustaining life. The gut plays a major role in this conservation, not only because it is the portal of entry for replenishment of the nutrients, but also because water and electrolytes in gastrointestinal secretions must be efficiently reclaimed to maintain body composition.

Digestion and Absorption of Fats

Lipids or fats present a special digestive problem to the animal because they do not dissolve in water, the medium in which digestion occur. The problem of solubility makes the mechanics of digestion and absorption of lipids somewhat different from that of proteins and carbohydrates. The dietary lipid molecules are triglyceride and phospholipids (these are from animal and plant origin), cholesterol and cholesteryl ester (from animal origin) and waxes (from plant source). Figures 5 and 6 illustrate the structures of lipids with polar groups and lipids without polar groups. In addition, the lipid-soluble vitamins A, D, E and K are absorbed along with the other dietary lipids.

Lipids with polar groups: phopspholipid, lysophospholipid, monoglyceride, NEFA, cholesterol

Lipid assimilation

Lipid assimilation can be divided into four phases: emulsification, hydrolysis, micelle formation and absorption. Emulsification is the process of reducing lipid droplets to a size that forms stable suspensions in

Phospholipid

$$H_2C-O-C(=O)-O\,(CH_2)_n-CH_3$$
$$H_2C-O-C(=O)-(CH_2)_n-CH_3$$
$$H_2C-O-P(-OH)-O-X$$

Lysophospholipid

$$H_2C-O-C(=O)-O\,(CH_2)_n-CH_3$$
$$HC-OH$$
$$H_2C-O-P(-OH)-O-X$$

Monoglyceride

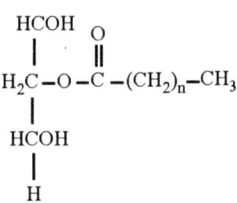

$$HCOH$$
$$H_2C-O-C(=O)-(CH_2)_n-CH_3$$
$$HCOH$$
$$H$$

Nonesterified fatty acid

$$HO-C(=O)-(CH_2)_n-CH_3$$

Cholesterol

$$HC-CH_2-CH_2-CH_2-C(CH_3)(H)-CH_3$$

CH$_3$

CH$_3$

CH$_3$

HO

**Bile acid
(cholic acid)**

CH$_3$ CH$_2$ C(=O)OH

HO CH$_3$ CH$_2$

CH$_3$

HO H OH

Figure 5 Chemical structures of lipid molecules with polar groups. n, Number of carbon atoms in fatty-acid chains; X, phospholipid head group, most often choline.

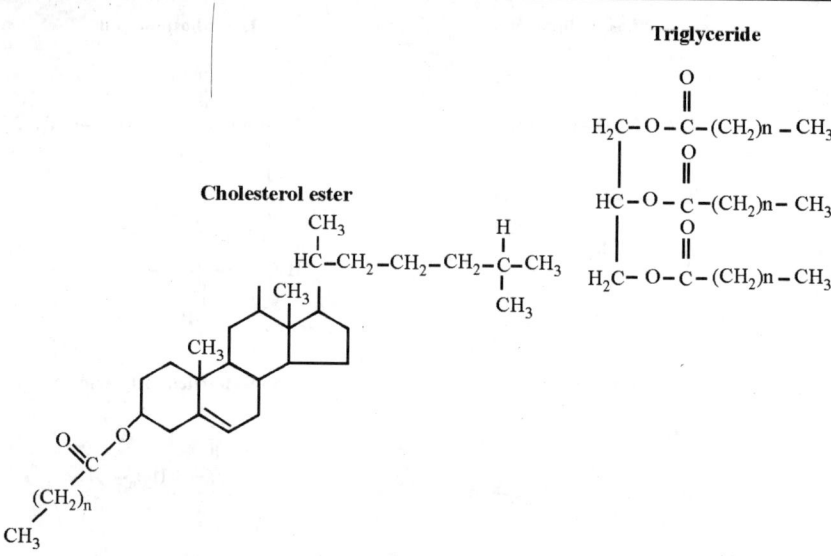

Figure 6 Chemical structures of lipid molecules without polar groups (triglyceride and cholesterol ester); n, Number of carbon atoms in fatty-acid chains.

water or water-based solutions. In the gut the emulsification phase begins in the stomach as the lipids are warmed to body temperature and subjected to the intense mixing, agitating and sieving actions of the distal stomach. The actions in the distal stomach tend to break lipid globules up into droplets that pass into the small intestine. In the small intestine, emulsification is completed by the detergent action of bile acids and phospholipids. The bile products reduce the surface tension of the lipids and allow the droplets to become even further divided and reduced in size (Figure 7).

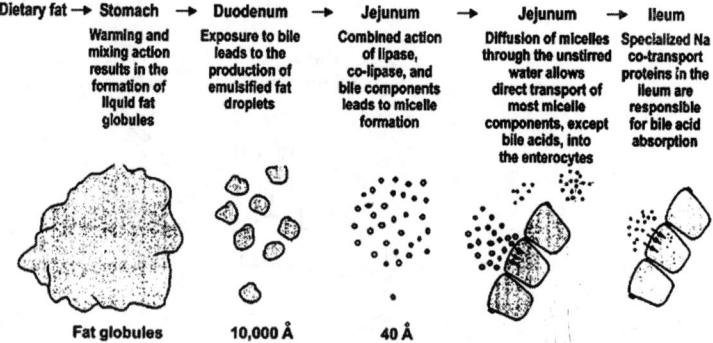

Figure 7 Sites and reactions involved in fat digestion and absorption. A°, Angstroms.
Source: Cunningham's textbook of Veterinary Physiology by Bradley G. Klein, 5th edition, 2013, pp314

Hydrolysis of triglycerides: Hydrolysis of triglycerides occurs by the combined action of lipase and co-lipase (pancreatic enzymes; see Table4). Lipase is secreted in its active form from the pancreas. However, lipase cannot penetrate the bile-coated or emulsified-droplet. The enzyme co-lipase (a relatively short peptide) 'clears the path' through the bile products and lipase enzyme get access to the triglycerides. Triglyceride molecule upon hydrolysis gives two free (or nonesterified) fatty acids and a monoglyceride. Other lipid-digesting pancreatic enzymes are cholesterol esterase and phospholipase. The products of these enzymes are nonesterified fatty acids, cholesterol and lysophospholipids.

TABLE 4   Lipids and endogenous enzymes of vertebrates
[Source: Modified from Stevens (1977)].

Substrate	Extracellular enzymes	Intestinal mucosal enzymes	End products
Triglycerides	Lipase Colipase		β-Monoglyceride 2Fatty acids
Phospholipids	Phospholipase	Phosphatase	Alcohol Fatty acids Phosphate
Cholesterol esters	Cholesterol estarase		Cholesterol Fatty acid
Waxes	Lipase Esterases		Monohydric alcohol Fatty acid

Micelle formation: The products of hydrolytic lipid digestion combine with bile acids and phospholipids to form micelles (small water-soluble aggregations of bile acids and lipids). The soluble micelles allow the lipids to diffuse through the gut lumen into the unstirred water layer and into close contact with the absorptive surface of the apical membrane.

Lipids are absorbed through the apical membrane by carrier proteins and simple diffusion

The process of lipid absorption into the enterocytes is incompletely understood. As the micelles come close to the surface of the enterocytes, the various lipid components diffuse the short distance through the glycocalyx to the apical membrane by means of special fatty acid-binding proteins. Other micellar components (which include monoglycerides, cholesterol and vitamin A) appear to simply diffuse into the apical membrane.

Bile acids are reabsorbed from the ileum by a sodium co-transport system

All components of the micelle diffuse into the enterocyte except the bile acids (see the figure 7). Bile acids remain in the lumen of the gut, and by the time bile acids reach the ileum, they are in a relatively free state, devoid of other lipids. Bile acids are absorbed by a specific bile acid transport system operated by sodium co-transport, and the absorbed ones are transported directly back to liver by the portal vasculature. The liver efficiently extracts bile acids from the portal blood, so normally the concentration of bile acids in the nonportal blood (systemic circulation) is small. The extracted bile acids are recycled into the bile. This recycling process occurs repeatedly, so the entire mass of bile acids within the body is circulated through the intestine several times per day.

Absorbed lipids are packaged into chylomicrons before leaving the enterocytes

After passing the apical membrane, the absorbed lipids are quickly picked up by carrier molecules and transported within the cell to the endoplasmic reticulum. When they are on the **smooth endoplasmic reticulum**, the major lipids are re-esterified to form triglyceride and phospholipids. The re-esterified lipids are then packaged with cholesterol, minor dietary lipids, and proteins from the **rough endoplasmic reticulum** into structures known as chylomicrons (Please see figure 22). Triglyceride and cholesterol esters are present in the core of the micelle, while the phospholipid and cholesterol on the surface with their hydrophobic (water repelling) ends facing the core lipids and hydrophilic (water attracting) ends facing the surface of the chylomicron particle. This arrangement of surface lipid makes the chylomicron water soluble. The presence of small number of special protein molecules on the surface of micelle help to stabilize it and to direct the metabolism of the particle.

After their formation, chylomicrons are expelled from the basolateral membrane into the lateral spaces. Unlike most other nutrients entering the lateral spaces, chylomicrons cannot be absorbed through the intestinal blood system. Chylomicrons are too large to pass through the basement membrane of the intestinal capillaries; rather they travel through the intestinal lymphatics, which eventually form a major abdominal lymph duct that passes through the diaphragm and into the thoracic duct. Chylomicrons finally reach the blood vascular system when this thoracic duct empties into the vena cava. After a fatty meal, the colour of intestinal lymph changes to milky white and this milky white colour can even be seen in blood plasma. In normal animals this white colour in blood plasma (lipemia) is transient, disappearing within 1 to 2 hours after digestion of the meal.

Digestion in the neonate

In the young livestock at birth, there are three primary alterations in the digestive tract. (1) Acid secretion from the stomach is delayed for several days after birth. (2) A similar delay appears in the development of pancreatic function, and thus acid and trypsin digestion of proteins is avoided. (3) A specialized intestinal epithelium present at birth only is capable of engulfing soluble proteins in the intestinal lumen and discharging them into the lateral spaces.

The fetal intestinal epithelium has the same villous structure as the mature epithelium, but the villi are covered with special enterocytes capable of protein absorption. Immediately birth, this special epithelium starts to disappear, and it is essentially gone after 24 hours. The loss of the protein absorptive function in the neonate is referred to as **gut closure**.

All mammals are born with high intestinal lactase activity because lactose from milk is the major carbohydrate in the diets of neonatal and young mammals. Maltase (enzyme for starch digestion) activity is weak or absent for several days after birth. As animals progress toward weaning, lactase activity wanes and maltase activity increases, allowing the animals to shift from milk diet to starch diets.

Digestion and Absorption: The Fermentative Processes

Fermentative and Glandular Digestion

In fermentative digestion, large molecules are broken down by the enzymes of microbial (bacteria and other microorganisms) origin in contrast to enzymes of host origin, which do the job in case of glandular digestion. Fermentative digestion is much slower than glandular digestion. The substrates are altered to a much greater degree in fermentative digestion.

The sites of fermentative digestion must be conducive to microbial growth Fermentative digestion occurs in specialized compartments that are positioned either before or after the stomach and small intestine. Forestomach- or pregut-fermentation is most developed in ruminants and camelids. Fermentation compartments positioned distal to the small intestine are the caecum and colon, often collectively called the hindgut; examples include horses, pigs. The forestomach and hindgut can support fermentative digestion because their pH (pH is close to neutral), moisture, ionic strength and oxidation-reduction conditions are maintained in a range compatible for the growth of suitable microbes. Further, the flow of ingesta through these areas is comparatively slow, allowing microbes sufficient time to maintain their population size.

In some species, including horse and rat, some fermentative digestion may occur in a nonglandular portion of the proximal stomach. In the stomach, bacterial numbers are kept low by the acid pH, whereas in the small intestine, bacterial numbers are kept in check by the constant flushing action of ingesta and secretions.

Rumen microbes

The microbes responsible for fermentative digestion include bacteria, fungi and protozoa. A vast bacterial population is associated with fermentative digestion with at least 28 functionally important species are present in the rumen (Figure 8). Please refer chapter 6 "Digestive Process in Different Species" for details on these rumen microbes.

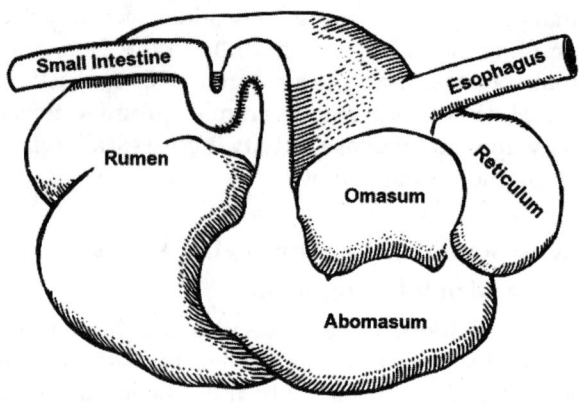

Figure 8   Ruminant stomach.

The essentiality of rumen protozoa

Either of rumen protozoa and bacteria can perform most of the fermentative functions of the rumen. Protozoa ingest large numbers of bacteria and hold rumen bacterial numbers in check. However, it is known that ruminants can survive well without protozoa (defaunation). Some reports gave positive results due to defaunation because protozoa cause intraruminal nitrogen degradation and thus wastage of nitrogen.

One potentially important function of protozoa involves their ability to slow down the digestion of rapidly fermentable starch. Protozoa are capable of ingesting particles of starch and storing them in their bodies, protected from bacterial action. This helps to maintain the rumen pH at optimum level through modulation or delay of the digestion of rapidly fermentable substrate. Also see page no 105 in chapter 6.

Cooperation and interplay among the many species of microbes give rise to a complex ecosystem in the forestomach and hindgut

The digestive process in the rumen or colon involves the interplay among the many species of bacteria and other microbes. For example, *Ruminococcus albus* and *Bacteroides ruminicola* appear to exist synergistically; the former digests only cellulose while the latter digests only protein. When the microbes are grown together, cellulose digestion by *R. albus* provides hexoses for the energy needs of *B. ruminicola*, and the ammonia and branch-chain fatty acids needed for the growth of *R. albus* are furnished by *B. ruminicola* from protein digestion. In addition to substrate needs, growth factor needs are also met synergistically within the rumen ecosystem. For example, B-vitamins are synthesized in the rumen and cross-feeding between the species obtain their needs.

Anaerobic conditions in the rumen result in metabolic activities leading to the production of volatile fatty acids

When carbohydrates enter the rumen or colon, they are attacked by hydrolytic microbial enzymes. Enzymatic action liberates glucose, other monosaccharides, and short-chain polysaccharides into the fluid phase, outside the microbial cell bodies. They are dissolved in the ruminal fluid and quickly subjected to further metabolism by the microbial mass. Glucose and other sugars are absorbed into the cell bodies of the microbes. Within the microbial cells, glucose enters the glycolytic, or Embden-Meyerhof, pathway. This is the same glycolytic pathway that exists in mammalian cells. As in mammalian tissues, catabolism of glucose through this pathway yields two molecules of pyruvate, NADH and ATP for each molecule of glucose metabolized. Because the rumen microorganisms do not have access to oxygen, they convert pyruvate to volatile (steam) fatty acids (VFA) instead of CO_2 and water. These pathways (Figure 9 illustrates the metabolic pathways of these reactions) lead to the major end products of the fermentative digestion of carbohydrate, the VFAs. The potential energy represented by the ATP formed in this reaction is the major source of energy for maintenance and growth of microbes

Oxidation of reduced cofactors

Under aerobic conditions, the pyruvate of glycolytic pathway would enter the citric acid (Krebs) cycle and would be metabolized to carbon dioxide and water in mammalian cells; the NADH produced would be oxidized in the cytochrome oxidase system with additional production of ATP and the regeneration of NAD^+.

However, the fermentative digestion in the rumen and colon proceeds in a reductive, highly anaerobic environment. Therefore a different mechanism must be provided for the oxidation of NADH and other reduced cofactors. If such mechanism were not available, all the oxidized cofactors present would soon be reduced, and metabolism would come to a halt. Because no atmospheric oxygen is available, some other compound must serve as an "electron sink" for the oxidation of enzyme cofactors. **(1) In fermentative digestion, pyruvate can act as an electron sink**, being further reduced to provide for regeneration of NAD$^+$ and the general removal of excess electrons, with an additional yield of ATP. Production of propionic acid from pyruvate results in the efficient regeneration of NAD+ with no net production of NADH. In fact, production of available oxygen by the 'randomizing branch of the propionic acid pathway' leads to oxidation of excess NADH originating from the acetic or butyric acid pathways (see figure 9). The production of acetic acid leads to the efficient generation of ATP but does not result in the regeneration of NAD$^+$ from NADH.

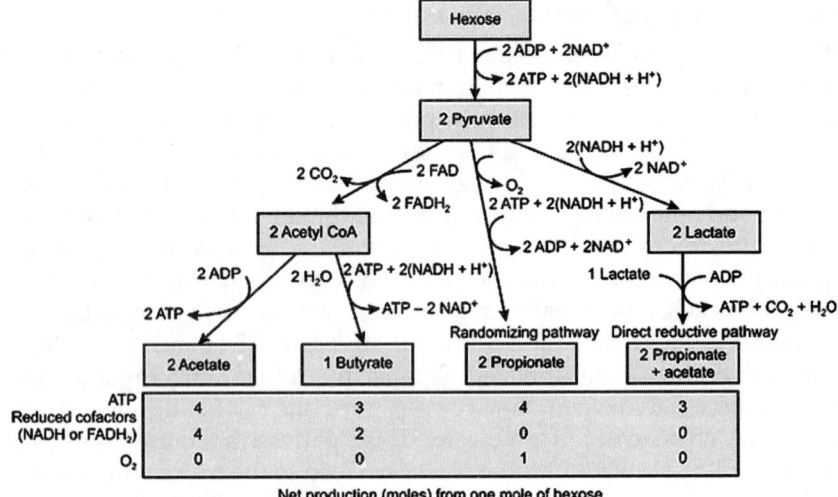

Figure 9   Pathways of volatile fatty acid (VFA) production by the rumen or colonic biomass. Source: Cunningham's textbook of Veterinary Physiology by Bradley G. Klein, 5th edition, 2013, pp324

(2) Methane as an electron sink: In the acetic acid pathway, excess NADH is produced. In this case, NAD$^+$ is regenerated by the formation of free hydrogen, which is subsequently used to reduce carbon dioxide to methane and water. The production of methane is necessary for the production of oxidized cofactors in the pathways leading to acetate and butyrate production. The production of oxygen by the randomizing pathway results in the net production of oxidized cofactors.

Generation of oxidized cofactors by reduction of carbon dioxide by methanogenic bacteria

$$NADH + H^+ \longrightarrow NAD^+ + H_2$$
$$4(H_2) + CO_2 \longrightarrow CH_4 + 2H_2O$$

Generation of oxidized cofactors by molecular oxygen arising from the randomizing pathway

$$2\,(NADH + H^+) + O_2 \longrightarrow NAD^+ + 2H_2O$$

(3) NADH can donate its electrons to reactions such as the synthesis of microbial protein and the saturation of unsaturated fatty acids.

Steam volatile and short-chain fatty acids

The VFAs are often referred to as their dissociated ions: acetate, propionate and butyrate; other quantitatively minor but metabolically important short chain fatty acids are valeric acid, isovaleric acid, isobutyric acid and 2-methylbutyric acid (Figure 10).

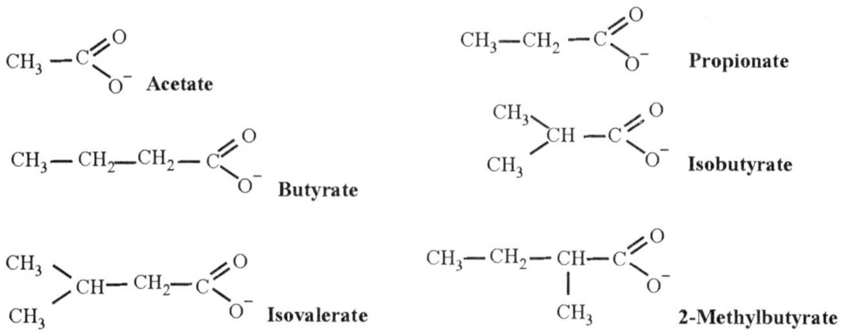

Figure 10   Chemical structures of the major volatile fatty acids (VFAs) produced by fermentative digestion

In ruminants and other large herbivores, the VFAs are the major energy fuels, to a large extent serving the role played by glucose in omnivorous monogastric animals.

Fermentative digestion of protein results in the deamination of a large portion of amino acids

As proteins enter fermentative areas of the gut, they are attacked by extracellular microbial proteases. The majority of these enzymes are "trypsin-like" endopeptidases that form short-chain peptides as end products. These peptides are formed extracellularly and are absorbed into the microbial cell bodies. Within the microbial cells, the peptides can be used to form microbial protein or can be further degraded for the production of energy through the VFA pathways.

Absorbed peptides contribute to intracellular pool of amino acids from which microbial proteins are synthesized. Another source of amino acids is frcm intracellular synthesis using ammonia and VFA. Many microbes appear capable of deriving their amino acids from either extracellular peptides or intracellular synthesis. However, several types of bacteria seem capable of using peptides for an amino acid source and are thus dependent on an extracellular source of ammonia for amino acid synthesis. Amino acids not used for protein synthesis can be metabolized to VFA and ammonia. The three branch-chain amino acids lead to the production of branch-chain VFAs by the following reactions:

Valine + 2 H_2O → Isobutyrate + NH_3 + CO_2

Leucine + 2H_2O → Isovalerate + NH_3 + CO_2

Isoleucine + 2H_2O → 2-Methylbutyrate + NH_3 + CO_2

These branch-chain fatty acids (and ammonia) are important growth factors for several species of bacteria, especially cellulose digesting bacteria.

Interorgan Nitrogen cycling in Ruminants

If sufficient carbohydrate/fermentable energy is available, most rumen microbes can synthesize protein from ammonia. Thus (microbial) protein can be synthesized in the rumen from such nonprotein nitrogen (NPN) sources as ammonia, nitrates and urea. This capability has been exploited by the inclusion of inexpensive NPN sources in ruminant diets allowing the microbes to synthesize protein for the amino acid needs of the host. This process also can be exploited physiologically by the recycling of endogenous urea.

Urea is formed in the liver. In ruminant animals, hepatic urea production is from two sources: (1) nitrogen arising from the deamination of endogenous amino acids and (2) nitrogen absorbed as ammonia from the rumen. Ammonia, which is toxic at moderate concentrations, is absorbed from the rumen and delivered to the liver through the hepatic-portal blood vascular system (The liver extracts ammonia from the portal blood efficiently). In monogastric animals, urea is excreted from the body almost exclusively by the kidneys. In ruminants, however, urea also may be excreted into the rumen. Such excretion can occur by direct absorption of urea into the rumen from the blood or by excretion of urea into saliva (Figure 11). In either case, the urea reaches the rumen, where it is quickly transformed to ammonia, and enters the general pool of rumen nitrogen sources for synthesis of microbial protein.

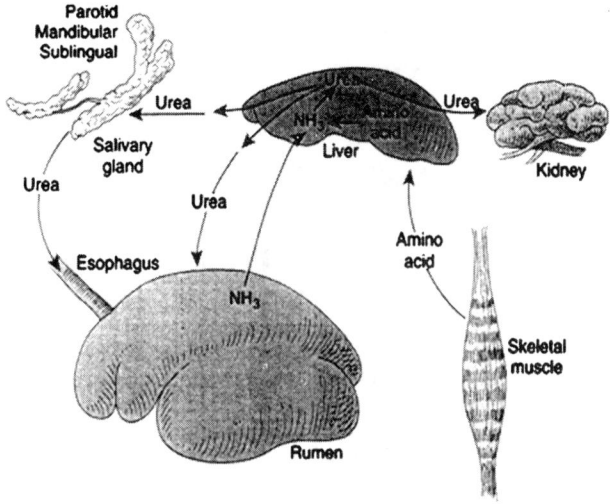

Figure 11 Interorgan nitrogen cycling in ruminants. Source: Cunningham's textbook of Veterinary Physiology by Bradley G. Klein, 5th edition, 2013, pp327.

Ruminants are efficient conservers of nitrogen on low-protein diets

During times of high nitrogen availability in the rumen (due to higher rumen degradable protein), relative to carbohydrate/fermentable energy availability, the microbial capacity to synthesize their cells is limited resulting in loss of precious nitrogen through urinary excretion. However, during times of high carbohydrate/fermentable energy availability relative to nitrogen availability, microbes could trap the nitrogen sources well and built their cells efficiently, and the major flow of urea nitrogen is from the blood into the rumen; under these circumstances, ruminal ammonia concentrations are low, most of the blood urea is from endogenous protein catabolism. Thus, under conditions of low-dietary protein, ruminants are efficient conservers of nitrogen.

Reticulorumen motility pattern - the effect of transit of feed through the rumen

The walls of the reticulorumen are muscular, possess an extensive intrinsic nervous system, and are capable of highly complex and coordinated motility patterns. These motility patterns are necessary for the critical function of the rumen, which is the selective retention of actively fermenting material accompanied by the simultaneous release of unfermentable residue. Reticulorumen is divided into compartments or sacs (see figure 12). These divisions are created by muscular pillars that

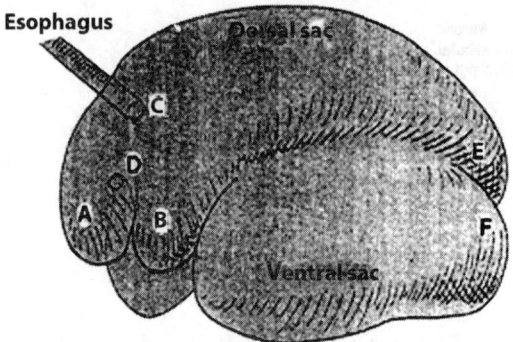

Figure 12 Rumen anatomy. A, Reticulum; B, cranial sac; C, cardia; D, reticulo-omasal
orifice; E, caudal-dorsal blind sac; F, caudal-ventral blind sac.

project into the lumen of the organ. The reticular fold and rumen pillars, in
addition to the walls themselves, are motile. During reticulorumen
contractions the pillars alternatively elevate and relax, accentuating or
reducing the divisions within the lumen of the reticulorumen. In general,
there are **two patterns of reticulorumen motility: primary or mixing
contractions and secondary or eructation contractions**. Figure 13
illustrates a view from the left side, the sagital section through the bovine
reticulo-rumen.

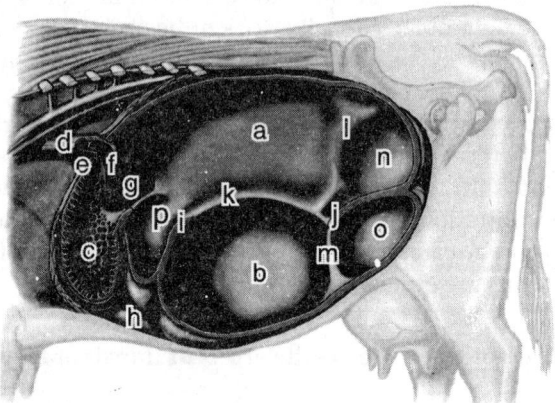

Figure 13 Sagital section through the bovine reticulo-rumen, viewed from the left side and
showing the internal structural relationships. [The reticulum lies against the diagram, while
the rumen extends almost to the pelvic cavity. The esophageal groove runs from the lower
esophageal sphincter to the reticulo-omasal orifice. a. dorsal sac, b. ventral sac, c. reticulum,
d. esophagus, e. diaghragm, f. esophageal groove, g. reticulo-omasal orifice, h. abomasums,
i. cranial pillar, j. caudal pillar, k. longitudinal pillar, i. dorsal coronary pillar, m. ventral
coronary pillar, n. dorsocaudal blind sac, o. ventrocaudal blind sac, p. craniodorsal blind sac].
Source: Physiology of Domestic Animals by Oystein V. Sjaastad et al., 2003, pp510

Primary (or mixing) pattern of motility: These are the most frequent contractions. They start at the reticulum at about one minute interval. To illustrate the primary pattern of motility and describe its effect on ingesta flow, consider the path of a single bolus of feed material as it passes through the rumen. Assume this material is forage such as grass, hay or silage. The animal chews the feed to create an initial reduction in particle size and form it into a bolus by mixing it with saliva. The swallowed bolus enters the rumen at the cardia, which is at the dorsal portion of reticulum near the junction of the reticulum and the cranial ventral sac (Figure 14A). Air bubbles trapped in the bolus give it a relatively low specific gravity, compared to surrounding ingesta, so it remains suspended in the area near the cardia (Figure 14B). As a primary rumen contraction begins, there is a biphasic, or double contraction of the reticulum. Material in the dorsal portion of the reticulum, including the recently swallowed bolus of feed, is washed back into the rumen by this flow of liquid ingesta (Figure 14C). A caudal-moving contraction of the dorsal sac follows the reticular contraction, continuing to move the recently swallowed bolus and other material further back into the dorsal sac. A subsequent cranial-moving contraction of the dorsal sac serves to mix the dorsal sac ingesta, creating a mass of tangled forage fibres representing a large collection of relatively recently swallowed material (Figure 14D).

The mass of material tends to remain in the dorsal rumen due to buoyancy (microbial action creates small bubbles of gas that adhere to the plant material; this accounts for its buoyancy and gives it a low functional specific gravity). As time passes, however, microbial action tends to cause the material to break apart (because of less fermentable substrate, less gas, less buoyancy leading to increase of functional specific gravity) and the material begins to sink in (ventral sac) the rumen as small particles (Figure 14E). The material in the dorsal sac is a solid mass of tangled forage fibres while the material in the ventral sac is a suspension of small particles that is much more fluid and water like. Contractions of the ventral sac tend to push the more buoyant material back up into the dorsal sac, while allowing the smallest and least buoyant particles to spill over the cranial ruminal pillar into the cranial ventral sac (Figure 14F).

Subsequent to the contractions of the ventral sac is a contraction of the cranial ventral sac, which further separates material based on functional specific gravity and results in small particles with the highest functional specific gravity flowing back into the reticulum (Figure 14G). By this time, the material has made a complete circuit of the rumen, entering at the cardia and passing through the dorsal, ventral and cranial ventral sacs and back to the reticulum. As the reticulum contracts at the beginning of a primary cycle, the reticulo-omasal orifice relaxes and dense (high functional specific gravity) material near the bottom of the reticulum is forced through the opening and into the omasum (Figure 14H). See figure 15 for a comprehensive occurrences related to transit of feed through the rumen.

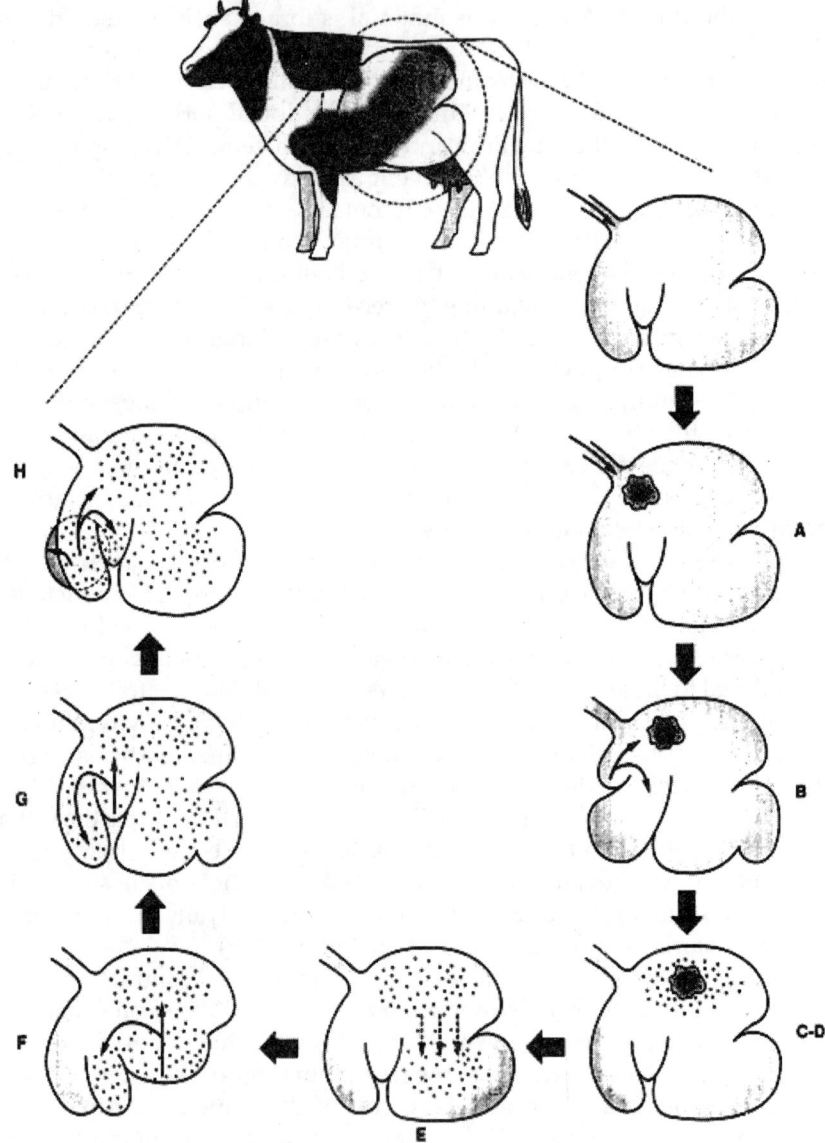

Figure 14   The sequential figures illustrate the pattern of flow of feed material through the reticulorumen from its arrival at the cardia (A) to its exit via the reticulo-omasal orifice (H). Source: Cunningham's textbook of Veterinary Physiology by Bradley G. Klein, 5th edition, 2013, pp332

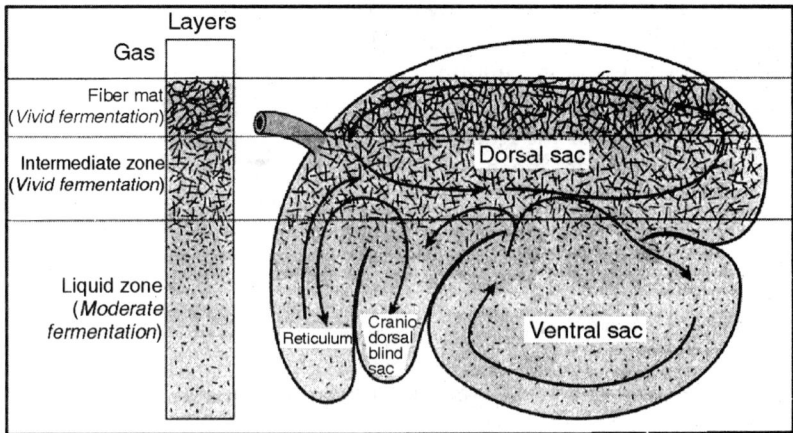

Figure 15 Layering of rumen content of cows consuming a diet with a high proportion of hay. The fibre mat contains coarse and relatively undigested material. As the content becomes digested, it sinks towards the lower parts of the rumen. During contractions of the ventral sac of the rumen, well-digested material from the lower part of the rumen is transferred to the craniodorsal blind sac. This material is then shuttled back and forth between the craniodorsal blind sac and reticulum until it is passed on to the omasum. Source: Physiology of Domestic Animals by Oystein V.Sjaastad et al., 2003, pp513

The overall effect of transit of feed: The overall effect of the transit of feed through the rumen is a reduction in particle size associated with the loss of fermentable matter of the feed. Long forage material is reduced by initial mastication to particles of 1 to 2 cm or shorter. Thereafter rumination reduces the particle size. Most of the material in the dorsal rumen is of similar particle size. Particle size diminishes in the more ventral portions of the rumen. As the particle size become reduced to 2 to 3 mm long, such particles move through the reticulo-omasal orifice. However, the reticulo-omasal orifice is probably about 2 cm in diameter (when dilated for feed passage). This indicates that selection of small particles for passage into the omasum is not based on the size of the reticulo-omasal orifice.

Secondary (or eructation) contractions: Secondary (or eructation) contractions occur as an added sequence of events at the end of a primary sequence of contractions. Secondary contractions consist of a cranial-moving wave that starts in the caudal-dorsal blind sac and continues over the dorsal sac. **The function** of the secondary contraction is to **force gas toward the cranial portion of the rumen**. The pattern begins with a contraction of the caudo-ventral blind sac, expressing trapped gas in that compartment into the dorsal sac. The secondary contraction continues with a forward-moving contraction of the dorsal sac that moves gas toward the cardia, while cranial sac relaxation and cranial pillar elevation allows liquid ingesta to move away from the cardia so that gas can enter the esophagus and be eructated. These secondary contractions are important because large amounts of gas, primarily carbon dioxide and methane that are formed during fermentation, are removed rapidly to prevent distension of the rumen. The readers may follow the figure 13 to understand expulsion of gas.

Reticulorumen Contraction: In general, one to three reticulorumen contractions occur per minute. Contractions occur more frequently during eating and disappear entirely during deep sleep. The rate and strength of contractions depend on the character of the diet - coarse and fibrous feeds stimulate the most frequent and strongest contractions. Although variable, secondary contractions usually occur in association with half the primary contractions and depend on the rate of gas formation.

Rate of passage of feed particles from the rumen and rate of feed intake

Feed does not leave the rumen until it is broken down into small particles. Microbial action and rumination are primarily responsible for particle size reduction in the rumen. The rate of breakdown of fibre is chiefly a function of its digestibility. Poorly digestible straws/stovers take longer time to be broken down sufficiently to sink into the ventral sac, compared to feeds of greater digestibility. This means that feeds of lesser digestibility remains in the rumen longer than feeds of greater digestibility. Since the volume/capacity of the rumen is fixed, the rate of feed intake cannot exceed the rate of ingesta outflow. Therefore, intake of poorly digestible feed is always less than intake of highly digestible feeds.

Feed preparation can influence this relationship. Chopping of such straws increases their rate of passage from the rumen because less particle size reduction is necessary to pass into the omasum. Thus, physical form (length) and digestibility each have an effect on rate of passage from the rumen and also on feed intake. In general, forage material of relatively high digestibility has a rumen half-life of approximately 30 hours, whereas poorly digestible material has a half-life of up to 50 hours.

Rumination or cud chewing has an important effect on the reduction of particle size

Rumination is the act of remasticating rumen ingesta. The initial act of rumination is regurgitation, which occurs just before the initiation of a primary rumen contraction. When regurgitation occurs, there is an extra contraction of the reticulum, which takes place just before the regular biphasic reticular contraction that initiates the primary cycle. This extra contraction removes newly-swallowed content from the opening of the esophagus, replacing it with a semi-liquid mass of feed which has already undergone some fermentation. Simultaneous with an extra reticular contraction, the cardia relaxes, and there is an inspiratory excursion of the ribs with the glottis closed. The latter action creates a negative pressure within the thorax, favouring the movement of food into the esophagus. When the food enters the esophagus, a reverse peristaltic wave propels the material cranially into the mouth. As soon as the food bolus reaches the mouth, excess water is expressed by action of the tongue, the water is swallowed, and remastication of the material begins. The duration of remastication depends on the character of the diet, with coarse material requiring more time for remastication than finely ground or highly digestible feeds.

The ingesta is subjected to microbial action during the initial phases of digestion in the dorsal sac. This partially fermented material is regurgitated and then subjected to remastication. This facilitates further comminution and exposure of additional fermentable substrate to microbial action leading to higher digestibility.

Rumination may also help the particle separation process - as the regurgitated bolus reaches the mouth, it is squeezed by the tongue and cheeks before mastication begins. Subsequently, water and small particles are swallowed while large particles are remasticated. The small particles sink into the reticulum where they are subject to passage to the omasum. The larger particles, when swallowed after remastication, are ejected back into the more cranial portions of the rumen.

Rumination occurs when the animal is not actively eating, usually during times of rest, but not during the deep sleep. The time spent for rumination ranges from almost none for high-grain diets to a maximum of about 10 hours per day for high-forage diets. The feed intake level also influences the amount of rumination time, with high intakes stimulating greater rumination.

Water moves through the Rumen at a much faster rate than particulate matter

The flow of water has important effects on rumen dynamics. For small particles and soluble material to exit the rumen, liquid must constantly be flowing through the mass of solid material through all sections of the rumen and moving through the reticulo-omasal orifice. In effect, the reticulorumen functions as a fermentation vat holding the mass of particulate matter while water flows through it and washes small particles and soluble material away. Therefore the transit rate of water must be considerably greater than the transit rate of particulate matter through the rumen. The relative differences in the rates of movement of solid-phase and liquid phase material through the rumen can be appreciated from their respective rumen half-lives: 30 to 50 hours for particulate matter and about 15 to 20 hours for liquid.

Dilution Rate

The rate of liquid flow through the rumen is often measured as the dilution rate, which is expressed as the percentage of total liquid that leaves the rumen in an hour. It should be remembered that water leaves the rumen only as it is replaced from some other source. The term dilution rate comes from the way liquid turnover is measured, some soluble marker substance (for example, Cr-EDTA, PEG, etc) is mixed into the rumen, and its concentration is measured as soon as it is thoroughly dispersed into the liquid phase. Samples are then taken over time, and the rate at which the marker substance becomes diluted is measured. The rate of dilution depends on the rate at which water that contains marker leaves the rumen and is replaced with new, unmarked water. The dilution rate is an indirect measure of the rate of water flow through the rumen. Normal dilution rate values vary with diet and feed intake and are usually in the range of 5% to 30% per hour.

Factors affecting Dilution rate: Almost all water that enters the rumen pass through the oesophagus, the sources being either from salivary flow, drinking, or succulent feeds. Thus the dilution rate depends on rates of salivation and drinking. The **salivation rate** is influenced by the chewing time and feed type: feeds such as long-stemmed dry roughages, which require relatively high rates of mastication, stimulate high rates of both salivary flow and dilution. Salivation occurs during rumination as well as during initial mastication; therefore those feeds that stimulate high rumination rates, such as forages, also stimulate high dilution rates. Conversely, feeds that do not stimulate extensive rumination (e.g., concentrates) result in relatively low dilution rates. The **rate of drinking** is influenced by (1) the rate of feed intake and (2) the salt, or electrolyte, content of the diet. Thus, high rates of intake or diets with high electrolyte contents stimulate high dilution rates.

Little water enters the rumen by way of the mucosa. The mucosa of the forestomachs is stratified squamous epithelium and is aglandular; thus there is no direct fluid secretion. Some water can enter the rumen through osmosis, but under normal conditions, the amount appears to be minimal. Normal rumen osmolality is about 280 mOsm/kg, slightly less than the 300 mOsm/kg osmolality of blood and extracellular fluid. Thus the usual osmotic flow of water is out of the rumen. After consumption of relatively digestible feeds, rumen osmolality increases briefly because of VFA production. However, it appears that osmolalities in excess of 340 mOsm/

kg are necessary for water to flow osmotically into the rumen. Under normal conditions, osmolalities this high are not sustained for long, and thus there is usually little osmotic flow of water into the rumen.

Influence of rumen dilution rate on fermentation and microbial cell yield

Small particles, including microbes, leave the rumen with the liquid phase. Therefore, high dilution rates result in rapid removal of microbes and reductions in microbial cell concentrations. Because high microbe concentrations suppress microbial cell division, the growth of microbes is stimulated by high dilution rates. High growth rates are nutritionally desirable because a larger portion of the energy available to the microbes is used for growth instead of for maintenance, as occurs in older, relatively stable microbial populations. Thus, high dilution rates usually increase Y_{ATP} values, provided that adequate protein is available to support cell growth.

In addition to its effect on Y_{ATP}, the dilution rate may affect the microbial makeup of the rumen biomass and also may have some influence on the fermentation pattern. The rate of microbial washout increases with the dilution rate. At high dilution rates, microbial species with slow growth rates diminish in population size because their replication rate is not great enough to match the rate at which they are removed. Thus, selection pressure favours species with faster growth rates during times of high rumen dilution rates. Exceptions to this pattern occur because some microbes are able to attach themselves to the particulate matter in the solid and slurry zones. Such microbes then exit the rumen according to the kinetics of particle size reduction rather than dilution rate. In general, the changes occuring in the rumen microbial population with high dilution rate appear to favour acetic acid production and to increase the acetic/propionic acid ratio.

Control of Reticulorumen Motility

Reticulorumen motility is controlled by the central nervous system and affected by intraluminal conditions

Vagus nerve and reticulorumen motility: In the dorsal vagal nucleus of the brainstem, there is a motility control center for the regulation of reticuloruminal motility. This center sends action potentials along fibres to the forestomach by way of the vagus nerve. There is an extensive enteric nervous system within the reticulorumen, but vagal innervation is necessary for coordination of normal motility patterns. Vagotomized ruminants do not survive because motility of the rumen musculature ceases.

The dorsal vagal nucleus receives afferent stimuli that affect the control of forestomach motility. Important afferent signals come from the lumen of the reticulorumen and monitor distention, ingesta consistency, pH, VFA concentration, and ionic strength. Rumen volume or distention, appears to be monitored by stretch receptors in the walls and especially in the pillars. Moderate distention increases rumen motility and rumination. Increased motility and rumination have the effect of raising the rate at which particles are broken down, leading to a higher passage rate. Thus, rumen throughput is enhanced when increased intake expands rumen volume. Severe distention, as occurs in bloat, causes cessation of rumen motility.

The consistency of ingesta also has an important influence on rumen motility. Consistency is determined largely by diet type. When the diet consists of succulent plants, grain, or finely chopped forage, there is little material in the solid zone, or rumen mat, and the slurry zone is fluid. This type of fluid ingesta offers little resistance to the movement of the rumen pillars and thus the rumen musculature has to apply relatively little force to mix and circulate the rumen contents. **Tension receptors** in the reticuloruminal muscle appear to monitor the force necessary to move the pillars through the ingesta. Highly fluid rumen ingesta are associated with low muscle tension and have a negative influence on reticulorumen motility. When animals are eating dry, long-stem hay, the rumen contents are solid and create a large and highly interwoven rumen mat. Resistance to movement of the pillars through the solid mass of ingesta is high and leads to stimulation of tension receptors, resulting in a positive feedback on motility. **The motility rate is directly related to the rate of particle breakdown.** This arrangement appears to be self-regulatory mechanism that increases the rate of particle comminution when animals consume diets with large particle size.

Chemoreceptors in the walls of the rumen and reticulum monitor pH, VFA concentration, and ionic strength (or osmolality). The pH of the reticulorumen is normally slightly acid, reflecting the acidity of the VFAs, but extreme acid conditions are undesirable. Increasing VFA concentrations or decreasing pH results in a suppression of rumen motility. The normal rumen pH is in the range of 5.5 to 6.8, depending on the type of diet. When the rumen pH falls much below 5.0, motility is severely depressed.

Osmolality may also influence rumen motility, although motility appears less sensitive to osmotic changes than it does to pH changes. Normal osmolality in the rumen is about 280 mOsm, but the osmolality increases during active fermentation. Osmotically active solutes in the rumen include organic acids as well as salivary and dietary electrolytes. As organic acid formation increases during fermentation, osmolality also increases, tending to reduce motility. The rumen epithelium creates a relatively impermeable barrier to water. However, at abnormally high osmolalities water can be drawn into the rumen.

Omasal Function

Passage of material from the Reticulum to the Omasum occurs during reticular contraction

The body of the omasum is filled with multiple muscular folds, or leaves, that project from the greater curvature into the lumen. The omasal canal connects the reticulum to the abomasum. Ingesta move into the omasum during reticular contractions. The reticulo-ómasal orifice usually remains open, but dilates especially during the second phase of the reticular contraction, during which ingesta flow rapidly into the omasal canal. After the reticular contraction, the reticulo-omasal orifice closes briefly as the canal contracts, forcing newly arrived ingesta up into the leaves. Intermittently, the body and leaves of the omasum contract, forcing the material from the omasal leaves into the canal and on into the abomasum.

Proper functioning of the omasum and reticulum appears to be particularly important to the passage of ingesta out of the rumen. Occasionally, when ingested foreign bodies cause **traumatic injury** resulting in damage to vagal fibres and adhesions in the wall of reticulum and omasum, the ability to move food out of the forestomachs is severely impaired. The rumen becomes greatly distended with finely comminuted feed, and the entire rumen becomes a slurry zone. Despite the distended rumen, little movement of ingesta occurs into the abomasum, and the animals eventually suffer severe inanition. This condition is variably known as **omasal transport failure and vagal indigestion**.

The structure of the omasum, with its many leaves and large mucosal surface area, suggests that it has an absorptive function, but the exact nature of this function is still incompletely understood. One important possibility is that it exists to remove residual VFAs and bicarbonate from ingesta before material is transported to the abomasum. Thus omasum prevents unfavourable reactions in the abomasum due to the passage of VFAs and bicarbonate.

VFA Absorption through the forestomach epithelium

VFAs are bacterial waste products and will suppress fermentation, if allowed to accumulate. But VFAs are extremely important energy substrates for the host animal and supply 60% to 80% of the dietary energy to ruminants with most types of diets. Therefore the presence of an efficient and high capacity mechanism for VFA absorption is important to both digestion and host metabolism. The forestomach epithelium supplies such a system, absorbing almost all the VFAs, with only small amounts escaping to the lower digestive tract. The absorptive process helps to maintain the rumen pH by removing acid from the forestomach ingesta and contributing bicarbonate in the process.

Epithelium of forestomach and small intestine: The forestomach surface is of the stratified squamous type (similar to the stratified squamous epithelium of the skin and other surfaces) and consists of several layers of cells of varying maturity. The deepest layer is the stratum basale, from which cells divide and migrate into the **stratum spinosum**. Cells of the stratum spinosum begin the process of keratinization and continue into the **stratum granulosum**, which is covered by the outermost and most keratinized layer, the **stratum corneum**. Although the forestomach epithelium seems completely different from the columnar epithelium of the small intestine, the nature of the rumen epithelium may give it functional characteristics similar to those of the absorptive epithelium of the small intestine and colon. An interesting similarity between forestomach and intestinal epithelia is noted when the cellular attachments and intercellular spaces of the forestomach are examined (see the figure 16).

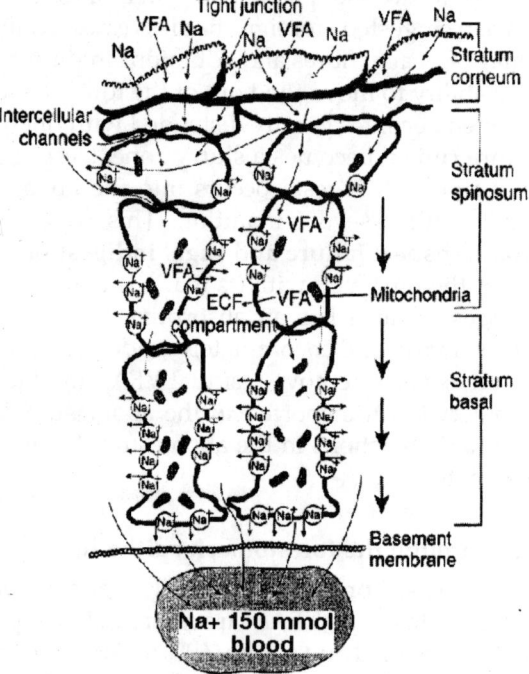

Figure 16   The stratified squamous epithelium of the rumen shares functional similarities with the columnar epithelium of the small intestine. Source: Cunningham's textbook of Veterinary Physiology by Bradley G. Klein, 5th edition, 2013, pp335

The cells of the stratum granulosum are tightly joined by junctions that may functionally resemble the tight junctions of the enterocytes. Deeper in the epithelium, the cells of the stratum spinosum and stratum basale are separated by intercellular spaces that increase in size as the basement membrane is approached. These intercellular spaces are reminiscent of the lateral spaces of columnar absorptive epithelia. If these observations are combined with the existence of the intercellular bridges that characterize the forestomach epithelium, an interesting analogy to columnar absorptive epithelia can be constructed. VFAs, electrolytes, and water apparently are initially absorbed through the stratum corneum and passed cell to cell by way of intercellular bridges to the cells of the stratum spinosum and stratum basale, from which the absorbed substances are passed into the intercellular spaces before entering the capillaries.

Because of the intercellular bridges, absorbed solute can be transferred directly from the outer keratinized cells (of the stratum corneum) to the deeper, more metabolically active cells (of the stratum spinosum and stratum basale). Thus the metabolic activity deep in the epithelium appears to maintain conditions for absorption at the epithelial surface.

Molecular mechanism of VFA absorption: Differences in pH (near the absorptive surface) can have an important influence on the molecular mechanism of VFA absorption because of shifts in the dissociation state of the VFA molecules. (1) The pKa of the VFA is approximately 4.8, well below the normal pH of the rumen. Thus most of the **VFAs exist in the rumen in the dissociated, or ionic, form**. However, at the absorptive surface, sodium-hydrogen ion exchange by the epithelial cells may decrease the local pH. Such a **drop in pH would lead to a shift in the VFA from the ionic (Ac⁻) to the free-acid state (HAc)**. (The outer, keratinized stratum corneum is permeable to the anions of the VFAs as well as the undissociated [or free-acid state] acids. The metabolically active middle layers [stratum spinosum and stratum basal] of the epithelium, on the other hand, act as a barrier to the negatively charged anions. At a normal reticulo-ruminal pH of 6.8, the concentration of acetate is 100 times higher than the concentration of the undissociated acetic acid). Cell membranes are permeable to VFA free acids, and absorption proceeds because of the concentration gradient between the lumen and cells. (2) The high CO_2 tension in the rumen, caused by the production of fermentation gases, may also enhance the conversion of VFA to the free-acid state. As shown in figure 17, when one VFA molecule is absorbed, one molecule of bicarbonate (HCO_3^-) is generated in the lumen. Thus VFA absorption helps buffer rumen pH both by generating base and by removing acid.

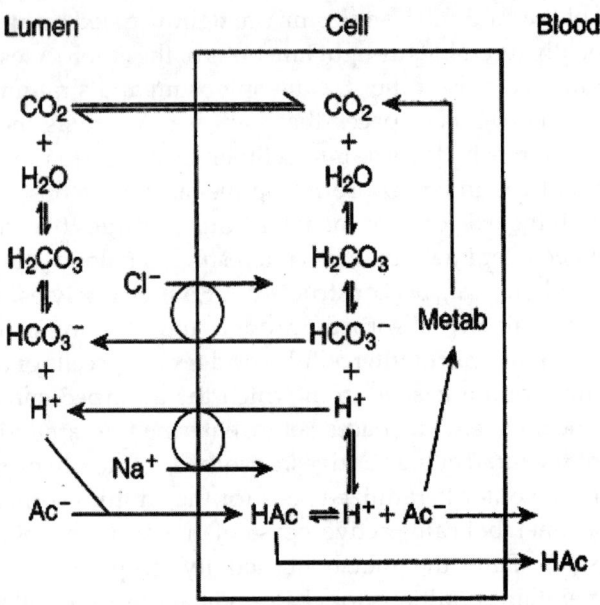

Figure 17   VFA absorption is promoted by the conversion of VFA anions (Ac⁻) to free
acids (HAc) in the microenvironment near the epithelial surface. Source: Cunningham's
textbook of Veterinary Physiology by Bradley G. Klein, 5th edition, 2013, pp335

All the VFAs appear to be absorbed by the same mechanism, but they
are handled differently within the epithelial cells. Some acetate seems to
be completely oxidized within the cells, with the remainder absorbed
unchanged. Most propionate is absorbed, but a small portion is converted
to lactate by the epithelial cells. Butyrate is modified extensively, and
essentially all molecules are changed to β-hydroxybutyrate (a ketone
body) before absorption. Ketone bodies are metabolites that frequently
have special medical significance. In ruminants the rumen itself is a
significant source of ketone bodies. However, ketone bodies arise
exclusively from the partial oxidation of long-chain fatty acids in
monogastric animals.

Size and shape of rumen papillae: The rumen epithelium is arranged
in papillae, fingerlike projections that increase the absorptive surface area.
These papillae serve to expand the area just like that of villi of the small
intestine. But the papillae are much larger and easily visible to the unaided
eye. The size and shape of the papillae are quite dynamic and responsive
to changes in diet. Papillary growth is stimulated by VFAs, especially
butyrate and propionate. Diets with high digestibility result in high rumen
VFA concentrations, which stimulate the growth of long papillae. In
contrast, short rumen papillae are observed in animals receiving little feed

or diets of low digestibility. It is important to adapt ruminants gradually when changing them from diets of low digestibility to high digestibility so as to allow time for sufficient adjustment of papillary size so that VFA absorption will match VFA production.

Rumen Development and Esophageal Groove Function

Significant changes in forestomach size and function occur with dietary changes in early life

In cattle the period of forestomach development is arbitrarily divided into the nonruminant period from birth to 3 weeks, and the transitional period from 3 to 8 weeks. The size of the forestomach is about equal to that of abomasum in young ruminants at birth, in contrast to that in adult animals wherein the forestomach accounts for more than 90% of the total stomach volume. Enlargement of the forestomach occurs rapidly after birth, but the rate depends on diet type. When young ruminants are given access to solid feeds soon after birth, the forestomach development rate is maximal. Stomach proportions of adults are achieved usually by 8 weeks, if the calves have access to solid feeds. Calves can be seen eating grain and forage as early as 2 weeks of age and frequently ruminate by 3 weeks, indicating considerable forestomach development by this time. Withholding solid feed dramatically reduces the rate of rumen development and forestomach development remains rudimentary for 14 to 15 weeks or longer in calves fed only milk.

Development of forestomach epithelium also follows the general development of the organ. At birth the epithelium is thin, with small or nonexistent papillae. Exposure of the epithelium to VFAs appears to stimulate papillary development and general organ development as well. Young ruminants in the transitional period should receive the calf starter/creep feed to meet their high nutrient needs in addition to high quality forage. Calf starter/creep feed contributes good amount of VFA production and fastest epithelial development. Dietary forage may aid in muscular development of the forestomachs.

Establishment of rumen microflora and fauna

The forestomach is sterile at birth but is quickly colonized by environmental bacteria, mostly facultative organisms. The reductive environment creates conditions necessary for the growth and establishment of the strict anaerobes. The development of forestomach bacterial flora occurs independently of any special inoculation process. It is impossible to prevent it from occurring except by raising calves under gnotobiotic conditions. However, protozoal inoculation seems to require some exposure to other cattle. Calves raised in complete isolation do not develop protozoal fauna. It appears that aerosol spread of protozoa can occur because no direct physical contact among cattle is necessary to establish a protozoal fauna.

The Esophageal Groove or Reticular groove and its functions

The esophageal groove is a gutterlike invagination traversing the wall of the reticulum from the cardia to the reticulo-omasal orifice. When stimulated, muscles of the groove contract, causing it to shorten and twisting, by which the lips of the groove close together to form a nearly complete tube from the cardia to the omasal canal. When milk enters the cardia, it is directed into the omasum (with 10% or less entering the rumen; milk in the rumen results in the formation of improper fermentation patterns) and milk quickly traverses the omasum and enters the abomasum bypassing the rumen and reticulum. This is important for proper rumen development in the suckling animal.

The reticular groove has its primary function in suckling animals. Activity of the reticular groove reflex appears to diminish after weaning and with advancing age. Reticular groove closure is a reflex action. Efferent impulses come from brainstem through the vagus nerve. Afferent stimuli arise centrally and from the pharynx. Anticipation of suckling invokes central stimulation of reticular groove closure, which may be considered a cephalic phase. (1) Milk (or sodium-containing fluid) in the pharynx stimulates afferent fibres that reinforce the cephalic phase of groove closure. (2) The posture of the calf or lamb when suckling does not appear to have much influence on reticular groove function. (3) Rapid drinking from an open pail, in contrast to suckling from a nipple, frequently results in inefficient groove function and spillage of milk in the rumen.

The esophageal groove reflex is also stimulated by antidiuretic hormone (ADH), indicating that it may have some physiological function in adult life. ADH is secreted by the posterior pituitary in response to dehydration or increases in plasma osmolality. ADH is associated with thirst, and because it stimulates the reticular groove, a large portion of the water consumed by the water-deprived animals may bypass the rumen and quickly arrives at the site of most rapid absorption, the small intestine

Function of the Equine (Large) Hindgut

A general function of the caecum and colon is to recover fluid and electrolytes from ingesta leaving the ileum. In many herbivorous species, this function has been expanded to include fermentative digestion. Absorptive and fermentation functions complement each other in the colons of nonruminant herbivores. However, this interdependence between the two processes may end up in problems of digestion and absorption.

Structural and nonstructural carbohydrates as well as proteins form the major substrates for hindgut fermentation. However, the passage of material through the stomach and small intestine before its arrival at the caecum and colon may have some important effects on fermentative digestion. (1) Hindgut fermentation may be aided by prior gastric action. The effects of soaking and acid exposure in the stomach may increase their susceptibility to microbial attack and thus raise their rate of digestion in the hindgut. (2) Some of the readily available carbohydrate, particularly sugars and starches, may be digested and absorbed before the other material arrives in the caecum. However, it is reported that glandular digestion of carbohydrate in the horse is not efficient and substantial amounts of starch and sugars reach the caecum. Further, cell-wall carbohydrate appears to interfere with the digestion or absorption of starch and sugars in the equine small intestine. Even with a high-grain diet, up to 29% of dietary starch may reach the caecum and colon.

Protein as well as carbohydrate is absorbed in the small intestine, potentially leading to a deficiency of nitrogen for colonic microbes. However, there is extensive urea recycling into the colon and caecum, similar to that occurring in the rumen. Thus, urea plus the protein that escapes small-intestinal digestion supplies the nitrogen needs of the microbes. In contrast to ruminants, horses do not have an efficient means of recovering the microbial protein synthesized in the hindgut, and most of it passes out in the faeces. Some experiments have shown a small amount of amino acid absorption from the equine caecum or colon.

The Equine Hindgut has a great capacity for fermentation

Functionally, the equine hindgut can be divided into four sections: caecum, ventral colon, dorsal colon, and small colon. Favourable conditions must be maintained in the hind gut to support optimal fermentation. As in the rumen, these conditions are (1) substrate supply, (2) control of pH and osmolality, (3) anaerobiosis, (4) retention of fermenting material, and (5) continual removal of waste products and the residue of spent fermentation substrate.

Separation of fermenting material from residue appears to be accomplished by selective retention of particles according to size, just as in the rumen. Anatomical characteristics and motility patterns in the caecum and colon are responsible for selective retention of long particles, allowing sufficient exposure for microbial digestion to occur. In general, the fermentative digestive process in the horse is not as efficient as that in the ruminant, and digestible energy values for forages are usually lower for horses than for cattle.

Figure 18 shows the equine digestive system, separated from its mesenteric attachments and laid out in linear fashion. The hindgut commences with the **caecum**, which is separated from the large colon by a well-defined orifice. The **large colon** is folded on itself three times, forming four major anatomical divisions: **the right ventral and left ventral and the left dorsal and right dorsal colon segments.** Ingesta enter the right ventral colon and pass to the left ventral colon, from which the material enters the left dorsal portion through the pelvic flexure. From the left dorsal colon, material moves to the right dorsal colon before entering the small colon. The tremendous size and volume of the caecum and colon compared with the small intestine are conspicuous. The differences in diameter that occur throughout the colon should also be noted, particularly the reductions in diameter that occur at the pelvic flexure and at the junction of the large and small colons. **The saclike evaginations that occur in the wall of the caecum and most segments of the colon are called haustra.**

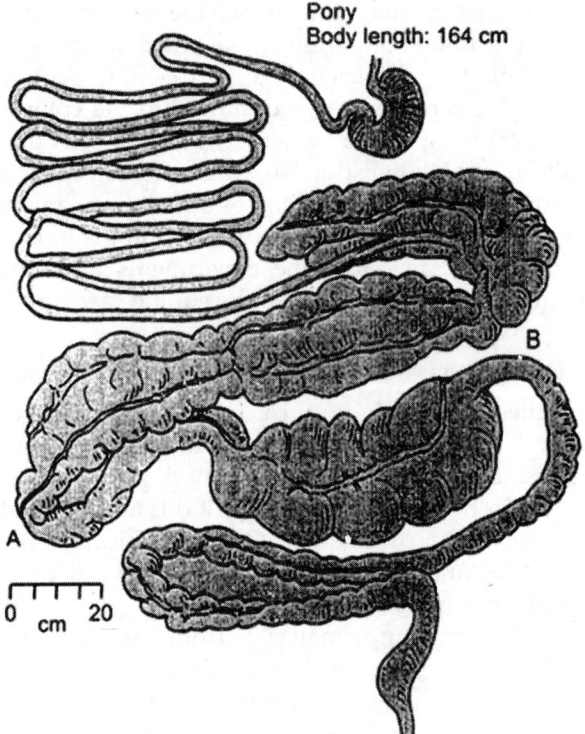

Pony
Body length: 164 cm

Figure 18 Equine gut [Note the tremendous development of the colon compared with the small intestine in a pony. Note also the relative areas of constriction at the junctions of the ventral and dorsal colons (A) and the large and small colons (B)]. Source: Cunningham's textbook of Veterinary Physiology by Bradley G. Klein, 5th edition, 2013, pp337.

Caecum

Ingesta reach the caecum after a relatively short time in the stomach and small intestine. A large portion of soluble ingesta usually reaches the caecum by 2 hours after ingestion, whereas solids take somewhat longer, depending on particle size and consistency. The material in the caecum and throughout the large colon has a high water content and a slurrylike consistency.

The majority of caecal motility is of a mixing nature and mixing action of the caecum maintains the caecal contents in a homagenous state. About once every 3 to 4 minutes, there is a strong contraction of caecal muscles in a mass movement type of action in which the body and apex of the organ shorten and constrict, lifting ingesta into the base. Constriction of the base forces material through the caecocolic orifice and into the right ventral colon. The motility pattern functionally separates the caecum from the ventral colon. In contrast to some other species, in horses there is no retrograde flow of material from the colon back into the caecum, so the composition of ingesta in these two organs usually differs.

Ventral colon

Three types of motility patterns exist in the right and left ventral colon: haustral segmentation, propulsive activity or aboral peristalsis, and retropulsive peristalsis or antiperistaltic movements. Segmentation serves a mixing function that aids in promoting fermentation and bringing VFAs in contact with the mucosa for absorption. Motility patterns result in the retention and mixing of material in the ventral colon, allowing time for microbial digestion and preventing the washout of microbes. The pumping action of caecal mass movements, combined with the propulsive action of the proximal ventral colon, continually moves ingesta toward the pelvic flexure. In the distal ventral colon, however, antiperistaltic activity and the narrow diameter of the pelvic flexure impede the movement of material, causing it to be retained in the ventral colon. As particle size is reduced by fermentative action and the mixing activity of the colon, particles eventually become small enough to flow with the fluid phase and leave the colon, although some large particles do escape the ventral colon. These factors allow the movement of particulate matter into the left dorsal colon.

Dorsal colon

The actions of the dorsal colon appear to mimic those of the ventral colon. Impedance to ingesta flow is created by the size restriction at the junction of the right dorsal colon and colon. In addition, retropulsive motility may originate in the area of the distal right dorsal colon, near the junction with the small colon. These actions tend to impede the movement of ingesta through the dorsal colon, subjecting the material to another round of fermentative digestion, as occurred in the ventral colon. The delay in the flow of ingesta created by the combined actions of the ventral and dorsal colons results in significant retention of material, with most particulate matter taking from 24 to 96 hours to pass the large colon.

Understanding the motility of the equine colon is important because problems of colon impaction in horses are common. Impactions usually occur near or within the pelvic flexure, probably because the pelvic flexure is a site of flow restriction and differential flow of solid and liquid material. One can easily appreciate how the normal motility pattern could allow solid material to accumulate in this area and cause obstructions.

Small colon

Although general understanding of small colon motility is limited, it appears to consist primarily of segmentation and propulsion. The characteristic faecal balls of horses are formed by segmentation within the small colon.

The Rate of Fermentation and VFA Production in the Equine Colon is similar to that in the rumen

In the equine colon, efficient means of buffering and VFA absorption must be present. (1) In the horse, large quantities of fluid, rich in bicarbonate and phosphate buffers, are secreted by the ileum and transferred to the caecum, thus mimicking the actions of the salivary glands in ruminants. (2) Additionally, because of the glandular nature of the colonic mucosa, bicarbonate and other electrolytes are added more directly to the lumen fluid in the caecum and colon.

Large fluxes of water traverse the caecal and colonic mucosa during the course of digestion. When horses consume feed, it starts to enter the caecum about 2 hours after eating, and VFA production rapidly commences. As ingesta are transported from the caecum, VFA production continues in the large colon. During the period of active VFA production, large quantities of water enter the hindgut from the blood through the mucosa. Although this water flux may be a response to increased osmolality created by the generation of osmotically active VFA molecules, it is more likely a response to direct fluid secretion from the crypts of the colonic epithelium. Secretion of fluid containing sodium, bicarbonate, and chloride from the colonic mucosa appears to occur in response to high concentrations of VFA in the lumen. This secretory response, in combination with the ileal secretions, is responsible for buffering of the lumen contents.

Figure 19 illustrates the magnitude of water fluxes that occur during hindgut digestion in the pony. Note that considerable inward and outward movement of water occurs across the mucosa in each of the major fermentation compartments, ventral and dorsal colons, and caecum. Inward (into the lumen) water movement results from mucosal secretion, whereas outward water movement occurs in association with absorption of VFA.

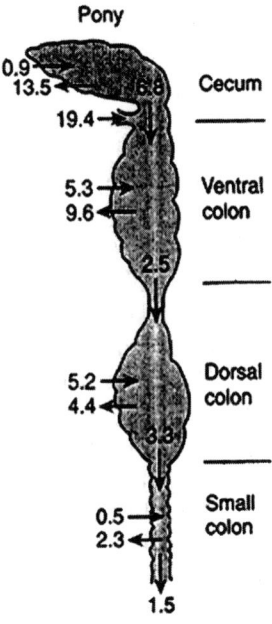

Figure 19 Net movement of water through the large intestine of a 160-kg pony. [Values are in liters per day; they represent the inward and outward movement of fluid in the various compartments of the pony's large intestine. Note 19.4 L/ day fluid is delivered to the pony's colon from the ileum. Source: Argenzio RA, Lowe JE, Pickard DW, Stevens CE: Digesta passage and water exchange in the equine large intestine, Am J Physiol 226(5): 1035-1042, 1974)].

The molecular mechanisms of VFA absorption in the equine colon appear to be identical to those in the rumen. As sodium absorption accompanies VFA absorption, bicarbonate is generated in the lumen. The absorption of VFA and sodium leads to osmotic absorption of water, probably through the transcellular pathway.

The function of the small colon is to recover water, electrolytes, and VFAs that were not absorbed in the large colon. VFA production appears minimal in the small colon, but considerable absorption of water, sodium, and phosphate occurs there.

The large water and electrolyte fluxes in the colon make horses vulnerable to colonic diseases, resulting in fluid and electrolyte losses that are more characteristic of small-intestinal disease in many other animals.

Hindgut fermentation meets the energy needs of rabbits, rats, guinea pigs, swine, and some large birds, in addition to Equidae to a significant extent. Also, ruminants have a reasonably extensive hindgut, and fermentative digestion occurs there, even after material has been through the rumen.

Postabsorptive Nutrient Utilization

The rate of absorption of nutrients from the gut is not constant, but rather fluctuates greatly with feed intake. Feeds are digested at a rate dependent on their chemical composition, regardless of the animal's nutrient needs. The nature of digestion dictates the nutrient absorption from the gut. The nutrient absorption is rapid during digestion and then ceases during interdigestive/intermeal periods. However, the cells continuously need nutrients to maintain the basal metabolic functions of the body. Therefore, animals must have a sophisticated system for maintaining the supply of nutrients, particularly energy-supplying nutrients, and buffering both the short-term and long-term "feast or famine" effects associated with the absorptive and postabsorptive periods of digestion.

Homeostatic mechanisms balance the supply and demand of almost all nutrients. All nutrients: energy-supplying, vitamins and minerals are subject to homeostatic regulatory mechanisms. This section focuses on supply regulations of the major energy-supplying nutrients.

Regulation of energy-supplying nutrients

Energy-supplying nutrients are referred to as metabolic fuels, and the physiological mechanisms for maintaining the supply of fuels and matching it to demand constitute fuel homeostasis. Fuel homeostasis is maintained by several mechanisms: the insulin-glucagon axis, the hypothalamic-pituitary axis, and the central nervous system (CNS). Let us know how the fuel is stored during the absorptive period of digestion, and how it is subsequently mobilized when needed to supply energy requirements.

The Tricarboxylic Acid (or Krebs) cycle is the major energy-yielding pathway of fuel utilization in the Body

Acetate sources: The Krebs cycle is the pathway through which all body fuels are eventually "burned." In this cycle carbon compounds from the various body fuels are completely oxidized to carbon dioxide and water.

Much of the energy released in this process is captured as ATP, the direct source of chemical energy for most physiological processes. The substrate for oxidation in the Krebs cycle is acetate, a two-carbon compound that enters the Krebs cycle in an activated form known as acetyl-CoA. Figure 20 illustrates that glucose and fatty acids are the sources of acetate for oxidation. Selecting between these two sources of acetate is a major function of fuel homeostasis.

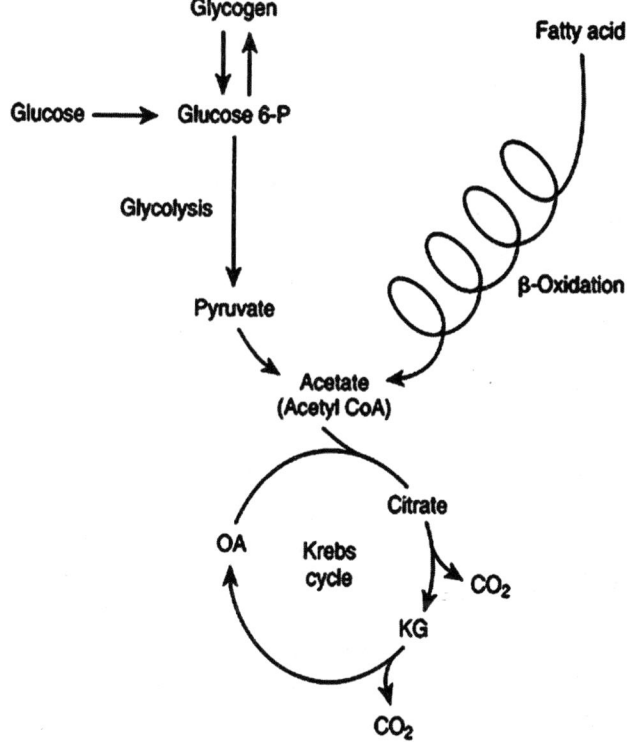

Figure 20   Relationship of the three major oxidative, catabolic pathways. P, Phosphate; OA, oxaloacetic acid; KG, α-ketoglutarate; CO_2, carbon dioxide.

The major metabolic fuels consist of glucose, amino acids, fatty acids, and ketone bodies

Glucose, amino acids, fatty acids, and ketone bodies are the compounds that can be directed into the Krebs cycle for energy production. **Fuel homeostasis** is the coordinated process by which these fuels are stored, mobilized, and interconverted to assure a continuous supply of energy for the body.

Glucose is the central fuel in the energy metabolism of most animals

Glucose is the digestion product of carbohydrate. It is the basic metabolic fuel during periods of adequate nutrition in omnivorous monogastric animals, such as swine, dogs and rats. Glucose has special significance because under most conditions it is the only fuel that is consumed by the CNS. Therefore, maintaining a steady supply of glucose for brain metabolism is of paramount importance to the body. An elegant system of homeostasis exists to regulate the availability of glucose to the brain and other tissues. See page no 207 for the regulatory hormones and their actions in controlling blood glucose concentration.

Glucose can be stored in the body as glycogen, a highly branched starch found in liver and skeletal muscle. Directing glucose to and from glycogen depots is a major function of fuel homeostasis. Glucose is released from glycogen through the process of **glycogenolysis**.

The first step through which glucose is used as a fuel is through **glycolysis**, the series of biochemical steps that initiate the oxidation of glucose. Through glycolysis, each molecule of glucose is converted to two molecules of pyruvate, a key molecule that stands at the junction of several metabolic pathways (see page no 575). When glucose is completely oxidized for fuel, pyruvate is converted to acetate (acetyl CoA) and passes into the Krebs cycle, the site of its complete oxidation. The conversion of glucose to pyruvate is reversible. Therefore any metabolic pathway that can lead to the production of pyruvate can also lead to the creation of glucose.

Figure 20 illustrates a key relationship between pyruvate, acetate, and oxaloacetic acid. The conversion of pyruvate to acetate is irreversible while the conversion of pyruvate to oxaloacetate can flow in either direction. Thus any metabolic pathway that can lead to the creation of pyruvate or oxaloacetate can lead to the synthesis of glucose. Creation of glucose through such pathways is called **gluconeogenesis**. The process of gluconeogenesis occurs in the liver and to a small extent also in the kidneys. It occurs in no other tissues.

Another pathway for glucose oxidation is the **pentose-phosphate pathway**. This is a quantitatively minor pathway that does not have great impact on fuel homeostasis. However, it is an important metabolic pathway in erythrocytes (RBCs), which have an absolute need for glucose, although these cells' overall need for energy is small compared with the rest of the body. This pathway is needed to synthesize ribose and NADPH that are needed for biosynthesis of nutrients. Metabolism of carbohydrates is dealt in detail in chapter 8.

Amino Acids are important fuels in addition to being the building blocks of protein

Amino acids are important fuels and can provide energy to the body. In addition, they are important substrates for gluconeogenesis, indicating that most amino acids can be converted to glucose when the available glucose supply is limited. Although it is sometimes said that there is no storage site of amino acids in the body, the protein of skeletal muscle could be considered to have an amino acid storage function in addition to its locomotor functions.

Fatty Acids are the major form of energy storage in the animal body

Fatty acids are stored in adipose tissue in the form of triglycerides (also called triacylglycerols). Triglycerides are an ideal form of energy storage for animals. They are highly reduced molecules (there is little oxygen compared with the amount of carbon and hydrogen), which means they are a concentrated energy source, having more than twice the caloric value per gram than carbohydrates or amino acids. In addition, adipose tissue contains little water compared with protein or glycogen, the storage forms of the other two potential fuels. Thus, adipose tissue is a concentrated form of energy storage in animals at a minimal amount of weight. However, fats have a metabolic disadvantage because they are not water soluble. Therefore, special transport systems are needed to enable fats to be distributed among the tissues through the blood and lymph systems. In addition, **fatty acids cannot be converted to glucose**, so they cannot, under usual circumstances, contribute to the energy supply of the CNS. However, **fatty acids can be converted to ketone bodies**.

Ketone Bodies are water-soluble metabolites that serve as glucose substitutes

Although glucose cannot be formed from fat, the fat-derived ketone bodies do have some glucoselike attributes. For example, ketone bodies can pass the blood-brain barrier. During prolonged periods of dietary energy deprivation, they can provide a large portion of the energy supply to the CNS, at least in some species. It does appear, however, that ketone bodies (Figure 21) cannot totally replace glucose in this function, and that a small amount of glucose is always needed by the CNS.

In monogastric species, ketone bodies are formed exclusively in the liver and are used by a wide variety of tissues. Some tissues, including cardiac muscle, use ketone bodies instead of glucose. In ruminants the ketone body β-hydroxybutyrate is formed from butyrate in the rumen epithelium. Thus, in ruminants, ketone bodies are not only products of fatty acid metabolism, but also products of normal digestion. Elevated

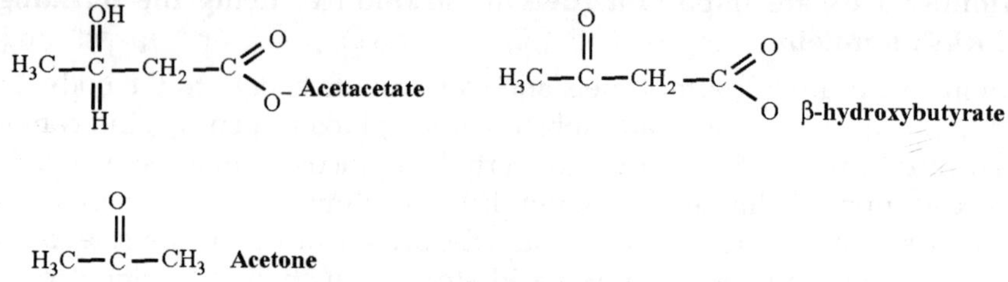

Figure 21 Physiological ketone bodies.

serum concentrations of ketone bodies are characteristic of several diseases associated with abnormalities of fuel homeostasis. This fact might lead one to conclude that ketone bodies are abnormal, or even toxic, metabolites. In fact, when present in physiological concentrations, ketone bodies are important fuels that occupy an integral part of the scheme of fuel homeostasis.

Fuel metabolism

Fuel metabolism discussion is divided into three phases: (1) an absorptive phase associated with the active digestion and absorption of nutrients from the gut, (2) a post-absorptive phase that occurs during the intervals when nutrients are not being absorbed from the gut, and (3) a prolonged energy deficiency or food deprivation phase.

General scheme of metabolism during the absorptive phase

The liver cells play a key role in the metabolism and conversion of nutrients. For example, amino acids can be converted to glucose or fatty acids. Because one type of nutrient can be converted to another, the relative amounts of carbohydrate, protein and fat in the feed can vary considerably without adverse consequences. During the absorptive phase, glucose and amino acids are first transported from the intestinal lumen to the intestinal capillaries, then via the portal vein to the liver capillaries. This permits the **liver to adjust the concentration of** the various nutrients (i.e. **glucose and amino acids**) in the blood **before the blood reaches the systemic circulation**. In contrast to glucose and amino acids, lipids are transported from the intestine by the lymph, which eventually empties into a large vein in the cranial part of the thorax, close to the heart. The pulmonary capillaries are the first capillary network through which the dietary lipids pass. Hence the **liver does not have an opportunity to process absorbed lipids before they are distributed throughout the body.**

As nutrient absorption takes place during the active digestion and absorption of nutrients from the gut, metabolic events in the liver and peripheral organs are coordinated to direct nutrients into storage molecules and storage sites (Figure 22). Liver takes up glucose and converts it into glycogen and triglyceride.

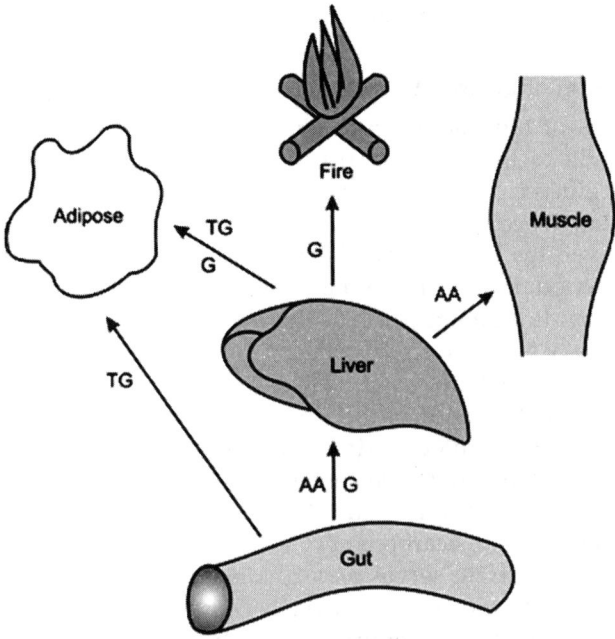

Figure 22 Metabolism during the absorptive period [absorbed glucose is converted into glycogen and fatty acids; G, glucose, AA; amino acid; TG, triglyceride]. Source: Cunningham's textbook of Veterinary Physiology by Bradley G. Klein, 5th edition, 2013, pp345

When feed is ingested, insulin secretion begins even before maximal absorption of glucose is achieved. This secretion is stimulated by the action of gastric inhibitory peptide and perhaps other enteric hormones. Early insulin secretion ensures that the liver and other tissues will be "primed" and ready for the arrival of glucose from the gut. A large portion of the glucose that has been absorbed postprandially is taken up by the liver as portal blood traverses the hepatic sinusoids. Under the influence of insulin, glucose in the liver is directed into **glycogen synthesis**.

The net effect is that glucose from the digestion and absorption of carbohydrate is stored in the liver during absorptive periods. Insulin exerts its stimulatory effect on hepatic glycogen synthesis by stimulating intracellular metabolic pathways that lead to the formation of glycogen. The amount of glycogen that can be stored in the liver is limited and, under normal conditions, probably never exceeds 10% of the total weight of the liver. This amount of glycogen does not account for all the glucose taken up by the liver during the digestion and absorption of a large carbohydrate meal. Therefore, some additional mechanism must exist for the disposal of excess glucose. **Fatty acid synthesis** offers an alternative mechanism for glucose removal.

The conversion of glucose to fatty acids is an irreversible process

The synthesis of fatty acids from glucose begins with glycolysis. This pathway leads to the production of two pyruvate molecules for each molecule of glucose consumed. Pyruvate can then enter the mitochondria to be activated to acetyl coenzyme A (acetyl CoA) for entry into the Krebs cycle. However, the Krebs cycle is for energy generation, and during the absorptive period, there is more than enough acetyl CoA for Krebs cycle activity to provide for energy needs. Therefore the excess acetyl CoA must be shunted away from the Krebs cycle.

The excess acetyl CoA combines with oxaloacetate to form citrate (essentially the first reaction of the Krebs cycle) and much of the citrate is transported out of the mitochondria into the cytosol. When in the cytosol, each citrate (6carbons) molecule contributes two carbons (as acetyl CoA) toward the synthesis of fatty acids. The remaining portion of the citrate molecule (oxaloacetate, 4carbons) cycles back into the mitochondria for further use. Thus citrate serves as a carrier molecule to transport two-carbon units out of the mitochondria because acetyl CoA cannot pass through the mitochondrial membrane directly (Figure 23).

Several important steps in this conversion of glucose to fatty acids are promoted by insulin. It is important to recognize that the conversion of glucose to fatty acids is irreversible. Thus carbohydrate can form fat, but fat cannot form carbohydrate. Liver is an important site of fatty acid synthesis in several species. Direct synthesis of fatty acids also occurs in adipose tissue. The relative importance of liver and adipose tissue as sites of fatty acid synthesis varies with species.

Transport of Fatty Acids out of the liver is through chylomicron-like particles known as VLDLs

When formed in the liver, fatty acids must be transported either to adipose tissue for storage or to other tissues (e.g., muscle) for direct utilization for energy production. Because fatty acids are insoluble in blood, some special transport mechanism for their distribution is necessary. This mechanism is through the hepatic formation of triglyceride-rich serum lipoproteins, also known as very-low-density lipoproteins (VLDLs). These triglyceride-rich lipoproteins are much less dense than other lipoproteins in blood serum. In the synthesis of VLDLs, fatty acids are first esterified to form triglycerides, and the triglycerides are wrapped in a coat of phospholipid, cholesterol, and specific proteins (Figure 24). This is essentially the same mechanism by which fatty acids are transported out of the enterocytes after absorption from the gut. In the latter case the lipoproteins are called **chylomicrons**. The VLDLs of the liver are smaller than chylomicrons but have a similar structure and function.

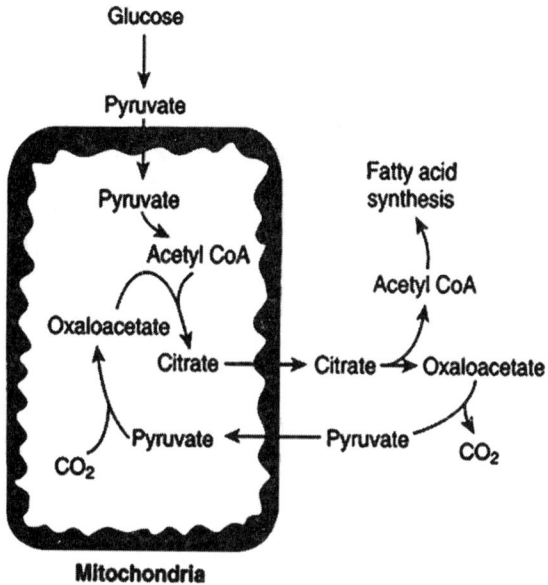

Figure 23   Hepatic synthesis of fatty acid from carbohydrate. Source: Cunningham's textbook of Veterinary Physiology by Bradley G. Klein, 5th edition, 2013, pp346

During the absorptive phase, triglyceride accumulation in adipose tissue occurs by two mechanisms: Uptake from VLDL and Direct Lipid Synthesis from Glucose

Triglyceride fatty acids are transferred from chylomicrons and VLDLs to adipose tissue by the action of lipoprotein lipase (LPL). This enzyme resides on endothelial surfaces of capillaries and, upon activation, binds to chylomicrons and VLDLs, catalyzing the hydrolysis of fatty acids from their core triglycerides and allowing the transfer of those fatty acids to the surrounding tissues. The sensitivity of LPL to specific hormones varies in different tissues. **Adipose tissue LPL** is stimulated by insulin; thus, during the absorptive phase, fatty acids from chylomicrons and VLDLs are selectively transferred to adipose tissue. Therefore, under the influence of insulin, excess carbohydrate and amino acids are converted to fatty acids in the liver, and those fatty acids are subsequently transported, via VLDLs, to the adipose tissue. Similarly, chylomicron triglyceride arising from intestinal fat'y acid absorption is also selectively transported to adipose tissue, under the influence of insulin.

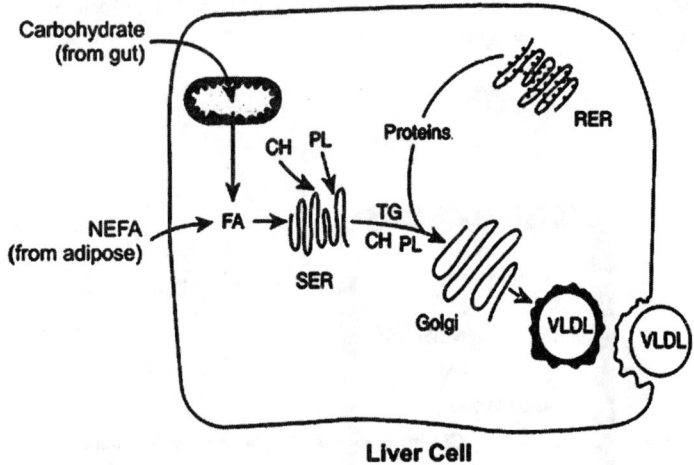

Liver Cell

Figure 24　Formation of very-low-density lipoprotein (VLDL) [CH, Cholesterol; PL, phospholipid; SER, smooth endoplasmic reticulum; RER, rough endoplasmic reticulum]. Source: Cunningham's textbook of Veterinary Physiology by Bradley G. Klein, 5th edition, 2013, pp346

Direct Lipid Synthesis from Glucose: Adipose tissue cells are metabolically active, and under the influence of insulin, they take up glucose. Within the adipocytes, glucose can be converted to fatty acids by the same metabolic mechanisms by which fatty acids were synthesized in the liver. In addition, acetate from fermentative digestion also can serve as a substrate for fatty acid synthesis in adipose tissue. Thus there are two major sites of fatty acid synthesis in the body: liver and adipose tissue. The relative importance of these sites varies with species.

Amino Acids can be classified into groups on the basis of metabolic characteristics

The discussion of amino acid absorption and metabolism becomes complicated because not all amino acids are subject to the same reactions. The amino acids are divided into two groups, each containing two subgroups (Table 5). The major groups are the **"nutritionally dispensable"** amino acids and the **"nutritionally indispensable"** amino acids. Within the dispensable amino acid group, glutamate, aspartate, alanine, glutamine, and asparagine are separated out as **'transport amino** acids'; within the indispensable amino acid group, leucine isoleucine, and valine form a special subgroup known as the 'branch-chain amino acids' (BCAAs). The transport amino acids are utilized in several reactions in which amino groups are transferred from molecule to molecule or organ to organ.

TABLE 5   Metabolic Classification of Amino Acids

Indispensible Amino Acids		Dispensible Amino acids	
Branch-Chain Amino Acids	Others	Transport Amino Acids	Others
Leucine	Arginine*	Alanine	Cysteine
Isoleucine	Histidine	Glutamine	Glycine
Valine	Lysine	Glutamate	Proline
	Methioninie	(Glutamic acid)	Tyrosine[1]
	Phenylalanine	Asparagine	Serine
	Threonine	Aspartate (Aspartic acid)	
	Tryptophan		

*Indispensable for cats, but not required in the diets of many other species;
[1]Dietary adequacy depends on a supply of phenylalanine.

Amino Acids are extensively modified during absorption

The profile of amino acids in the portal vein is considerably different from that of the diet, indicating that amino acid destruction and transformation occur during the absorptive process. Essentially all the glutamate and much of the aspartate in the diet are removed by the intestinal epithelial cells during absorption, so the portal blood is almost devoid of glutamate and contains little aspartate. Much of the nitrogen from glutamate and aspartate is transferred to pyruvate to form the amino acid alanine, which is present in high concentrations in portal blood. The metabolism of the 'transport amino acids' in the intestinal epithelium is a good example of both the way in which amino groups can be gained and lost and how the metabolism of amino acids interfaces with the metabolism of carbohydrate.

Glutamate and aspartate are similar to two Krebs cycle intermediates, α-ketoglutarate and oxaloacetate, differing only by the presence of an amino group or a keto oxygen. Carbohydrates and amino acids having this relationship are said to be analogues. Thus α-ketoglutarate is the keto-analogue of glutamate, and pyruvate is the keto-analogue of alanine (Figure 25). All amino acids can form keto-analogues, and all keto-analogues can be readily converted back to their parent amino acids.

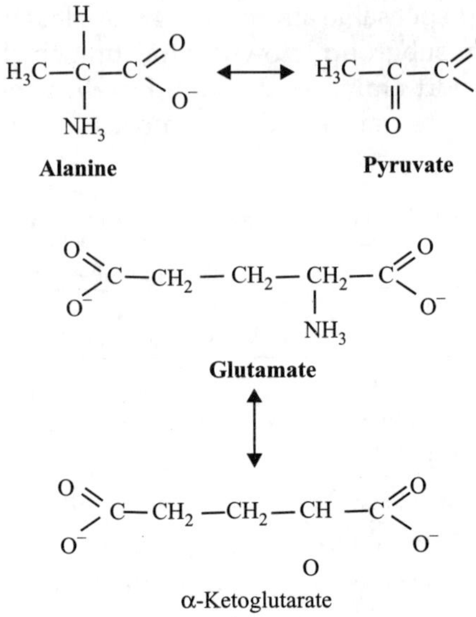

Figure 25 Examples of amino acids and their keto-analogues. All amino acids can reversibly form ketoanalogues.

Many Amino Acids are removed by the liver, hence never reaching the systemic circulation

The hepatic-portal circulation is arranged in such a way that all nutrients leaving the gut via the blood pass through the liver before entering the systemic circulation. This arrangement places the liver in a "sentinel" position, from which it can modify the nutrient composition of portal blood before the blood is distributed to other tissues. Many of the amino acids absorbed into portal blood are removed as the blood passes the liver, so they never reach the general circulation. It was reported that in the dog, only about 23% of the amino acids reaching the liver during the absorptive period pass into the general circulation. The liver thus helps keep blood amino acid concentrations stable during periods of amino acid absorption. The blood amino acid concentration, as with the blood glucose concentration, is usually kept relatively constant.

Some Amino Acids taken up by the liver are used for protein synthesis

The liver is an important site of protein synthesis, and thus its priority position for amino acid uptake seems reasonable. It was shown (in case of canines) that approximately 20% of the portal blood amino acid supply is used for protein synthesis in the liver, although this proportion varies with dietary protein intake. Almost all the serum proteins are synthesized in the liver, including such critical proteins as albumin and the blood-clotting factors. The direct amino acid supply for protein synthesis in non-hepatic tissue comes from free amino acids in the blood, not from pre-formed serum proteins.

Most Amino Acids taken up by the liver are converted to carbohydrates

Most amino acids entering the liver undergo deamination, which means the amino groups are removed and the molecules get converted to their keto-analogues. The keto-analogues enter the pathways of carbohydrate metabolism, from which they may be completely metabolized for energy, converted to glucose or glycogen, or shunted to fatty acid synthesis. Figure 26 illustrates the sites at which the various amino acids enter the carbohydrate pathways.

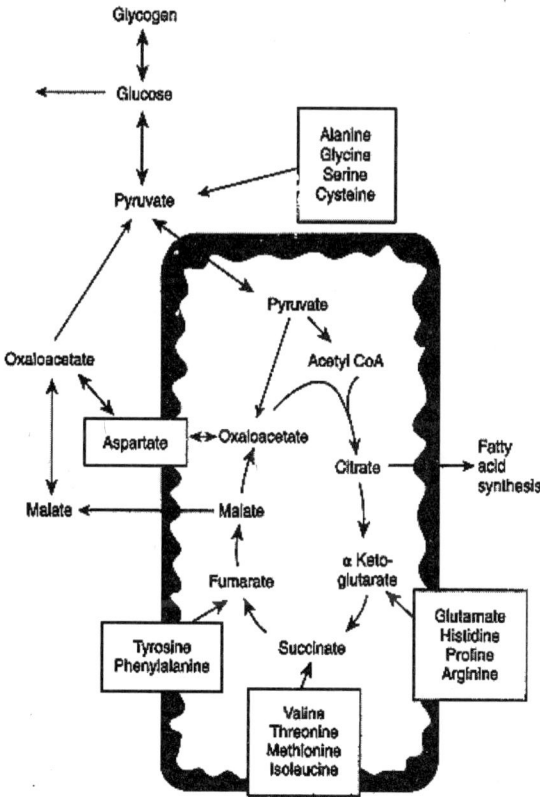

Figure 26 Sites of entry of various amino acids into the scheme of carbohydrate metabolism. Source: Cunningham's textbook of Veterinary Physiology by Bradley G. Klein, 5th edition, 2013, pp348

Deamination of amino acids for the production of carbohydrate or energy may seem like a waste of expensive dietary protein. In some species, however, the deamination of amino acids is important for homeostasis of glucose and other fuels. For example, the natural diets of the true carnivores (e.g., cats, mink) contain a large portion of protein and little carbohydrate, but their glucose needs are no less than those of other animals, so it is extremely important that they synthesize glucose from amino acids. Ruminants are in a similar situation because most of the carbohydrates they consume undergo fermentative digestion and are absorbed as volatile fatty acids rather than glucose. As with carnivores, ruminants depend on amino acids for some of their glucose needs, although a large portion of ruminant glucose requirements may be met through conversion of propionate.

To allow carbohydrate production and the deamination of excess amino acids, the endocrine reactions to high-protein meals are somewhat different from those to meals containing substantial amounts of carbohydrate. During the digestion of high-protein meals, insulin and glucagon secretion does not occur in its usual reciprocal pattern. **Insulin secretion is stimulated by amino acids as well as by glucose. Glucagon secretion**, which is inhibited by glucose, **is stimulated by amino acids as long as glucose concentrations are moderately low.** This relationship means that during the digestion of a high-protein, low-carbohydrate meal, there is simultaneous secretion of insulin and glucagon. One of the effects of insulin is the greater cellular uptake of amino acids as well as glucose. Thus the effect of insulin in this situation is to increase transport of amino acids into tissues.

If insulin secretion were the only action stimulated by amino acid absorption, however, the animal would risk insulin-stimulated hypoglycemia when it consumed a high-protein, low-carbohydrate diet. An important action of glucagon is to stimulate gluconeogenesis through the deamination of amino acids in the liver. This process ensures that adequate glucose will be available to counterbalance the effects of amino acid - stimulated insulin secretion.

Protein synthesis in non-hepatic tissue

Amino acids for peripheral (non-hepatic) protein synthesis must come from that portion of amino acids that escape hepatic destruction, during the absorptive period. In one study, it was reported only 23% of the amino acids are to be allocated for protein synthesis by all body tissues except liver. The indispensable amino acids, especially the BCAAs, are not avidly extracted by the liver, whereas some of the dispensable amino acids like alanine are extensively taken up by hepatic tissue. The dispensable amino acids can be synthesized by protein-producing tissues. Hence the relatively low concentration of serum amino acids resulting from hepatic amino acid removal is not a rate-limiting for tissue protein synthesis. Low-protein diets lead to reductions in hepatic amino acid uptake, protein synthesis and amino acid destruction by the liver.

The overall effects of hepatic metabolism during the absorption of a meal are the removal of glucose and amino acids and the synthesis of protein and fat. Complementary changes occur in peripheral tissues, so additional glucose and amino acids are removed by skeletal muscle and adipose tissue. In addition, fatty acids secreted by the liver as VLDL triglycerides are deposited in adipose tissue, as are the triglycerides of chylomicrons.

Insulin promotes the synthesis of protein and the deposition of glycogen in muscle

The absorptive period is dominated by the effects of insulin. In skeletal muscle (the largest tissue mass of the body) insulin promotes the uptake of glucose and amino acids and thus tends to moderate the increase in blood concentration of these nutrients during absorption of a meal. The uptake of glucose by muscle is associated with glycogen synthesis, just as in the liver. Muscle glycogen, in contrast to liver glycogen, cannot be made directly available to augment blood glucose concentrations during periods of low glucose availability. Muscle glycogen is primarily for metabolism in the muscle.

Insulin-stimulated uptake of amino acids by muscle results in a net increase in muscle protein synthesis

Muscle protein is in a state of dynamic equilibrium, that is, in a constant state of flux; that is why the term net increase is used with reference to muscle protein synthesis. Protein molecules are continuously being broken down and their amino acids added to an intracellular amino acid pool. Simultaneously, new proteins are constantly being made, deriving their amino acids from the same pool. The size of the amino acid pool depends on the relative rates of entry and exit of amino acids. Amino acids enter the pool from the blood during the absorptive phase and at all times from the breakdown of body protein. Exit of amino acids from the pool results from protein synthesis and oxidative catabolism.

In the absorptive phase of digestion, the amino acid pool is large because amino acids are being taken up from the blood. In addition, few of the amino acids leaving the pool are directed toward oxidative catabolism because sufficient glucose is available for oxidation and energy generation. Therefore the amino acid pool is large, and a high proportion of amino acids is directed to protein synthesis. When the rate of protein synthesis exceeds the rate of protein breakdown, there is a net increase in the amount of muscle protein. Thus, during the absorptive phase, amino acids are stored in muscle protein, protein that has a functional role not only for locomotion and posture, but also for amino acid storage.

General scheme of metabolism during the postabsorptive phase

The postabsorptive phase occurs during interdigestive/intermeal period when nutrients are not being absorbed from the gut and is usually lasts a few hours in well-fed animals. It is characterized by short-term changes that mobilize nutrients from storage pools (adipose tissue, skeletal tissue, liver) to maintain fuel availability for metabolically active tissue (Figure 27).

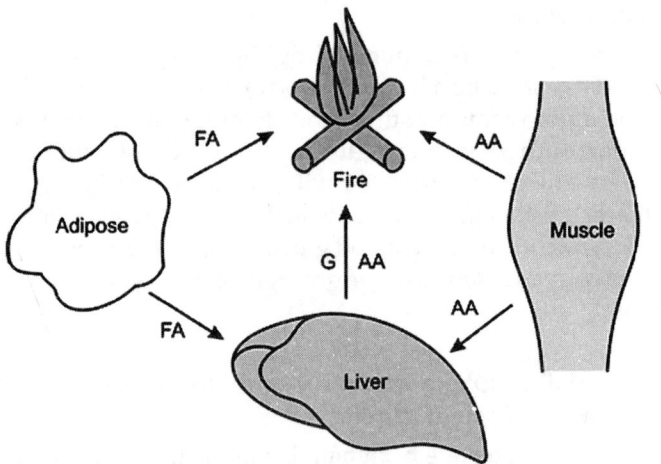

Figure 27   Postabsorptive metabolism [FA, fatty acid; G, glucose; AA, amino acid].
Source: Cunningham's textbook of Veterinary Physiology by Bradley G. Klein,
5th edition, 2013, pp350

Hepatic metabolism switches to glucose production during the postabsorptive phase

As the absorption of a meal is completed, the rate of glucose absorption from the gut wanes, and the blood glucose concentration diminishes, removing the stimulus for insulin production. As blood glucose concentrations decline, glucagon secretion is stimulated. The primary target organ of glucagon is the liver, in which glucagon creates marked metabolic changes. Through stimulation of specific cell surface receptors on hepatocytes, glucagon activates adenyl cyclase, leading to the phosphorylation of numerous cellular enzymes

The enzymes that stimulate mobilization and utilization of fuels are activated by phosphorylation, while those stimulating storage of fuels are inactivated by phosphorylation. It must be understood that many enzymes of intermediary metabolism serve a passive role, catalyzing reactions that can go in either direction, depending on substrate concentrations. A relatively small number of regulatory enzymes usually stand at the head of metabolic pathways and determine the substrate concentrations to which the other, unregulated enzymes are exposed. Through its effect on several key regulatory enzymes, glucagon (a stimulator of phosphorylation) places the liver in a fuel-mobilization state. In contrast, insulin (an inhibitor of phosphorylation) promotes a hepatic metabolic pattern that favours fuel storage.

Effect of phosphorylation on four key enzymes of glucose production and utilization

The opposing actions of insulin and glucagon on hepatic metabolism are evident from their actions on two **key regulatary enzyme pairs**: glycogen synthase and glycogen phosphatase, and phosphofructokinase and fructose-1,6-bisphosphatase. The first of these pairs regulates glycogen synthesis and breakdown, whereas the second regulates glycolysis and gluconeogenesis, respectively. All four enzymes are phosphorylated under the influence of cyclic adenosine monophosphate (cAMP). Figure 28 illustrates the actions of these enzymes and their regulatory effects.

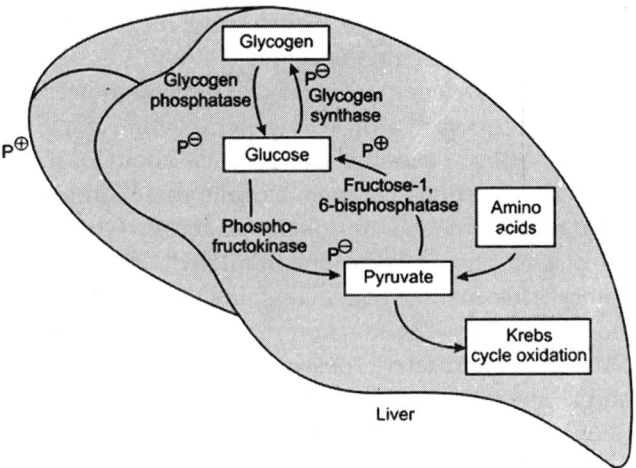

Figure 28   Glucose production and utilization. [Note that the enzymes that favour glucose formation are stimulated by phosphorylation (P^+), whereas those that favour glucose utilization and storage are inhibited by phosphorylation (P^-)]. Source: Cunningham's textbook of Veterinary Physiology by Bradley G. Klein, 5th edition, 2013, pp 351

Glycogen synthase and phosphofructokinase are inhibited by phosphorylation and thus are stimulated by insulin. Glycogen phosphatase and fructose-1,6-bisphosphatase are stimulated by phosphorylation and thus stimulated by glucagon. The actions of insulin and glucagon on these antagonistic enzyme pairs emphasize the importance of the insulin/glucagon ratio to which the liver is exposed. Neither hormone elicits an "all-or-none" reaction, but rather alters the balance of opposing reactions by influencing the relative activity of antagonistic enzymes. Thus the fuel-mobilizing or fuel-storing activity of the liver depends on which hormone is most dominant. For this reason, the **insulin/glucagon ratio** appears to be more important to liver metabolism than the absolute concentration of either hormone.

Under the influence of glucagon, glycogen phosphatase is activated by phosphorylation, promoting **glycogenolysis** and the elevation of intracellular glucose concentrations. As glucose accumulates, it is prevented from cycling back into glycogen because the major enzyme catalyzing that reaction, glycogen synthase, is blocked by phosphorylation. In addition, the flow of glucose into glycolysis is also blocked by phosphorylation inhibition of phosphofructokinase (see Figure 28). Thus the normal pathways for glucose utilization within the hepatocyte are all inhibited by glucagon, allowing glucose from glycogen breakdown to accumulate in the cells. Eventually, intracellular glucose escapes into the extracellular fluid and on into the blood. In this manner, hepatic glycogen is mobilized to elevate and maintain blood glucose concentrations when they begin to decline.

The liver stores of glycogen are relatively limited and cannot maintain blood glucose concentrations for a long period (only for 6 to 12 hours under conditions of light exertion and for only about 20 minutes under conditions of heavy exertion in humans). Under these conditions of greater demand, glucose is provided by gluconeogenesis. **Gluconeogenesis** is promoted by the phosphorylation-stimulated enzyme **fructose-1,6-bisphosphatase**. This enzyme essentially puts the glycolytic pathway into reverse, leading to glucose production from the same molecules that are intermediates in its oxidative destruction. Important substrates are pyruvate and all the intermediates of the Krebs cycle.

At this point, it is important to remember that most of the Krebs cycle intermediates or pyruvate can be supplied by the deamination of amino acids. Pyruvate and all the Krebs cycle intermediates can flow backward through the oxidative pathway (not all the reactions of gluconeogenesis are the exact reverse of the corresponding reactions in glycolysis, but the net result of gluconeogenesis is the reverse of glycolysis), resulting in the production of glucose. Thus, amino acids provide a large store of precursors for glucose formation. **The end result of glucagon stimulation is to promote the production of glucose through glycogenolysis and gluconeogenesis, turning the liver into a glucose-synthesizing organ.**

Fuel mobilization in peripheral tissues occurs when the blood insulin concentration declines

The pattern of metabolism in the peripheral tissues changes in the postabsorptive phase to support the liver's capacity to maintain fuel supplies.

Mobilizing amino acids to support hepatic gluconeogenesis

Mobilization of amino acid from muscle appears to be stimulated largely by a relative lack of insulin. Thus mobilization occurs when blood glucose concentrations are low.

The postabsorptive decline in the serum insulin concentration has a twofold effect on muscle: the entry of amino acids from the serum into the intracellular amino acid pool is diminished, and the entry of glucose into muscle cells for energy production declines. Reduced amino acid entry results in conditions favouring net protein degradation to maintain the cellular amino acid pool size. Reduced glucose entry results in increased utilization of amino acids from the pool for energy production.

The pattern of utilization of amino acids for energy by muscle may at first seem unnecessarily complex, involving selective use and extensive transformation of amino acids. **Branch-chain amino acids (BCAAs)** serve as primary sources of energy in muscle cells during the postabsorptive phase because these amino acids account for approximately one third of all muscle amino acid. Catabolism of BCAAs begins with deamination and the formation of the α-keto acid of the BCAA. The α-keto acids then enter the Krebs cycle for energy production. Deamination of the BCAA requires that some acceptor be available to receive the amino group, and this acceptor is ultimately pyruvate, resulting in the formation of alanine. The source of pyruvate can be muscle glycogen, blood glucose, or the metabolic products of BCAA α-keto acids. When metabolism of BCAA α-keto acids serves as the supply of pyruvate for alanine synthesis, the net reaction is conversion of BCAA to alanine (Figure 29). Thus the overall metabolic activity in muscle during the postabsorptive phase is the destruction of BCAAs and the formation of alanine. The alanine formed is released from the muscle cells into the blood, from which it may be taken up by the liver for gluconeogenesis.

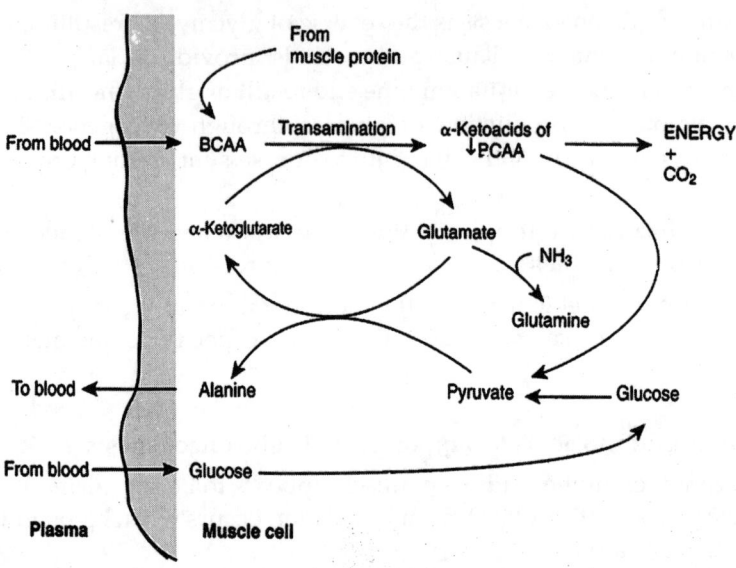

Figure 29   Catabolism of branch-chain amino acids (BCAAs) by muscle cells. Source: Cunningham's textbook of Veterinary Physiology by Bradley G. Klein, 5th edition, 2013, pp352

The transamination reaction may be depicted as follows

$$\text{Alanine} + \alpha\text{-Ketoglutaric acid} \xleftrightarrow{\text{B6}} \text{Pyruvic acid} + \text{Glutamic acid}$$
Alanine transaminase or Glutamic pyruvic transaminase

The cycle of alanine to glucose forms a shuttle to transport nitrogen from the muscle to the liver for urea synthesis

It might appear that a simpler system of amino acid transfer to the liver would suffice. However, liver has limited uptake capacity for BCAAs and these are the predominant amino acids of skeletal muscle. Thus, if BCAAs were not transformed to alanine, amino nitrogen transfer to the liver would be limited.

In addition, alanine is a convenient means by which nitrogen from the deamination of muscle amino acid can be transported to the liver. This is important because free amino groups liberated by the catabolism of amino acids in muscle, if not removed, could lead to the formation of toxic levels of ammonia. Ammonia is detoxified in the body by the formation of urea, but urea formation occurs only in the liver. Thus, alanine forms a gluconeogenic precursor that also transports nitrogen to the liver for urea synthesis, Figures 29 and 30 illustrate the role of alanine in the transport of amino acid nitrogen and carbon to the liver for synthesis of urea and glucose, respectively.

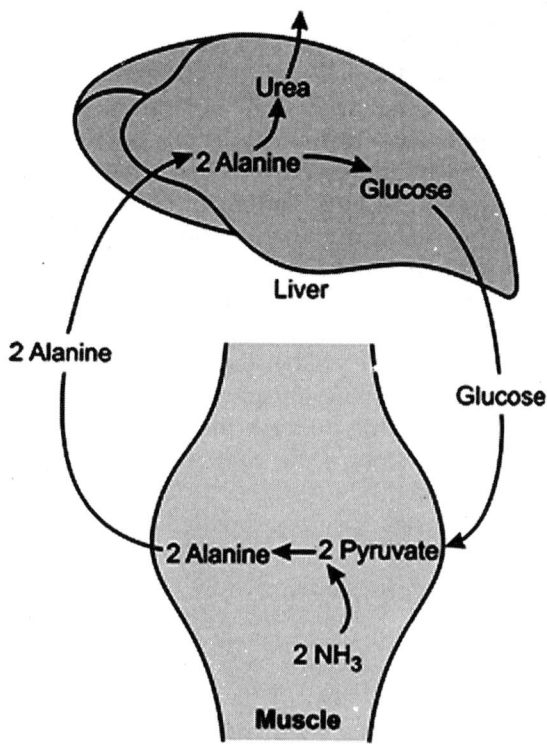

Figure 30   Alanine arising from BCAA catabolism in muscle is converted to glucose and urea in the liver. NH_3, Ammonia. Source: Cunningham's textbook of Veterinary Physiology by Bradley G. Klein, 5th edition, 2013, pp353

   The regulation of muscle protein mobilization is influenced to a large extent by the lack of insulin. However, the adrenocortical hormone **cortisol** has an important effect of stimulating protein break down and amino acid mobilization. Through the mobilization of muscle protein and stimulation of hepatic gluconeogenesis, cortisol exerts one of its major effects raising blood glucose concentration. Under normal conditions, glucagon (the other major gluconeogenic hormone) exerts its effects on the liver and does not appear to have a direct effect on muscle.

The Reaction of adipose tissue during the postabsorptive phase is to mobilize fatty acids

Fatty acids are released from adipose tissue because of the action of the phosphorylation-stimulated enzyme **'hormone-sensitive lipase' (HSL)**. This enzyme is stimulated by the relative lack of insulin in the postabsorptive period. Insulin suppresses the action of HSL by promoting its dephosphorylation. Glucagon may have some adipose tissue activity in promoting triglyceride breakdown by stimulating the phosphorylation and activation of HSL. However, in all likelihood, glucagon's effects are restricted to the liver, and the normal stimulation of HSL comes from **epinephrine or norepinephrine**, which originates from sympathetic nerves in the adipose tissue. The exact means by which sympathetic nerve activity in adipose tissue is coordinated with body fuel availability is not well established, but the catecholamine hormones and neuroregulators appear to be the primary positive stimulus for breakdown of adipose triglyceride. However, the negative stimulus provided by the absence of insulin may be the most important regulator of adipose fat mobilization.

Stimulation of HSL in the postabsorptive state leads to the release of fatty acids from adipose tissue into the blood. Fatty acids in blood are reversibly bound to albumin because they are not otherwise soluble in water. Albumin-bound fatty acids in blood are usually referred to as **nonesterified fatty acids** (NEFAs) to distinguish them from triglyceride fatty acids in chylomicrons and lipoproteins. NEFAs in blood may be used directly for energy by many tissues. However, many NEFAs are taken up by the liver and used for either ketone body production or VLDL synthesis.

General scheme of metabolism during prolonged catabolic periods

During prolonged periods of fasting, glucose and amino acids are conserved by extensive utilization of fats and ketone bodies for energy production

During the postabsorptive metabolism, it is noted that amino acids form an important depot for glucose precursors and energy-producing substrate. However, it would not be advantageous for animals to rely heavily on their skeletal muscle for energy and glucose production during prolonged fasting or undernutrition. If used, it would soon lead to severe weakness as the skeletal muscle protein was consumed. During prolonged periods of feed deprivation or energy deficiency, the ketone bodies, fatty acids and triacylglycerols become the major fuels.

A large portion of the fatty acids released from adipose tissue is taken up directly by the liver

During prolonged periods of undernutrition, low glucose availability leads to rapid mobilization of adipose fatty acids in the form of NEFAs. Although NEFAs are metabolized by various tissues, many are extracted from the blood by the liver, which receives much of the total blood flow and has an efficient hepatic NEFA extraction mechanism. **When the NEFAs are in the hepatocytes, they may follow any of three potential**

metabolic paths. The first is complete oxidation for energy production. However, the hepatic requirements for energy are such that only a small amount of the total fatty acid supply during adipose mobilization needs to be used for complete oxidation. The second pathway is esterification leading to triglyceride formation, and the third is production of ketone bodies.

Hepatic ketone body formation is promoted by low glucose availability, a high glucagon/insulin ratio, and a ready supply of fatty acids

Ketone body formation occurs within the hepatic mitochondria, and the rate of ketone body synthesis is controlled by the regulated transport of fatty acids across the mitochondrial membrane. Under conditions when **CPT-I is active**, most available fatty acid is transported into the mitochondria for ketone body synthesis. This well-orchestrated but somewhat complex regulatory system is important because the liver can both produce and consume fatty acids (Figure 31).

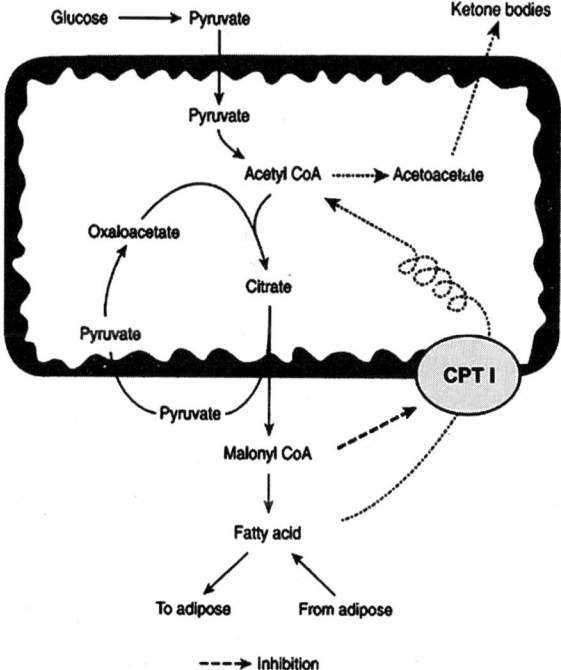

Figure 31 The liver is a site of both destruction and synthesis of fatty acids. To keep both processes from occurring simultaneously, fatty acid destruction is inhibited during periods of fatty acid synthesis. Solid lines, pathway of fatty acid synthesis; irregular broken line, fatty acid destruction. Source: Cunningham's textbook of Veterinary Physiology by Bradley G. Klein, 5th edition, 2013, pp354

Fatty acids enter mitochondria in combination with carnitine, and transport depends on an enzyme known as carnitine palmitoyltransferase I (CPT-I). The activity of this enzyme, along with the availability of fatty acid, is the primary determinant of the rate of ketone body formation. CPT-I activity is inhibited by an intermediate of the fatty acid synthesis pathway, malonyl CoA. Malonyl CoA concentrations are high when the liver is responding to insulin and glucose is being used for fatty acid synthesis. When glucagon concentrations are high relative to insulin, little fatty acid is synthesized in the liver. Thus, **malonyl CoA concentrations are low**, and CPT-I is fully active when the insulin/glucagon ratio is low. Ketone body synthesis is stimulated under these hormonal conditions.

The inhibition of CPT-I by malonyl CoA provides a system that blocks the metabolic destruction of newly synthesized fatty acid while still providing a mechanism for the utilization of fatty acids derived from adipose tissue. The overall pattern of metabolism results in a reciprocal relationship between glucose availability and ketone body production. Although ketone bodies are produced in the liver, they cannot be used there for energy production. Therefore, **all ketone bodies are transported to peripheral tissues for utilization**. When the concentration of ketone bodies in the blood becomes abnormally high, some are excreted in urine.

Glucagon plays an important role in the excessive production of ketone bodies in diabetes mellitus in Dogs

In diabetes mellitus in animals, especially dogs, untreated disease lead to high concentrations of ketone bodies in the blood. Diabetes mellitus occurs because of a lack of insulin, but the hepatic production of ketone bodies results from the unrestrained action of glucagon. Even though serum concentrations of glucose are high in diabetes mellitus, the inability of the pancreas to secrete insulin leads to a low insulin/glucagon ratio. Thus the liver functions solely under the direction of glucagon. Glucagon inhibits fatty acid production from glucose, so malonyl CoA concentrations are low and CPT-I activity is high. **Because of the lack of insulin to suppress adipose HSL, blood NEFA concentrations are high.** The combination of high NEFA availability and unrestrained CPT-I activity results in rapid transport of fatty acids into the mitochondria with extensive ketone body production, even though blood glucose concentrations are high.

Fatty acids cannot be used for glucose synthesis

It is important to understand that the metabolism of fat within the mitochondria cannot contribute directly to gluconeogenesis. When they cross the mitochondrial membrane, fatty acids undergo β-oxidation, which leads to the successive removal of two-carbon acetyl CoA units from the carbon chains of the fatty acids. The resulting acetyl CoA (see figure 20) can enter the Krebs cycle through condensation with oxaloacetate. Existing oxaloacetate combines with acetyl CoA to form citrate in the initial step of the cycle. At the end of the cycle, the original oxaloacetate is reformed as the two carbons from the acetyl CoA are converted to carbon dioxide. No new oxaloacetate can be produced by this process (Figure 32). That is there is no net production of oxaloacetate associated with the consumption of acetyl CoA by the Krebs cycle.

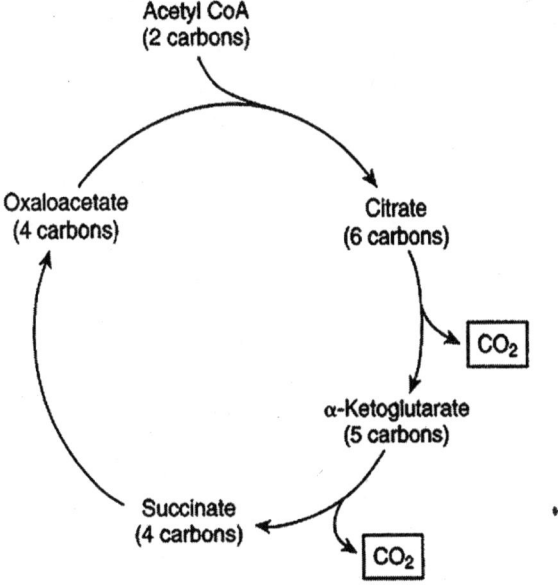

Figure 32   Oxidation of acetyl CoA by the Krebs cycle

Ketone bodies reduce the need for gluconeogenesis: Ketone bodies are formed in the mitochondria from the excess acetyl coenzyme A because all mitochondrial acetyl CoA need not enter the Krebs cycle. Ketone bodies are able to leave the mitochondria freely. Ketone bodies affect fuel homeostasis in peripheral tissues, where they serve as a substitute for glucose. In this way, they conserve available glucose and reduce the need for gluconeogensis.

Hepatic VLDLs may be synthesized from adipose-derived fatty acid as well as from newly synthesized fatty acid

VLDLs provide a transport system for fatty acids that is independent of serum albumin: The section on absorptive-phase metabolism discussed the hepatic production of VLDL (see page no 160). During the absorptive phase, triglyceride for VLDL synthesis comes from fatty acids synthesized from glucose. During catabolic periods, VLDLs may continue to be produced, but fatty acids derived from serum NEFAs are used for VLDL synthesis (see Figure 24). It may initially appear to be an unnecessary and inefficient metabolic step. One may feel that the fatty acids can directly be utilized for energy by the tissues locally rather than transporting them to liver for VLDL formation. Here the answer lies: The need for VLDL synthesis occurs because of the need for a better transport system. The capacity of the serum to transport NEFA is limited because NEFA must circulate bound to albumin. The NEFA-binding capacity of albumin is finite and may become almost saturated during periods of rapid adipose mobilization. VLDLs provide a transport system for fatty acids that is independent of serum albumin.

Hormonal conditions direct the distribution of VLDL fatty acids in the body

During the absorptive phase, VLDLs are directed to adipose tissue by the action of adipose tissue LPL (an insulin-stimulated enzyme) (see page no 161). LPL also exists in muscle tissue, but does not depend on insulin stimulation for activity. Thus, during periods of low glucose availability, adipose tissue LPL is inhibited because of a lack of insulin, but muscle tissue LPL is fully active. This situation leads to the selective direction of VLDL fatty acids to muscle tissue during times of adipose mobilization.

Changes in growth hormone concentrations may aid in shifting peripheral fuel utilization from glucose and amino acids to ketone bodies and fatty acids

The fat mobilization-induced changes in hepatic metabolism are effective in conserving protein only because of changes that occur in glucose and amino acid utilization in peripheral tissues. As ketone bodies, NEFAs, and VLDL triglycerides become the major energy supplies, there is less tissue demand for glucose or amino acids as energy substrates. Endocrine alterations, in addition to low insulin concentrations, may aid in promoting this switch in peripheral fuel utilization. In several species, growth hormone concentrations rise during a prolonged period of energy deprivation. Growth hormone is antagonistic to insulin, thus promoting an increase in the serum glucose concentration even in the presence of normal or near-normal serum insulin levels. In addition, growth hormone may have some direct effect on conserving protein and mobilizing lipid.

Special fuel considerations of ruminants

Ruminants exist in a perpetual state of gluconeogenesis because of their unique digestive process

Most carbohydrate digestion in ruminants occurs in the forestomach through fermentative digestion. The result is that almost no digestible carbohydrate enters (except bypass starch) the intestine for glandular digestion and absorption as glucose. Therefore, ruminants exist in a constant state of potential glucose deficiency. To cope with this situation, ruminants have developed efficient systems of both production and conservation of glucose.

Essentially, all the glucose available to ruminants with typical diets originates from gluconeogenesis. Quantitatively, the most important glucose precursor is the volatile fatty acid (VFA) propionate. Propionate contributes to glucose synthesis after entering the Krebs cycle at the level of succinate (Figure 33). Note that succinate is a four-carbon Krebs cycle intermediate that can lead to net formation of oxaloacetate (OA), the entry metabolite for gluconeogenesis. The other VFAs, acetate and butyrate, also enter the Krebs cycle, although they enter as acetyl CoA. As previously discussed (see page no 177), acetyl CoA cannot lead to the net production of oxaloacetate or glucose. Therefore, among the ruminant's major energy sources (acetate, propionate, and butyrate) only propionate can support glucose production.

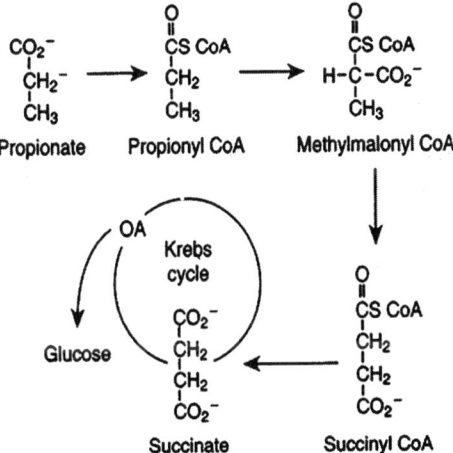

Figure 33 Gluconeogenesis from propionate involves its initial conversion to succinate.

Efficient conservation of glucose in ruminants

Almost all propionate absorbed from the rumen is extracted from the portal blood by the liver, never entering the systemic circulation.

In addition to constant gluconeogenesis, ruminants also support their glucose needs by efficiently conserving glucose. Fatty acids are synthesized in the liver of some animals (e.g., primates, rats, dogs) but in case of ruminants they are synthesized only in the adipose tissue. Furthermore, glucose is essentially not used for fatty acid synthesis. Rather, fatty acids are synthesized from acetate, which is the most abundant energy source in ruminants. The only glucose used by adipose tissue is for the synthesis of the glycerol backbone for triglycerides. In lactating animals, fatty acids produced in the udder for milk fat are synthesized from either acetate or ketone bodies, but never from glucose.

Lactational ketosis in dairy cows and pregnancy toxemia in ewes and does: Some important metabolic diseases of ruminants occur during periods when their system of glucose homeostasis is stressed. Dairy cows are especially vulnerable in early lactation because the synthesis of lactose (milk sugar) requires glucose. In high-producing cows, nearly all the glucose they produce goes to lactose synthesis, whereas the remaining tissues function on alternative fuels. Sheep and goat experience a similar stress on glucose synthesis in late gestation. The energy needs of the fetus and placenta can be met only by glucose (or glucose-derived lactate) and amino acids. Compared with many other animals, sheep and goat have a high ratio of fetal mass to body size and thus their fuel homeostatic mechanisms are particularly stressed by pregnancy. Failure of the glucose homeostatic mechanism that frequently occurs under these circumstances result in conditions known as lactational ketosis in dairy cows and pregnancy toxemia in ewes and does.

Chapter 8

Carbohydrates — Their Digestion, Absorption and Metabolism in Nonruminants, Birds and Ruminants

Nonruminants and Birds: Digestion and Absorption

Salivary amylase or ptyalin initiates the digestion of the polysaccharide, starch and its derivative, dextrin, and continues the digestion in the stomach (for only 15 to 30 min.) until inactivated by the acid in the gastric juice. During this time up to 60% to 75% of the starches and dextrins may be converted to maltose. The enzyme acts only on a-1, 4 linkages. So oligo-1, 6-glucosidase is needed to act at the 1, 6 branch points of amylopectins.

Next, enzymes from the pancreas and the intestinal glands act on the carbohydrates. Pancreatic amylase requires inorganic ions (chloride, primarily) for activity. Maltase, lactase, sucrase in the intestinal juice hydrolyze the respective disaccharides mostly during the process of their absorption in the brush border or microvilli surrounding each villus.

Absorption of monosaccharides may result by either passive diffusion or active transport. Fructose, mannose and other pentoses are absorbed passively. Glucose, and galactose are absorbed by active transport which require energy and sodium ions. Rate of absorption of hexoses: galactose, the fastest, then glucose and fructose.

The rate of absorption of carbohydrates by birds is rapid. Feed passes rapidly through the digestive tract, reaching the crop and the gizzard, within seconds. It may only take a few minutes to reach the duodenum, and undigested residues may begin voided within a couple of hours. Glucose absorption is indeed rapid and can occur even from the crop. The rate of glucose absorption from the chick intestine is double that of rats and four times that of dogs. Glucose is absorbed more rapidly than xylose, which in turn is absorbed faster than arabinose.

Metabolism of Carbohydrates

Digestion of carbohydrates yields primarily glucose, fructose, mannose and galactose. In the liver, fructose and galactose are converted to glucose.

There is always a basal requirement for glucose. A continued supply is needed, especially for red blood cells and the nervous system. It alone can supply energy to the skeletal muscle under anaerobic conditions. Glucose is precursor of lactose in the mammary glands. It is needed by adipose tissue to produce glycerol. It is needed to continually produce intermediates in the citric acid cycle. So glucose may be used as an immediate source of energy or may be used to store as glycogen in liver/ muscle or may be used to produce glycerol for triglyceride synthesis.

Glucose catabolism: Glucose is phosphorylated to glucose-6-phosphate and it is oxidized by one of the three pathways:

1. It is catabolized primarily, especially in skeletal muscle, through the Embden-Meyerhof-Parnas scheme (to commemorate the work of Gustav Embden, Otto Meyerhof and Jacob Parnas in its elucidation) of glycolysis to pyruvic acid and through citric acid cycle (tricarboxylic acid cycle or Krebs cycle) and oxidative phosphorylation (cytochrome system), pyruvate is oxidized to CO_2 and H_2O. Glycolytic cycle exists in the cytosol while citric acid cycle and oxidative phosphorylation require oxygen and are thus aerobic. The latter take place within the mitochondrion. Glycolysis is one of the most completely understood biochemical pathways. It is a sequence of 10 enzyme catalyzed reactions in which one molecule of glucose is converted to two molecules of pyruvate with net production of 2 ATP and the reduction of 2 NAD^+ to 2 NADH. Under anaerobic conditions, *glycolysis terminates in many cases with the formation of lactic acid* from pyruvic acid (Fig. 1). Efficiency of energy conservation of glucose is about 39% with the loss appearing as waste heat.

2. Hexose-monophosphate shunt or pentose cycle (pentose shunt or phosphogluconate oxidative shunt): It is important in liver, mammary gland and adipose tissue. Enzymes for this pathway are

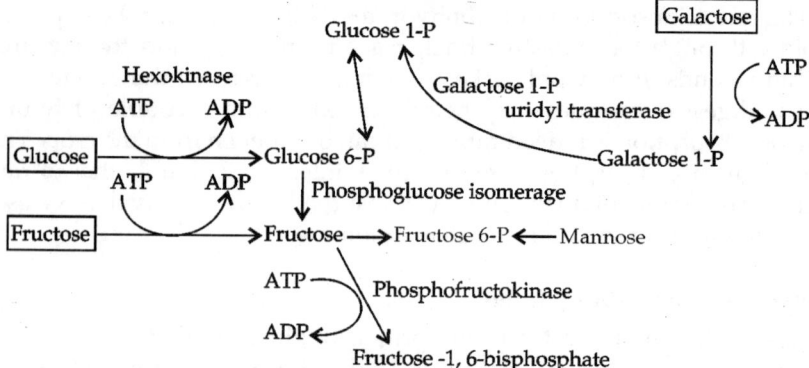

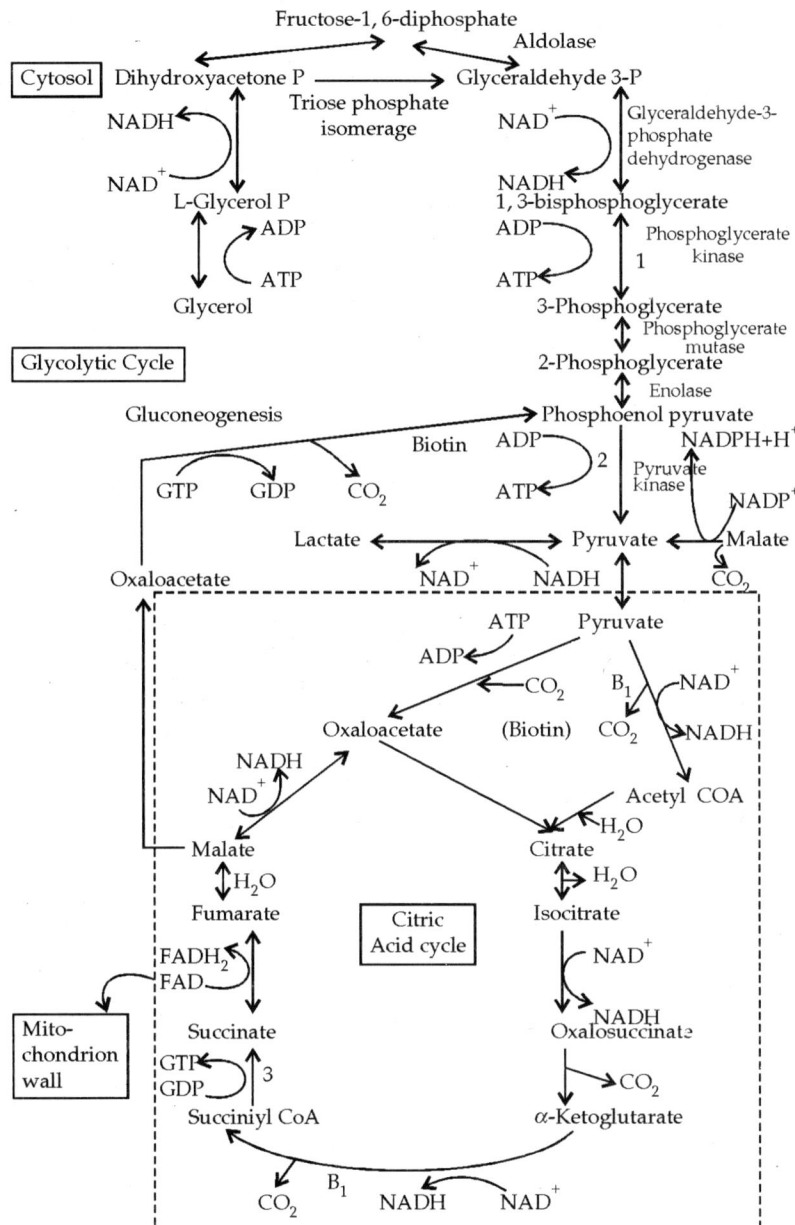

Figure 1. Glycolysis and TCA Cycle. 1, 2 and 3 are good examples of substrate level phosphorylation since ATP is synthesized from the substrate without the involvement of electron transport chain.

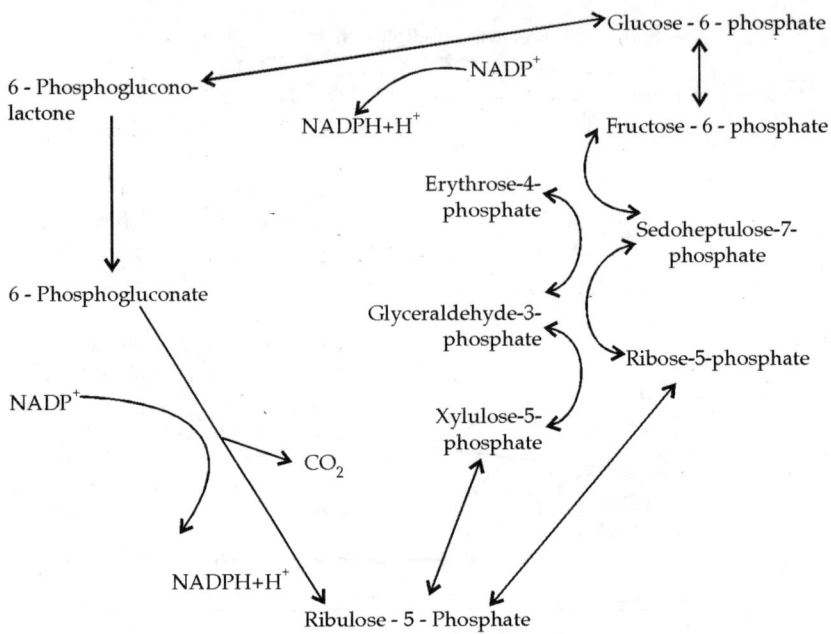

Figure 2. Pentose Shunt or Pentose Phosphate Pathway.

in the cytosol of the cells. This is more complex pathway than glycolysis.

NADPH is required for several reductive processes in addition to biosynthesis. As much as 30% of glucose oxidation to CO_2 in the liver occurs by way of the pentose phosphate pathway during highly lipogenic situations; the percentage can be even greater in adipocytes. Enzymes of the pathway are virtually absent in skeletal muscles. This pathway is needed to synthesize 5-carbon sugar (ribose), ribose-5-phosphate and reduced coenzyme NADPH (Fig. 2).

3. Uronic acid pathway: The product of this pathway include uridine diphosphoglucuronic acid, which is involved in a number of conjugating reactions that contain glucuronic acid, such as mucopolysaccharides. The pathway is also important in xylulose metabolism and ascorbic acid synthesis.

The Reactions of Glycolysis

In the first stage of glycolysis, glucose is phosphorylated by hexokinase, isomerized by phosphoglucose isomerase (PGI), phosphorylated by phosphofructokinase (PFK), and cleaved by aldolase to yield the trioses glyceraldehyde-3-phosphate (GAP) and dihydroxyacetone phosphate (DHAP), which are interconverted by triose phosphate isomerase (TIM). These reactions consume 2 ATP per glucose.

In the second stage of glycolysis, GAP is oxidatively phosphorylated by glyceraldehyde-3-phosphate dehydrogenase (GAPDH), dephosphorylated by phosphoglycerate kinase (PGK) to produce ATP, isomerized by phosphoglycerate mutase (PGM), dehydrated by enolase, and dephosphorylated by pyruvate kinase to produce a second ATP and pyruvate. This stage produces 4 ATP per glucose for a net yield of 2 ATP per glucose.

Fermentation: The Anaerobic Fate of Pyruvate

Under anaerobic conditions, pyruvate is reduced to regenerate NAD^+ for glycolysis. In homolactic fermentation, pyruvate is reversibly reduced to lactate.

Regulation of Glycolysis

The glycolytic reactions catalyzed by hexokinase, phosphofructokinase, and pyruvate kinase are metabolically irreversible. Phosphofructokinase is the primary flux control point for glycolysis. ATP inhibition of this allosteric enzyme is relieved by AMP and ADP, whose concentrations change more dramatically than those of ATP. The opposing reactions of the fructose-6-phosphate (F6P), fructose-1, 6-bisphosphate (FBP) substrate cycle allow large changes in glycolytic flux.

Metabolism of Hexoses other than Glucose

Fructose, galactose, and mannose are enzymatically converted to glycolytic intermediates for catabolism.

The citric acid cycle

The citric acid cycle (Fig. 1) is the major route for the formation of ATP and it takes place in the matrix of mitochondria adjacent to the enzymes of the respiratory chain and oxidative phosphorylation. The citric acid cycle is an ingenious series of eight reactions that oxidizes the acetyl group of acetyl-CoA to two CO_2 molecules with the concomitant generation of three NADH, one $FADH_2$ and one GTP. The pyruvate dehydrogenase multienzyme complex generates acetyl-CoA from the glycolytic product pyruvate. The eight enzymes are citrate synthase, aconitase, isocitrate dehydrogenase, α-ketoglutarate dehydrogenase, succinyl-CoA synthetase, succinate dehydrogenase, fumarase and malate dehydrogenase.

The net reaction of citric acid cycle is

$$3NAD^+ + FAD + GDP + Pi + acetyl\text{-}CoA \rightarrow 3NADH + FADH_2 + GTP +$$
$$CoA + 2\,CO_2$$

The oxaloacetate that is consumed in the first step of the Krebs cycle is regenerated in the last step of the cycle. Thus, the citric acid cycle acts as a multistep catalyst that can oxidize an unlimited number of acetyl groups. Neither of the CO_2 molecules released in a given turn of the citric acid cycle is derived from the acetyl group that entered the same turn of the cycle. Instead, they are derived from the oxaloacetate that was synthesized from the acetyl groups that entered previous turns of the cycle.

Citric acid cycle is amphibolic

The citric acid cycle is catabolic because it is the final pathway for the oxidation of carbohydrates, lipid and protein. Cycle intermediates are required in only catalytic amounts to maintain the degradative function of the cycle. However, several biosynthetic pathways use citric acid cycle intermediates as starting materials for anabolic reactions. The citric acid cycle is therefore amphibolic (both anabolic and catabolic).

Pathways that Use Citric Acid Cycle Intermediates

Sometimes inappropriate buildup of citric acid cycle intermediates in the mitochondrion occurs, for example, when there is a high rate of breakdown of amino acids to citric acid cycle intermediates. **Cataplerotic reactions** (reactions that utilize and drain such intermediates) occur in the following pathways:

Glucose biosynthesis (gluconeogenesis) utilizes oxaloacetate. Because gluconeogenesis takes place in the cytosol, oxaloacetate must be converted to malate or aspartate for transport out of the mitochondrion. Since the citric acid cycle is a cyclical pathway, any of its intermediates can be converted to oxaloacetate and used for gluconeogenesis.

Fatty acid biosynthesis is a cytosolic process that requires acetyl-CoA. Acetyl-CoA is generated in the mitochondrion and is not transported across the mitochondrial membrane. Cytosolic acetyl-CoA is therefore generated by the breakdown of citrate, which can cross the membrane, in a reaction catalysed by **ATP-citrate lyase**. This reaction uses the free energy of ATP to "undo" the citrate synthase reaction: ATP + citrate + CoA → ADP + P_i + oxaloacetate + acetyl-CoA

Amino acid biosynthesis uses α-ketoglutarate and oxaloacetate as starting materials. For example, α-ketoglutarate is converted to glutamate by reductive amination catalyzed by a **glutamate dehydrogenase** that utilizes either NADH or NADPH. Oxaloacetate undergoes transamination with alanine to produce aspartate and pyruvate.

Reactions that Replenish Citric Acid Cycle Intermediates

In aerobic organisms, the citric acid cycle is the major source of free energy, and hence the catabolic function of the citric acid cycle cannot be interrupted: Cycle intermediates that have been siphoned off must be replenished. The replenishing reactions are called **anaplerotic reactions**. The most important of these reactions is catalyzed by pyruvate carboxylase, which produces oxaloacetate from pyruvate: This is also one of the first steps of gluconeogenesis.

$$\text{Pyruvate} + CO_2 + ATP + H_2O \rightarrow \text{oxaloacetate} + ADP + P_i$$

During exercise, some of the pyruvate generated by increased glycolytic flux is directed toward oxaloacetate synthesis as catalyzed by pyruvate carboxylase. Pyruvate can also accept an amino group from glutamate (a transamination reaction) to generate alanine (the amino acid counterpart of pyruvate) and the citric acid cycle intermediate α-ketoglutarate (the ketone counterpart of glutamate). Both of these mechanisms help the citric acid cycle efficiently catabolize the acetyl groups derived (also from pyruvate) by the reactions of the pyruvate dehydrogenase complex. The end result is increased production of ATP to power muscle contraction.

Methods of ATP synthesis

Substrate-level phosphorylation: Two ATP synthetic reactions in glycolysis and one reaction in citric acid cycle involve the direct transfer of a phosphate to ADP. These reactions are examples of substrate-level phosphorylation.

Oxidative phosphorylation: Synthesis of ATP occurs when NADH and $FADH_2$ are oxidized (to NAD+ and FAD, respectively) by electron transport through the respiratory chain. Electrons flow from NADH to oxygen through three of these complexes as shown in Figure 3. Each complex contains several electron carriers that work sequentially to carry electrons down the chain. Two small electron carriers are also needed to link these large complexes; ubiquinone, which is also called coenzyme Q and cytochrome c.

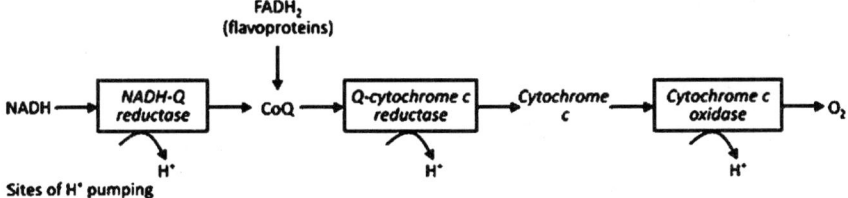

Figure 3   Overview of the electron transport chain (respiratory chain).

ATP Generated from Complete Oxidation of Glucose

1. Glycolysis   2ATP
2. Citric acid Cycle   2ATP
3. Oxidative Phosphorylation (*)
   a. NADH from glycolysis $1 \times 2 = 2$ (**) or $1 \times 3 = 3$
   b. NADH pyruvate to acetyl CoA $1 \times 3 = 3$
   c. NADH from citric acid cycle $3 \times 3 = 9$
   d. FADH$_2$ from citric acid cycle $1 \times 2 = 2$

$$16 \times 2 = 32 \text{ ATP}; \quad 17 \times 2 = 34$$

Total   = 36 ATP or 38 ATP

(*) 1 glucose yields 2 moles of glyceraldehyde-3-phosphate which proceed to pyruvate.

(**) Intact mitochondria are impermeable to NADH and NAD$^+$. How then does cytoplasmic NADH gets oxidized by electron-transport chain the respiration chain? The solution is that electrons from NADH, rather than NADH itself, are carried across the mitochondrial membrane. One carrier is glycerol-3-phosphate (Figure 4) which use FAD prosthetic group of a dehydrogenase and hence only two ATP are formed. Another carrier is malate-aspartate shuttle (Figure 5) which is seen in liver and heart and three ATP are formed per NADH.

ATP yield from complete oxidation of glucose is 36 or 38. The number depends on which shuttle system is used to transfer reducing equivalents into the mitochondrial matrix.

Recent research shows 1 NADH = 2.5 ATP; 1FADH = 1.5 ATP.

The updated ATP generation may be depicted as follows

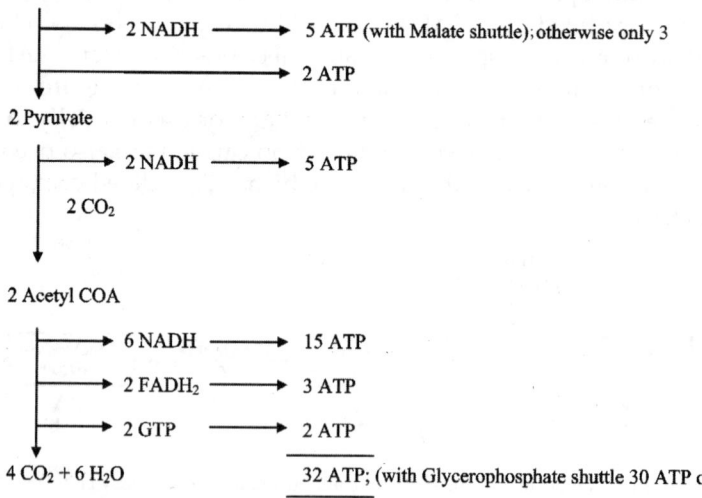

Glucose

→ 2 NADH → 5 ATP (with Malate shuttle); otherwise only 3
→ 2 ATP

2 Pyruvate

→ 2 NADH → 5 ATP
2 CO$_2$

2 Acetyl COA

→ 6 NADH → 15 ATP
→ 2 FADH$_2$ → 3 ATP
→ 2 GTP → 2 ATP

4 CO$_2$ + 6 H$_2$O   32 ATP; (with Glycerophosphate shuttle 30 ATP only)

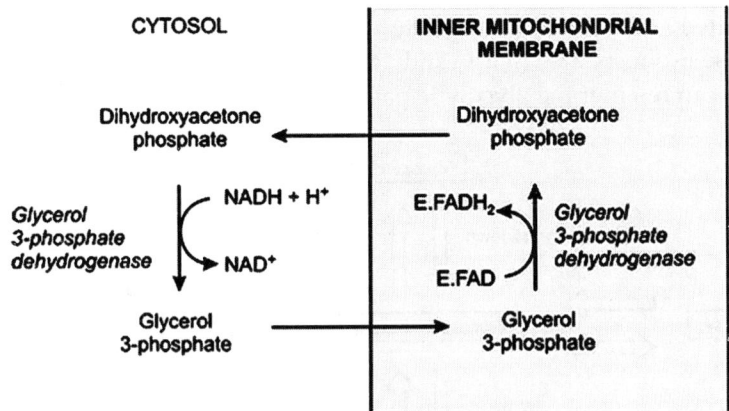

Figure 4   The glycerol 3-phosphate shuttle

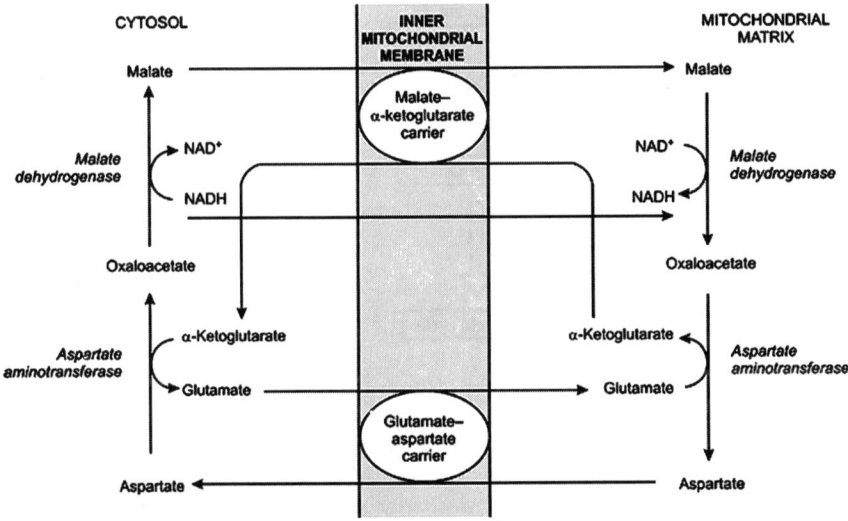

Figure 5   The malate-aspartate shuttle

The Pentose Phosphate Pathway

The pathway has an oxidative phase, which is irreversible and generates NADPH, and a nonoxidative phase, which is reversible and provides ribose precursors for nucleotide synthesis (Figure 2). In the pentose phosphate pathway, glucose-6-phosphate (G6P) is oxidized and decarboxylated to produce two NADPH, CO_2 and ribulose-5-phosphate (Ru5P). Depending on the cell's needs, ribulose-5-phosphate may be isomerized to ribose-5-phosphate (R5P) for nucleotide synthesis or converted, via ribose-5-phosphate and xylulose-5-phosphate (Xu5P), to fructose-6-phosphate (F6P) and glyceraldehydes-3-phosphate (GAP) which can re-enter the glycolytic pathway.

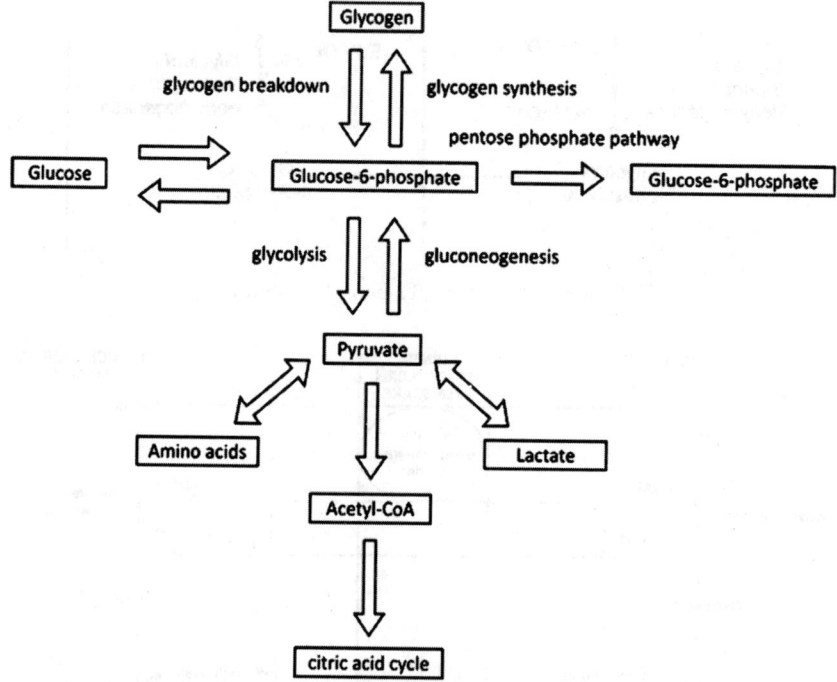

Figure 6   Overview of glucose metabolism. Glucose-6-phosphate (G6P) is produced by the phosphorylation of free glucose, by glycogen degradation, and by gluconeogenesis. It is also a precursor for glycogen synthesis and the pentose phosphate pathway. The liver (and kidney) can hydrolyze G6P to glucose. Glucose is metabolized by glycolysis to pyruvate, which can be further broken down to acetyl-CoA for oxidation by the citric acid cycle. Lactate and amino acids, which are reversibly converted to pyruvate, are precursors for gluconeogenesis. Source: Principles of Biochemistry, International Student Version, 4th edition, Wiley Plus; 2013, pp518

Glucose to Glycogen (Animal starch): Glycogen synthesis

The excess energy consumed is stored as either liver or muscle glycogen or as fat for future needs. When blood glucose is elevated following a meal containing carbohydrate, insulin is secreted which triggers the formation of glycogen. Uridine triphosphate (UTP) is used for synthesis.

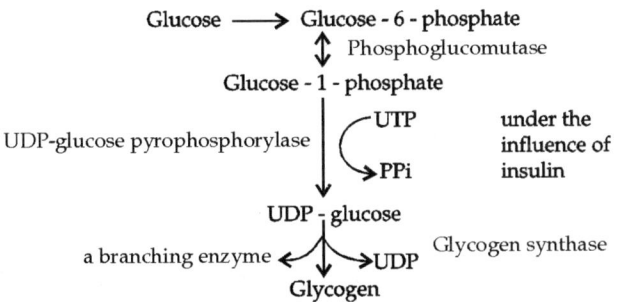

Liver glycogen synthesis involves a series of conversions from glucose to glucose-6-phosphate, to UDP-glucose and finally to glycogen. The synthesis of glycogen from glucose-1-phosphate under physiological conditions is thermodynamically unfavourable. Consequently, **glycogen synthesis and breakdown must occur by separate pathways.**

The mechanism of insulin action is very complex. In liver, insulin stimulates glycogen synthesis. An increase in glucose concentration promotes inactivation of glycogen phosphorylase 'a' through its conversion to phosphorylase 'b'. The subsequent release of phosphoprotein phosphotase-1 activates **glycogen synthase.** Thus when glucose in plentiful, the liver stores the excess as glycogen.

Blood glucose levels: Ruminants 40 to 60mg/100ml; Nonruminants 80 to 120 mg %. Birds have higher blood-sugar (250 mg%) values than do mammals. Cold-blooded animals (frog) have 20 mg %.

Glycogen to Glucose : Glycogen breakdown or glycogenolysis

1. In the muscles, under the influence of epinephrine, glycogen is converted to glucose-6-p and enters the glycolytic cycle to provide ATP. As muscle has no glucose-6-phosphatase and the glucose-6-phosphate can't diffuse out of the cells, this metabolite can only be used at the cell for energy. Normally mammalian muscle contains glycogen in between 0.5-1.0% whereas in horse it is up to 2.26%. **Liver cells contains up to 10% by weight.**

   Glycogen is a polymer of α(1 → 4)-linked D-glucose with α(1 → 6)-linked branches every 8-14 residues. Glycogenolysis requires three enzymes: (1) Glycogen phosphorylase (or simply phosphorylase) catalyzes glycogen phosphorolysis (bond cleavage by the substitution of a phosphate group) to yield glucose-1-phosphate. The enzyme releases a glucose unit only if it is at least five units away from a branch point. (2) Glycogen debranching enzyme removes glycogen's branches, thereby making additional glucose residues accessible to glycogen phosphorylase. (3) Phosphoglucomutase converts glucose-1-phosphate to glucose-6-phosphate.

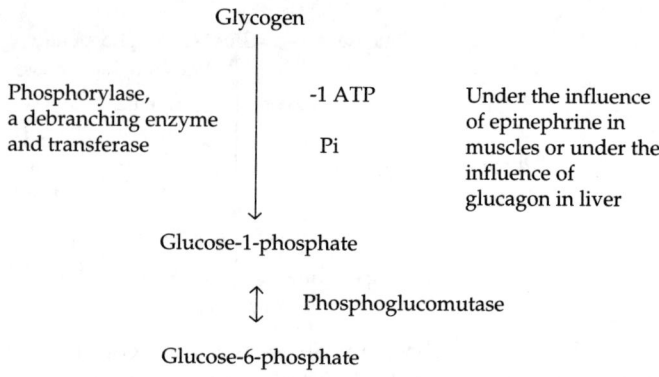

Glycogen

Phosphorylase,
a debranching enzyme
and transferase

-1 ATP

Pi

Under the influence
of epinephrine in
muscles or under the
influence of
glucagon in liver

Glucose-1-phosphate

$\updownarrow$ Phosphoglucomutase

Glucose-6-phosphate

2. In the liver, however, glycogenolysis occurs due to the hormone *glucagon* secreted by the pancreas in response to the low blood glucose level. The resulting glucose-6-phosphate is hydrolyzed by *glucose-6-phosphatase* present in the liver cells releasing glucose into the circulation where it can be utilized by the brain and muscle for energy.

Glucose-6-phosphatase is absent in muscle and brain.

Using glycogen as a storage element is 97% as efficient as using glucose directly.

Glycogen reserve is shortlived. A 24-hour fast will reduce the levels to nearly zero. Glycogen stores have to be constantly replenished.

Glucose to Fat

The ability of the liver and other tissues to store sugar as glycogen is limited. When the carbohydrate intake regularly exceeds the current need of the body for energy purposes, sugar is transformed into fat. The formation of body fat from carbohydrate food was first demonstrated by J.B. Lawes and J.H. Gilbert in 1859 by means of slaughter experiments. Formation of fat from glucose involves the synthesis of two components, fatty acids and glycerol.

Dihydroxy acetone P $\xrightarrow{\hspace{1cm}}$ Glycerol
$\qquad\qquad\qquad$ - 1 ATP

Pyruvate $\xrightarrow{\hspace{1cm}}$ Acetyl CoA
$\qquad\qquad\qquad\searrow CO_2$

However, synthesis of fatty acid from glucose in ruminants is not possible.

Oxygen Debt During Prolonged Strenuous Exercise

Under the limiting oxygen conditions experienced during vigorous exercise, the need for ATP exceeds the ability of the animal to provide

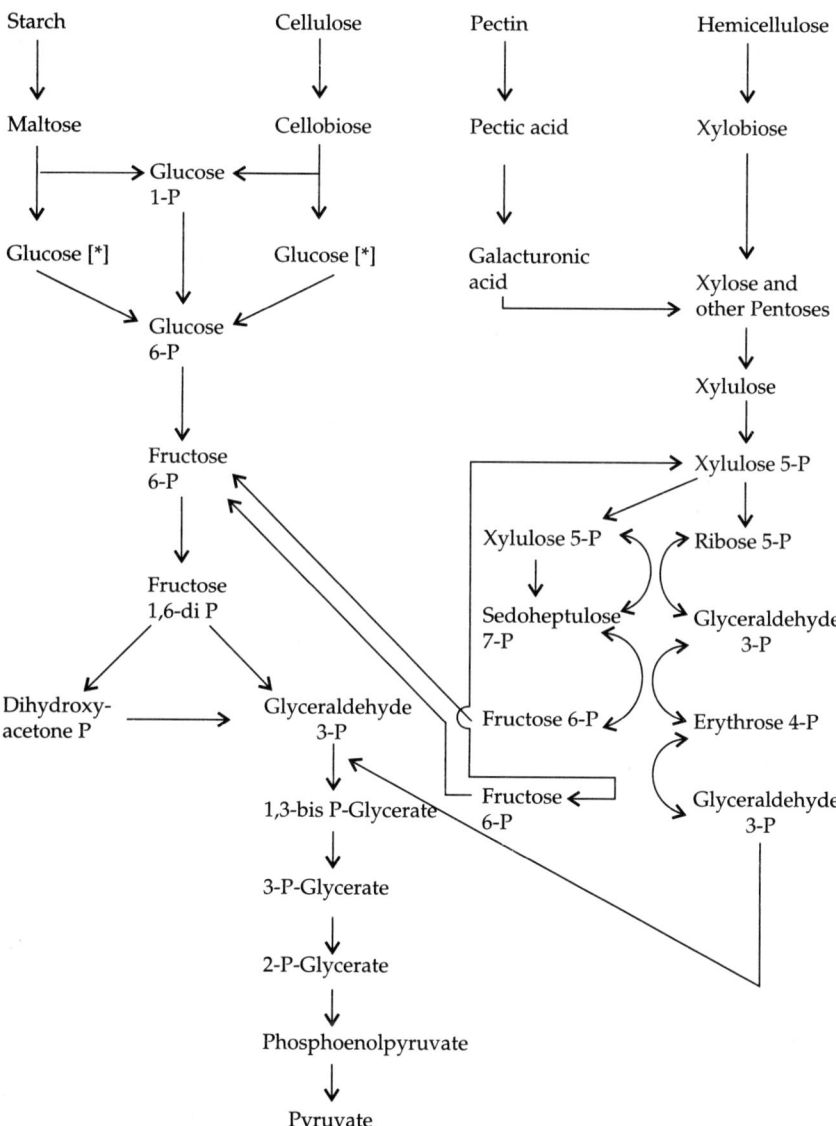

Figure 8. Metabolic Pathways of the Major Carbohydrates of
Plants to 3C Units in the rumen.
([*] Glucose is present only transiently).

oxygen to the tissues to keep the oxidative phosphorylation and TCA cycle operative. As a result glucose metabolism stops at pyruvate and pyruvate concentration increases in muscle. However, in the presence of lactate dehydrogenase, pyruvate is promptly reduced to lactate and NADH (which was produced in the reaction glyceraldehyde-3-P to 1-3-diphosphoglycerate) is oxidized back to NAD⁺.

This oxidized cofactor can then be returned to react with glyceraldehyde-3-P and allow glycolysis to continue.

$$\text{Glucose} \rightarrow \text{Pyruvate} + 2\text{ATP}$$

NADH

NAD⁺   Lactate dehydrogenase

Lactate

Lactate diffuses from the muscle cell into the blood, carried to the liver. Here it is converted back to pyruvate by lactate dehydrogenase. The pyruvate is then converted to glucose by gluconeogenesis and the released gluclose then diffuses back into the circulation to return to the skeletal muscle (and brain) (to be reduced again to lactate via the glycolytic cycle). This cycle of reactions is called the Cori cycle. In this way, ATP continues to be generated to a limited degree in spite of a dearth of oxygen. The organism has thus been able to function in spite of a limited tissue oxygen supply. (See figure 7).

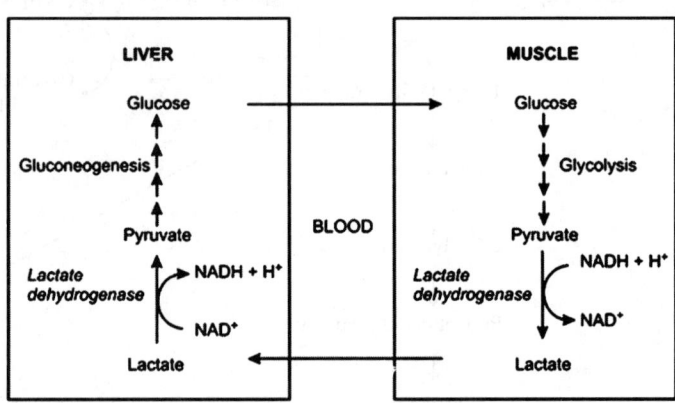

Figure 7   The Cori cycle.

Carbohydrates-their Digestion, Absorption and Metabolism in Ruminants

Microbial digestion of carbohydrates has been studied earlier. The complex feed carbohydrates, cellulose, hemicellulose, pectin and starch are hydrolysed to their respective monomeric units, which are then fermented to pyruvate primarily by the Embden Mayerhof and the pentose phosphate pathways (Fig. 8). Pyruvate is then converted to a number of end products, depending on the microorganisms and feed nutrients (Fig. 9). See Appendix II also.

Feed composition is important both for the total amounts of VFA formed and for the relative amounts of the various acids. When feed contains large amounts of starch, the total production of VFA per kg feed is greater than when feed contains large amounts of fibre is fed. At the same time, the amount of propionic acid relative to the amounts of the other acids, also increases when the diet is rich in starch. Relative amounts of different VFAs are variable based on the ratio between hay and concentrate in the diet (Table 1).

TABLE 1   Molar percentage of VFAs and other short-chain fatty acids in cows fed on total mixed rations (Modified from Bondi, 1987)

Ratio of hay to concentrate	Acetate	Propionate	Butyrate	Other acids
60:40	66	20	10	4
30:70	56	30	10	4
10:90	46	40	09	5

Proportion of VFA: On a predominantly hay diet the fermentation products are (on a molar basis): Acetic 65%, propionic 20%, butyric 9%, branch chain fatty acids (isovaleric, isobutyric and 2-methyl butyric) 5% and n-valeric acid 1%. The total concentration of VFAs in rumen liquor varies between 2 and 15 g/litre according to the animal's diet and the time that has elapsed since the previous meal. The total weight of acids produced may be as high as 4 kg per day in cows. Small quantities of additional fatty acids such as isobutyric, valeric, 2-methyl butyric and 3-methyl butyric are also formed by deamination of amino acids such as valine, proline, isoleucine and leucine, respectively.

Propionic acid appears to be formed primarily from the decarboxylation of succinate when fibrous carbohydrates are fermented. High starch or sugar diets produce lactic acid and it may accumulate if grain diets are suddenly introduced to ruminants. Further, lactic acid is a stronger acid (pK 3.8) than the VFAs and is absorbed at a rate that is only 5-10% of the absorption for VFA. Consequently, lactic acid accumulates easily in the rumen. This will lower the pH and may precipitate severe acidosis. Lactic acidaemia may occur. However, if starch diets are gradually introduced the necessary bacteria develop (*Megasphaera elsdenii, Bacteroides ruminicola*) to ferment the lactic acid rapidly and propionic acid is produced via acrylate pathway. The oxaloacetate and succinate pathway predominates under most conditions (Fig. 9). The lactate and acrylate pathway become important in ruminants fed grain, even predominant during sulphur deficiency.

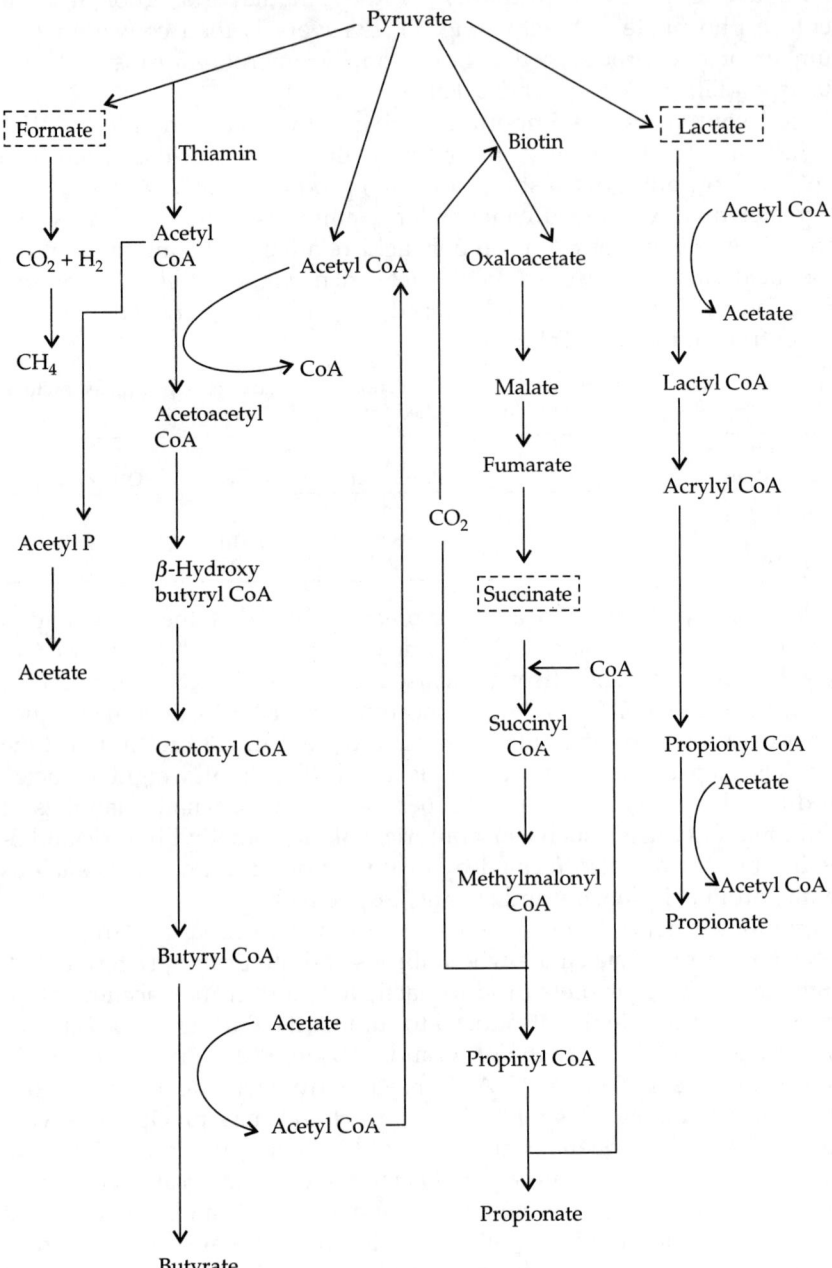

Figure 9. Metabolic Pathways of Degradation of 3C Units.

Acetate is formed from pyruvate in two ways. One is decarboxylation, yielding carbon dioxide and hydrogen. The other is a phosphoroclastic reaction yielding formate as well as acetate. Methane is formed from carbon dioxide, formate and hydrogen. Butyrate is formed from pyruvate via acetyl CoA, malonyl CoA and acetoacetyl CoA. It may interconvert with acetate.

Production of Hydrogen in the Rumen

Van Soest (1977) has adapted the concepts reported by Wolin (1974).

1. Acetate = $C_6H_{12}O_6 + 2H_2O \rightarrow C_2H_4O_2 + 2CO_2 + 8H$
2. Propionate = $C_6H_{12}O_6 \rightarrow 2C_3H_6O_2 + 2(O)$ (acrylate pathway)
3. Butyrate = $C_6H_{12}O_6 \rightarrow C_4H_8O_2 + 2CO_2 + 4H$

So there will be an excess of 8H per mole acetate, 4H per mole butyrate and a deficiency of 4H for each mole of propionate formed via the acrylate pathway. Thus in a normal fermentation there is an excess of [H] and the rumen contents constitute a highly reduced medium.

Methanogenesis

To stay in balance, extra hydrogen must be removed. Methane is the hydrogen sink. Organic acids can be used as alternative hydrogen sinks. It can't be metabolized by the animal. Most of it is lost by eructation. Thus it is a net loss of feed energy. Further, hydrogen functions to reduce sulfate and nitrate and hydrogenate unsaturated fatty acids in the rumen. Carbon dioxide usually forms about 40% of the rumen gas and methane 30% to 40%; 5% hydrogen, and small and variable proportions of oxygen and nitrogen (from ingested air). Methanogenesis is a complicated process that involves folic acid and vitamin B_{12}. About 4.5g of methane is produced per 100g of carbohydrate digested. Methane is a major greenhouse gas contributing heavily to global warming.

Reductive Acetogenesis is an Alternative to Methanogenesis

Methane is generated in the rumen by methanogenic archaea that utilise hydrogen to reduce carbon dioxide, and is a significant electron sink in the rumen ecosystem. However, there are other mechanisms for removing excess hydrogen that have been suggested as alternatives to methanogenesis, including sulfate, nitrate, fumarate reduction and reductive acetogenesis. Of all these, reductive acetogenesis appears to be more likely alternative to methanogenesis.

Reductive acetogenesis combines hydrogen with carbon dioxide to form acetate, which is then utilised by the host animal as a source of energy. Reductive acetogenesis is undertaken by a broad range of genetically diverse bacteria (Mackie and Bryant 1994) and replaces methanogenesis as the dominant mechanism for hydrogen removal, with considerable energetic advantages, in many anaerobic ecosystems.

Absorption of VFA: Pioneering studies of Barcroft and associates revealed that VFA are directly absorbed from the rumen, reticulum, omasum and large intestine. The absorption of VFA from the rumen is prompt. Elevated levels in the portal blood have been noted within 10 min. after eating. Absorption is by simple diffusion with the disassociated acid passing through at the normal pH of the rumen of about 6.7 and less. In acid pH, absorption is fastest for butyric acid, then propionic and acetic. See chapter 7.

Metabolic activity of rumen epithelium: The rumen epithelium is not a simple sieve. It has the capacity to metabolize VFA as they are absorbed. It is reported that 80 to 90% of the butyrate is converted to ketone bodies. Thus portal and systemic blood levels of butyrate are extremely low. Up to 50% of the propionate may be metabolized to lactate and pyruvate during absorption. Relatively little acetate is used other than as a source of energy by ruminal epithelium.

Production and fate of VFA: On a high roughage low concentrate ration, acetic acid production is more while on high levels of grains/concentrates or adding monensin in the ration, the production of propionic acid is more accompanied by reduction of methane level. Fermentation favouring propionate production usually results in improved feed efficiency in growing-fattening animals. Depressed acetate production may result in milk with a lowered percentage of fat.

Both fattening and milking animals are more efficient in the utilization of propionic acid than acetic acid though acetic acid is required for the synthesis of milk. About 40% of the fasting energy requirements of ruminants are supplied by VFA. In rabbits, the relative amount of butyric acid is usually greater than that of propionic acid.

Metabolism of VFA: These acid provide 60-80% of the ME of ruminants on most diets. Molar proportions of 7:2:1 for acetic, propionic and butyric acids, respectively, are equivalent to energy proportions of 6:3:2, the relative proportion of butyric acid is doubled when converted from a molar to an energy basis.

Volatile fatty acids and other short chain acids reach liver through the portal blood. Acetate largely passes through to enter the bloodstream and it is the only VFA found in appreciable quantities in the peripheral circulation. Acetate is phosphorylated (–2 ATP) to acetyl CoA and then oxidized via citric acid cycle yielding 10 ATP. The net gain is 8 ATP per mole of acetic acid absorbed. It can also be used for the synthesis of milk fat, especially the short chain fatty acids.

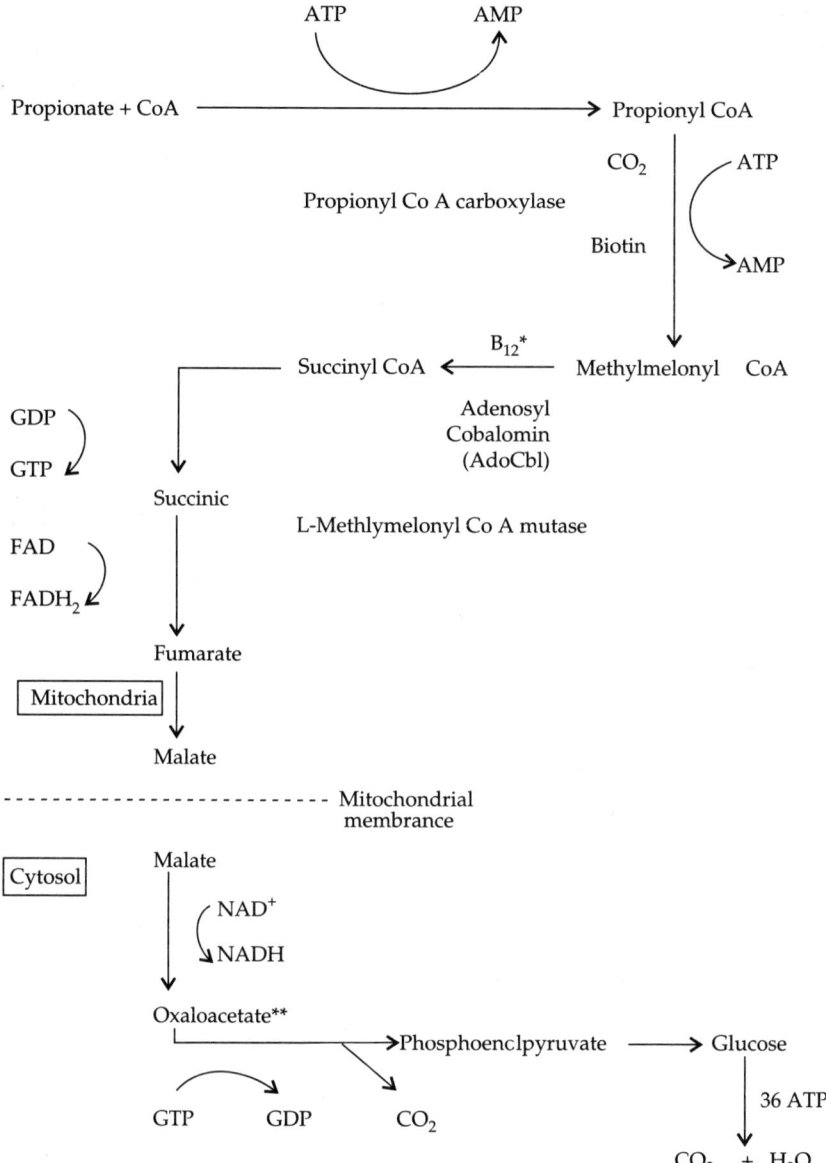

Figure 10. Metabolism of Propionate in Ruminants.

* Deficiency of vitamin B_{12} virtually elevates levels of propionic acid/accumulation of methylmelonyl CoA and contributes towards ketosis.

** Oxaloacetate may also lead to form glucogenic amino acids like aspartic acid, glutamic acid or alanine.

Metabolism of Propionate in Ruminants

Although some propionic acid may be oxidized to lactic acid in the rumen wall during absorption, the remainder is absorbed and carried to the liver, where it is converted to glucose (Fig. 10). It is the primary source of glucose for the ruminant.

If propionate is converted to glucose and then metabolised to CO_2 and H_2O there is a net gain of 17 ATP per mole (one report say 18 ATP per mole) or 34 per glucose equivalent. (See the updated ATP yield). This contrasts with 36 from glucose alone. One gram propionic acid can theoretically provide 1.23 g of glucose.

Butyric acid is absorbed as a ketone body, being eventually metabolized as acetyl CoA. The net ATP production is 20 per mole.

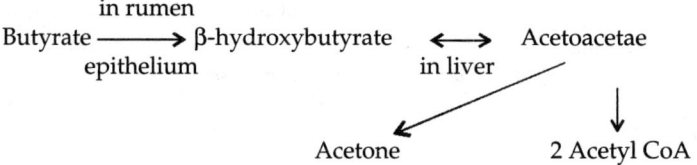

ATP yield from one mole of acetic acid

Attributes	ATP +	ATP −
1 mole of acetate to 1 mole of acetyl-CoA	--------	2
From cell cytoplasm, it reached mitochondrial matrix in a complex with carnitine; acetyl CoA enters the TCA cycle and is oxidized	10	-----
Net gain of ATP per mole of acetate	8	------

ATP yield from one mole of propionic acid

Attributes	ATP +	ATP-
2 moles propionate to 2 moles succinyl-CoA	-----	6
2 moles succinyl-CoA to 2 moles malate	5	-----
2 moles malate to 2 moles phosphoenolpyruvate	5	2
2 moles phosphoenolpyruvate to 1 mole glucose	------	5
1 mole glucose to CO_2 + H_2O	30 or 32	------
Total	40 or 42	13
Net gain of ATP	27 or 29	

There is a net gain of 13.5 or 14.5 moles of ATP per mole of propionic acid.

Small amounts of propionic acid are present in the peripheral blood supply. Such propionate could be used directly for energy production. Here the phosphoenolpyruvate would follow glycolysis via pyruvate, acetyl-coenzyme A and the TCA cycle. In this case the ATP yield may be as mentioned below. Therefore, this pathway is marginally more efficient than that via glucose. There is a net gain of 14.5 moles of ATP per mole of propionic acid.

Attributes	ATP +	ATP-
1 mole propionate to 1 mole succinyl-CoA	-----	3
1 mole succinyl-CoA to 1 mole malate	2.5	-----
1 mole malate to 1 mole phosphoenolpyruvate	2.5	1
1 mole phosphoenolpyruvate to 1 mole acetyl CoA	3.5	-----
1 mole acetyl CoA to CO_2 + H_2O	10	------
Total	18.5	4
Net gain of ATP	14.5	

ATP yield from one mole of butyric acid

Attributes	ATP +	ATP-
1 mole butyrate to 1 mole D-3-hydroxybutyrate	4	4.5
1 mole D-3-hydroxybutyrate to 2 moles acetyl-CoA	2.5	2
2 moles acetyl-CoA to CO_2 + H_2O	20	-----
Total	26.5	6.5
Net gain of ATP per mole of butyrate	20	------

Ruminants utilise ketones as one of the energy sources. The normal concentration in the blood is between 5 and 10 mg per cent. But at times when mobilisation of body fat is required to compensate carbohydrate deficiency for energy, ketone concentration may rise to about 50 mg/100 ml or more thus may lead to ketosis (Fig. 11).

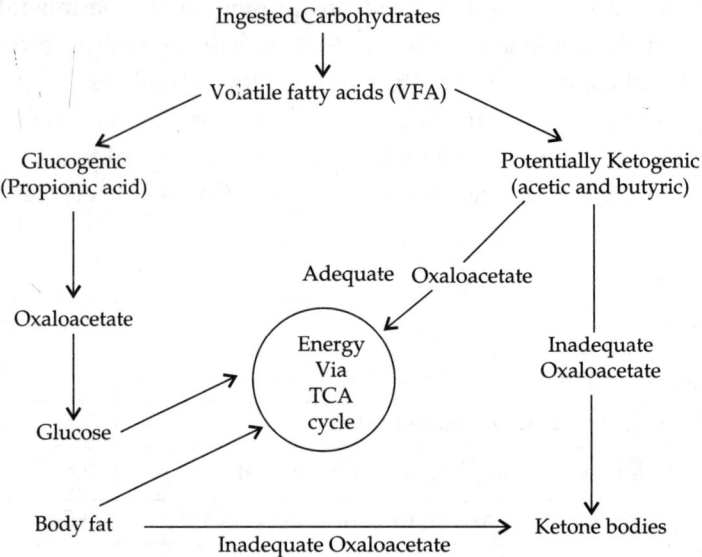

Figure 11. Carbohydrate metabolism in Ruminants.

Ketone bodies are important fuels in extrahepatic tissues (eg, muscles)

Enzymes responsible for ketone body formation are associated mainly with the mitochondria. Ketogenesis occurs solely in liver and rumen epithelium. While an active enzymatic mechanism produces acetoacetate from acetoacetyl-CoA in the liver, acetoacetate once formed cannot be reactivated directly except in the cytosol.

In extrahepatic tissues, acetoacetate is activated to acetoacetyl-CoA, which is split to acetyl-CoA and is oxidized in the citric acid cycle. In most cases, ketonemia is due to increased production of ketone bodies by the liver rather than to a deficiency in their utilization by extrahepatic tissues. While acetoacetate and β-hydroxybutyrate are readily oxidized by extrahepatic tissues, acetone is difficult to oxidize in *vivo* and to a large extent is volatilized in the lungs.

Gluconeogenesis: Gluconeogenesis, in simple terms, is production of glucose from noncarbohydrate substances. The liver and kidney are the only organs that are capable of any significant gluconeogenesis, and the kidneys do so only in states of chronic acidosis. Very little gluconeogenesis occurs in brain or muscle. In gluconeogenesis pyruvate is metabolized to glucose and gluconeogenesis is not a simple reversal of glycolysis. Precursors for gluconeogenesis are glycerol, lactate, pyruvate, citric acid cycle intermediates and the carbon skeletons of most amino acids.

Gluconeogenesis: Ruminants: Little glucose *per se* is absorbed directly. Ruminants must depend upon rumen propionate, amino acids, lactate, pyruvate or glycerol for its glucose (Fig. 12). When feed intake is high, propionate and amino acids will be the primary source (A high producing cow can derive no more than 60% of its glucose from propionate). When feed intake is below the maintenance level, glycerol from mobilized fat and amino acids from mobilized protein will become the predominant precursors. About 85% of the glucose is produced in the liver and 15% in the kidney.

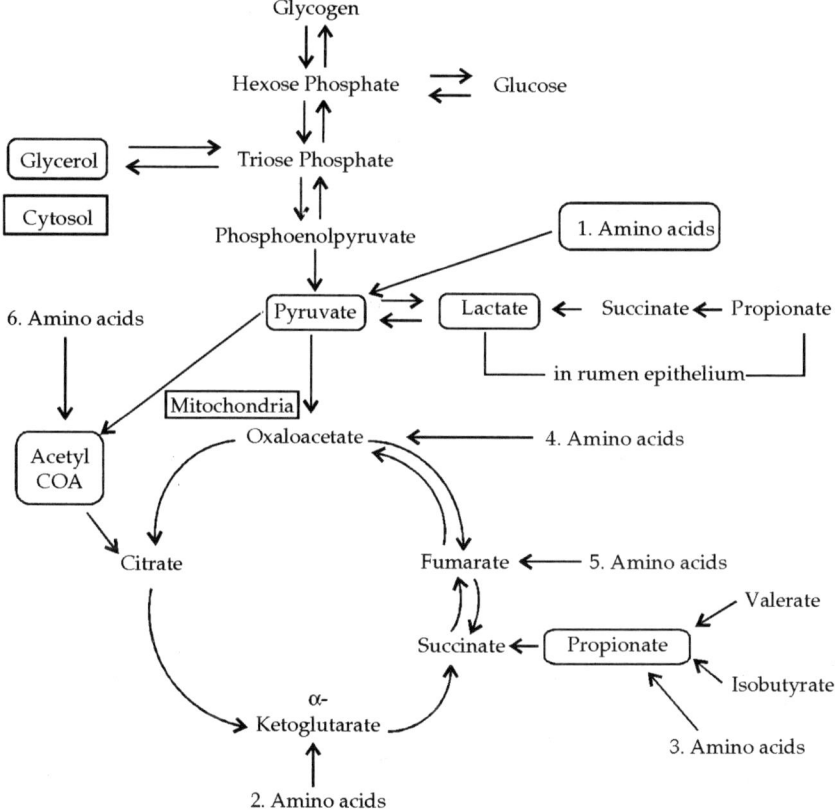

Figure 12. Scheme showing the metabolic pathway for gluconeogenesis in the liver of ruminants and the relationship of glucose precursors that become available from the digestive tract (R.A. Leng, 1970). Glucogenic amino acids: 1. cysteine, glycine, serine, alanine; 2. glutamate, histidine, proline, arginine; 3. valine, threonine, methionine, isoleucine (part); 4. aspartate; 5. tyrosine (part), phenylalanine (part); Ketogenic amino acids; 6. isoleucine (part), phenylalanine (part), tyrosine (part), lysine, leucine.

Ruminants must have a continuous and a relatively high rate of gluconeogenesis in the liver to maintain the blood glucose level. Glucagon appears to be an important endocrine stimulant to maintain this rate of gluconeogenesis. Rising levels of amino acids and propionic acid can stimulate glucagon release.

Gluconeogenesis in Ruminants and Monogastric Animals

There are two basic differences in the substrate availability to ruminant and monogastric animals. Maximal gluconeogenesis occurs during feeding in ruminants in contrast to monogastric animals where gluconeogenesis occurs during starvation or on low carbohydrate diets. A further consideration is that normally gluconeogenesis by monogastric animals is stimulated in starvation, and lipogenesis is depressed and the reverse occurs on refeeding. Generally when gluconeogenesis is high, lipogenesis is low and vice versa. However, when gluconeogenesis is high in the ruminant animal, lipogenesis may also be high and, thus, there may be a need for differences in the control of gluconeogenesis in these animals.

In non-ruminants, the rate of gluconeogenesis is lowest after feeding when glucose is being absorbed and is highest during fasting when no exogenous glucose is provided. Gluconeogenesis is a continual process that is of great importance to ruminants because almost all dietary carbohydrates are fermented to volatile fatty acids in the rumen. In turn, propionate is the only major VFA that contributes to gluconeogenesis.

Oxaloacetate is produced in cytosol by direct diffusion from the mitochondria and by enzyme action from pyruvate, aspartate, and possibly malate. Cytosol oxaloacetate may enter the lipogenesis or gluconeogenesis pathways (Figure. 13). Oxaloacetate would tend to be drawn into the lipogenesis pathway when malate dehydrogenase is active and an excess of NADH exists. Gluconeogenesis will compete effectively for oxaloacetate when malate dehydrogenase activity is low, NADH concentration is low, and phosphoenolpyruvate carboxykinase activity is high. Enzymic activities in cow livers suggest that oxaloacetate is effectively channeled into gluconeogenesis in ruminants.

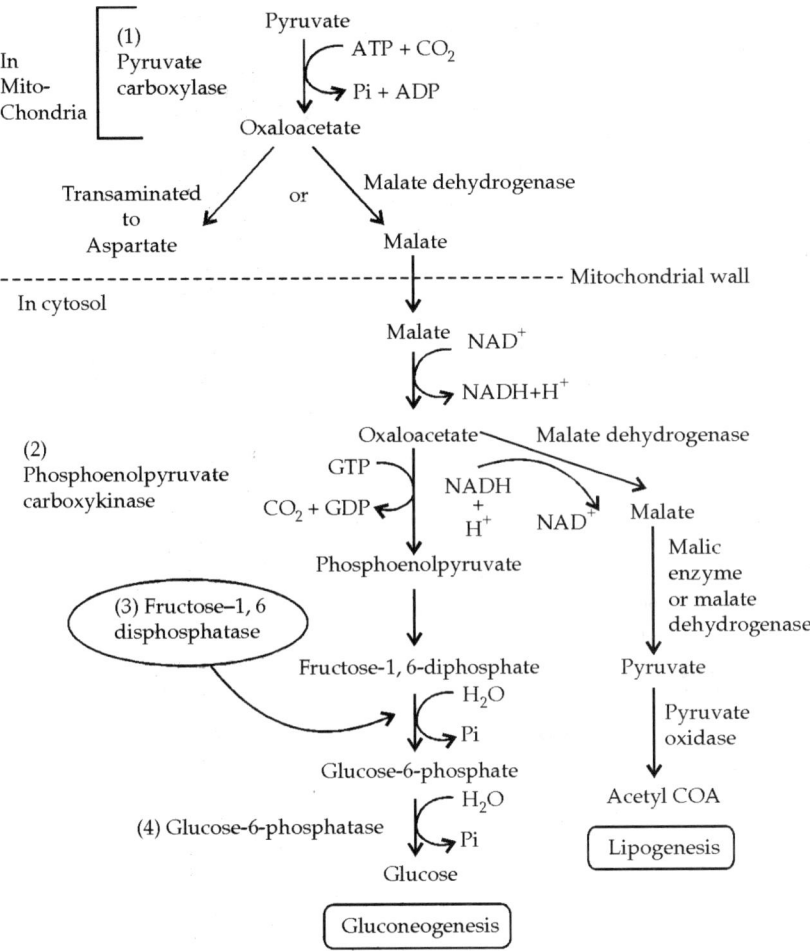

Figure 13. Two pathways of oxaloacetate utilization in the liver of ruminants
(F.J. Ballard et. al, 1969).

Comparison of gluconeogenesis and glycolysis is illustrated (Figure 14) for better comprehension. The three steps of glycolysis numbered are irreversible. The first step in the gluconeogenesis is the conversion of pyruvate to oxaloacetate, which is converted to phosphoenolpyruvate. Both these conversions need 1ATP each. Conversion of 3-Phosphoglycerate to 1,3-Bisphosphoglycerate also need 1 ATP. Thus 3×2 moles of pyruvate = **6 ATP are required to synthesize one molecule of glucose.** This compares with only two ATPs as the net ATP yield from glycolysis. In fact, two molecules of NADH are consumed in the glyceraldehyde 3-phosphate dehydrogenase reaction. Each cytosolic

NADH generates about two ATP molecules and this is equivalent to the input of another four ATPs per glucose synthesized.

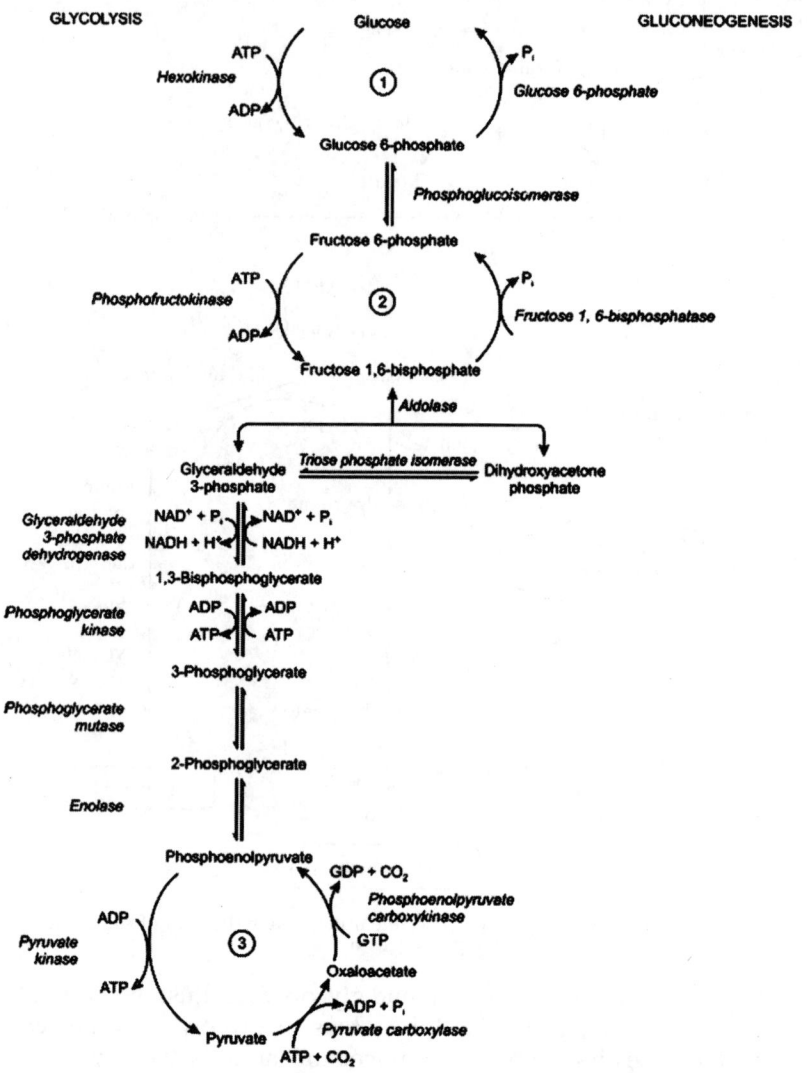

Figure 14   Comparison of gluconeogenesis and glycolysis.

Control of glucose metabolism

Glucose is always required by the central nervous system and erythrocytes

Erythrocytes lack mitochondria and hence are wholly reliant on (anaerobic) glycolysis and the pentose phosphate pathway at all times.

The brain can metabolize ketone bodies to meet about 20% of its energy requirements; the remainder must be supplied by glucose. Hence blood glucose and limited reserves of liver and muscle glycogen are preserved for use by the brain and red blood cells while ensuring the supply of alternative metabolic fuels for other tissues. In pregnancy the fetus requires a significant amount of glucose, as does the synthesis of lactose in lactation.

Homeostasis of blood glucose concentration

Homeostasis of blood glucose concentration is maintained by hormones and neural devices. At least five endocrine glands (pancreatic islets, anterior pituitary gland, adrenal cortex, adrenal medulla and thyroid gland) and at least eight hormones secreted by these glands function as key elements of the glucose homeostatic mechanism (Figure 15). It is to be kept in mind that these hormones have many different kinds of regulatory effects in the body and not just limited to their effects on glucose metabolism.

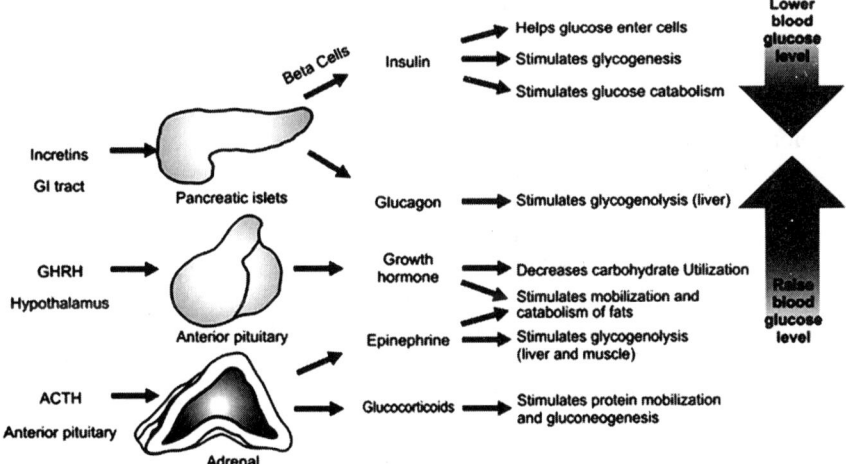

Figure 15 Hormonal control of blood glucose level - simplified view of some of the major glucose-regulating hormones. Source: Essentials of Anatomy and Physiology by K.T.Patton et al., 2012, pp522

Beta cells of the pancreatic islets secrete the most well-known sugar-regulating hormone - insulin. Insulin decreases blood glucose level (1) by moving them out of blood into cells. (2) It increases the activity of glucose kinase, which catalyzes glucose for phosphorylation. This phosphorylation is a must for either glycogenesis or glucose catabolism to take place. Thus insulin moves glucose into cells and increases glycogenesis and increases catabolism of glucose - all of which decrease blood glucose levels.

Alpha cells of the pancreatic islets secrete the sugar-regulating hormone glucagon. Glucagon tends to increase the blood glucose by way of increasing the activity of phosphorylase enzyme. This enzyme promotes liver glycogenolysis leading to release of more glucose into the bloodstream.

Hormones **incretins** (these include glucagon-like peptide I [GLP-I] and gastric inhibitory peptide [GIP]) are released by endocrine gastrointestinal cells in response to the presence of glucose. Incretins act to increase insulin level and decrease glucagon level, thereby tend to decrease blood glucose levels. Incretins may also reduce the rate of gastric emptying and decrease desire for more food.

Adrenal medulla secretes hormone **epinephrine** in times of emotional or physical stress. It increases phosphorylase activity, which promotes both liver and muscle glycogenolysis. Epinephrine and glucagon increase the blood glucose level. Epinephrine is the only hormone whose release into the systemic circulation is directly under the control of the nervous system.

Adrenocorticotropic hormone (ACTH) stimulates the adrenal cortex to increase its secretion of glucocorticoids (e.g., cortisone). Glucocorticoids accelerate gluconeogenesis by mobilizing proteins to amino acids to glucose. Glucocorticoids also stimulate enzymatic reversal of glycolysis helping the cell to manufacture more glucose. ACTH and glucocorticoids, thus, increase the blood glucose concentration.

Growth hormone (GH) made by the anterior pituitary, also increases blood glucose. GH causes a shift from carbohydrate to fat catabolism; more fats are mobilized and catabolized. Thyroid-stimulating hormone (TSH) from the anterior pituitary gland and its target secretion, thyroid **hormone (T_3 and T_4)**, have complex effects on metabolism; some of these raise, and some lower, the glucose level.

Most of the hormones cause the blood glucose level to rise. These hormones (glucagon, epinephrine, ACTH, glucocorticoids, GH) are called hyperglycemic. The one notable exception is insulin, which is hypoglycemic because it tends to decrease the blood glucose level. Incretins also tend to decrease blood glucose levels.

Chapter 9

Digestion and Absorption of Proteins and Nitrogen Compounds in Nonruminants and Birds and Ruminants; Metabolism of Absorbed Nitrogen

Nonruminants and Birds

Dietary proteins are hydrolyzed to their constituent amino acids, absorbed and transported to the liver via the hepatic portal vein. Some amino acids appear in the lymph but the amounts are small.

But in certain newborn mammals, for instance, calf during the first 24 hours of life 'intact immune globulins' are directly absorbed into the lymphatic system (thoracic duct). The intestinal villi of the newborn are able to absorb the globulins by **pinocytosis** and this enables the newborn to acquire 'instant immunity' by ingesting colostrum high in immunoglobulins.

Protein digestion begins in the stomach with significant denaturation by hydrochloric acid followed by peptic digestion (Gastricsin in human body, Rennin in young calves; pepsin). Pepsin cleaves bonds adjacent to aromatic amino acids and splits the polypeptide into large peptides and relatively few amino acids. In duodenum the ingesta come in contact with the pancreatic and bile secretion. The pancreatic enzymes (trypsin, chymotrypsin and carboxypeptidase) and enzymes of the intestinal mucosa (amino peptidase and dipeptidase) complete the digestion of proteins to free amino acids.

Pancreatic nucleases (ribonuclease, deoxyribonuclease) perform the digestion of dietary nucleic acids present in every plant and animal cell.

Amino acids are absorbed into blood and reached the portal circulation. No peptide appear in the portal blood. **Rate of absorption of amino acids** is maximum in the proximal two-thirds of the small intestine. It is an active type, similar to glucose, in which the transport of sodium is involved.

Tripeptides are absorbed more rapidly than dipeptides, which are in turn faster than free amino acids and these peptides are hydrolyzed by peptidases. There appears to be a competition for absorption of free amino acids within groups i.e. acidic, basic, neutral and imino acids. Natural L-forms are absorbed more rapidly than D-forms. Neutral amino acids are absorbed rapidly than basic amino acids. Vitamin B_6 also appears to greatly enhance intestinal transport of amino acids. This competition disappears, when amino acids are absorbed as **oligopeptides**. All essential amino acids are not absorbed with equal efficiency-54% for isoleucine, 80% for histidine in the pig consuming fish meal. Generally, amino acid concentration in tissues is 5 to 10 times of that in plasma.

In most cases, the contribution of stomach to the total digestive process is about 20%. Removal of **peptic digestion** is rapidly accommodated for in the small intestine, but removal of **pancreatic digestion** seriously reduces total protein digestibility. For the young animals receiving milk, the stomach is substantially more important.

Digestion and Absorption of Protein and Nonprotein Nitrogenous Compounds in Ruminants

The key to nitrogen metabolism in the ruminant is the ability of the microbial population to utilize ammonia in the presence of adequate energy to synthesize the amino acids for their growth. Most (80%) of the rumen bacterial species, especially cellulolytic, can utilize ammonia as the sole source of nitrogen for growth while 26% require it absolutely and 55% could use either ammonia or amino acids. A few species can use peptides as well. Protozoa can not use ammonia but derive their nitrogen needs by consuming bacteria and particulate matter.

The bulk of the dietary nitrogen is in the form of protein (under ordinary conditions of feeding) though pasture grasses contain about 20-30% of their total nitrogen as NPN which include amino acids, nitrate, nucleic acids and various amines. The NPN compounds are rapidly degraded in the rumen and ammonia is produced. Ingested true protein may be degraded by microorganisms to the extent of 60% and the remaining 40% escapes ruminal degradation (Fig. 1). VFA are also produced. However, rate of proteolysis is closely related to the solubility of the protein in the rumen fluid. The **ingesta moving into the abomasum** and small intestine thus contains feed protein which has not been degraded as well as bacterial and protozoal bodies. 20% of absorbed microbial N is in the form of nucleic acids and efficiency of their utilization is poor.

In the small intestine enzymatic hydrolysis produces amino acids from the chyme plus the endogenous secretions. These are in turn absorbed via

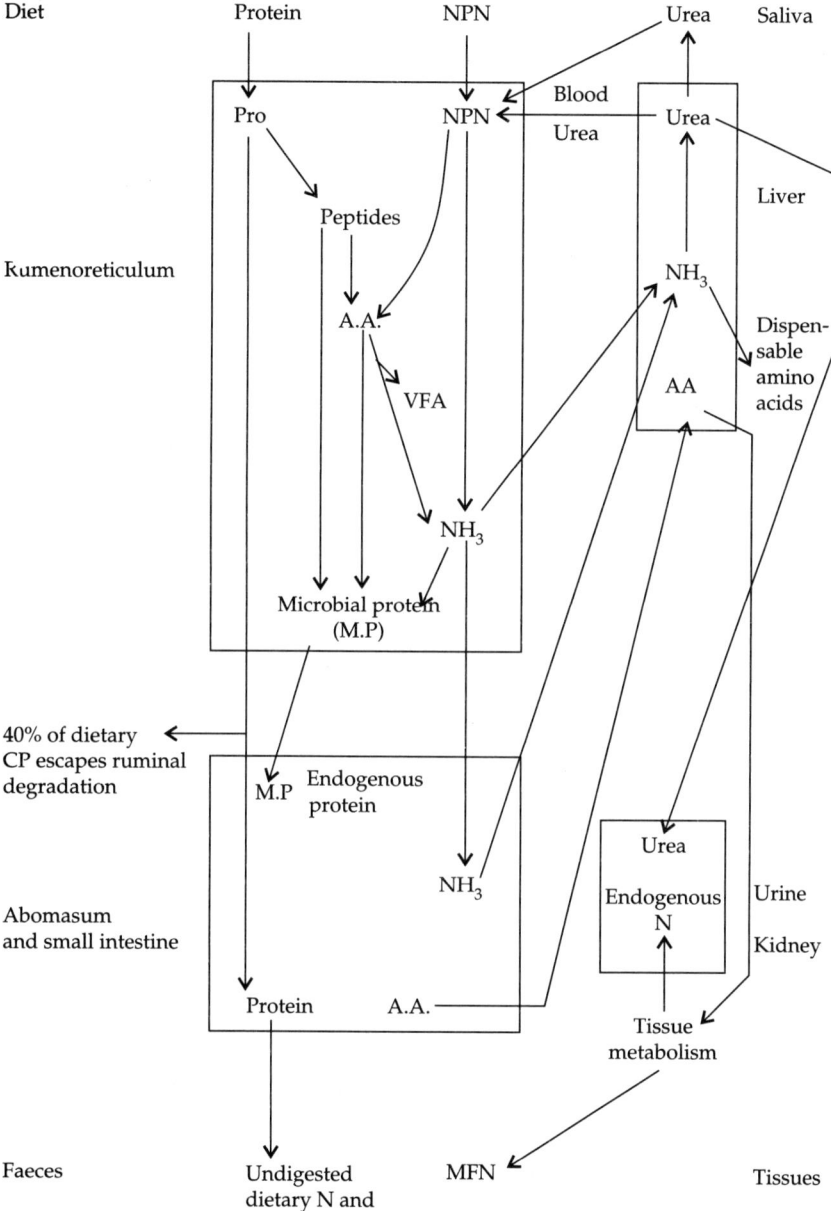

Figure 1. Pathways of Digestion and Metabolism of Nitrogenous Compounds in the Ruminant.

the portal circulation in a similar way as it occurs in nonruminants. However, it has been reported that ileum is an excellent site for digestion and absorption of protein in sheep.

The caecum and large intestine receive the undigested protein from the small intestine plus urea from the blood. This urea supports an active microbial fermentation. The faeces contain the indigestible feed nitrogen, and microbial nitrogen and metabolic nitrogen.

Movement (flux) of ammonia and urea is unique to the system. In the rumen when ammonia is produced in excess of the ability of the microbes to use it (i.e. ammonia overflow), it can be absorbed into the portal circulation, transported to the liver and converted to urea. The urea can then be either excreted by the kidneys into the urine or recycled into the rumen by way of the saliva or through blood. Thus synthesis of urea facilitates to get rid of excess ammonia when needed or to conserve it when the excess in the rumen is only transitory.

On low protein diets, the kidney reabsorbs a greater quantity of urea and thus is recycled into the rumen to provide added N for microbial fermentation. While ammonia is toxic in excess, it can be used as a source of N for the synthesis of dispensable amino acids. Also see page No. 133

Rumen Ammonia Level for Microbial Protein Synthesis/Straw Degradability

The optimal ammonia concentration of rumen fluid may be defined as that which results either in the maximum rate of fermentation in the rumen or that which allows the maximum production of microbial protein per unit of substrate fermented. However, these two statements may not always coincide. **Maximal microbial growth** was observed in the rumen when the ammonia nitrogen concentration was 5 mg per 100 ml rumen fluid while **maximum fractional rates of digestion** of cotton wool and oaten chaff (incubated in nylon bags) were observed with a concentration of 21 mg (range 13-30 mg) per 100 ml rumen fluid. It is theorized that the ammonia concentration required by the adherent, fibre-digesting organisms might be greater than the requirements of the free-floating organisms in the rumen fluid.

Microbial Protein

The rumen bacteria contain approximately 65% protein based on total nitrogen content. The nitrogen content of the protozoa is low as compared to the bacteria because of a higher polysaccharide content. Microbial yield of protein is variable but ranges between 90 to 230 g per kilogram of organic matter digested. This amount is adequate to provide the protein for growing animals over about 100 kg and to maintain levels of milk production up to 10 kg per day. Feed protein *per se* obviously must be provided for high producing cows.

Metabolism of Absorbed Nitrogen

Few animals are continuous eaters. So influx of nutrients into the body is sporadic rather than uniform. The metabolic machinery of the animal must be equipped to handle these sharp increases in nutrients, arrange for their temporary storage and then supply to the tissues during leaner times. Protein reserves are not distinct like glycogen for carbohydrates and depot fat for dietary fat. But protein reserves are available from practically all body tissues for the purpose of meeting emergent situations. Liver is the key organ that synthesizes proteins, supplies amino acids to the circulation when needed and process nitrogen for excretion when in excess.

As studied earlier, the nitrogenous products are digested and enter the blood stream mostly as amino acids in all ruminants and nonruminants. Body tissue proteins continually undergo catabolism to amino acids. The amino acids in the blood constitute the amino acid pool.

Metabolism of amino acids: Amino acids undergo transamination, oxidative and nonoxidative deamination and decarboxylation. These reactions provide for interconversion, synthesis of dispensable amino acids, utilization of amino acids for energy and the utilization or excretion of excess ammonia.

Transamination: It refers to the process whereby amino groups are transferred from an amino acid to a keto acid without the intermediate formation of ammonia. It requires enzymes called transaminases or **aminotransferases**. Transaminases are involved directly in the biosynthesis of a number of dispensable amino acids. They link protein and carbohydrate metabolism. They are also involved in amino acid degradation and in the synthesis of such compounds as urea and γ-amino butyric acid. The functional coenzyme of transaminases is pyridoxal phosphate, and all reactions are freely reversible. The two most widespread transaminases are alanine transaminase (formerly glutamic-pyruvic transaminase) and aspartic transaminase (formerly glutamic-oxaloacetic transaminase).

General transaminase reaction:

$$\alpha\text{-amino acid} + \alpha\text{-keto acid} \xrightarrow{\ B_6\ } \alpha\text{-keto acid} + \alpha\text{-amino acid}$$

Important transaminase reactions:

$$\text{Alanine} + \alpha\text{-Ketoglutaric acid} \xrightleftharpoons{\text{B}_6} \text{Pyruvic acid} + \text{Glutamic acid}$$

Alanine
transaminase (ALT) or GPT

$$\text{Aspartic acid} + \alpha\text{-Ketoglutaric acid} \xrightleftharpoons{\text{B}_6} \text{Oxaloacetic acid} + \text{Glutamic acid}$$

Aspartic
transaminase (AST) or GOT

Liver contains transaminases that are specific for the formation of each amino acid in natural proteins except glycine, lysine and threonine. Glutamine and asparagine, the two common amides, participate in the transamination of more than 30 α-keto acids. The rate of transamination differs among the amino acids. Transamination of lysine takes place with difficulty, if at all. Transamination of histidine and arginine are difficult because of the imidazole ring and the imino group, respectively.

Deamination: Deamination is the removal of amino group from an amino acid which may be oxidative or nonoxidative.

Oxidative deamination: It is insignificant compared to transamination. A deamination reaction proceeds with a simultaneous oxidation as in the conversion of an α-amino acid to an α-keto acid and the amino group to ammonia. The reaction is catalysed by amino acid oxidase, an enzyme which contains the oxidising coenzyme, FAD.

$$\text{Alanine} + \text{FAD} + \text{H}_2\text{O} \longrightarrow \text{Pyruvic acid} + \text{NH}_3 + \text{FADH}_2$$

The reduced coenzyme (FADH$_2$) is oxidized by molecular oxygen to form hydrogen peroxide which is decomposed to water by catalase. A specific enzyme, glutamic dehydrogenase deaminates L-glutamic acid.

$$\text{Glutamate} + \text{NAD}^+ \xrightarrow{\text{L-Glutamate dehydrogenase}} \alpha\text{-Ketoglutarate} + \text{NH}_3 + \text{NADH}$$

The NADH is oxidized by the mitochondrial electron transport system and 2.5 moles of ATP are formed by oxidative phosphorylation.

Nonoxidative deamination: These reactions are catalyzed by amino acid dehydratase and also require vitamin B$_6$.

Serine $\longrightarrow$ Pyruvate + NH_4^+

Threonine $\longrightarrow$ α-Ketoglutarate + NH_4^+

Aspartic acid $\longrightarrow$ Fumaric acid + NH_4^+

Decarboxylation of amino acids: It involves enzymes found especially in liver, kidney and brain, that decarboxylate amino acids. The reaction produces carbon dioxide and primary amines called **biogenic amines**. A general aromatic L-amino acid decarboxylase can decarboxylate histidine to histamine, tyrosine to tyramine, dopa (3, 4-dihydroxy phenylalanine) to dopamine (hydroxytyramine), 5-hydroxy tryptophan to 5-hydroxy-tryptamine (serotonin), although there appear to be specific decarboxylases also.

Synthesis of Dispensable Amino Acids

The most abundant free amino acids in cells are alanine, aspartic acid and glutamic acid. Glutamic acid makes an effective source of nonspecific nitrogen. Alanine is chiefly formed by transamination of pyruvate and decarboxylation of aspartate. Aspartic acid is formed by transamination of oxaloacetate and hydrolysis of asparagine. Transamination of α-ketoglutarate yields glutamic acid. It is a precursor of proline, hydroxyproline and ornithine.

Serine $\leftrightarrow$ Glycine

Because of this efficient interconversion, the dietary requirement for glycine can be fulfilled by serine and vice versa. Thus the requirement is expressed as glycine plus serine. They can also be synthesized during threonine catabolism.

Serine + methionine yields cysteine. Glutamate + 3-phosphoglycerate yields serine. Tyrosine and cysteine are derived from phenylalanine and methionine, respectively. If the diet contains sufficient tyrosine and cysteine, the levels of phenylalanine and methionine (indispensable amino acids) in the diet can be reduced. With an adequate supply of amino nitrogen and a source of carbon and energy, the dispensable amino acids (which make up almost 40% of tissue protein) in short supply are synthesized to make up the deficit.

Disposal of Excess Amino Acids

The extra amino acids are promptly metabolized often within hours. The ammonia is converted to urea in the liver and excreted. Most **terrestrial vertebrates** excrete ammonia as urea in the urine, **fowl and land-based reptiles** excrete it as uric acid, **most fishes** excrete ammonia directly through the gill tissue into their water environment. In **fowl**, uric acid is synthesized, from glutamine, glycine and aspartic acid with the help of xanthine oxidase. Urea is not synthesized in birds. The only urea in chicken urine comes from the breakdown of dietary arginine.

Urea is formed in the liver through Krebs-Henseleit cycle. This is an energy requiring process. Note that both the amino groups found in the urea molecule came from glutamate one from oxidative deamination and

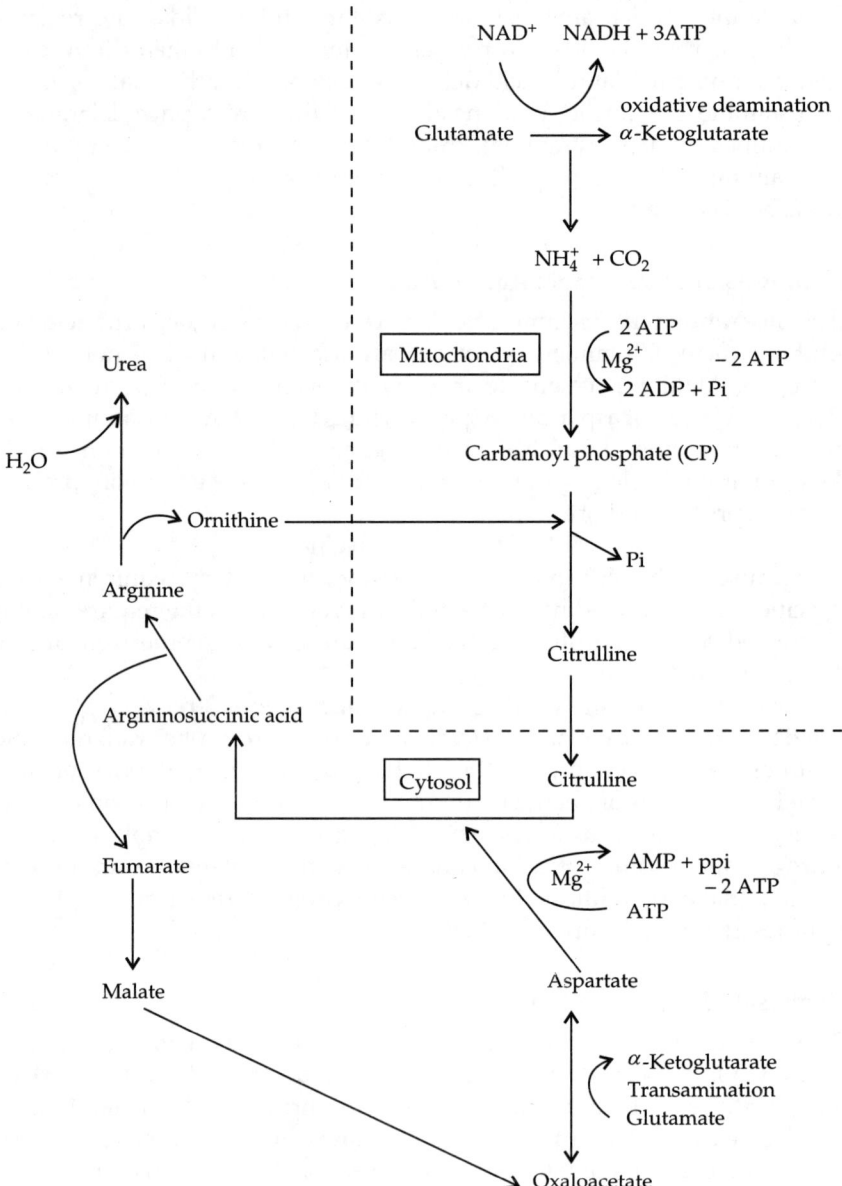

Figure 2. Formation of Urea and integration of Urea cycle & TCA cycle.

the other from transamination (Fig. 2).

The following steps are involved in the urea cycle.

1. Formation of carbamoyl phosphate (CP). Enzyme required is carbamoyl phosphate synthetase.
2. Formation of citrulline from CP and ornithine. Enzyme is ornithine— carbamoyl transferase.
3. Formation of argininosuccinate and arginine. A second amino group is transferred from aspartic acid to carbamoyl keto group of citrulline, to produce argininosuccinate. Enzyme needed is argininosuccinate synthetase. Argininosuccinase cleaves argininosuccinate to give arginine and fumarate.
4. In the presence of an enzyme, arginase and magnesium, arginine yields one molecule of urea and of ornithine. The regenerated ornithine can participate in the next turn of the cycle. There is a net loss of 1 ATP per mole of urea synthesized from glutamic acid.

Ornithine and citrulline are basic amino acids (They are never found in protein structure due to lack of codons).

Metabolic precursors of the nitrogen in the purine ring of uric acid-two of these arise from the amide N of glutamine and the other two from the amine groups of glycine and aspartic acid. Glutamine is the carrier of ammonia from deamination of amino acids.

The purines and pyrimidines absorbed from the intestines can be used for the synthesis of nucleotides and nucleic acids. Purine compounds which are degraded in the tissue are readily reused. When excreted they are converted to uric acid in primates, to allontoin in most mammals, and to urea in fish. Pyrimidines are excreted as urea and ammonia.

Fate of Carbon Skeletons of Amino Acids

The carbon skeletons of the amino acids which have lost their amino groups enter the citric acid cycle. All the amino acid residues which do not enter at either acetyl CoA or acetoacetate have the potential of being converted to glucose in the process of gluconeogenesis. These are called **glucogenic**. Those entering at acetyl CoA or acetoacetate could provide ketones. Those are referred to as **ketogenic**. Some are referred to as both glucogenic and ketogenic (Table 1).

Catabolism of Tissue Protein and Amino Acids

The protein mass of the body, like the adipose mass, is in a continuous state of flux, with tissues constantly being catabolized and resynthesized. As amino acids are released they become available to the general amino

TABLE 1. Fates of Carbon Skeletons of Common Amino Acids.

Glucogenic	Ketogenic	Both glucogenic and ketogenic
Alanine	Leucine	Isoleucine
Arginine	Lysine	Leucine
Aspartic acid		Lysine
Cystine		Phenylalanine
Glutamic acid		Tyrosine
Glycine		
Histidine		
Hydroxy proline, proline		
Methionine		
Serine		
Threonine		
Tryptophan		
Valine		

acid pool and can either be reused for protein synthesis or utilized as a source of energy. Two types of catabolism are observed-one a normal function of tissue maintenance and renewal, and the other that follows periods of undernutrition/starvation.

Why Should there be a Continuous Turnover or Protein renewal?

As protein synthesis requires energy, it would appear that the protein renewal to be wasteful. Yet this continuous turnover of tissue protein represents changing environment. With a continuing protein turnover capability, **the animal has the means, flexibility** and **speed to adapt to certain subtle or gross changes in its environment** which, in the long run, may affect its ability to survive. The rate of turnover is not similar for all tissues. **Renewal of intestinal mucosa is extremely rapid.** During periods of undernutrition/starvation, tissues lose their protein and release amino acids. About one fourth of the body protein especially liver, muscle are depleted and repleted. In general the integrity of brain and kidney are maintained. Thus, due to this property, the vital functions may be protected up to 30-50 days of total starvation.

During starvation or fasting, the primary need is energy, particularly glucose. This is met through glucogenic amino acids such as alanine and glutamine.

Utilization of Nonprotein Nitrogen (NPN) by Ruminants and Nonruminants

The place of nonprotein nitrogen (NPN) in ruminant nutrition had its origin in 1879 in Germany and entered the United States with conduct of feeding trials at Wisconsin in 1939. In 1891 **Zuntz** reported that rumen bacteria use, by preference, amides, amino acids and ammonium salts instead of protein. Later, **Fingerling and coworkers** in 1937 produced clear evidence that urea can be utilized to supply a part of the protein needs for growth of ruminants. Some important NPN compounds are listed in Table 2.

TABLE 2. Some Important NPN Compounds other than Amino Acids.

Amides	Amines	Alkaloids	Others
Asparagine	Betaine	Cocaine	Ammonia
Glutamine	Histamine	Morphine	Nitrates
		Nicotine	Nucleic acids
Urea	Tryptamine	Solanine	Purines
	Tyramine	Strychnine	Pyrimidines
			Uric acid

Ruminants do not need to compete with humans or nonruminants for protein because they have the unique ability, thanks to presence of millions of microbes in the rumen, to convert NPN compounds in the feed to microbial protein. The NPN compounds include urea, biuret, dicyanodiamide, ammonium salts. Dicyanodiamide has 66 per cent N or 412 per cent CP. But it is not well utilized by ruminants. Biuret contains not less than 35% N. It is quite costly although it is palatable and less toxic. Urea is the most widely used NPN compound in ruminant rations. **Fertilizer grade urea** is used in feeding since **feed grade urea** is not available in India.

Characteristics of Urea

1. It is deficient in all minerals.
2. It contains no methionine and cystine and thus it is deficient in sulphur in contrast to natural protein.
3. It has no energy value of its own.
4. It is extremely soluble and is converted to ammonia in the rumen quickly. If fed in large amounts, it results in sufficient ammonia release to cause a fatal toxicity.

How is Urea Utilized by Ruminants?

1. Urea is hydrolyzed to ammonia and carbon dioxide by the urease enzyme.
2. Microbial fermentation of carbohydrates (primarily) yield volatile fatty acids and keto acids.
3. Rumen bacteria use ammonia and keto acids to synthesize amino acids which are linked through peptide bonds and thus proteins are synthesized.

4. This microbial protein is digested in abomasum and small intestine and the host animal obtains amino acids.
5. The host ruminant builds body protein from the microbial amino acids.

Optimum utilization of urea requires source of sulphur, phosphorus, etc. and these factors are described hereunder.

Factors Affecting Urea Utilization

1. Addition of sulphur to urea supplemented diets to make the N : S ratio as 10 : 1 improves utilization of urea.
2. Addition of methionine also improves the urea utilization.
3. The nature and quantities of carbohydrates in the ration:
   The rumen bacteria must have a readily available source of energy synchronizing the release of ammonia from urea hydrolysis. Molasses, starch and cellulose were tested for their efficiency as energy source. Starch has been found to be the best though molasses as a source of soluble carbohydrates provide energy instantly. A level of 1 kg of starch per 100 g of urea is often suggested as a guide line.
4. Low levels of urea are better.
5. Feeding frequently improves the utilization of urea.
6. Using urea in complete diet dilutes the total amount of urea in the diet and thus helps in preventing development of a high peak of rumen ammonia. This increases the efficiency of urea utilization.
7. It is also important that the other ingredients of the diet are not too high in NPN compounds which otherwise total ammonia release could be excessive for maximum efficiency.
8. When the amount of protein in the basal ration is increased, the ability to utilize urea nitrogen decreases. The urea is very poorly utilized when it is added to concentrate mixtures containing greater than 18% CP and complete diets containing greater than 13% CP.
9. The nature of the protein in the ration may affect the utilization of urea nitrogen. The presence of highly soluble and easily hydrolyzable protein in the diet depresses urea utilization.

   Bacteria are unable to use ammonia effectively if rumen ammonia concentrations exceed 5 to 8 mg per 100 ml, a level generated by a 13% protein diet (Satter and Roffler, 1975). However, practical feeding trials indicate that urea may be well utilized in diets with above 13% CP.

10. Adaptation period: Rumen microorganisms must become adapted to dietary urea for a period of 2 to 4 weeks.

11. Age of the ruminant animal: The extent of development of the rumen and its bacterial population is related to the age of the animal. This undoubtedly influences the animal's ability to utilize urea. The usual period for the development of an effective flora in the rumen is from 6-12 weeks. The nature of the diet has a great influence on the development of the functional rumen.

NPN is of little practical value for nonruminants. It is ineffective for swine. It is used to some extent by mature horses on lowprotein diets. It can be used for synthesis of dispensable amino acids for hen fed diets well balanced in the essential amino acids.

Use of Molasses in Feeding of Livestock and Poultry

Molasses is used for animal feeding mainly in three different ways:

1. As part of concentrate mixture as an energy source and sweetening agent to enhance palatability of feeds (masking the bitter taste of unconventional feeds), molasses is added up to 10% in concentrate mixtures for livestock and up to 5% in case of poultry. Molasses is used as binder for pelleting of feeds.
2. As a liquid feed supplement offered directly with urea and minerals or after spraying on roughages to ruminants.
3. As blocks where the molasses is solidified with a limited quantity of bran, protein supplement, urea and minerals.

Use of Urea in the Feeding of Ruminants

When urea is consumed by ruminants along with other feed ingredients, the urease enzyme from the rumen microbes and ensiled feeds or from legume seeds hydrolyze it to carbon dioxide and ammonia. The reaction is so quick that almost all of the urea may be hydrolyzed within a couple of hours. This reaction can be shown in the following way:

$$\text{Urea} + \text{Water} \xrightarrow{\text{Urease}} \text{Ammonia} + \text{Carbon dioxide}$$

Some part of the ammonia thus produced is used by the rumen microorganisms (primarily by rumen bacteria) for amino acid and protein synthesis which would be available to the host ruminant as microbial protein. Much of the ammonia may be absorbed from the rumen wall or pass down the tract before the microbes can incorporate it into their cell protein. The absorbed ammonia either goes into the synthesis of essential amino acids or is converted to urea again in the liver and excreted in urine or recycled into the rumen through saliva or directly through rumen wall.

Urea and crude protein: With 46% nitrogen, one kg urea is taken equivalent to 2.87 kg protein assuming complete conversion. The cost of one kg CP from urea is much cheaper than conventional protein supplements. It is, however, to be recognised that urea supplies only nitrogen whereas protein supplements such as GNC, cottonseed cake contain carbohydrates, true protein, fats, minerals, etc.

Level of urea: Results of research work have shown that urea can be successfully incorporated to the extent of 2-3% of the concentrate mixture (BIS recommended at 1% level) or 1% of the total dry matter fed (complete feed) or $\frac{1}{3}$ of protein requirement can be met by urea.

Methods to improve urea utilization: A large number of experiments have been conducted to find out ways to slow down the release of ammonia from urea inside the rumen in order to regulate the ammonia release and to minimise its losses. Some of the methods to improve urea utilization are as follows:

1. Inhibition of Urease Activity

Urea hydrolysis is decreased by inhibiting urease activity inside the rumen by using substances like barbituric acid, copper sulphate, neomycin sulphate, bacitracin. But none has proved entirely satisfactory.

2. Establishing Urease Immunity

Subcutaneous injection of jackbean urease has been tried by some workers to produce urease immunity. Urease antibodies in serum of animals 4 weeks after the first injection of jackbean urease have been demonstrated. This seems to be a promising method of inhibiting urease activity.

3. Use of Processing Techniques

(a) Extrusion cooking technology was used to produce slow release urea products.
(b) Uromol
(c) Urea-molasses blocks
(d) Urea-molasses liquid feed.

a. Slow Release Urea Products

These are prepared by cooking a mixture of starch and urea at optimum temperature, moisture and pressure and extruding the gelatinized product in the form of pellets. **Starea** is a product that was developed by **Bartley and coworkers** at Kansas State University, (USA) to improve urea utilization by ruminants. Starea is produced by mixing finely ground grains with urea. Other economical starch sources may also be used. Examples: Salseed meal, mangoseed kernel, tamarindseed meal. The ammonia release from such products (in the rumen) is lowered so that the ammonia is utilized by rumen microbes effectively. Several slow release products have been produced using SL-40 Cooker Extruder and evaluated *in vitro* and *in vivo* at College of Veterinary Science, Tirupati (A.P) under the leadership of Dr. D. Anjaneya Prasad.

b. Uromol

A urea-molasses complex named 'uromol' has been prepared by heating the two together for half an hour (chopra *et al.*, 1974).

c. Urea-molasses Blocks

The animals lick such block and meet part of their daily nutrient requirements. The level of urea used in these blocks is generally 10%, although higher levels have also been tried. Main problem with such blocks is the maintenance of consistency. If it is soft, animal consumes more material which may result in toxicity. If it is hard, animal may not get the required nutrients. Different binding materials have been tried such as quicklime, cement, dolomite, magnesium oxide and starch.

Cement and calcium oxide appear to be good binding materials. National Dairy Development Board, Anand, has popularised the blocks. They are called 'Buffalo Chocolates'.

Urea-molasses-mineral blocks: These can be prepared by hot process or cold process. The composition is as follows:

Molasses	-	45%
Urea	-	15
Min. mix	-	15
Cottonseed meal	-	10	Size = 245 × 150 × 65 mm
Salt	-	8	Weight = 3 kg
Calcite powder	-	4
Sod. bentonite	-	3
		100

d. Urea-molasses Liquid Feed

Preston *et al.* (1967) demonstrated that urea levels at 2 to 3% of molasses was safe for *ad libitum* feeding to cattle with restricted forage. Liquid molasses containing 2 to 3% of uniformly mixed urea fortified with minerals and vitamins is named as 'liquid feed'.

Preparation of liquid feed: The principle of urea-molasses liquid feed preparation is the homogenous mixing of urea in the liquid molasses.

Composition of 100 kg liquid feed:

Urea	-	2.5 parts
Fresh Water	-	2.5
Min. Mixture	-	2.0
Salt	-	1.0
Molasses	-	92.0
Vitablend (Vit. A and D_2)		25 g

Procedure: The urea is completely dissolved in the water and poured gradually over molasses with a simultaneous mixing. Powdered salt and mineral mixture and other additives are sprinkled over the molasses while mixing to ensure uniform distribution of all the additives in the liquid molasses. Special attention is required for the uniform mixing of urea solution. Heating of molasses is required during the winter season (due to higher viscosity) for thorough mixing. Undiluted urea-molasses liquid feed containing 65% and more of dry matter can be safely stored for long.

Urea-molasses feeding is a new system and sudden shift of animals from conventional feeding to liquid feeding may cause some digestive disturbances and animals may go off feed, or due to excessive intake molasses toxicity may take place. It is therefore advisable to introduce liquid feed gradually in the ration in about 15 days.

Economic Ration for a Milk Cow

Crossbred cows giving 7 to 8 litres of milk per day were fed on *ad lib.* urea-molasses liquid feed and 500g of fish meal (to supply intact protein) and chaffed green oats at the rate of 1 kg dry matter per 100 kg body weight. An example of urea-molasses liquid diet:

Molasses	84%
Bypass protein (Cottonseed meal)	10%
Urea	3%
Min. mixture	1%
Phosphoric acid	2%
Vitablend A, D_2	20 g

This was fed to buffaloes as a sustenance ration. This liquid diet was developed in I.V.R.I., Izatnagar (UP).

Use of Urea to Improve Nutritive Value of Straws

The straws and stovers are usually poor in nutritive value mainly due to their low crude protein content. Urea has been used extensively to improve the nitrogen content of these roughages.

1. Enrichment with Urea Alone

The recommended level of urea for enrichment of straw is 2 to 3%. Straw is spread on cemented floor or on a thick polythene sheet to a thickness of 3-4 inches. With the help of a gardener's sprayer, 2% solution of urea in water (2 kg urea in 98 litres of water) is sprayed on straw and the sprayed straw is given turning every time. This enriched material is offered to ruminants. A major proportion of urea is in the free form and without readily available source of energy, it may result in toxicity.

2. Enrichment with Urea-molasses

Urea of 2 kg and 10 kg molasses are mixed together and dissolved in 100 litres of water. This mixture is sprayed on 100 kg of straw/bagasse and dried in the sun. This method provides nitrogen and a readily available source of energy to the rumen microbes for utilization of urea.

3. Urea-ammonia Treatment

One of the most promising methods of ammoniation is to use fertilizer grade urea as a solution (4-5% W/W) and preserve the sprayed material under air tight conditions for 3-4 weeks. (refer page no 504 for the detailed technique). Ammonia is an alternative to sodium hydroxide for treatment of poor quality roughages.

1. It does not leave residual alkali as NaOH.
2. It increases the N content of straw by 0.8 to 1.0 percentage units.

In the presence of moisture and the enzyme urease, urea is decomposed to form ammonia and carbon dioxide. The ammonia, as a weak alkali acts on alkali labile ester bonds of lignin-hemicellulose-cellulose linkages making cellulose and hemicellulose available. Further cellulose crystallinity is also decreased. Thus digestibility of straw is increased. With impregnated nitrogen from ammonia, the intake of treated straws is increased. Substantial increases in body weight gain and milk production have been reported in cattle and buffaloes fed with urea-ammonia treated straw.

Urea Toxicity

Excess urea is always toxic. The toxicity is mainly due to rapid formation of excess amounts of ammonia. This is due to sudden ingestion of about 116 g of urea by cattle or 10 g of urea by sheep. Eventually, the pH of the ruminal fluid increases, thus facilitating the passage of ammonia across the rumen wall. It has been reported that urea toxicity results from a grossly elevated rumen ammonia level (80 mg per 100 ml) which in turn causes blood ammonia to rise. If the level of ammonia absorbed is greater than the capacity of the liver to convert ammonia to urea, ammonia accumulates in the blood. When the level of ammonia exceeds 1 mg / 100 ml blood, the animal is under toxic condition.

Symptoms of ammonia toxicity may include tetany, respiratory difficulty, bloat, excessive salivation, ataxia, convulsions and bellowing. If it is not promptly treated, death will follow in 30 min. to 2.5 hours. The common treatment is drenching 20 to 40 litres of cold water which inhibits ureolytic activity in the rumen. Another approach is by drenching 4 to 5 litres of 10% acetic acid to neutralize the releasing ammonia.

Accidental Ingestion of Urea Kept in the Field for its Application

Clinical examination revealed subnormal body temperature, dyspnea, arrythmia, severe abdominal pain, incoordination accompanied with violent struggling and bellowing.

Serum urea N = 67 mg/dl and serum creatine = 4 mg/dl, a 3-fold rise is observed; rumen pH = 8.0. Treatment included oral administration of 2.5 litre of 5% acetic acid in the form of vinegar and after half an hour another one litre was administered with which animal recovered from the illness.

Chapter 10

Lipids-Their Digestion and Absorption in Nonruminants and Ruminants; Metabolism of Lipids

Digestion and Absorption of Lipids in Nonruminants and Birds

Following the nursing stage, the lipids make up only a small part of the diet of most animals, except humans and carnivores.

Dietary lipids consumed include triglycerides primarily, phospholipids and cholesterol. There appear to be no digestion of these lipids in the mouth. Although gastric juice contains a lipase, it is essentially inactive because of low pH of the stomach. This lipase may be much more important in the young ones where the gastric pH is higher and the fat of milk is highly emulsified. However, proteolytic activity in the stomach helps to release lipids from feed matrices; acid conditions and churning activity due to gastric motility serve to dispose the lipids into a **coarse emulsion**. Thus, dietary fat leaves the stomach in the form of relatively large globules that are difficult to hydrolyse rapidly. Fat hydrolysis is helped by emulsification and the emulsification is completed by the detergent action of bile acids and phospholipids.

The principal site of lipid digestion is the small intestine. Under the influence of the peristaltic action of the stomach, duodenum and presence of bile (bile salts and phospholipids) fat exists in the duodenum as a coarse emulsion of triglycerides. The contents are alkaline. Pancreatic lipase (Ca++ ions and bile salts increase its activity) and colipase hydrolyze the triglycerides into fatty acids and monoglycerides and reduce the lipid to a finer and **finer emulsion**.

Phospholipids (lecithins and cephalins) are preferentially hydrolyzed at the 2- position by phospholipase A_2 (from pancreas and small intestine) and lysophospholipase (from small intestine) to yield lysolecithins and free fatty acids. Cholesterol esterases (from pancreas and small intestine) catalyses the splitting of cholesterol esters. The nucleic acids DNA and RNA are hydrolysed by the polynucleotidases: deoxyribonuclease

(DNase; from pancreas and small intestine) and ribonuclease 1 (RNase; from pancreas and small intestine), respectively. These enzymes catalyse the cleavage of the ester bonds between the sugar and phosphoric acid in the nucleic acids. The end products are the component nucleotides. Nucleosidases (from small intestine) attack the linkage between the sugar and the nitrogenous bases, liberating the free purines and pyrimidines. Phosphatases (from small intestine) complete the hydrolysis by separating the orthophosphoric acid from the ribose or deoxyribose.

The primary object of lipid digestion and absorption is to arrange the lipid in a form that is water miscible since the microvilli of the small intestine are often covered with an aqueous layer. The products of hydrolytic lipid digestion combine with bile acids and phospholipids to form micelles. See 'lipid assimilation' in the new chapter 7.

The diameter of fat droplet is 5000 A° while micelle is 30 to 100 A°. Micelle, thus greatly increases the surface area for enzyme action. The micelle migrates to the brush border where it is disrupted. These micelle are readily absorbed by the approximately 1000 microvilli (brush border) of each villus in the intestinal mucosa.

All but the bile is absorbed into the mucosa by the time the ingesta reaches the mid jejunum. The bile remains in the lumen and eventually moves down the intestine to be reabsorbed in the ileum by an active transport. The bile be returned to the liver by the blood stream and resecreted. This cycle is known as **enterohepatic circulation.**

Small quantities of bile salts are not reabsorbed but enter the large intestine, where they are converted into products known as 'secondary bile salts' by anaerobic gut bacteria. Loss of this quantity of bile salts in the faeces is the only route for cholesterol excretion from the body. These non-polar lipids are surrounded by free cholesterol, phospholipids and specific proteins called apoproteins (apo-B48, apo-AZ and apo-AIV).

Within the mucosa (endoplasmic reticulum of intestinal wall), the fatty acids and beta monoglycerides are resynthesized into triglycerides.

These triglycerides combine with cholesterol and phospholipid, "encased" in a thin layer of protein and secreted into the central lacteal of the villus as either chylomicron or very low density lipoproteins (VLDL) particles. The central lacteal drains into the lymph vessels and enters the general blood circulation via the thoracic duct at the right atrium. **Fatty acids of chain lengths below C_{12} are directly absorbed into the hepatic portal circulation.** Chylomicrons do not enter the portal blood directly because they are too large to pass through the endothelial membranes of blood capillaries. About 22-50% free glycerol, being soluble in water, is easily absorbed into the portal blood and carried to the liver. On a highfat meal, the lymph drainage appears milky due to the turbidity of the VLDL and chylomicrons.

The hydrolysis and resynthesis of triglycerides during the process of digestion and absorption produces similar but not identical triglyceride molecules in the lymph. For example, 78% of the glycerol is from the diet and 22% is synthesized *de novo*. About 88% of the fatty acids on the 1 and 3 carbon atoms and 75% on the 2 carbon atom were the same one as in the diet. The minor shifts result from translocation to and from the other positions

Both phospholipid and cholesterol are secreted in the bile in substantial quantities (In fact in humans, the amount is equivalent to 5 or 6 eggs per day). About 20% of the phospholipid is synthesized *de novo* within the intestinal mucosa.

In general, **absorbability (digestion and absorption) of fat depends upon its ability to participate in micelle formation**. Fat absorption is increased by phospholipid. Absorbability is superior with shorter chain length fatty acids, more unsaturated fatty acids and as triglycerides rather than free fatty acids.

Absorption of saturated fatty acids is greater when they are in the sn-2 position of triacylglycerols, because they are absorbed as the 2-monoacylglycerol after pancreatic lipase action. **Fatty acid digestibility increases somewhat with age** in both pigs and poultry; fat digestibility in young chicks in particular is quite poor because of the limited production of bile salts.

In avian species there is no lymphatic system. Lipid absorption occurs via the portal vein. and most of the fat is transported in the portal blood as low-density lipoproteins.

Most plant sterols such as ergosterol are not absorbed by animals. Vitamin D_2 (ergocalciferol) is readily absorbed. Dietary vitamin A esters are dehydrolyzed to the free vitamin and fatty acids in the small intestine. The vitamin appears to be reesterified within the intestinal wall and is absorbed in the lymph. Carotene that is not converted to vitamin A within the intestinal wall reaches the liver through the portal vein. Bile salts aid in the absorption of vitamin A esters, vitamins D, E and K.

Digestion and Absorption of Lipids in Ruminants

The presence of a **pregastric esterase** (secreted at the base of the tongue) gives the preruminant animal (calf, lamb, etc) a head start on lipid hydrolysis. Later part of assimilation of milk fat by the preruminant animal is considered to be essentially the same as that of a nonruminant.

The ruminant diet consists of a high proportion of unsaturated fatty acids (linolenic 53%, linoleic 13% and oleic acid 10%) found in the galactolipids of forage and in the triglycerides of cereal grains, oilseed cakes, etc. The rumen microbial population (*Anaerovibrio lipolytica, Butyrivibrio fibrisolvens, Selenomonas ruminantium*, etc.) promptly hydrolyze the galactolipids and triglycerides, release free fatty acids and allow the glycerol and galactose to be fermented to VFA.

The capacity of rumen microorganisms to digest lipids is strictly limited. **The lipid content of average ruminant diets is 3-5% on DMB.** If it is increased above 10% the activities of rumen microbes are reduced, the fermentation of fibre is retarded (since fatty acids are adsorbed on their surface) and feed intake falls.

Change of Lipids in the Rumen (Hydrogenation and Rumen Synthesis of Fatty Acids)

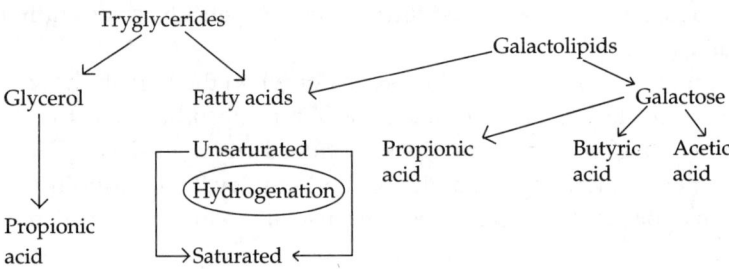

The intraruminal environment is a highly reduced one and hence the liberated unsaturated fatty acids (linolenic, linoleic, oleic) may settle on surfaces of bacteria and feed particles (probably as calcium salts) and get hydrogenated to stearic acid. Some of the 'cis' double bonds are converted to 'trans' form. There is an accumulation of 'trans' forms relative to 'cis' and a portion of trans unsaturated acids (have higher melting points) are absorbed by the animal contributing to the generally higher melting point of ruminant fats.

As a consequence of ruminal hydrolysis and saturation of dietary unsaturated fatty acids, absorbed fatty acids do not resemble those consumed by the ruminant animal. The proportions of C 18:1 indicate that this is a major end product.

The rumen bacteria and protozoa are also capable of synthesizing a number of odd chain fatty acids from propionate and branch chain fatty acids from the carbon skeletons of amino acids-valine, leucine and isoleucine. Thus biohydrogenation of unsaturated fatty acids and rumen synthesis of fatty acids are responsible for higher stearic and oleic acids of ruminant depot fats and presence of branch chain and odd numbered (15-17 carbons) **fatty acids in tissues and milk of ruminants.**

All short chain fatty acids and VFA are largely absorbed through the rumen wall. Long chain fatty acids, mostly saturated pass along with rumen contents into abomasum where also the dead bodies of microbes reach and disintegrate releasing their lipids before the digesta enters the duodenum. **In the ruminant animal gastric lipolysis plays a negligible role** in hydrolysis of fatty acid esters, because numerous strains of ruminal microorganisms produce lipases that hydrolyse fatty acids before the esters reach the abomasum. **The contents of the duodenum and upper jejunum are more acidic in the ruminant,** not becoming alkaline until about three quarters of the way down the jejunum. These conditions indicate that there is little triglyceride available to be converted to monoglyceride (a potent emulsifying agent) and pancreatic lipase is less active in the duodenum and upper jejunum. However, active micelle formation of fatty acids does occur under the influence of bile salts primarily taurocholate and biliary and ingesta phospholipid, largely lecithin.

Although absorption of lipid does occur in the upper jejunum (about 20%), the large percentage is absorbed in the lower three quarters of the jejunum where the pancreatic phospholipase hydrolyze lecithin into a fatty acid and the highly polar lysolecithin, which further enhances micelle formation. Monoacylglycerols, which play an important role in the formation of mixed micelles in nonruminants, are replaced in ruminants by **lysophosphatidyl choline.** The bile salts are not absorbed in the jejunum, but continue to form micelles. Most bile salts are absorbed in the ileum and are returned to the liver to be reincorporated into the bile. In the intestinal mucosa, resynthesis of triglycerides and phospholipids occurs, so that the chylomicrons produced contain about three-fourths triglycerides, with the rest being largely phospholipid. The triglycerides contain largely stearic acid bound to α and α^1 positions of glycerol. Since the flow of fatty acids is more or less continuous with rumen outflow, the lymph draining the intestine is invariably milky. The particles are made up of about 75% in the VLDL fraction and 25% of chylomicrons which is about the reverse for the nonruminant.

As with the nonruminant the rate of absorption of fatty acids is less for the saturated acids. The lipid in the form of chylomicrons and VLDL is carried by the capillaries to the adipose tissue under the skin, in kidneys, in membranes surrounding the intestines, in muscle, etc. **The adipose tissue is extremely dynamic.** It has blood and nerve supply and thus the body fat is in a state of flux.

Fat Transport from Lymph to Tissues

The lipid in the form of chylomicrons and VLDL reaches blood from the lymph and it is carried by the capillaries to the adipose tissue. The VLDLs and chylomicrons do not penetrate the capillary wall. Hence, in plasma the tryglycerides of chylomicrons are hydrolyzed by the **lipoprotein lipase**, an enzyme bound to endothelial cells. The free fatty acids, glycerol, and cholesterol esters are released by the disintegration of the chylomicrons and the VLDL. The free fatty acids then either diffuse into the cells, where they combine with glycerol phosphate to form triacylglycerols once again in adipose, mammary and other cells, or they are transported in the plasma bound to albumin. The free fatty acids in plasma are taken up by many tissues and ultimately used as energy source.

   The lipids come from two sources: Chylomicrons and VLDLs that have entered the blood from the lymph, and from lipids produced in the liver (The liver cells in non-ruminants produce triacylglycerols from glucose, if its level is elevated even after formation of glycogen stores. In ruminants, **less glucose** is available for lipid synthesis in the liver).

Lipoproteins

Lipoproteins are macromolecules with a central core of triglycerides surrounded by cholesterol and its esters, phospholipid, mainly phosphatidyl choline and sphingomyelin, and a little protein the apoprotein. The three types of lipoprotein are designated as very low density lipoprotein (VLDL), low density lipoprotein (LDL) and high density lipoprotein (HDL). Lipoproteins are looked upon as transporters of triglycerides and cholesterol. LDL cholesterol is considered as bad cholesterol and HDL cholesterol is considered as good cholesterol.

   Dietary lipids are transported from the intestinal epithelial cells in the form of chylomicrons, and stored in adipose tissue as triacylglycerols. During the processing of chylomicrons, most of the dietary triacylglycerols are transferred to adipose tissue and dietary cholesterol is transferred to the liver. VLDL are so named because their lipid content is high relative to their protein content.

Characteristics of the Lipoproteins

Lipoprotein	Density g/ml	% protein
Chylomicrons	<0.95	1.5-2.0
VLDLs	<1.006	5-10
LDLs	1.006-1.063	10-25
HDLs	1.063-1.210	40-55

Biosynthesis of Fatty Acids: Precursors: Nonruminants

Whenever excess calories are consumed they are preferably converted to form liver and muscle glycogen. When these stores are full, fat is synthesized. In case of the nonruminant, the primary substance for fat synthesis is glucose which enters the glycolytic cycle and eventually becomes pyruvate. In times of sufficient food, there is ample oxaloacetate and pyruvate is diverted to acetyl CoA which is used for fat synthesis (Figure 1).

Acetyl CoA cannot penetrate the mitochondrial wall, whereas citrate can. Thus acetyl CoA condenses with oxaloacetate to form citrate, which then passes into the cytosol, where oxaloacetate is removed (enzyme is ATP citrate lyase) and thus acetyl CoA is available for fatty acid synthesis (Figure 1). The oxaloacetate is converted to malate (enzyme is NADP malate dehydrogenase) and to pyruvate and returns to the citric acid cycle.

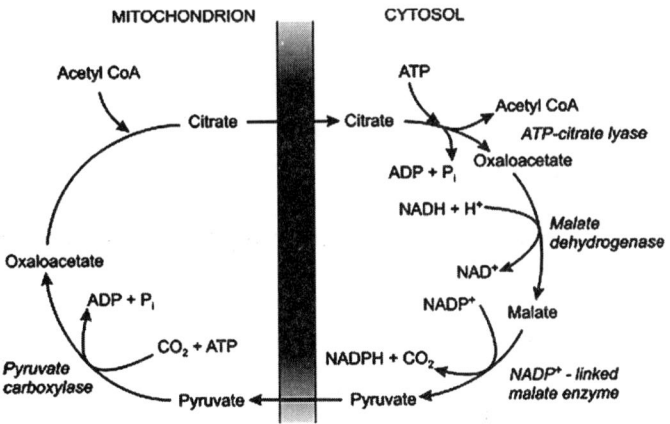

Figure 1 Transport of acety CoA from the mitochondrial matrix into the cytosol

Ruminants: In case of the ruminant, excess energy from the rumen exists primarily as acetate and butyrate. Propionate is preferentially diverted to glucose. The ruminant is unique in that it can not convert glucose to fat, the reason being ruminants do not have the two key enzymes (very low activity)-ATP citrate lyase and NADP malate dehydrogenase (malic enzyme).

Lipid Metabolism

Lipid catabolism

Triglycerides are first hydrolysed to yield fatty acids and glycerol. Glycerol is then converted to glyceraldehyde-3-phosphate, which may then be converted to glucose or it may enter the glycolytic pathway directly. Fatty acids are broken down by a process called β-oxidation into two-carbon pieces, the familiar acetyl-CoA. These molecules are then catabolized via the citric acid cycle. The final process of lipid catabolism therefore consists of the same reactions as does carbohydrate catabolism. Catabolism of lipids, however, yields considerably more energy than does catabolism of carbohydrates.

Lipid anabolism

Lipid anabolism (lipogenesis) consists of the synthesis of various types of lipids notably triglycerides, cholesterol, phospholipids and prostaglandins. Triglycerides and structural lipids (e.g., phospholipids) are synthesized from fatty acids and glycerol or from excess glucose or amino acids. So it is possible to "get fat" from foods other than fat. Triglycerides are stored mainly in adipose tissue cells. Most fatty acids can be synthesized by the body. Essential fatty acids must be provided by the diet.

Fat Synthesis

The glycerides (triacylglycerols) of the depot fat are derived from preformed glycerides or may be synthesized in the body from fatty acyl-CoAs and L-glycero-3-phosphate. This can takes place in most tissues but is confined mostly to the liver and adipose tissue.

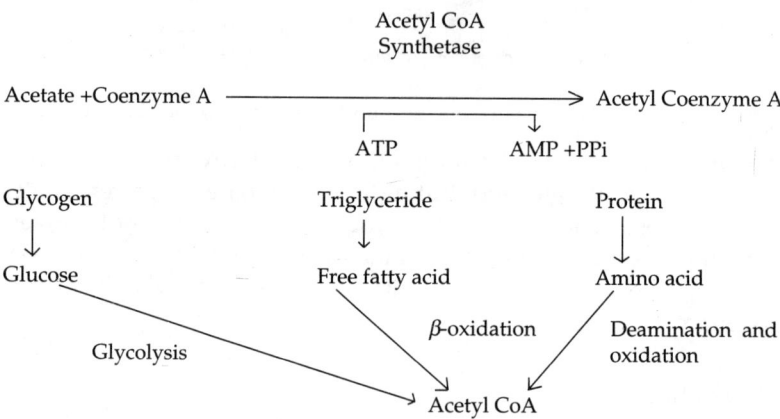

Thus acetyl CoA is the starting point and the chief source is pyruvate from carbohydrate metabolism in the nonruminants and acetate in the ruminants. There are three systems of fatty acid synthesis.

Three Systems of Fatty Acid Synthesis

1. **Cytosolic synthesis of palmitate from acetyl coenzyme A :** It is active in liver, kidney, brain, lungs, mammary gland and adipose tissue. The synthesis of long-chain fatty acids (lipogenesis) is carried out by **two enzyme systems:** Acetyl-CoA carboxylase and fatty acid synthase. Acetyl-CoA carboxylase converts acetyl-CoA to malonyl-CoA. Cofactors required are NADPH, ATP, Mn^{+2} and HCO_3^- (as a source of CO_2).

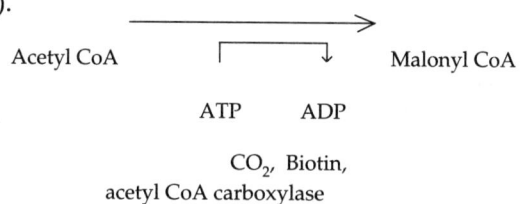

Fatty acid synthase is a multienzyme complex of one polypeptide chain with seven separate enzymatic activities that extends acyl-ACP chains by two carbons at a time. It catalyses the formation of palmitate from one acetyl-CoA and seven malonyl-CoA molecules.

Malonyl-CoA reacts with acyl-carrier protein (ACP), in the presence of malonyl-CoA-ACP transacylase, to give the malonyl-ACP complex. Acetyl-CoA is then coupled with ACP in the presence of acetyl-CoA-ACP transacylase, and this (Acetyl-ACP) reacts with the malonyl-ACP, the chain length being increased by two carbon atoms to give the butyryl-ACP complex. The butyryl-ACP complex then reacts with malonyl-ACP complex, resulting in further elongation of the chain by two carbon atoms to give caproyl-ACP. Chain elongation takes place by successive reactions of the fattyacyl-ACP complexes with malonyl-CoA until the palmitoyl-ACP complex is produced and the chain elongation ceases. These steps resemble the reverse of β-oxidation but are catalyzed by separate enzymes in the cytosol. Palmitic acid is liberated by the action of a specific deacylases. The overall reaction is as follows:

1 mole acetyl CoA + 7 moles malonyl CoA + 14 NADPH + $14H^+$
$\rightarrow$ Palmitate + 7 CO_2 + 14 $NADP^+$ + 6 H_2O + 8 coenzyme A

(2) Elongation and (3) Desaturation of Fatty Acids

Mitochondrial elongation Vs endoplasmic reticulum elongation: Palmitate (a saturated C16 fatty acid) is converted to longer chain saturated and unsaturated fatty acids through the actions of elongases and desaturases. Elongases are present in both the mitochondria and the endoplasmic reticulum, but the mechanisms of elongation at the two sites differ.

Mitochondrial elongation (a process independent of the fatty acid synthase pathway in the cytosol) occurs by the successive addition and reduction of acetyl units in a reversal of fatty acid oxidation; the only chemical difference between the two pathways occurs in the final reduction step in which NADPH takes the place of $FADH_2$ as the terminal redox coenzyme. Elongation in the endoplasmic reticulum involves the successive condensations of malonyl-CoA with acyl-CoA. These reactions are each followed by NADPH-dependent reductions similar to those catalyzed by fatty acid synthase, the only difference being that the fatty acid is elongated as its CoA derivative rather than as its ACP derivative.

Unsaturated fatty acids are produced by terminal desaturases. Mammalian systems contain four terminal desaturases of broad chain-length specificities designated Δ^9-, Δ^6-, Δ^5-, and Δ^4-**fatty acyl-CoA desaturases.** Stearic acid is converted to oleic acid; $\Delta9$ desaturase is the enzyme. In animals, double bonds are never inserted at positions beyond C9. Since animals have a $\Delta9$ desaturase, they are able to synthesize the ω9 (oleic acid) family of unsaturated fatty acids completely by a combination of chain elongation and desaturation. However, linoleic (ω6) or α-linolenic (ω3) acids required for the synthesis of other members of the ω6 or ω3 families must be supplied in the diet.

Sources of NADPH

(1) NADPH are obtained from Pentose Phosphate Pathway; chief source of hydrogen required for the reductive synthesis of fatty acids. Both the processes occur in cytosol.

(2) Reaction that converts malate to pyruvate catalyzed by the 'malic enzyme' (NADP malate dehydrogenase) and

(3) the extramitochondrial isocitrate dehydrogenase reaction (important in ruminants). There are means to transfer reducing equivalents from extramitochondrial NADH to NADP.

NADPH for the dienoyl-CoA reductase step is supplied by intramitichondrial sources such as glutamate dehydrogenase, isocitrate dehydrogenase and NAD(P)H transhydrogenase.

Fat Synthesis from fatty acyl-CoAs and L-glycero-3-phosphate

Direct synthesis of triacylglycerols (triglycerides) from monoacyl-glycerols takes place in the intestinal mucosa of higher animals.

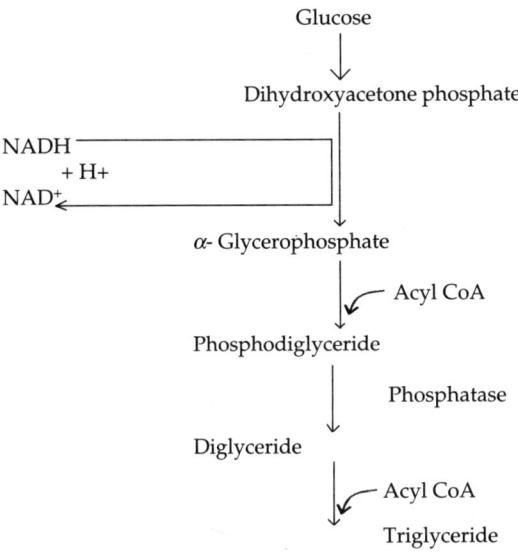

Glyceroneogenesis is important for Triacylglycerol Biosynthesis. The dihydroxyacetone phosphate used to make glycerol-3-phosphate for triacylglycerol synthesis comes either from glucose via the glycolytic pathway or from oxaloacetate via an abbreviated version of gluconeogenesis termed glyceroneogenesis.

Glyceroneogenesis is necessary in times of starvation, since approximately 30% of the fatty acids that enter the liver during fasting are re-esterified to triacylglycerol and exported in VLDL. Adipocytes also carry out glyceroneogenesis in times of starvation. They do not carry out gluconeogenesis but contain the gluconeogenic enzyme phosphoenolpyruvate carboxykinase (PEPCK), which is upregulated when the glucose concentration is low and participates in the glyceroneogenesis required for triacylglycerol biosynthesis.

At this point, we can appreciate how triacylglycerols synthesized from fatty acids built from two-carbon acetyl units can be broken back down into acetyl units. In the liver, the resulting acetyl-CoA may be shunted to the formation of ketone bodies and later converted back to acetyl-CoA by another tissue. The acetyl-CoA can then either be used to build fatty acids that are stored as triaclglycerols or be oxidized by the citric acid cycle to generate considerable ATP by oxidative phosphorylation. As we will see, the flux of material in the direction of triacylglycerol synthesis or triacylglycerol degradation depends on the metabolic energy needs of the organism and the need for synthesis of other compounds, such as membrane lipids and cholesterol. These key features of lipid metabolism are summarized in Figure 2.

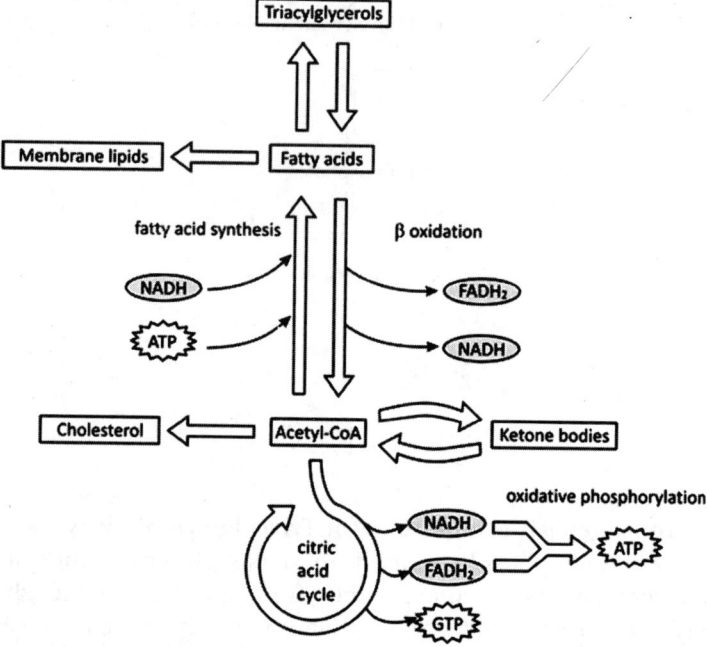

Figure 2   A summary of lipid metabolism. Source: Principles of Biochemistry, International Student Version, 4th edition, Wiley Plus; 2013, pp691

Effect of Food fat on Body fat

The fat in animals synthesized from carbohydrates contains about two-thirds unsaturated fatty acids. However, the fat deposited in the adipose tissue arises not only from carbohydrates, but also from the fatty acids of dietary fat. Thus, in nonruminants, the composition of the depot fat can be considerably altered by the character of the dietary fat while it is not in ruminants. **Let us examine the effect of food fat on the nature of body fat deposited in these two categories of animals.**

Nonruminants

Depot fats are formed from ingested fats and carbohydrates. That is why the nature of the fat deposited can be markedly affected by the character of its food source. The influence of the kind of the food fat upon the character of the body fat is striking-iodine number of food fat is proportional to that of body fat. When the ration contains much unsaturated fatty acids in the form of oils, the body fat is also soft, i.e. of low melting point (higher iodine number).

Adipose tissue is not static and there is a constant exchange of fatty acids between the body fat and fat in the blood. Hence deposits of soft fat can be modified by a change in diet. When a ration which will produce a hard fat is given after a period on feeds rich in unsaturated fat, the deposited fat gradually becomes harder. This process is called "**hardening off**". It is noted that rations containing cottonsed oil produce lard (pig fat) graded as hard, and those rich in highly unsaturated fats, e.g. maize oil or soybean oil produce soft lard. The "hardening off" process is taken advantage of in feeding practice in finishing pigs for market. Anderson and Mendel (1928) showed that the process takes place more rapidly where the animal was fasted for a period before the hardening ration was given.

Ruminants

In contrast to nonruminants, the fatty acid composition of adipose tissue in ruminants is not markedly affected by the fatty acid composition of the diet. There is intense biohydrogenation of dietary unsaturated fatty acids in the rumen due to its highly reduced environment. Less than 10% of the PUFA usually escape hydrogenation. Any attempt to increase the level of unsaturated fatty acids in the milk fat or adipose tissue by feeding them at high levels would not be fruitful. However, nothing is rarely 100% in biology. The rumen microflora are apparently rapidly able to hydrogenate only one double bond. That is complete hydrogenation is not there. Incomplete biohydrogenation of dietary PUFA also produce conjugated linoleic acid (see page 67) isomers. Ruminant body fat is rich in stearic acid, oleic acid and CLA. Ruminant body fat has high melting point and higher 'trans' fatty acids.

Conjugated linoleic acid has potentially beneficial attributes on human health. Humans do not have the ability to synthesize CLA and must obtain it from the diet. Ruminant milk and meat are good sources of CLA containing about 0.5–1.5% of total fatty acids. In recent years there have been numerous studies in ruminants on increasing CLA content using a dietary supplement of vegetable oils rich in C 18:2 (sunflower oil) and other PUFA-rich oils, such as rapeseed oil and linseed oil. Supplementation with vegetable oils reduced milk fat concentration of saturated fatty acids. Supplementation with sunflower and linseed oils increased both rumenic (18:2 cis-9, trans-11) and vaccenic acids (18:1 trans-11) in milk of cows and linseed oil appeared better.

Concept of Feeding Protected Lipids to Ruminants

It may be needed to feed high level of fat to ruminant animals especially high yielding dairy cows to meet their high energy requirements. But as it has been discussed elsewhere (p. 230), high level of fat depress fibre digestion and affect rumen fermentation. So to avoid such undesirable effects fat has been 'protected' in the rumen from getting fermented and thus made rumen 'inert'.

Australian workers (Scott and Cook, 1975) developed a procedure of encapsulating small droplets of lipid in a thin layer of protein. By treating the protein with formaldehyde, the droplet avoids attack by rumen microorganisms but is released by the acidic and proteolytic conditions of the abomasum. The lipid is thus available for digestion and absorption as with the nonruminant. In spite of the conditions of the duodenum which mediate against fat hydrolysis, digestion and absorption of 'protected lipid' is highly efficient.

Methods to produce rumen inert fatty acids

Over the year several methods have been developed to produce rumen inert fatty acids. Example: Prilled fatty acids, calcium salt of fatty acids. Calcium salts of fatty acids are the most commonly used as they are cheaper and more effective.

Prilled fatty acids: Saturated fatty acids are liquified and by spraying the solution under pressure into a cooled atmosphere dried prilled fatty acids are produced.

Calcium salts of fatty acids: These are produced by double decomposition method and fusion method. Double decomposition method was used by T.C. Jenkins and D.L. Palmquist in 1984 and the technique was standardized in 1999 by Dr. N. Krishna, Dr. Y. Ramana Reddy and coworkers at College of Veterinary Science, Hyderabad, Andhra Pradesh using locally available vegetable oil sources.

Double decomposition method: Here the fat source is heated in a metal container and aqueous sodium hydroxide solution is added to the melted fat source with constant stirring till the fatty acids are dissolved. Calcium chloride solution is added slowly with constant stirring, while the contents are still warm. This causes precipitation of calcium soaps. The calcium soap is dried at low temperature and is ground before mixing in the ration.

Fusion method: Oils and fatty acids are heated with calcium oxide or calcium hydroxide in the presence of catalyst in a closed vessel at a required temperature and pressure. It is a single step method. A hard mass of calcium saponified salt is obtained. Prafulla Kumar Naik et al (2007) developed a simple technology for the preparation of calcium salts of long chain fatty acids.

Following feeding of unsaturated fats in a protected form there is a prompt rise in the degree of unsaturation of the serum lipids, tissue fat and milk fat. In many cases milk yield is increased.

Clearly, the means for altering the fatty acid composition of animal fats (ruminant and nonruminant) are available should it be economically feasible to do so for the benefit of health conscious consumers.

Catabolism of Fat and Fatty Acids

The end result of catabolism of fats and fatty acids is the production of ATP, CO_2 and H_2O with the liberation of excess heat. The initial degradation of fat leads to the formation of glycerol and acetyl CoA. In the ruminant, absorbed acetate, butyrate and ketone bodies are also available for immediate catabolism. When the triacylglyceros are hydrolysed within adipose tissue, the free fatty acids (FFA) or non-esterified fatty acid (NEFA) are available to adipose cells for the resynthesis and storage of lipids as triacylglycerol. In other organs, such as skeletal muscle, cells use the FFA for energy.

Mobilization and Oxidation of Fat

It is well known that between meals the blood free fatty acid levels are elevated as a result of the mobilization of fat. Upon eating, they drop promptly. Triglycerides are released from the adipose tissue under hormonal control by triacylglycerol lipase enzyme. This enzyme is named **as hormone-sensitive triacylglycerol lipase** because it is susceptible to regulation by phosphorylation and dephosphorylation in response to hormonally controlled cAMP levels. Triglyceride gives glycerol and fatty acid.

Glycerol Metabolism

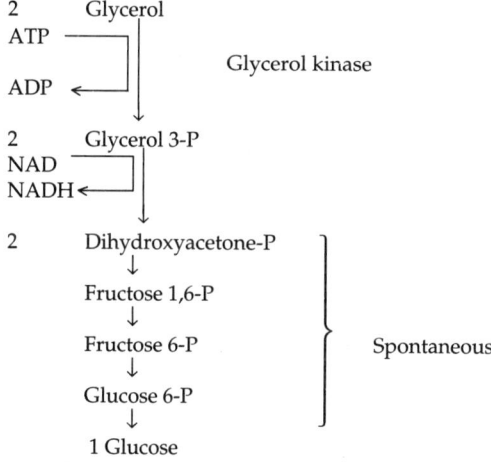

ATP yield from one mole of glycerol

Attributes	ATP +	ATP-
2 moles glycerol to 2 moles dihydroxyacetone phosphate	5	2
2 moles dihydroxyacetone phosphate to 1 mole glucose	-------	-------
1 mole glucose to $CO_2 + H_2O$	30 or 32	-------
Total	35 or 37	2
Net gain of ATP per mole of glycerol	16.5 or 17.5	------

If dihydroxyacetone phosphate enters the glycolytic pathway and metabolized via pyruvate and the TCA cycle to carbon dioxide and water, the ATP yields differs. See below

Attributes	ATP +	ATP-
1 mole glycerol to 1 mole dihydroxyacetone phosphate	2.5	1
1 mole dihydroxyacetone phosphate to 1 mole pyruvate	4.5	-------
1 mole pyruvate to $CO_2 + H_2O$	12.5	-------
Total	19.5	1
Net gain of ATP per mole of glycerol	18.5	-------

β-Oxidation of Fatty Acids occurs in Mitochondria

The fatty acids in the body are mostly oxidized by β-oxidation. β-oxidation may be defined as the oxidation of fatty acids on the β-carbon atom. Franz Knoop proposed this in 1904 and the Knoop's hypothesis was confirmed only by 1950. Shorter-chain fatty acids are more water soluble and exist as the un-ionized acid or as a fatty acid anion. Longer-chain free fatty acids are combined with an albumin and circulate as an albumin-fatty acid complex.

In the cell, fatty acid oxidation begins in the extramitochondrial cytoplasm with the formation of fatty acyl CoA (Fatty acid + coenzyme A → fatty acyl CoA). This fatty acid activation needs the enzyme **acyl-CoA synthetase (thiokinase)** and uses one high-energy phosphate with the formation of AMP and PPi. Acyl-CoA synthetases are found in the endoplasmic reticulum, peroxisomes, and inside and on the outer membrane of mitochondria. Longer-chain acyl-CoA will not penetrate the inner membrane of mitochondria. Fatty acyl CoA needs a special carrier mechanism in the form of carnitine to pass into the mitochondrion.

Carnitine (β-hydroxyl-γ-trimethylammonium butyrate) is widely distributed and is particularly abundant in muscle. Carnitine palmitoyl transferase-I (present in outer mitochondrial membrane) and carnitine palmitoyltransferase-II (inner mitochondrial membrane) help in transit of acetyl-CoA to mitochondrial matrix, where it is reesterified to CoA (and carnitine is liberated).

In the mitochondria, β oxidation occurs in four reactions: (1) formation of an α, β double blond, (2) hydration of the double bond, (3) dehydrogenation to form a β-ketoacyl-CoA, and (4) thiolysis by CoA to produce acetyl-CoA and an acyl-CoA shortened by two carbons. This process is repeated until fatty acids with even numbers of carbon atoms are converted to acetyl-CoA. The acetyl-CoA is oxidized by the citric acid cycle and oxidative phosphorylation to generate ATP. The steps in case of palmitic acid are as follows:

	Earlier ATP	Updated ATP yield
Palmitic to Palmityl CoA	–2	–2
Palmityl CoA → 8 acetyl CoA		
(7 cleavages × 5)	+35	7×4 = 28
8 acetyl CoA → 16 H_2O + 16 CO_2		
8 × 12	+96	8×10= 80
	129/mole	106*

*as per the recent findings

The acetyl CoA that is formed here may also follow the below mentioned fates.

1. It may condense to form acetoacetate and ketone bodies.
2. It may be converted to malonyl CoA as in fatty acid synthesis.
   or
3. It may react with acetoacetyl units in sterol synthesis.

Fatty acids with odd numbers of carbon atoms are converted to acetyl-CoAs and one molecule of propionyl-CoA. Propionyl-CoA is converted to the citric acid cycle intermediate succinyl-CoA, in part, by the coenzyme B_{12}-containing enzyme methylmalonyl-CoA mutase; or it may follow the lipid pathway by converting into melonyl CoA.

Importance of Carnitine in Fatty Acid Oxidation

Dairy ruminants are susceptible to a number of metabolic disorders and infectious diseases during the periparturient period. An increased understanding of lipid metabolism may allow the development of nutritional and management approaches to prevent the development of metabolic disorders in dairy cows. Hepatic oxidation of long-chain fatty acids occurs in mitochondria and peroxisomes (Drackley et al., 2001). L-Carnitine is required for mitochondrial fatty acid oxidation.

J.K. Drackley and coworkers from Department of Animal Sciences, University of Illinois, Urbana (USA) conducted several studies in dairy cows. In cows fed for *ad libitum* intake, carnitine abomasal infusion (20 g/d) influenced hepatic and peripheral nutrient metabolism. L-Carnitine abomasal infusion effectively decreased liver lipid accumulation during feed restriction as a result of greater capacity for hepatic fatty acid oxidation.

Peroxisomal β Oxidation

In mammalian cells, the bulk of oxidation occurs in the mitochondria, but peroxisomes also oxidize fatty acids, particularly those with very long chains or branched chains. Peroxisomal oxidation shortens very long chain fatty acids (> 22 carbon atoms), which are then fully degraded by the mitochondrial pathway. In plants, fatty acid oxidation occurs exclusively in the peroxisomes and glyoxysomes (which are specialized peroxisomes). In addition to lipid catabolism, mammalian peroxisomes participate in the synthesis of certain lipids, including bile acids.

Peroxisomal β Oxidation differs only slightly from mitochondrial Oxidation. Very long chain fatty acids are transported into the peroxisomes by a mechanism that does not require carnitine. These fatty acids are activated by a long chain acyl-CoA synthetase. Peroxisomal oxidation results in the same chemical changes to fatty acids as in the mitochondrial pathway but requires only three enzymes: 1. Acyl-CoA oxidase catalyzes the reaction

$$\text{Fatty acyl-CoA} + O_2 \; trans\text{-} \; \Delta^2\text{-enoyl-CoA} + H_2O_2$$

The enzyme uses an FAD cofactor, but the abstracted electrons are transferred directly to O_2 rather than passing through the electron transport chain with its concomitant oxidative phosphorylation. Peroxisomal fatty acid oxidation therefore generates 1.5 fewer ATP per C_2

cycle than mitochondrial fatty acid oxidation. Catalase converts the H_2O_2 produced in the oxidase reaction to $H_2O + O_2$.

2.   Peroxisomal enoyl-CoA hydratase and 3-L-hydroxyacyl-CoA dehydrogenase activities occur on a single polypeptide. The reactions catalyzed are identical to those of the mitochondrial system.

3.   Peroxisomal thiolase catalyzes the final step of oxidation. This enzyme is almost inactive with acyl-CoAs of length C_8 or less, so peroxisomes incompletely oxidize fatty acids.

The peroxisome contains both a carnitine acetyltransferase and a transferase specific for longer chain acyl groups. Acyl-CoAs that have been chain-shortened by peroxisomal β oxidation are thereby converted to their carnitine esters. These substances, for the most part, passively diffuse out of the peroxisome to the mitochondrion, where they are oxidized further.

Oxidation of unsaturated fatty acids

Oxidation of unsaturated fatty acids occurs by a modified β-oxidation pathway. The oxidation of unsaturated fatty acids requires an isomerase to convert Δ^3 double bonds to Δ^2 double bonds and a reductase to remove Δ^4 double bonds. The oxidation of odd-chain fatty acids yields propionyl-CoA, which is converted to succinyl-CoA through a cobalamin (B_{12})-dependent pathway. Very long chain fatty acids are partially oxidized by a three-enzyme system in peroxisomes.

Comparison of fatty acid synthesis and oxidation

Fatty acids are oxidized to acetyl-CoA and synthesized from acetyl-CoA. However, fatty acid oxidation is not the simple reverse of fatty acid biosynthesis. It is an entirely different process taking place in a separate compartment of the cell. See the table 1 for comparison of synthesis and oxidation.

The opposing pathways of fatty acid degradation and synthesis are hormonally regulated. Glucagon and epinephrine and norepinephrine activate **hormone-sensitive lipase**, which causes lipolysis in adipose tissue, thereby increasing the supply of fatty acids for oxidation in other tissues (such as liver and muscle), and inactivate acetyl-CoA carboxylase. Here fatty acid oxidation is stimulated while inhibiting fatty acid synthesis. Insulin has the opposite effect; it stimulates the formation of glycogen and triacylglycerols. Insulin also regulates the levels of acetyl-

CoA carboxylase and fatty acid synthase by controlling their rates of synthesis. **The glucagon:insulin ratio therefore determines the rate and direction of fatty acid metabolism.**

TABLE 1   Comparison of fatty acid synthesis and oxidation

Site and process	Fatty acid synthesis	β-Oxidation
Major tissues	Liver, adipose tissue	Muscle, liver
Subcellular site	Cytosol	Mitochondria
Precursor / substrate	Acetyl CoA	Acyl CoA
End product	Palmitate	Acetyl CoA
Intermediates are bound to	Acyl carrier protein	Coenzyme A
Coenzyme requirement	NADPH (supplying reducing equivalents)	FAD and NAD$^+$ (get reduced)
Carbon units added/degraded	Malonyl CoA	Acetyl CoA
Transport system	Citrate (mitochondria to cytosol)	Carnitine (cytosol to mitochondria)
Inhibitor	Long chain acyl CoA (inhibits acetyl CoA carboxylase)	Malony CoA (inhibits carnitine acyl transferase I)
The pathway increased	After rich carbohydrate diet	In starvation
Hormonal status that promotes	High ratio of insulin/glucagon	Low rates of insulin/glucagon
Status of enzyme(s)	Multifunctional enzyme complex	Individual enzymes

Conversion of Fat into Glucose

Animals cannot convert fatty acids into glucose. Specifically, acetyl CoA cannot be converted into pyruvate or oxaloacetate in animals. The two carbon atoms of the acetyl group of **acetyl CoA enter the citric acid cycle, but two carbon atoms leave the cycle in the decarboxylations** catalyzed by isocitrate dehydrogenase and α-ketoglutarate dehydrogenase. Consequently, oxaloacetate is regenerated but it is not formed *de novo* when the acetyl unit of acetyl CoA is oxidized by the citric acid cycle. In contrast, plants have two additional enzymes enabling them to convert the carbon atoms of acetyl CoA into oxaloacetate via **glyoxylate cycle**. Anyway the glycerol moiety of fat can yield glucose and thus 'fat' can contribute somewhat to the glucose pool.

Interrelations among Fats, Proteins and Carbohydrates

The metabolism of fatty acids and that of carbohydrates and proteins are intimately related. The constituents are in a constant state of flux. Even the structural proteins, carbohydrates and storage lipids are constantly broken down and rebuilt (Figure. 3).

The status of a particular animal is the net result between the rates of synthesis and of breakdown of its body constituents. Glycerol is the only component of lipids that is involved in the synthesis of carbohydrates. On the other hand, lipids can be formed from carbohydrate in many ways. Indeed, the metabolism of lipids, carbohydrates and proteins is metabolically dynamic.

Some of the facts about metabolism of carbohydrates, fats and proteins set forth in the earlier chapters are summarized in Table 2 and Figure 3.

TABLE 2   Metabolism

Nutrient	Anabolism	Catabolism
Carbohydrates	Temporary excess changed into glycogen by liver cells in presence of insulin; stored in liver and skeletal muscles until needed and then changed back to glucose	Oxidized, in the presence of insulin, to yield energy and wastes (CO_2 and H_2O)
Fats	Built into adipose tissue; stored in fat depots of body	Fatty acids are beta-oxidized to acetyl CoA; glycerol is converted into acetyl CoA through glycolysis
Proteins	Synthesized into tissue proteins, blood proteins, enzymes, hormones, etc.	Deaminated by liver, forming ammonia (which is converted to urea) and keto acids (which are either oxidized or changed to glucose or fat)

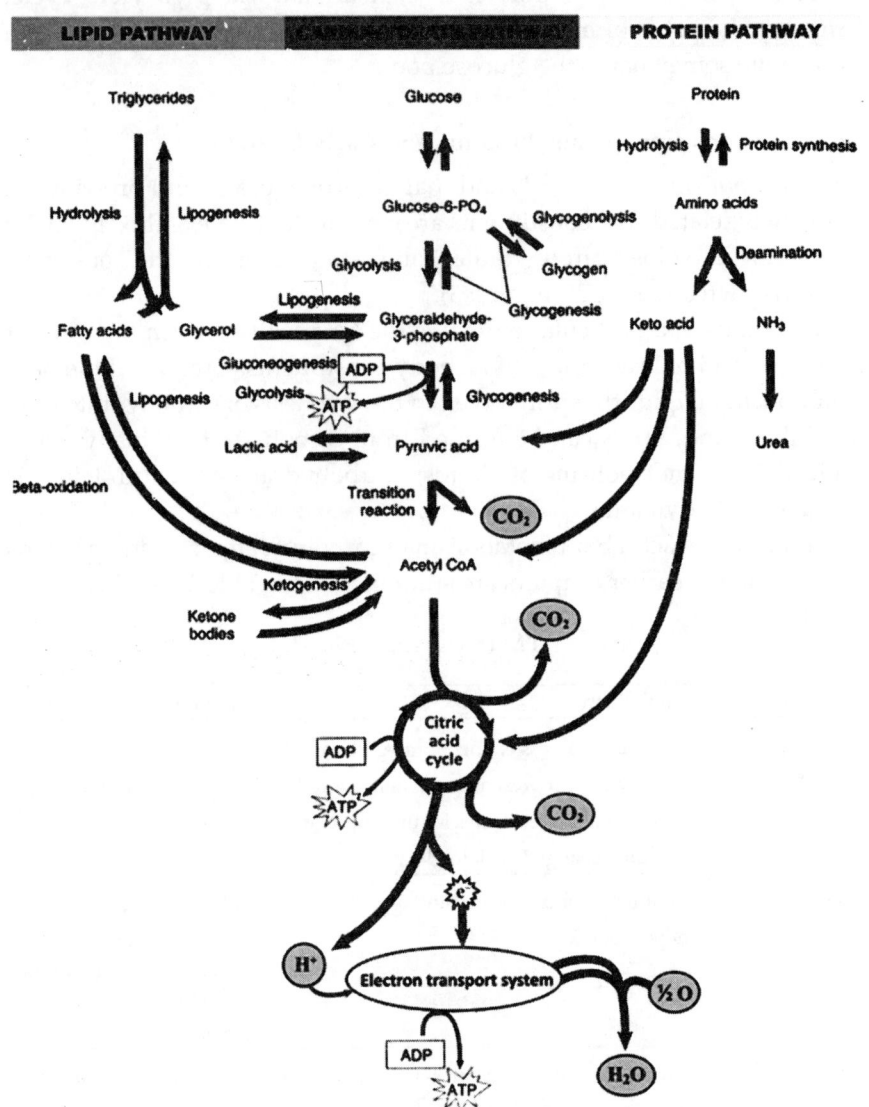

Figure 3   Summary of metabolism [Notice the central role played by the citric acid cycle and electron transport system. Notice also how different molecules can be converted to forms that may enter other pathways.] Source: Anthony's Textbook of Anatomy & Physiology 20th edition, 2013; pp951

Chapter 11

The Inorganic Elements and their Metabolism

Introduction

The following mineral elements are recognized to perform essential functions in the body and thus must be present in the food. These are calcium, phosphorus, magnesium, sodium, potassium, chlorine, sulphur, iron, copper, cobalt, iodine, manganese, selenium, zinc, fluorine, molybdenum, nickel, arsenic, vanadium, silicon, chromium and tin. Thus 22 mineral elements (7 major minerals and 15 trace minerals) were believed to be essential for the higher forms of animal life (Underwood, 1981). Lithium, boron, aluminium, lead and rubidium have been shown to be beneficial in some circumstances. The essentiality of tin, vanadium, fluorine, silicon, nickel, arsenic, aluminium, lead and rubidium (often referred to as the 'newer' trace elements) is based largely on growth effects with laboratory animals reared in highly specialized conditions. So far, these have not been shown to have any practical significance in the nutrition of domestic livestock.

The occurrence of minerals is as follows: calcium 46, phosphorus 29, potassium, sulphur, sodium, chloride and magnesium put together 25 and other microminerals 0.3% of total body minerals. Although aluminium, barium, boron, bromine, cadmium and strontium occur in animal tissues, their significance is unknown.

Minerals Versus Elements

In practical nutrition, the term mineral is generally used to denote all the mineral inorganic elements. However, not all the elements are minerals (e.g. C, H, O and N), and minerals frequently found as salts can be a combination of different inorganic elements. In some books, the terms mineral, element and mineral element are used interchangeably.

Major Elements and Trace Elements

Many of the minerals in the body function primarily as specific organic and inorganic combinations. In case of the food, the combination is important for certain elements. For example, the primary need for sulphur in the food is a constituent of the amino acids cysteine and methionine and in the ruminants it is important for urea utilization. In the estimation of total ash the organic matter is oxidized and the minerals present in organic combination are changed to an inorganic form. The acid soluble fraction of this total ash contains the minerals. The elements are classified as 'major' and 'trace (micro)' elements according to their requirements by plants and animals or according to the concentrations in which they are present in plant or animal tissues.

Mineral Nutrition of Livestock and Poultry

Livestock and poultry derive their mineral nutrients from the feeds, forages and the water that they consume. **The concentration of minerals in the forages depends** on the following several interdependent factors—the genus, species or strain (variety), the type of soil on which the plant grows, the climate or seasonal conditions (tropical/temperate), stage of maturity of the plant at harvesting, application of fertilizers and soil amendments and use of irrigation water.

Leguminous species are generally substantially richer in macroelements than grasses irrespective of whether they are temperate forages or tropical forages. The seeds of leguminous plants and the oil seeds used, as dietary protein supplements are richer in most minerals than are the seeds of grasses and cereals.

Mineral uptake by plants is greatly influenced by soil pH. This is particularly so in legumes. Soils derived from clays, shales and limestones are alkaline or calcarious. Molybdenum uptake by plants is increased in such soils and 'conditioned' copper deficiency occurs in animals due to high concentration of molybdenum in the forages.

Soil pH can be raised or lowered by the application of lime and sulphur, respectively. This changes the availability of minerals to plants: concentrations of cobalt and manganese decrease markedly and those of molybdenum increases while the concentrations of copper and zinc show little change, as soil pH increases; the absorption of nickel, cobalt and manganese by plants is favoured by acid conditions.

Growth requirements of plants for iodine, selenium and cobalt are negligible. Hence there is a need to raise the concentration of these elements in the forage plants to meet the requirements of animals. Applications of magnesium compounds are sometimes necessary to raise the magnesium concentration in the pasture to meet the intense needs of cows during early lactation. Similarly application of phosphatic fertilizers at 20-50 kg per hectare has been advocated to increase the herbage phosphorus concentration in the tropics.

The zinc and selenium content of grains and pastures reflect the soil status of these minerals and the use of fertilizers. The selenium concentration in sugarcane tops was 6-14 times higher in seleniferous areas than in nonseleniferous areas in certain parts of India, but was reduced by applying gypsum at 1 ton/ha (Dhillon and Dhillon, 1991). But sulphur levels in pastures can be raised by using much small applications of gypsum.

Geophagia: Elements such as cobalt, fluorine, iodine and selenium occurs in soils in concentrations usually much higher than those of the plants growing on them. Soil ingestion can be beneficial to the animal in such cases. However, ingestion of iron, molybdenum and zinc (copper antagonists), which are biologically active in soil, may reflect in diseases of copper deficiency in sheep and cattle.

Application of small quantities of molybdenum to deficient soils markedly increase the legume yields and herbage molybdenum and protein concentration. However, increased molybdenum induces copper deficiency. Increased molybdenum is helpful where copper intakes are high because copper retention is depressed and chances of copper poisoning are reduced.

Factors Affecting Requirements for Minerals

1. Dietary requirements for minerals are more difficult to accurately define (than those for organic nutrients) because many factors

Approximate Concentration of Minerals in the Animal body (excluding digesta)

Major Element		g/kg	Trace Element		mg/kg
Calcium	Ca	15	Iron	Fe	20-80
Phosphorus	P	10	Copper	Cu	1-5
Magnesium	Mg	0.4	Cobalt	Co	0.02-0.1
			Manganese	Mn	0.2-0.5
Sodium	Na	1.6	Iodine	I	0.3-0.6
Potassium	K	2.0	Zinc	Zn	10-50
Chlorine	Cl	1.1	Molybdenum	Mo	1-4
Sulphur	S	1.5	Selenium	Se	1-2

determine the utilization of minerals. For example, interrelationships among the minerals or relationships between minerals and organic fractions may result in enhanced or decreased mineral utilization. Presence of **antimetals** e.g. phytates, oxalates affect the availability of minerals.

2. The actual amount of mineral in the diet may also influence utilization. For example, if the diet contains more calcium than required, the efficiency of absorption is usually decreased.
3. The mineral status of the animal may also influence absorption. An iron deficient animal is more efficient in the absorption of iron than an animal with adequate iron stores.
4. The form of the mineral: Iron oxide is not available but ferrous sulfate can be readily utilized.
5. Genetic-nutrition relationships: One strain of mice showed higher requirement for copper, another strain showed for manganese.
6. Changes in management practices may also influence the mineral requirement.
7. Age, sex, productivity level of the animal and bird.

General Functions of Mineral Elements

I Protective functions: 1. Calcium and phosphorus together with fluorine form the hard enamel and thus protect the teeth from rapid wear. Enamel is the hardest substance in the body and has the lowest water content (5%) and contains only 3.5% organic matter. 2. Calcium has a protective function in helping blood clot formation.

II Structural functions: 1. As constituents of bones and teeth, they give rigidity and strength to the skeletal structures e.g., Ca, P, Mg, F, Si. 2. Minerals are constituents of the organic compounds such as protein and lipids, which make up the muscles, organs, blood cells and other soft tissues of the body e.g., P, S, Zn.

III Regulatory functions: Minerals occur in body fluids and tissues as electrolytes concerned with the maintenance of osmotic pressure, acid base balance, membrane permeability and tissue irritability. 1. Sodium and chlorine maintain osmotic pressure of body fluids. 2. Sodium, potassium, calcium, magnesium and chlorine regulate the acid base balance in the body. 3. Sodium, potassium and calcium regulate heart beat. 4. Iodine controls the general metabolic rate. 5. Minerals have been found to regulate cell replication and differentiation. For example, calcium influences signal transduction and zinc influences transcription.

IV General metabolic functions: 1. Minerals exert characteristic effects on the irritability of muscles and nerves. 2. They are important in the activation of many enzymes. For example, magnesium activates enzyme reactions involving phosphates, manganese activates certain digestive enzymes. 3. Sodium and chlorine are also required for digestive processes. 4. Phosphorus is essential for carbohydrate, fat and protein digestion and is responsible for the storage of energy by forming high energy phosphate bonds. 5. Iron in the form of haemoglobin transports oxygen. 6. Copper is required for haemoglobin formation. 7. Cobalt is necessary for vitamin B_{12} synthesis.

Minerals can act as catalysts in enzyme and hormone systems as components of metalloenzymes/hormones.

Some important metalloenzymes

Metal	Enzyme	Function
Copper	Cytochrome oxidase (1 Cu) Lysyl oxidase Ceruloplasmin (ferroxidase) Monoamine oxidase (1 Cu) Uricase (1 Cu)	Terminal oxidase Lysine oxidation Iron utilization (copper transport)
Copper+ zinc or manganese	Superoxide dismutase	Dismutation of the superoxide free radical
Iron	Succinate dehydrogenase (4 Fe) Cytochrome a, b and c Catalase NADH-dehydrogenase (4 Fe)	Aerobic oxidation of carbohydrates Electron transfer Protection against H_2O_2
Manganese	Pyruvate carboxylase (4 Mn) Glycosylaminotransferases	Pyruvate metabolism Proteoglycan synthesis
Molybdenum	Xanthine dehydrogenase (8 Fe, 1.5 Mo) Sulphite oxidase Aldehyde oxidase (8 Fe, 2 Mo)	Purine metabolism Sulphite oxidation Purine metabolism
Selenium	Glutathione peroxidase (4 Se) Type I and II deiodinases	Removal of hydrogen peroxide and hydroperoxides Conversion of thyroxine to active form
Zinc	Carbonic anhydrase (1 Zn) Alcohol dehydrogenase (4 Zn) Carboxypeptidase A (1 Zn) Alkaline phosphatase Nuclear poly (A) polymerase Leucine aminopeptidase (4-6 Zn)	Carbon dioxide formation Alcohol metabolism Protein digestion Hydrolysis of phosphate esters Cell replication

Calcium and Phosphorus

Calcium is the second most abundant nutrient element (after N) in the animal body.

Functions of Calcium: Calcium performs skeletal and nonskeletal functions:

1. Calcium provides a strong skeleton for supporting and protecting delicate organs, jointed to allow movement and malleable to allow

growth. Bones grow in length by the proliferation of cartilaginous plates at the ends of bones. Bones grow in width as well.
2. The ionized plasma calcium performs several nonskeletal functions.

Functions of Phosphorus:
1. The most important function is the formation and maintenance of bone, similar to calcium. However, phosphorus is required for the formation of the organic bone matrix as well as the mineralization of that matrix.
2. The 20% of phosphorus widely distributed in the fluids and soft tissues of the body serves a range of essential functions.

Ca and P in Bones

About 3% of the animal body consists of minerals. Over 70% of the ash of the body consists of calcium and phosphorus. Majority of the calcium (99%) and phosphorus (80%) are present in bones and teeth. In bones calcium and phosphorus occur in the ratio of 2:1 and the elements are closely related to each other. Bones serve as a store house for calcium and phosphorus. That is why the requirements for growing, pregnant and milch animals are high.

Normal adult bone has water 45%, ash 25%, protein 20% and fat 10%. On fat free and moisture free basis bone contains 36% calcium, 17% P and 0.8% Mg.

Calcium and Phosphorus in Soft Tissues

The 1% of body calcium which occurs outside the bones is widely distributed throughout the organs and tissues and has many important functions. Calcium is required for normal blood clotting as it is a must for the formation of thrombin from prothrombin. Calcium is necessary for muscle contraction, myocardial function, normal neuromuscular excitability, activation of several enzymes and secretion of several hormones and hormone-releasing factors.

Pathological deposits of calcium in certain soft tissues sometimes occur as a result of upset in mineral relations such as a low magnesium intake relative to calcium and phosphorus.

Large amounts of phosphorus are present mostly in organic combinations such as phosphoprotein, nucleoprotein, phospholipids, phosphocreatine and hexose phosphate. Phosphate is a component of many enzyme systems. Phosphorus makes up 0.15 to 0.2% of the soft tissues of the body.

Calcium and Phosphorus in Blood

The blood cells are entirely devoid of calcium. The plasma calcium occurs in two forms, one the soluble ionized form (60% of the total) and the other fraction is bound with protein, primarily albumen and plasma proteins. The level of blood calcium (9-11 mg/100ml) is maintained at constant level despite high intakes or marked body losses or otherwise. The blood levels of calcium regulate secretion of hormones and they in turn regulate deposition and release of calcium from bone. Low levels stimulate **parathormone** secretion, which promote the release of Ca and P from bone. The calcium is utilized to meet the calcium needs of the animal and phosphorus is excreted. Another hormone that controls blood calcium is **calcitonin** (from thyroid), which decreases the rate of calcium mobilization from bone and therefore, decreases serum calcium level.

Whole blood contains from 35 to 45 mg of phosphorus per 100 ml, most of which is in the cells. The element occurs in a variety of forms, principally organic combinations. Plasma has inorganic phosphorus (4 to 9 mg/100 ml). It is evident that an interchange of phosphate between organic and inorganic forms continually occurs. The level is higher at birth than at maturity, the most rapid decline occurring early in life. The plasma phosphorus level is more easily changed by dietary means than the calcium levels. A dietary deficiency of phosphorus could produce hypophosphatemia and higher dietary intakes produce hyperphosphatemia.

Absorption and Excretion of Calcium and Phosphorus

Calcium is absorbed in the small intestine. Calcium is transported in the blood in an ionized and protein-bound form. The absorption is dependent upon the solubility at the point of contact with the absorbing membranes.

1. Vit. D is necessary for the synthesis of a protein that is necessary for the transport of calcium in the intestinal mucosa. (calcium binding proteins-cadmolin and osteopontin).
2. Very high dietary levels of inorganic phosphorus, phytin phosphorus, and magnesium interfere with calcium absorption.
3. Lactose, a sugar that is slowly absorbed, improves calcium absorption. Oxalates and phytates decrease the absorption of calcium.
4. Dietary levels of Ca and P, vitamin D, parathyroid hormone (PTH), and calcitonin all seem to play a role in calcium homeostasis.
5. High dietary levels of calcium depress efficiency of absorption.
6. A great excess of either Ca or P interferes with the absorption of the other. Ratio of Ca and P is important. This ratio is more important for nonruminants than for ruminants.

Phosphorus is absorbed in the phosphate form from the small intestine. It is necessary that the phosphate be in solution at the point of contact with the intestinal mucosa. Therefore, any compound or cation that will form an insoluble complex with the phosphate ion will decrease its absorption. Large amounts of Ca, Mg, aluminium, or iron may cause the formation of insoluble salts and thus reduce absorption.

A determination of apparent digestibility of ash is of no value. The reason is that the faeces are a path of excretion of minerals which have been absorbed and metabolized and thus served the body, as well as those which have escaped absorption.

Modern isotope (Ca^{45}, P^{32}) techniques provide for a distinction between the faecal fraction which is a metabolic excretion (the endogenous fraction) and the fraction of the diet which was not absorbed. Major portion of the calcium found in the faeces is endogenous. The true digestibility which is arrived at by correcting for the faecal endogenous loss is commonly referred to as availability. In all species, the faeces is a primary path for calcium excretion.

The faeces is the primary path for phosphorus excretion in the case of herbivora, but urine is the principal path for carnivora and the output is equally divided between two channels in the case of humans.

The Effects of High Intakes of Calcium

High dietary intakes of calcium well above requirements without concurrently increasing the zinc results in a severe parakeratosis in swine. High levels of calcium and/or phosphorus in the rations of swine and poultry intensify the effect of manganese deficiency. High calcium intakes are reported to cause the formation of kidney stones. Chronic intakes of high dietary calcium may also cause a hypersecretion of calcitonin and bone abnormalities such as osteopetrosis (dense bone).

Calcium toxicity: Calcium is not generally regarded as a toxic element, because of excellent homeostatic mechanisms. However, doubling the dietary calcium concentration of chicks to 2.05 g/kg DM caused hypercalcaemia and growth retardation, fast-growing strains being more vulnerable than slow-growing strains (Hurwitz et al., 1995). Feeding excess calcium results in impairment of absorption of other elements; thus deficiencies of P and Zn are readily induced in nonruminants. Hypercalcaemia can cause life-threatening tissue calcification but usually occurs as a secondary consequence of P deficiency or overexposure to vitamin D_3 and its analogues.

Symptoms of Deficiency of Calcium: Young Animals

Calcium deficiency in the young animal is characterized by poor bone development and the condition is known as rickets. The bones of the young animal are usually soft, bend easily, and are often misshapen.

The joints are enlarged and the animal often exhibits lameness. When examined in the laboratory, the bones are found to contain very low levels of ash. In some young animals, such as the chicken, calcium deficiency causes reduced growth rate; in swine, it has little influence on growth rate; in the rat, serum calcium drops, and it is susceptible to internal haemorrhage and may go into tetany.

In broilers tibial dyschondroplasia (TD) has been reported; it is inducible by feeding diets low in calcium. "Osteofibrosis" is the term used to the bone dystrophy that occurs in young horses.

Adults

In adult animals a chronic calcium deficiency leads to osteomalacia, a condition in which the calcium of the bone is withdrawn and not replaced. There is a constant mobilization of calcium and phosphorus in bone; it is in a dynamic state.

If sufficient dietary calcium or phosphorus is not available to replace that mobilized from the bone, there is a net loss of Ca and P and a general softening of the bone. Most acute cases of osteomalacia occur during gestation and lactation in mammals and during egg laying in birds. It is important to realize that, while osteomalacia may be due to simple Ca deficiency, it may also be caused by P deficiency, by abnormal Ca to P ratio in the feed, and by vitamin D deficiency. Cases of calcium tetany occur when the serum calcium level falls below the optimum. Bone fractures are common in cases of osteomalacia due to over functioning of the parathyroid glands.

Low Ca intake is sometimes a problem in ageing humans, and either osteomalacia or osteoporosis may result. Osteoporosis is used to denote a failure of normal bone metabolism in the adult. In osteoporosis the mineral content of the bone is normal but the absolute amount of bone has decreased. Osteoporosis is a skeletal disorder that compromises bone strength and predisposes one to increased fracture risk. According to WHO, the best criteria for the diagnosis of osteoporosis is the measurement of 'bone mineral density' (BMD). DEXA (see p. 373 of 3 ed. Applied Nutrition Livestock, ...;) scan is used in measuring BMD. Calcium problems in older people are often complex and may represent low calcium intake, poor calcium absorption, or abnormal metabolism, or a combination of these factors. Osteoporosis condition is prevalent in the human population after the age of 50, particularly in women. A long continued low intake of calcium plays a role in its development. It can be corrected, in some cases, by an intake of calcium double the recommended adult allowance. Osteomalacia and osteoporosis are sometimes used interchangeably in referring to bone troubles in the adult.

Osteopenia: It is often used to describe bone pathology and simply means too little bone.

Birds have a tremendous need for calcium immediately after commencing egg production, and bone reserves are mobilized to meet this tremendous demand for calcium to make egg shells. The pullet is supplied with an extra supply of calcium in the medullary bone, which occupies almost the whole marrow cavity of such long bones as the femur. This reserve of labile calcium is utilized during the time of egg shell formation. However, if adequate dietary calcium is not supplied in a matter of 5 to 7 days the egg shells became thin and fragile, and the hen develops osteomalacia. Withdrawal of calcium from the skeletal reserves in response to the demand of egg laying result in most of the hens end lay in an osteoporotic state (Whitehead, 1995).

As bone calcium and P are mobilized for calcium for shell formation there is considerable loss of phosphorus from the hen's body.

Nutritional Secondary Hyperparathyroidism

When animals are fed diets containing low or marginal levels of calcium but excessive amounts of phosphorus, a condition called nutritional secondary hyperparathyroidism (NSH) may develop.

1. Excess phosphorus depresses calcium absorption. The resulting hypocalcemia triggers the parathyroid to release parathormone which mobilizes Ca from bone to replenish the blood level.
2. A high level of dietary phosphorus also causes a greater turnover rate in the bone. In horses and monkeys the fibrous connective tissue invades the area and enlarged facial bones result. Hence the disease is also called osteodystrophia fibrosa and big-head disease.

Field cases of NSH have been reported in horses and rabbits fed high grain intakes, birds fed all-grain diets, primates fed only fruit and nuts, and carnivores (dogs, cats, lions and tigers) fed all meat diets. NSH causes periodontal disease (loss of bone around the teeth) in the dogs and humans.

Phosphorus Deficiency and Appetite

Free-choice feeding of calcium and phosphorus is often recommended but several recent studies demonstrate that ruminants don't have the nutritional wisdom to select the amount of these nutrients needed. Therefore, the addition of proper amounts of calcium and phosphorus to the diet of domestic livestock appears to be a prudent practice.

Pica: Deficiency of phosphorus is characterised by a loss of appetite and even a depraved appetite, which is exhibited in the eating of bones, wood, clothing and other materials (soil, plastic, etc.) to which the animal may have access. The animal becomes very emaciated. The depraved appetite (pica) may be known as either allotriophagia (a generalized form) or as osteophagia (craving for bones) and as sarcophagia (craving for flesh). These forms of pica are expression of deficiency of not only P but also Na and K.

Reduced fertility and **reduced or delayed conception** are signs of the deficiency. Abnormal bones and teeth are apparent signs of P deficiency and may be manifested by stiffness of gait, enlarged and painful joints, bending or deformation of bones, arching of the back, and fracture of bones. These symptoms are the same whether the deficiency state arises from a deficiency of Ca, P or Vit. D. Rickets, osteomalacia and osteoporosis may all occur depending upon the age of the animal and the conditions under which the deficiency is produced.

Calcium rich feeds	*Phosphorus rich feeds*
Legume seeds	Vegetable protein supplements
Legume roughages	Cereal grains and their
Animal byproducts	byproducts (brans)
(bone meal, tankage,	Animal protein supplements
meat scrap, fish meal)	
Milk and milk products	
Plant leaf meals	

Phosphoric acid is a highly available source of phosphorus for the animals. Rock phosphate has fluorine and hence it is defluorinated. Defluorinated phosphate/superphosphate is a good source of Ca and P. Phosphorus from animal byproducts is available completely in comparison to plant byproducts. Availability of calcium and phosphorus are affected by the presence of **oxalic acid** and **phytic acid**, respectively. This aspect has been discussed elsewhere (see page no. 552).

Supplements of Ca and P

	%	
	Ca	P
Limestone, calcium carbonate, oyster shell.	34-35	-
Sterilized bone meal	29	14
Dicalcium phosphate	26	21
Defluorinated phosphate	29-36	12-18
Calcium phosphate	17	21
Sodium phosphate	-	22

Magnesium

Distribution: Magnesium is closely related to calcium and phosphorus in its distribution and metabolism. About 70% is in the skeleton and the rest is distributed in other soft tissues (29%) and various fluids (1%). The ratio of Ca:Mg in bone is about 50:1. Approximately one-third of the supply in the bones is subject to mobilization for soft-tissue use when the intake is inadequate. But in the young animal up to 60% of the total bone magnesium may be mobilized during times of inadequate intake. Blood serum contains about 2.5 mg/100 ml and its level varies with the phosphorus content. The soft tissues contain more Mg than calcium. Within animal cells, Mg is the second most abundant cation, after potassium.

Essential functions: Magnesium is essential for all plant and animal life.

1. It is an essential constituent of bones and teeth.
2. It is regarded as an activator of various enzymes transferring phosphate from ATP to ADP.
3. It is a cofactor for decarboxylation for certain peptidases and for alkaline and acid phosphatases.
4. It is a constituent of chlorophyll, a metalloprotein complex essential for photosynthesis.
5. It is required for oxidative phosphorylation, β-oxidation of fatty acids and transketolase reaction of the pentose monophosphate shunt.

Absorption

Forages from soils fertilized with high levels of nitrogen and potassium often contain reduced levels of magnesium and sodium. Potassium apparently depresses the absorption of magnesium from the rumen, a primary site of magnesium absorption. The susceptibility of ruminants to Mg deficiency hinges upon the fact that the primary site of absorption is usually the rumen, whereas in the nonruminant it is the small intestine. The absorptive level of efficiency in ruminants is roughly half that of nonruminants (35 vs 70% of intake).

The Ca and P content of the diet have been shown to have an effect on the Mg requirement. When the diet contains adequate amounts of Ca and P in the proper ratio, there is no interference due to magnesium. On a low-phosphorus diet, magnesium interfers with calcium absorption. High phosphorus diets not only decrease the absorption of dietary magnesium but increase the rate of loss of endogenous magnesium through the gut and faeces. High dietary magnesium levels may increase calcium requirements when the phosphorus level of the diet is also high.

Deficiency of Magnesium

Magnesium deficiency has been shown to cause calcium deposition in the kidney. Renal calculi may be formed both in magnesium deficiency or excess. The deficiency disease is known as **grass tetany** or **grass staggers** or **wheat staggers** or **wheat poisoning**. This is observed in calves reared for long periods on milk alone and in cows fed on lush green pasture.

The signs of grass tetany include excessive nervousness, twitching of muscles, laboured breathing, rapid pulse, convulsions and death. The affected cattle are nervous, with their heads held high, ears pricked and eyes staring. The animal may move in a stiff manner and stagger when walking. The animal becomes extremely excited and violent convulsions develop, with animal lying on its side, the forelegs pedalling and jaws working, making the teeth grate. If treatment is not given, the animal usually goes into a coma and dies.

Lactation tetany (hypomagnesaemic tetany) is a disease of lactating cows and is characterized by hypomagnesaemia (less than 1 mg%) (usually accompanied with hypocalcaemia), muscular spasms and convulsions and death due to respiratory failure. Temperature, pulse and respiration rate are high. Tetany can be produced by feeding excess potassium and citric acid or transaconitic acid (blood Mg depressant).

In the young chick deficiency of Mg causes slow growth rate. The chick often pant and gasp, they are lethargic and when disturbed exhibit convulsions from which they may go into a comatose state that is often fatal. In pigs, a magnesium deficiency is manifested in a peculiar stepping syndrome.

Sources: Most of the commonly fed roughages and concentrates contain at least 0.1% of magnesium on DMB. Magnesium deficiency is of rare occurrence under field conditions.

Sodium, Potassium and Chlorine

These highly soluble minerals are found mainly in body fluids and soft tissues. **Functions** of them are to maintain osmotic pressure and acid-base equilibrium, to regulate the passage of nutrients through cell walls and help water metabolism in general. There is a regular dietary need for these minerals because of limited storage. A deficiency of any of these elements results in lack of appetite, a decline of growth, loss of weight and production, and decreased blood levels.

Sodium

The body contains 0.2% sodium. It is **major cation**. It is mostly extracellular and makes up 93% of the bases of the blood serum, (i.e. major cation in ECF) but little is present in the blood cells. Sodium occurs in considerable amounts in the muscles, where it is associated with their contraction.

Amino acid and glucose uptake are dependent on sodium. Adequate sodium in the diet is important because of its role in 'sodium pump' and its concentration being more in extracellular compartment. The 'sodium pump' is vital to the maintenance of electrochemical differences across membranes and the cellular uptake of glucose through the action of a Na^+-K^+ dependent ATPase, but activity is sustained at a significant energy cost (Underwood and Suttle, 1999).

Sources: Most cereal grains are fairly low in sodium (0.01 to 0.06%). Vegetable protein concentrates are also very low (0.01 to 0.05%). Feeds of animal origin usually contain relatively high concentration of sodium (0.01% to 0.8%).

The **hormone aldosterone**, secreted from the adrenal cortex, regulates the reabsorption of sodium from the kidney tubules. In the absence of this hormone, sodium, is excreted in the urine. Excessive losses of sodium may occur from vomiting, diarrhoea, or profuse sweating.

Symptoms of Deficiency

General symptoms of nutritional deficiency of sodium are slow growth, softening of the bones, keratinization of the corneal epithelium, impotency in the male, and delayed sexual maturity and impaired estrus rhythm and reproductive processes in the female. A lack of the element lowers the utilization of digested protein and energy. Cardiac output decreases, blood drops, and the hematocrit increases.

The animal will eventually go into shock and die. In laying hens, a deficiency results in lowered production, loss of weight and cannibalism.

Toxicity

Levels of salt in the diet over 0.5% usually cause increased water consumption and watery faeces. Salts that are present in high saline water are sodium chloride, magnesium sulphate and carbonates. Of these sodium chloride is least injurious.

Potassium

It exists primarily **as cellular constituent**. Potassium rank one and magnesium rank two in quantity in intracellular fluids and organelles. It plays a vital role in muscle, where its content is six times that of sodium. Human blood cells contain over 20 times as much of the potassium as does the plasma. During nerve transmission and muscle contraction, potassium moves out of the cell and sodium enters. The potassium then moves back into the cell when the sodium is removed. Thus Na and K are interrelated in metabolism.

Sources: Most foods contain rather high levels of potassium; the grains 0.3 to 0.8%, the vegetable proteins 1 to 2% and animal products 0.3 to 2%.

Potassium, like sodium, is readily absorbed, and the excess over body needs is immediately excreted. This excretion normally takes place in the urine to the extent of 90%. Adrenal hormones cause the kidney to conserve sodium but increase the excretion of potassium. The kidney has only limited capacity to conserve potassium even when the diet is deficient.

Deficiency

Potassium deficiency is not usually observed in farm animals, as plant products contain 10 to 20 times more of this element than sodium. Experimentally produced potassium deficiency in most animals causes decreased growth rate, general weakness, and in acute cases, tetany, followed by death.

Decreased use of hay and increased use of grain may result in deficiency of potassium. Replacement of protein supplements such as soybean meal or groundnut cake by urea may also decrease dietary potassium intake.

Chlorine

Chlorine is found both within the cells and in the body fluids, including the gastric secretions. Less than 15% of the chlorine in the body is found in the cells. Chloride ion is **the major anion of the extracellular fluids** (ECF).

About 15 to 20% of the chlorine of the body appears to be in organic combination. The gastric secretion contains chlorine as free acid and in the form of salts. The requirement is half of that for sodium. The body has certain capacity to store chlorine in the skin and subcutaneous tissues.

Chlorides play a key role in regulating the pH of body fluids. The movement of chlorine from body fluid to erythrocytes in what is known as "chloride shift" is a primary mechanism in regulating pH and osmolarity of tissue fluids. The chlorides of the blood make up two-thirds of its acidic ions. This indicates their large role in acid base relations. Respiration is based on 'the chloride shift', whereby the potassium salt of oxyhaemoglobin exchanges oxygen for carbon dioxide via bicarbonate in the tissue and reverses that process in the lung, where reciprocal chloride exchanges maintain the anion balance (Block, 1994). Most plant foods are fairly low in chlorine content. Animal and fish products contain reasonable levels of chlorine.

Chlorine metabolism and the animals requirement for chlorine is related to Na and K intake, and the form in which these cations are obtained by the animal. For instance, if large amounts of Na and K are taken in as the salt of glutamic acid, they may be detrimental unless balanced with sufficient chloride or other anions. Conversely, if large amounts of chlorides are taken in as organic salts that are easily metabolized by the body, it is necessary to balance the ration with sodium and potassium.

Common Salt

As early as in 1847, Boussingault demonstrated the supplementary value of salt in cattle followed by the classical studies of Babcock (1905) on the effect of salt deprivation on lactating dairy cows and in 1957, Aines and Smith identified that the sodium was the critically limiting element in the sodium chloride salt.

Salt serves as a condiment. It stimulates secretion of saliva. Sodium content of plant feedstuffs is usually low and excess potassium content affects adversely the retention of sodium. Hence the **ration of herbivorous animals is always supplemented with salt** at the rate of 1% of the concentrate mixture. Salt supplementation of most animal rations is necessary unless large amounts of animal and fish products are consumed. Heavy milk production during lactation and high rate of egg production can put a strain on sodium and chlorine reserves. So salt supplementation is necessary.

Effects of Deficiency of Salt

These include 1. loss of appetite and marked decline in weight and milk yield. 2. retarded growth 3. lowered fertility 4. cannibalism in chicks.

Absorption and Excretion of Salt

When the intake is at minimum, the body makes an adjustment whereby the output of sodium and chlorine in the urine ceases. In contrast, large intakes of salt involve a correspondingly large excretion, the water requirement being increased accordingly. The kidney is the regulating organ which controls the concentration of electrolytes in the blood. With healthy kidneys and an appropriate water intake, large amounts of salt taken for short periods can be excreted without any harmful effects.

Effects of Excess Salt Intake

Excessive intakes can, however, result in water retention in the body resulting in edema. **Excessive intakes cause salt poisoning in pigs and poultry.** The primary mode of action of salt poisoning is through a disturbance of water balance. Ruminants have a higher tolerance. But with low water intake salt toxicity has been produced with 2.2% level.

Human kidney can excrete as little as 1g or as much as 40 g of common salt per day, depending on the intake. Chronic intakes of high levels of salt have been reported to raise blood pressure in some people. Low-sodium, high-potassium diets are often recommended. The salt requirement is greatly increased under conditions which cause heavy sweating because of the large loss in the sweat. It has been reported that miners lose 2.5 kg of sweat per hour, containing 2 g of NaCl. If large amount of water is drunk under these conditions, cramps result. The cramps disappear on drinking water containing salt. On a low-salt diet, however, the body gradually makes an adjustment whereby the concentration in the sweat and the urine is gradually decreased. Equilibrium between intake and outgo is thus established at a much lower level than is possible initially.

Sulphur

Sulphur occurs entirely in organic compounds, notably in proteins in which it is present as the sulphur containing amino acids cysteine and methionine. Wool contains approximately 4% of sulphur. Thiamin and biotin contain sulphur. Sulphur is present in inorganic form in chondroitin sulphate, a constituent of cartilage. Glutathione, oxytocin, lipoic acid and insulin contain sulphur. Blood contains small amount of sulphate. Thiocyanate ions are also present in blood, saliva, etc.

Sulphur is excreted through the faeces and urine. There is evidence that the excretion of neutral sulphur (cystine, taurine, thiosulfates) is proportional to the basal metabolism.

Rumen bacteria can utilize inorganic sulphur to build the sulphur containing amino acids. Sulphate ion is of importance in molybdenum toxicity: increasing the sulphate intake enhances molybdenum excretion.

Sulphur deficiency in ruminant diets may result in reduced feed intake and reduced cellulose digestion. It is recommended that the nitrogen sulphur ratio of ruminant diets should be approximately 10:1 to 15:1.

Iron

It is a constituent of blood pigment, haemoglobin, muscle protein, myoglobin, and enzymes, cytochrome c, peroxidase and catalase. In addition, it is stored in liver, spleen and kidney as ferritin (20%) and haemosiderin (35%). It occurs in blood serum in a protein called transferrin (siderophillin) which is concerned with the transport of iron. Over half of the iron (60 to 70%) present in the body is in the form of haemoglobin. The normal haemoglobin content of blood for most mammals lies within the range of 10 to 18 g per 100 ml blood depending on species, sex and age (11 to 12 g per 100 ml in pigs, poultry and cattle and 10 to 11 g per 100 ml in sheep, goat and horses). Sex differences are insignificant except in poultry, where slightly higher haemoglobin values occur in cocks than in hens and in nonlaying hens than in laying hens.

In other words **body iron is mostly organic (hemal and nonhemal)** and very small percentage is found as free inorganic ions. Hemal iron, forms part of a porphyrin group, represents 70-75% of total iron and includes hemoglobin, myoglobin, cytochromes, cytochrome oxidase, catalase and peroxidase. Nonhemal iron includes iron transport and storage forms such as transferrin, ferritin, hemosiderin and other iron proteinates.

Anaemia

Red blood cells (RBC) and their haemoglobin are constantly being destroyed and replaced and hence iron undergoes very active metabolism. The RBC are formed in the bone marrow (haematopoises) and their average lifespan is 127 days. In the course of their destruction, the hematin of the haemoglobin is split into an iron compound, bilirubin and other pigments which are carried to the liver and secreted in the bile. Iron released by the normal blood cell destruction can be used again to form haemoglobin, practically without loss. However, in certain diseases this destruction may be accelerated and iron formed by toxic destruction can not be reutilized.

If the cells are not renewed as rapidly as they are destroyed, or if the increase in the number of cells which are required to enlarge the blood supply with growth does not occur, anaemia results. Anaemia may occur at any time of life when the available supply of the mineral becomes deficient relative to the needs for haemoglobin formation. **Anaemia is defined** as reduction in the concentration of haemoglobin in the blood below the normal for age and sex of the animal.

In iron deprivation, the onset of anaemia is early in contrast to the late development of anaemia in cobalt and copper deprivation.

Different types of anaemia: Reduced haemoglobin content of the blood in anaemia is due to **reduction in the number of red cells** and **changes in the size and haemoglobin content of the cells.** Thus anaemias are microcytic, normocytic or macrocytic in accordance with the cell size and hypochromic, normochromic or hyperchromic in accordance with their colour index. Deficiencies of protein, iron, copper and certain vitamins can result in anaemias, most of which differ in morphological type. Anaemia may result from an interference with or cessation of the production of haemoglobin, a block in cell maturation, increased destruction or from blood loss. Various specific nutrients play a role in haemoglobin production and cell maturation and thus the term 'nutritional anaemia' has a broader significance. Hereditary anaemia e.g. 'sickle cell anaemia' occurs in humans.

The general symptoms of anaemia are poor growth, lethargy, blanching of visible mucous membranes, increased heart and respiratory rate, and a decreased resistance to disease. Iron deficiency results in hypochromic, microcytic anaemia in pigs and chicken while in calves it is microcytic and normochromic type. In chicken with pigmented feathers there is a depigmentation of feathers (achromotrichia) which is reversible with iron supplementation.

Most unprocessed foods other than milk and milk products contain levels of iron adequate to supply the iron needs of animals under usual conditions. **Iron deficiency in animals** has been associated with suckling animals in confinement rearing and restricted to milk alone and animals suffering blood loss and receiving diets marginal in iron. Iron deficiency anaemia is not observed in lambs and calves because they begin to eat supplementary food/forage which supplies the needed iron. Iron deficiency in mink may cause "cotton fur". Other effects of iron deficiency may include reduced growth rate, elevated serum triglyceride levels and depressed folic acid levels.

Piglet Anaemia

Among the farm animals, suckling pigs are highly susceptible for iron deficiency. Piglets kept in confinement to concrete stalls are more susceptible due to their nonaccessibility to greens or soil. Piglet anaemia is characterized by

1. Low haemoglobin content of blood (3 to 4g/100 ml).
2. Lack of healthy pink colour of the visible mucous membranes,
3. Poor growth rate,

4. Wrinkled skin and rough coat,
5. Laboured, spasmodic breathing, often popularly described as 'thumps' and
6. A dilated heart and oedematous lungs on postmortem examination.

Mortality is high. Piglet anaemia usually occurs within 2 to 4 weeks of birth. It does no good to feed the mineral to the lactating mother, for the iron content of milk can not be increased. The young piglet must retain about 7 to 16 mg of iron per day to grow at a normal rate without becoming anaemic. Milk may provide 1 mg per day.

Nutrition Physiology of Iron Peculiar to Pigs

1. The placental transfer of iron is so poor that the piglet is born with unusually small store of body iron, compared with newborn of most other species. The ash of a newborn puppy has six times higher iron content compared to that to bitch's milk. The liver of newborn has 5 to 8 times as much iron as liver of mature dogs.
2. The polycythaemia of birth seen in other species is absent in the piglet, so that a source of iron from breakdown of the excess haemoglobin is denied to it.
3. Low levels of iron in sow's milk.
4. Rapid early growth rate compared with that of the lamb or calf. If adequately fed, a young pig can reach 5 times its birth weight at the end of 3 weeks and 10 times its birth weight in 5 weeks.
5. Large litter size. All these features contribute to piglet anaemia.

Piglet anaemia can be prevented or cured in its early stages by drenching the suckling pigs with a saturated solution of ferrous sulphate. Pasting the ferrous sulphate salt on the udder of the mother also help piglets to ingest iron. The popular method of prevention is injection of 100 mg iron-dextran intramuscularly/subcutaneously at 4th and 14th day after birth. This maintains normal haemoglobin level.

Iron Absorption and Conservation

Iron is absorbed primarily from the small intestine, mostly duodenum. Iron in haeme compounds is absorbed directly into the intestinal mucosal cells, while inorganic forms of iron and iron protein compounds are broken and the iron reduced to the ferrous state (in the acidic conditions) before it is absorbed.

McCance and Widdowson (1937) established the new concept that the amount of iron in the body was regulated by controlling absorption of iron and not by excretion of excess iron into the urine or faeces. That is iron absorption is quantitatively controlled by body needs. Once iron is absorbed, it is tenaciously held by the body and not excreted to any appreciable extent. There are two theories proposed to explain absorption of iron.

1. 'Mucosal block' theory was pronounced in 1943 by P.F. Hahn and coworkers and elaborated by S. Granick (1951). The intestinal mucosa absorbs iron during periods of need and rejects it when stores are adequate. Mucosal cells of the GI tract absorb iron and convert it into ferritin. When the cells become physiologically saturated with ferritin, further absorption is impeded until the iron is released and transferred to plasma.

2. Another theory recently proposed explains that the main regulator of iron uptake is the iron concentration in the epithelial cells of the duodenal mucosa (Conrad and Crosby 1963 and 1964). The mechanisms by which the body regulates iron absorption in accordance with body iron needs are not completely understood (Morris, 1987).

Absorption of iron is poor, to a large extent, independent of the dietary source. However, acidic condition in the G.I. tract, ascorbic acid in the diet improves iron absorption while phytic acid in the diet reduces iron absorption. The efficiency of iron absorption is increased during periods of iron need (growth, pregnancy) and decreased during periods of iron overload.

Toxicity of Iron

Very high levels of iron may cause nutritional problems by decreasing phosphate absorption. Rather high levels of ferrous salts have been used in poultry rations when cottonseed meal containing gossypol is fed. The ferrous iron forms a complex with the otherwise toxic gossypol, making it nontoxic to the animal. **Iron toxicity** is characterized by excessive deposition of storage forms of iron in tissues (siderosis) accompanied by high plasma iron (hypersideremia) and damage to the intestinal mucosal cells.

High iron intakes associated with grazing pastures irrigated with iron-rich bore water and contaminated with (iron-rich) soil may inhibit copper absorption or may even cause copper toxicity if sulphur content of the diet is low.

Sources: All green feeds, liver, egg yolk are rich in iron. The outer coating (brans) and germ of cereal grains are rich in iron. Colostrum contains 3-5 times more of iron than milk.

Copper

In 1928, Hart and his associates of USA discovered that a small amount of copper is necessary along with iron, for haemoglobin formation. It is not a constituent of haemoglobin but it does occur as haemocuprein in blood cells. It is required in red cell maturation. It appears copper exerts an influence on iron metabolism at the cellular level. Copper is also important for normal bone formation as it is essential for osteoblastic activity and for normal collagen and elastin formation. Copper is an integral part of many metalloenzymes such as cytochrome C oxidase, uricase, tyrosinase, lysyl oxidase, benzylamine oxidase, diamine oxidase, ascorbic acid oxidase, etc. It also occurs in certain respiratory pigments as well as hair and feather pigments. These include haemocyanin of marine organisms and turacin, a feather pigment from the turaco bird.

After absorption primarily from the upper section of the small intestine, copper becomes loosely bound to serum albumin and amino acids and transported throughout the body. Liver is the major storage organ. Copper is released from the liver primarily for hepatic synthesis of ceruloplasmin (Cu-metalloprotein), for synthesis of erythrocuprein and for incorporation into many enzymes. Copper is believed to regulate lipid metabolism and has bactericidal properties at the intestinal level (See chapter on Feed Additives).

About half of the total body supply of copper is found in the muscle mass. Stores are also found in the bone marrow, liver, etc. The body supply of copper is greatly reduced when the diet is deficient. Milk is deficient in copper just like iron. Copper deficiency can be detected by the estimation of this mineral in blood. Normal copper concentration is 0.1 mg/100 ml. The copper content of the soil is very poor in various parts of the world. The forages grown do not contain sufficient copper. Animals kept on forages containing copper below 7 mg per kg of DM exhibit copper deficiency. In some places, deficiency has been noted even though the forages contain sufficient amount of copper. This is due to the presence of excess of molybdenum or inorganic sulphate in the fodders. Such deficiency is known as **'conditional' or 'induced' deficiency**.

Symptoms of Copper Deficiency

Symptoms of deficiency vary among species. Anaemia is a general symptom. The other symptoms are depressed growth, bone abnormalities, de-pigmentation of hair, feathers and wool, defective keratinization of wool, fibrosis of the myocardium, scouring or diarrhoea, and myelin aplasia of the spinal card. Copper content of blood, liver, spleen and hair is decreased.

Effects of Deficiency and Deficiency Diseases

1. When copper is deficient in the diet, there is a decreased absorption of iron, a decrease in its mobilization from the tissues and development of microcytic and hypochromic anaemia in pigs and chickens and microcytic and normochromic anaemia in calves.
2. Depigmentation of coloured hair and black wool due to a defect in melanin synthesis because of a reduced tirosinase activity.
3. Decreased wool growth, development of 'stringy' or 'steely' wool characterised by limp (not stiff or firm), glossy (smooth and shiny) fibres lacking the normal crimp (wavy or curly).
4. Enzootic ataxia (in Australia) or swayback (in England). Enzootic ataxia (neonatal ataxia) occurs in lambs, kids and calves. Ataxia is caused by myelin aplasia rather than myelin degeneration and is associated with degeneration of the motor neurons of the brain and spinal cord.

    Uncoordinated movements of the hind legs, a stiff and staggering gait with a swaying of the hind quarters, is characteristic of animals as the deficiency develops in the few weeks following birth. Some become completely paralyzed and locomotion becomes impossible. Blood copper levels are usually low in both the mother and the affected offspring. On postmortem examination degenerative changes can be seen in the brain and spinal cord. Nervous symptoms are due to demyelination of the spinal cord.
5. Falling disease: A chronic copper deficiency cause this disease in grazing cattle in Australia. This is characterized by staggering, falling, and instantaneous death due to the heart failure because of atrophy of myocardium.
6. Lechsucht or scouring disease is wasting disease of cattle and sheep observed in Northern Europe. Symptoms are diarrhoea, loss of appetite and anaemia. It is also known as copper pine.
7. Bone troubles have been described in lambs, cattle, pigs, chickens and dogs. Symptoms include lameness and swelling of the joints. The bone cortices may be thin and spontaneous fractures may occur. A copper deficiency can affect bone formation in at least two ways.
    (a) Decreased osteoblastic activity which means a lack of bone matrix formation or
    (b) A reduction in lysyl oxidase activity which leads to diminished stability and strength of bone collagen because cross linkage is impaired.
8. Copper deficiency in chickens also causes dissecting aneurysm of the aorta. Deficient chicks show an absence of amine oxidase in the aorta and liver. This enzyme has been shown to be necessary for the

incorporation of lysine into elastins of the aorta. Thus the copper deficiency produces a lack of amine oxidase, an enzyme required for the formation of normal elastin in the aorta, and the resulting weak aorta, is subject to rupture of the inner coat and formation of the aneurysm.

9. Impaired reproduction: Low fertility characterized by delayed or depressed oestrus occurs.

Interaction Among Cu-Mo-S

There is interaction among copper, molybdenum and sulphur. Copper antagonists such as molybdenum and zinc may also be obtained by ingestion of soil rich in these minerals. High molybdenum and sulfate content of forage causes copper deficiency in grazing animals, even when the forage contains more than adequate levels of copper. High levels of zinc and cadmium depress copper absorption. Silver, calcium carbonate, ferrous sulphide and calcium phytate interfere with copper absorption.

Copper from cupric sulfate, nitrate, chloride and carbonate were available when fed to sheep. Copper from cuprous oxide was less available.

Copper Toxicity

It is rare in most animals when adequate iron and zinc are present in the diet. Copper poisoning can occur in humans where there is continous ingestion of copper from an industrial hazard. Sheep are more susceptible to copper toxicity than any other farm animal. Pigs are highly tolerant while cattle and goats are less tolereant. **Palm kernal cake** (PKC) feeding causes copper toxicity in sheep. Dietary zinc supplementation can inhibit the accumulation of hepatic and renal copper concentrations as well as whole blood copper content in sheep fed with excess PKC. In Australia feeding of sheep with 30 mg/day caused **haemolytic jaundice**. Administration of molybdenum salts is effective in alleviating symptoms of copper toxicity. Copper toxicosis occurs as a familial copper storage disorder with liver and kidney injury as in Wilson's disease in man.

Cobalt

The discovery of a lack of cobalt, in the soil and the herbage grown was responsible for the diseases of sheep and cattle-**coast disease** and **wasting disease or enzootic marasmus** (rapid muscular wasting) or **pine** and cobalt was needed to cure or prevent those diseases, was reported independently in 1935 by Filmer and Underwood and Marston and Lines, working in Australia. In 1948, two groups of workers independently discovered that the **antipernicious anaemia** (APA) factor (subsequently designated as vitamin B_{12}) contained cobalt at 4.4% (Rickes et al., 1948; Smith, 1948).

* Cobalt deficiency has not been shown in monogastric animals.

* It was demonstrated that parenteral injections of vit. B_{12} would give complete remission of all signs of cobalt deficiency in lambs.

* The nonruminant animal requires vitamin B_{12}, but due to the low level of vit. B_{12} synthesis in its intestine by microorganisms, cobalt will not substitute for vitamin B_{12} in the diet.

* Ruminants require cobalt in their rations. Rumen microorganisms synthesize vitamin B_{12} utilizing the cobalt ingested in the feed. So only oral administration of cobalt is effective in deficiency. Parenteral administration is ineffective.

* Rumen microbes partition cobalt between active (cobalamines) and physiologically inactive vitamin B_{12}-like compounds (corrinoids) that the ruminant can neither absorb nor use.

* **Vitamin B_{12} is metabolic essential for all species** but it is not dietary essential for ruminants.

* In contrast to iron and copper, body has very limited capacity to store cobalt.

The essentiality of cobalt for mammals is linked to two distinct forms of vitamin B_{12}. As methyl-cobalamin (MeCbl), cobalt assists a number of methyltransferase enzymes by acting as a donor of methyl groups and is thus involved in one-carbon metabolism, i.e. the building up of carbon chains. As adenosyl-cobalamin (AdoCbl), cobalt influences energy metabolism (propionate metabolism), facilitating the formation of glucose by assisting methylmelonyl-coenzyme A mutase to form succinate from propionate, chiefly in the liver. The enzyme leucine 2, 3-mutase is also AdoCbl-dependent and a breakdown in this pathway has been implicated in pernicious anaemeia in humans (Poston, 1980).

Sources

Healthy pastures contain 0.1 ppm of cobalt whereas sick pastures contain about 0.004 to 0.07 ppm. In cobalt deficient areas 150 g of cobalt sulphate per 100 kg of salt fed free-choice should suffice. For milking cows cobalt sulphate can be added to the concentrate mixture at the rate of 2 g per 1000 kg. Cobalt 'bullets' which can be placed in the rumen and slowly release cobalt over a long period of time have also been used.

Requirements of cobalt are roughly 1/10th of that of copper and is similar to iodine requirement.

Symptoms of Cobalt Deficiency (Effects of Deficiency)

Cobalt deficiency is the most severe mineral limitation to grazing livestock in tropical countries besides phosphorus and copper.

1. The symptoms in cattle and sheep are similar to those of general malnutrition (extreme emaciation, wasting of musculature). The animals become listless, lose of appetite and weight, become weak and anaemic and finally die. **The anemia is of the normocytic and normochromic**. In humans, it **is megaloblastic anaemia**.
2. General inanition, a fatty degeneration of the liver, and deposits of hemosiderin in the spleen are commonly found changes.
3. Wool growth is retarded and the fibres are weak.
4. A lowering of vitamin B_{12} content of the blood.
    Response to cobalt feeding, or vitamin B_{12} injections is rapid. Daily administration of 0.1 mg cobalt salts to sheep and 1 mg to cattle prevents its deficiency. About 10 times more of this element for each species is the dose to cure the disease, unless the symptoms are far advanced. Appetite picks up in about a week, and weight gains follow, but the remission of the anaemia occurs more slowly, indicating that it may be a secondary effect.

Iodine

Body contains a very minute quantity of iodine. Half to two-thirds of this total is found in the thyroid gland. The **primary function** of thyroid gland is to control the basal metabolic rate (BMR) through the output of its hormone, thyroxine. The gland consists of two parts lying on each side of the trachea at its upper end. The iodine content of thyroid gland on DMB is 0.1%. The iodine in the thyroid gland exists as inorganic iodide, mono- and diidotyrosine, triidothyronine, polypeptides containing thyroxine and thyroglobulin. Thyroglobulin (glycoprotein) is the main storage form of the iodine in the thyroid gland. **Thyroxine** (3, 5, 3′, 5′- tetra-idothyronine) is the most active form of thyroid secretion from the thyroid gland. It contains about 65% of iodine.

The removal of the thyroid gland early in life results in all species in a stunting of physical, mental and sexual development; in adult animals the hair and skin show premature ageing. Mental and physical sluggishness may develop. In all cases there is a lowered BMR. The administration of thyroxine and of iodine containing proteins stimulates body processes, notably milk and egg production. On the otherhand, certain specific compounds such as thiourea and thiouracil suppress the gland's action and metabolic processes, thus promote increased fattening (see p. 184).

Sources of iodine: Sea salt, sea weed, sea fish (all marine feedstuffs) are rich in iodine. Iodised salt is used to provide iodine as a supplement.

Iodised salt loses its iodine due to the catalytic action of sunlight, moisture, etc. Hence suitable stabilizers are often used. In mixed feeds, protein and unsaturated fats prevent loss of iodine (from iodised salt) to large extent. Sodium thiosulphate should be added to prevent loss of iodine on storage.

The iodine content of water and forage is dependent on the content and availability of iodine in the soil and the amount and iodine content of fertilizer applied to the soil. Iodine concentration in crops and grasses are greatly influenced by marine deposition and therefore decrease with distance from the sea.

Iodine content of milk and eggs can be enormously increased by feeding cows or hens with large quantities of seaweed.

Symptoms of Deficiency

Severe goiter or **enlargement of the thyroid gland** can often be seen or palpated in animals suffering from iodine deficiency. The skin and its appendages are often affected by iodine deficiency. Calves and piglets from iodine-deficient cows and sows are often hairless with thick, pulpy skin. The molting process and pigmentation of feathers can be affected by iodine deficiency in birds.

Iodine deficiency in the young lamb may influence the quality of the fleece when it is mature. Infertility problems, such as male sterility and a decline in libido, may occur in the adult sheep suffering from iodine deficiency. **Hairless pups** may be produced by bitches on iodine deficient diets.

Goiter is the enlargement of thyroid gland. Simple goiter is the most common type. Simple goiter is caused primarily by lack of iodine. Hyperplastic changes begin as a result of a failure of the thyroid tissue to supply enough secretion, owing either to a reduced supply of iodine for its manufacture or to an increased demand for the secretion by the body. The demand for thyroxine varies.

Simple goiter is most likely to develop in the humans during pregnancy and puberty when the requirement for iodine is more. (Thyroid gland weighs about 30 g in adult man). The discovery that iodine deficiency impaired brain development in humans replaced the term goiter with **iodine deficiency disorders (IDD)**. In farm animals, goiter is seen in the young at birth as a result of a deficiency of iodine in the rations of the mother during gestation. The young thus affected are born weak or dead. Though a lack of iodine is the primary cause of simple goiter, it is recognized that **other factors** may contribute.

1. High-calcium content of the water in many goitrous regions.
2. Specific goitrogenic substances in certain foods, notably various members of the Brassica family (cabbage), peanuts and soybeans.

These foods contain specific substances which slow down the thyroxin-secreting activity of the gland. Peanuts are goitrogenic for the rat. Active principle is glucoside, arachidoside.

Goitrogens interfere with thyroid hormone synthesis by limiting the capacity of the gland either to 'trap' iodine or to incorporate this iodine into thyroactive substances. These are of two types:

1. organic goitrogens e.g. cruciferous plants (thiouracil type-progoitrin), most brassics and white clover (cyanogenetic glycosides → thiocyanate), rapeseed meal (glucosinolates → isothiocyanates, thiocyanate and goitrin).
2. inorganic goitrogens e.g. high arsenic and high fluoride intake, excess ingestion of bivalent cobalt, rubidium, etc.

Toxicity

Prolonged consumption of large amounts of iodine can cause a markedly reduced thyroidal iodine uptake, causing iodide goiter. This is not a common occurrence in animals. The tolerance for iodine appears to be high relative to normal dietary iodine intakes, indicating a wide margin of safety for this element. Most animals appear to start showing ill effects when fed rations containing from 200 to 500 ppm of iodine.

Manganese

Manganese is required to activate several enzymes such as arginase, cystine desulfydrase, thiaminase. It is also thought to be involved in oxidative phosphorylation. It is necessary for the synthesis of chondroitin sulfate, a major constituent of the cartilage of bone. Manganese is needed in glucosyl transferase activity which is needed for the formation of mucopolysaccharides and glycoproteins. A deficiency of these products leads to decreased chondrogenesis (cartilage formation). High levels of iron, potassium, calcium and phosphorus in the diet appear to interfere with manganese absorption. Higher manganese levels appear to interfere with iron absorption.

Manganese deficiency is extremely rare in farm animals, except perhaps in poultry whose requirements are much higher than that of other species. This is because manganese is fairly well distributed in the common feeds available for farm animals.

Sources: Most of the manganese in the animal body is present in the bones. Most roughages contain 40 to 140 mg per kg and seeds and byproducts contain 15 to 45 mg per kg.

Symptoms of deficiency: **Manganese deficiency** as a practical production problem is **largely confined to avian species**. A major symptom of manganese deficiency in most animals is bone abnormality.

Swine: Manganese deficiency in swine causes slow skeletal growth, irregular estrus cycles, reabsorption of foetus or birth of small, weak pigs, poor udder development and inability to produce milk. **Crooked legs** and **enlarged hocks** have been produced on manganese deficient rations.

Poultry: In the young growing chicken the primary symptom is **perosis** or **'slipped tendon'**, a malformation of the leg bones of growing chicks. The hock joints become swollen and the Achilles tendon slips from its condyle. A shortening of the leg bones was involved. In severe form the birds are reluctant to move, walk upon their hocks and soon die. When hens are fed manganese deficient diets, abnormalities show up in the embryo (chondrodystrophy) and in the newly hatched chick (ataxia characterized by a star-gazing position). Embryo chicks develop **"parrot beaks"**. The most striking signs of deficiency, biochemically, is the reduced content of chondroitin sulphate in the epiphyseal cartilage. Crooked front legs are produced in rabbits by feeding a diet low in manganese.

Toxicity: Manganese is considered to be among the least toxic of the trace elements to birds and mammals. There is no problem of toxicity from moderate excesses of manganese, but 125 ppm have been found to depress haemoglobin synthesis in baby pigs. This apparently represented a manganese-iron antagonism since additional iron overcame the depression. Growth was depressed by 1250 ppm in growing pigs.

Manganese between 50 and 125 ppm affected haemoglobin formation in lambs and mature rabbits. Rats and hens have been reported to tolerate 1000 ppm without obvious ill effects.

Zinc

Zinc is required for the activity of over 300 enzymes and participates in many enzymatic and metabolic functions in avian and mammalian species. One of the most important functions of zinc is related to its antioxidant role and its participation in the antioxidant defense system. Dietary zinc is required for normal immune function as well as proper skeletal development and maintenance. Carbonic anhydrase (found in RBC) contain 0.3% Zn and plays an essential role in eliminating CO_2. It can serve as an activator of alkaline phosphatase. Zinc has antagonising effect on calcium. High dietary calcium levels cause a tremendous increase in the zinc requirements. **'Conditioned' zinc deficiency** may be caused by including a high amount of calcium in the ration.

The highest concentrations are found in the epidermal tissues, such as skin, hair and wool, but traces also occur in the bones, muscles, blood and various organs.

Absorption and Excretion

Zinc is absorbed in the small intestine and an intestinal pool of zinc may be formed by binding the metal to the intestinal metallothionein or zinc may be transported by albumin in plasma to the liver. More than one isoform of metallothionein is found in different tissues in animal species. Metallothionein is synthesized in tissues in response to dietary zinc and can bind 7 atoms of zinc per molecule of protein. Metallothinein can also bind copper with a higher affinity. It is a cysteine-rich protein that acts as a free radical scavenger. **High levels of Ca, phosphate, phytate, copper and cadmium in the ration decrease zinc absorption**.

Zinc is primarily excreted from the body in the faeces. Most animals exhibit considerable tolerance to high levels of zinc in the diet; however, cattle and sheep are less tolerant than most nonruminants.

Effects of Zinc Deficiency

Zinc deficiency causes loss of appetite and reduced efficiency of feed utilization and thus leads to growth retardation. Zinc deficiency increases oxidative damage of cell membranes caused by free radicals. Zinc deficiency causes a decrease in cellular immunity and adversely affects thymus, spleen, and interleukin production.

Pigs have been shown to suffer from zinc deficiency called **"parakeratosis"**. The disease is characterized by specific skin lesions, retarded growth and lowered feed utilization. Skin gives the appearance of severe 'mange'. Diarrhoea and anorexia are also observed.

In chicks zinc deficiency symptoms include, slow growth, shortened and thickened long bones and poor feathering, with keratosis resulting when the deficiency is severe. Lower egg production and hatchability and embryonic anomalies are also observed. Mortality has been observed in severe cases.

Zinc deficiency has been reported in humans. Dwarfism and absence of sexual maturation have been reported in severe deficiencies. On less severe deficiency of zinc, poor growth, poor appetite and impaired taste acuity (acuteness) in children are reported.

Sources: Animal protein and feed products, such as distiller's solubles, contain rather large amounts of zinc, while the endosperm of most cereal grains is low in zinc content. Zinc supplementation of swine and poultry diets is usually necessary. This is especially true when these diets contain large amounts of corn and SBM and high calcium levels. The large amounts of phytate in such rations tie up zinc and makes it unavailable for absorption in the presence of high calcium concentrations. Zinc supplements include Zn-methionine (organic source), ZnO and $ZnSO_4$.

Fluorine

Fluorine occurs in an apatite form as an integral part of the structure of bones and teeth to the extent of 0.04 to 0.06% in the adult.

Is Fluorine an Essential Element ?

Tooth decay in man and experimental animals: Both epidemiological and experimental studies revealed that the incidence of dental caries is decreased during the period of tooth development where the water supply contains 1 ppm, in contrast to lower levels. Thus, as a public health measure, many muncipalities in USA are adding 0.7 to 1 ppm of fluorine as fluoride to water supplies which otherwise contain much smaller traces. This added level does not result in mottled enamel or any other deleterious effect observable in longterm studies. Clearly it has been proven that **fluorine in traces is a useful mineral for the prevention of dental caries** in children, and some workers have considered it an essential dietary constituent on this basis.

Fluorosis

Though fluorine gives rigidity to bones and teeth, intakes of rather minute amounts have been shown harmful cumulatively. **Fluorosis** is a condition caused by drinking water containing more than 1 ppm of fluorine. It is also observed in animals fed rations supplemented with natural mineral phosphates (containing high amount of fluorine) for a long period. Similarly ingestion of forage contaminated with fluorine from fumes released by smelting plants cause fluorosis.

Effect of Fluorosis (Fluorine Toxicity) and Symptoms

Fluorine is a cumulative poison. Most of the fluorine ingested is deposited in the skeleton and teeth. The level of fluorine in bone and teeth then reaches ten times the normal values. It is at this stage metabolic disorders and certain pathological syndromes are clearly manifested. Thus **skeletal system acts as a buffer**. The avidity of the bones and teeth for fluorine tends to protect the soft tissues against excessive concentrations. Chicken will tolerate a considerably higher level than farm animals.

1. The bones and teeth lose their natural colour and turn yellow due to gradual excessive accumulation. The bones become thickened and softened and the breaking strength is decreased. Joints may be swollen and painful.
2. Bone outgrowths from the surface, called **exostoses**, occur from jaw bones and long bones. A varient of severe skeletal fluorosis in humans is termed as 'Genuvalgum' or knocked knee syndrome.

3. **Elongation of incisor teeth and molars**. The enamel loses its glistening yellow colour and becomes chalky and brittle. The teeth are mottled, molars get worn out, and the animal experiences difficulty in chewing. Teeth may become stained, showing a colouration which varies from yellow to black. Mottled teeth are structurally weak. Mottling occurs in children who regularly drink water containing as little as 2 to 5 ppm of fluorine.

4. It interferes with feed/food consumption and eventually growth and production are decreased.

BIS specified the maximum level of fluorine in bone meal and mineral mixtures as 0.05 to 0.07%. Sodium fluoride is more toxic than calcium fluoride.

Molybdenum

Molybdenum as an Essential Element

Molybdenum has been found to be essential in traces. It is a constituent of the enzyme xanthine oxidase/dehydrogenase (XDH), a metallo-flavoprotein. This enzyme plays a useful role in purine metabolism. Molybdenum is also a cofactor in aldehyde oxidase (AO) and sulfite oxidase (SOX). These enzymes catalyse redox reactions. Molybdenum is essential for the growth of chicks and poults hatched from eggs from molybdenum-depleted hens or in chicks fed diets containing tungsten, which is an antagonist of molybdenum. Chick has a large need for xanthine oxidase for uric acid formation in contrast to the rat.

Molybdenum Toxicity

Ruminants especially young calves and milch cows are particularly susceptible to the intake of pasture containing molybdenum more than 10 ppm. Molybdenum toxicity in cattle is called '**teartness**'. The prominent physical symptoms were extreme diarrhoea with consequent loss in weight and milk production and loss of coat colour. A healthy pasture does not contain more than 3 to 5 ppm. Horses and pigs are the most tolerant and cattle and sheep are least tolerant to molybdenum toxicity. Rats, rabbits, guinea pigs and poultry are intermediate in their tolerance.

In laboratory animal experiments the **symptoms of chronic molybdenum poisoning and of copper deficiency were found similar**. This copper-sulphate-molybdenum interrelationship has already been discussed.

Selenium

In North America it was shown that the livestock diseases 'blind staggers' and 'alkali disease' were caused by acute and chronic selenium poisoning, respectively, after Franke and Potter identified selenium as the toxic factor in forage in 1935. **Degnala disease** in India, **Saliman disease** in Mexico are similar to alkali disease. Selenium is grouped under ultratrace minerals along with iodine, cobalt, and molybdenum.

Selenium as an Essential Nutrient

Beginning in 1950, evidence accumulated suggesting that selenium in traces is an essential nutrient despite its toxicity in larger intakes. Liver necrosis in rats and pigs, **exudative diathesis** (a haemorrhagic disease) in chickens, degeneration of the pancreas in chicks, dystrophy of heart muscles and gizzard (**gizzard myopathy**) in turkeys, white muscle disease (**muscular dystrophy**), sometimes heart necrosis in lambs and calves are caused by selenium deficiency. Retarded growth rate is commonly seen. All these diseases are prevented by either selenium or vitamin E supplementation.

In 1973 it was discovered that selenium is a component of glutathione peroxidase. This enzyme catalyzes the removal of peroxides which explain the antioxidant role of selenium and why vitamin E (which is also a biological antioxidant) may have similar effects to selenium in certain situations.

Selenium plays an important role in animal reproduction. Selenium deficiency results in impaired reproductive performance in males (reduced viability of semen) and females. **Reproductive problems associated with selenium deficiency** included retained placenta, abortions, birth of premature, weak or dead ones, cystic ovaries, metritis, erratic or silent heats and poor fertilization.

Sel-Plex (Alltech) selenium yeast is the only organic selenium source that has been approved for broilers, layers, pig and turkey feeds by the FDA in the US.

Selenium supplementation (0.1 ppm) improved the reproductive efficiency of sheep and reduced the incidence of retained placenta in dairy cattle.

Chemistry and Distribution

After absorption, selenium in excess of that needed in glutathione peroxidase and other enzymes is usually methylated to trimethyl selenide and excreted from the body. However, when the body load becomes so great that it cannot be made into the trimethyl form, the dimethyl selenide, a volatile compound, is excreted via the lungs in the expired air. This compound imparts a garlic odour to the breath that has long been associated with selenium toxicity.

Selenium-deficient areas: These have less than 0.03 ppm. Seleniferous areas will contain high levels of selenium (0.5 to 6 ppm). Animal and fish products usually contain fairly high levels of selenium; however, the selenium from these products may not be as available to animals as is selenium in plant products. The inorganic sodium selenite is the predominant form of selenium supplement added to animal feeds.

Toxicity

Dietary levels of 10 to 20 ppm of selenium are toxic for most species of animals. This is at least 100 times the level needed by the animal. Selenium toxicity is associated with animals grazing seleniferous areas. Selenium-accumulator plants (Astragalus species of plants) growing on these soils may accumulate selenium to give levels of 100 ppm to 14,920 ppm, the highest level recorded till now. Selenium content of the plant declines with maturity.

When grazing animals eat such plants, they rapidly become unthrifty, dull and listless, their appetite decline, and they become emaciated. They become lame, develop an atrophy of the heart, cirrhosis of the liver, anaemia and eventually die of starvation. Young animals are especially susceptible and growth is retarded with levels too low to cause other evident symptoms. In swine, conception rates are lowered and result in a higher percentage of pigs dead at birth or weak and smaller in size. Reproduction troubles have also been noted in sheep and poultry.

Selenium occurs in the milk and eggs from cows and hens fed rations containing the element. In chronic cases, there is a loss of hair from the mane and tail in horses, from the tail in cattle and a general loss of hair in swine. The hoofs slough off, lameness occurs, food consumption decreases, and death may occur by starvation.

In some parts of Haryana and Punjab, the animals suffer with selenosis, the disease is known as 'Degnala'. Toxic effects can be mitigated by high protein intake (linseed oil meal exert some protective action) and inorganic sulfate and arsenic supplementation. Sulfate used as fertilizer also lessens selenium uptake by plants.

Selenium Assimilation in Plants

Where soil conditions allow, plants take up soil selenite, selenate and selenomethionine, though no requirement by higher plants for selenium has yet been found.

The similarities between sulphur and selenium cause a number of interactions. Sulphate and selenate compete for common uptake sites in plant roots; therefore selenate uptake can be inhibited by high sulphate supplies.

Plants are considered in three categories with respect to selenium content: accumulator plants, selenium indicator plants and non-accumulator plants. The former two groups absorb high quantities of selenium when grown on high selenium soils (seleniferous soils). The latter group does not accumulate selenium in levels toxic to animals when grown on seleniferous soils. Most common species of plants, marine algae, bacteria and yeast (non-accumulator species) can synthesize both methionine and selenomithionine; however animals can form neither. For this reason methionine is listed among the dietary essential amino acids for higher animals.

Accumulator plants and non-accumulator plants metabolize selenium differently. In non-accumulator plants soil selenite or selenate is converted primarily into selenomethionine, which is then incorporated into plant protein in place of methionine (see Figure 1). In accumulator plants such as many Austragalus spp, selenocysteine is transformed into small, water-soluble NPN compounds such as selenomethylcysteine.

Selenium metabolism in animals

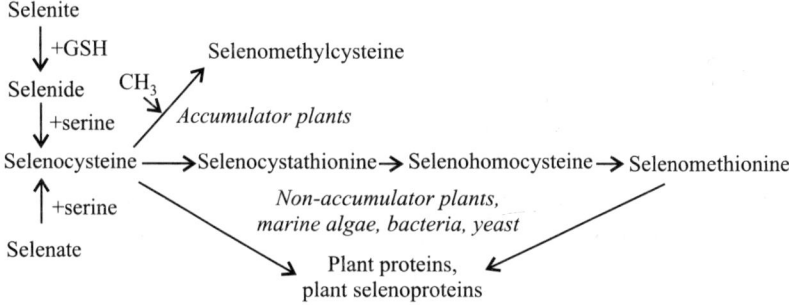

Figure 1 Selenium assimilation in accumulator plants versus assimilation in non-accumulator species (Source: K.A.Jacques, 2001).

Absorption of selenium by animals and availability of selenium in feedstuffs

Animal diets contain variable amounts of organic selenium (predominantly selenomethionine) and whatever amounts of inorganic selenium we add at diet formulation. Inorganic and organic forms of selenium in animal diets are absorbed by different mechanisms. Selenite is absorbed from the intestine by a simple diffusion process, whereas selenate is actively absorbed in the ileum by co-transport with sodium ions. Selenomethionine is derived primarily from plants and it is absorbed in the small intestine via the Na+-dependent neutral amino acid transport system. The difference in the metabolism of plant-derived selenium (selenomethionine) and inorganic selenium (for example, sodium selenate) sources by animals is a pointed example of the importance of nutrient form in physiological function. Selenomethionine is the main source of easily metabolized and easily retained form of selenium for animals, including humans.

The amount of absorbable inorganic selenium presented at absorption sites depends on interactions with a range of interfering substances in the diet or drinking water including iron, sulphur, phytate and antioxidants, among others. The amount of selenomethionine in forage or grain available for absorption will depend on the digestibility of the source. Highly available sources of selenium include selenium yeast, wheat and alfalfa; moderately available sources being the most plant materials, while the selenium in meat and fish-byproducts are poorly available (Combs and Combs, 1986).

Newly Discovered and Other Trace Elements

There are 15 definitely known essential trace elements—these are:

Iron Fe, Copper Cu, Manganese Mn, Zinc Zn, Cobalt Co, Iodine I, Molybdenum Mo, Selenium Se, Fluorine F, Chromium Cr, Boron B, Lithium Li, Nickel Ni, Vanadium V, and Silicon Si.

Tin (Sn) was suggested to be essential in 1970. But confirmation of essentiality is still lacking. Aluminium (Al), Arsenic (As), Cadmium (Cd), Lead (Pb) and Mercury (Hg) are frequently classified as toxic elements because their biological activity is largely confined to toxic reactions.

Al, Cd, Pb, and As have been suggested as possibly essential.

Cd, Hg, Pb, and As are frequently encountered in insecticides, fungicides, batteries, paints, gasoline additives, phosphate fertilizers, etc.

Selenium, fluorine, molybdenum, lead and arsenic cause poisoning in ruminants.

High levels of Hg and Cd are particularly antagonistic to Ca, Cu, Zn, Se, Fe. Aluminium complexes with P, making it unavailable for plants, thereby increasing the incidence and severity of P deficiencies in livestock. A further 20 to 30 trace elements occur regularly in feeds and animal tissue, and it is unknown whether they serve some useful purpose or are merely contaminants.

Improved procedures for diet purification, use of metal—free isolator system for raising animals, and advances in trace-element analytical techniques are helpful in identifying the essentiality of trace elements. The advent of multielement analyses using neutron activation, inductively coupled plasma emission atomic absorption spectroscopy (AAS), and spark-source mass spectrometry have stimulated biological interest in a large number of trace elements.

Aluminium

Abundant elements in the earth's crust rank wise are 1. oxygen 2. silicon 3. aluminium. But aluminium is found only in trace amounts in biological organisms. Kaolin and bentonite clays used as pellet binders, forages, as contaminant from dust, sewage-grown algae (up to 8% Al), mineral supplements, certain plants of aluminium accumulators are sources of Al to animal diets.

Chromium

The chromium that occurs in brewer's yeast is now known to be a chelated complex between chromium, two nicotinic acid molecules, and several amino acids. It now appears that humans can use this preformed **glucose tolerance factor (GTF)** or slowly synthesize the factor from inorganic chromium, niacin, and amino acids. **Chromium deficiency** leads to a decreased sensitivity of peripheral tissues to insulin. In response to sudden increases of insulin in the blood the glucose tolerance factor is released and exerts its action, potentiation of insulin at the target tissues.

GTF complex actually might possibly qualify as a vitamin since it contains Cr, organic components of nicotinic acid, glycine, glutamic acid and cystine, and has a much greater biological activity than do inorganic sources of Cr alone. This would be comparable to vitamin B_{12} being more metabolically effective than the element Co.

Chromium and Human Health

Chromium is an essential trace element because it potentiates insulin action. Studies conducted in 1990 reported that sub-optimal chromium intake in humans led to detrimental changes in glucose, insulin and glucagon with slightly impaired glucose tolerance. That is chromium deficiency is associated with diabetic like symptoms and its supplementation enhances glucose tolerance and insulin sensitivity.

It is reported that chromium deficiency is prevalent in North America because most diets contain too little organic chromium and high sugar intakes, strenuous exercise and emotional and physical trauma, cause loss of body stores of it in urine.

Beneficial effects of chromium supplementation in malnourished children suggest that this is essential and that deficiencies exist. Chromium supplementation almost immediately restored glucose tolerance to normal in these children.

It is also reported that chromium can reduce zinc absorption just as phytate, calcium plus phytate, fibre, phosphorus, copper and cadmium. In experimental animals and humans, some studies have shown decreased cholesterol and increased high density lipoprotein (HDL) cholesterol (good cholesterol), while others have shown no effect of chromium supplementation.

Chromium and Pigs

Studies in pigs fed with supplemental chromium as **chromium picolinate at 200 ppb** level from 20 kg to 105 kg body weight showed increased muscle and decreased lipid deposition and the supplemental pigs had greater longissimus muscle area and greater absorption and retention of nitrogen. This kind of carcass modifying effect of chromium is a welcome feature which is otherwise possible with hormone injections, implants or feed supplements which attract resistance from the consumers.

Similarly sows fed diets with supplemental chromium picolinate from 40 kg through two parities had larger litters than sows that had never received supplemental chromium. The sows received supplemental chromium had lower insulin concentrations and a lower insulin: glucagon ratio in mid gestation, indicating greater efficiency of insulin action.

Chromium and Stress

Studies conducted in 1995 indicated that cattle also may be susceptible to chromium deficiency, particularly during stress. Supplementation of organic chromium to transit–stressed calves, and early lactation dairy cows, improved the immune status and milk yield. Chromium seemed to reduce blood cortisol concentrations during stress and promoted improved insulin or insulin-like growth factor (IGF-1) sensitivity in target tissues such as muscle, mammary gland, and the immune system. It was concluded that occurrence of infectious diseases could be reduced and production potential increased if the diets of high-producing or intensively reared cattle were supplemented with chromium. It is suggested that supplemental organic chromium is immunomodulatory in high-producing dairy cows. Studies conducted in primiparous and multiparous cows revealed that supplementation (0.5 ppm Cr as amino acid chelated chromium) from 6 week prepartum to 16 week postpartum (after calving) increased the milk yield of primiparous cows by 7 to 13% along with higher lactose concentration in milk. Serum concentrations of beta hydroxy butyric acid (BHBA) were lower in supplemented cows. These results suggest that supplemental chromium may improve lactation performance and reduce incidence of some metabolic disorders (e.g. Milk fever) in early lactation.

Chromium Toxicity

In chrome tanning, which is widely used, as many as 276 chemicals including 14 heavy metals are used and the chromium concentration in the discharge of effluent from tanneries ranged from 2000 to 5000 ppm. These pollutants tended to accumulate in the soil and levels in the water rise. These high levels naturally affect the animal and human health in those tracts.

We are fortunate that by nature the plant uptake and absorption of chromium by animal is very limited; otherwise the effect would have been disastrous. Very high oral intakes are necessary to attain toxic levels because of poor absorption of trivalent chromium. Hexavalent chromium is much more toxic than is the trivalent form.

Cats tolerate 1000 mg/day, and rats showed no adverse effects from 100 mg/kg diet.

Chromic oxide (Cr_2O_3) (III) has been used as a faecal marker in cattle and sheep for periods of several weeks at levels as high as 3000 ppm Cr with no adverse effects.

Chicks fed with 1000 ppm Cr as chromic chloride had no effect while a dose of 2000 ppm resulted in reduced growth.

In animals **chronic chromium toxicosis** result in skin-contact dermatitis, irritation of respiratory passages, ulceration and perforation of the nasal septum, and lung cancer. Acute systemic chromium intoxication is rare but was produced with a single oral dose of 700 mg/kg of body weight using chromium (IV) in mature cattle and 30-40 mg/kg of body weight in young calves. Signs of acute toxicosis included inflamation and congestion of the stomach and ulceraticn of the rumen and abomasum.

Chromium Toxicity in Humans

In humans, symptoms of industrial exposure to chromium include allergic dermatitis, skin ulcers, and increased incidence of bronchogenic carcinoma. Airborne hexavalent chromium is responsible for this to a greater extent because trivalent chromium is less well absorbed and less irritating.

Chronic exposure to chromate dust has been correlated with increased incidence of lung cancer, and oral administration of 50 ppm of chromium has been associated with growth depression and liver and kidney damage in experimental animals. Chromium exposure is a common skin sensitizer in allergic eczema; chromium in detergents and bleaches also causes dermatitis among the users of such material.

Boron: Boron has been known to be essential for higher plants since the 1920s, but only recently has a possible role in animal and human nutrition been suggested.

Essentiality: A study in day-old chicks indicated a relationship among B, Ca, Mg and vitamin D_3 (Req. about 1 ppm in the diet). **Boron** (somehow) **regulates parathormone action**, and therefore, indirectly influences metabolism of Ca, P, Mg and cholecalciferol.

Boron is needed by the parathyroid and has been shown to prevent loss of Ca and bone demineralization in postmenopausal women (Humans might require near 1 mg/day).

Toxicity: High dietary B has been shown to be **detrimental to riboflavin inducing riboflavinuria**. Newly hatched chicks treated with boric acid at 96 hr of incubation exhibited curled-toe-paralysis.

Lithium: It ranks 27th in abundance among the elements. **It is used in the therapy of manic-depressive psychosis**. It has been shown to be an effective agent in the recovery of animals with **bovine spastic paresis** (BSP), a disease of the central nervous system.

Nickel (Ni)

It is present in RNA in rather high concentrations. The average Ni concentration in the earth's crust is about 80 ppm. Levels of nickel greater than 1000 ppm in the diet are toxic to most animals.

Nickel is essential for urease activity of rumen microbes. It is also essential for the rat, pig and goat. Chicks fed a diet containing less than 14 ppb nickel exhibited several abnormalities. These include impaired liver metabolism such as reduced ability to oxidize alpha glycerophosphate, increased lipid content and decreased phospholipid content, and ultrastructural degeneration of the liver cells. Gross changes included a dermatitis and change in pigmentation of shank skin and a decrease in friability of the liver.

Plant foods are generally higher in nickel than are foods of animal origin.

Tin (Sn): Tin increased the average daily gain of rats when supplemented at 2 ppm of tin in the form of stannic sulphate. It has been suggested that tin could be an oxidation-reduction catalyst and function at the active site of metalloenzymes.

Vanadium (V): Vanadium is believed to be essential for the chick and rat. It is present in human enamel and dentin. It has been reported that vanadium decreases the incidence of caries in rats, hamsters and guinea pigs.

A deficiency of vanadium results in reduced body weight and feather growth, impaired reproduction, altered red blood cells and iron metabolism, impairement of bone tissue metabolism and altered blood lipid levels. Vanadium might have a role in the regulation of Na^+, K^+-ATPase, phosphoryl transfer enzymes, adenylate cyclase, and protein kinase (Nielsen, 1990).

EDTA appears to act as an antidote in vanadium toxicosis, possibly by preventing absorption from the intestinal tract. Vanadium forms up to 110 to 150 ppm of the earth's crust, and its prevalence probably equals that of Cu, Pb or Zn. Levels of 25 to 30 ppm in the diet is toxic to most animals while the dietary requirement is less than 500 ppb.

Whole grains, seafood, meats and dairy products have a range of 5 to 30 ppb vanadium. Fats and oils and fresh fruits and vegetables contain the least (< 1 to 5 ppb).

Silicon: Next to oxygen, silicon is the most abundant element on earth, and quartz (crystalline silica) is the most abundant mineral in the earth's crust. Carlisle (1970) demonstrated that silicon (Si) was **essential for normal calcification of chick bone**. Silicon may have a role in mucopolysaccharide synthesis and may function as a biological cross-linking agent contributing to the structural integrity of connective tissue.

Symptoms of Deficiency

1. Growth depression has been reported in rats and chicks fed silicon-deficient diets.
2. Rats also demonstrated impaired incisor pigmentation.
3. Deficient chicks had no wattles and their combs were very small.
4. Lack of Si may be involved in several human disorders, including atherosclerosis, osteoarthritis and hypertension as well as the ageing process (Nielson, 1988).

High levels of silicon in the diet of farm animals may be detrimental but nontoxic. The digestibility of plants containing high levels of silicon as silicates is greately decreased. In mature forage plants, Si is in the form of solid mineral particles known as **opal phytoliths** ($SiO_2.H_2O$). Ruminants may develop **siliceous renal calculi**. Such calculi may become large enough to block passage of urine. However, this urolithiasis is not simply due to high intakes of silicon alone. In human urolithiasis, oxalates, urates or phosphates play the predominant role.

Sources: Cereal grains contain much lower concentration of Si than do leaves and stems of the same species.

Lead: It is one of the most common causes of accidental poisoning in man and domestic animals. It is not an instantaneous killer but an insidious, slow and steady killer, through, "plumbism". Sources of lead include ingestion-drinking water from lead pipe, lead-base paint, toys, newspaper and newsprint ink; surma, sindoor and azarcon which are used as cosmetics; food sources include cooking utensils, vegetables grown in lead-rich soil, acid foods like vinegar and fruit juices stored in containers, canned foods, adulterated turmaric; used motor oil and storage batteries and vehicular emission. Lead poisoning may also occur when animals eat forage contaminated by lead from fumes and dusts emitted from industrial lead operations. Lead concentration of 80 ppm in forage could be toxic to horses but cattle could tolerate 200 ppm or more. High levels of calcium may decrease lead toxicity.

New Delhi (India) is declared as the fourth most polluted city in the world. Many diplomatic missions in the capital are fortifying themselves against its effects by fitting the premises with oxygenators, and depollution equipment,

Lead and benzene content in the vehicular emission in Delhi are high. Benzene is carcinogenic. Petrol is the single most important cause for the increase in lead in the atmosphere worldwide. There is a high level of particulate lead in the ambient air of Delhi.

Effects of Lead Poisoning and Symptoms

Lead poisoning causes permanent brain damage, and reduction in normal intelligence quotient in children, even in low concentrations of lead, and increased lead absorption in cases of deficiency of iron, calcium and zinc are reported. Higher concentrations of lead result in anaemia, seizures, coma and death in children. The study has also established that lead in the blood could aggravate or cause anaemia, colic and abdominal pain, neurological problems, hypertension and heart disease, behavioural disturbances, kidney damage, multisystem damage, among other things in adults.

Populations at great risk of lead absorption are malnourished, anaemic children, industrial workers, traffic police, street vendors and auto drivers.

The most important target of lead in the body is the brain. In the polluted areas level of lead in the blood is 35-40 µg/dl. Children with blood lead levels of 25 µg/dl at birth had impaired cognitive abilities and their intelligence quotient is dropped. Levels over 10 µg/dl blood are considered bad. Young children absorb lead more easily than adults. Children between six and 72 months are four to five times more vulnerable than adults in absorbing lead. The permissible limits of lead in air are about 0.75 to 1.5 µg/cu M, and in drinking water, it is 0.05 µg/litre.

Lead once ingested, it enters the blood stream. Although some of it is routinely excreted, excess amounts accumulate in the bones resulting in its ossification. Pregnant women with high blood levels could pass this on to the foetus *in utero* and thereafter when they breast feed the child. Lead competes with calcium. As a result, the breast milk of such women could contain high levels of lead.

Organic Minerals

Minerals in an organic form (chelated) are becoming more widely used. These organometallic complexes are also called chelates. The AAFCO identifies complexes/chelates in different classes: a metal specific amino acid complex (Figure 2), a metal amino acid chelates, metal proteinates and metal polysaccharide complex.

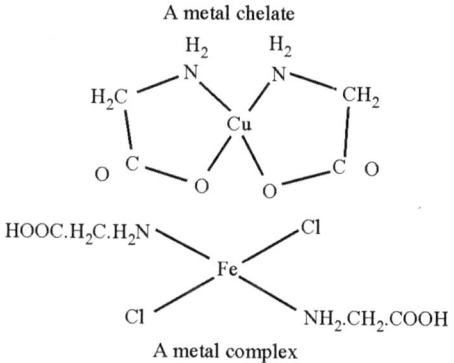

Figure 2 Metal chelate and metal complex.

A metal amino acid complex is obtained by combining a soluble metal salt with any amino acid(s). The minimum metal content must be declared on the product, but no mention of the particular amino acid is made. Metals used are calcium, copper, iron, magnesium, manganese, potassium and zinc. **A metal amino acid chelate** is the product formed by the reaction of one mole of a soluble metal ion with 1-3 moles of amino acids. An example is given in Figure 3, which shows the formation of ferrous bis-glucinate chelate from two ligands of glycine and a ferrous (+2) iron atom. The minimum metal content is finally declared when used as a commercial feed ingredient. The various amino acids used for chelation of mineral elements are lysine, threonine, tryptophan, methionine and glycine. **A metal proteinate** is a product obtained from the chelation of a soluble mineral salt with an amino acid and /or a particular hydrolyzed protein. The final product is called a specific metal proteinate.

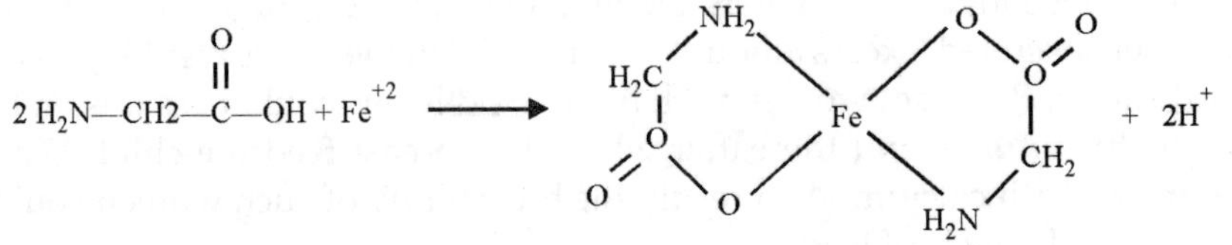

$$
2\ H_2N-CH2-\overset{\overset{\displaystyle O}{\|}}{C}-OH + Fe^{+2} \longrightarrow
$$

Figure 3   Metal amino acid chelates.

Organic mineral supplements have been shown to improve serum and tissue levels of micronutrients compared to inorganic sources where complex interactions may occur. Organic forms of minerals help in better absorption of other minerals as well. Organic forms of minerals have higher bioavailability. They improve the immune response of animals, decrease the susceptibility to diseases and give better performance in respect of prcduction as well as reproduction, e.g., chelated zinc versus zinc oxide; copper proteinate versus copper sulphate; selenomethionine versus sodium selenite or sodium selenate.

Chelation

A chelate is a cyclic compound which is formed between an organic molecule and a metallic ion, the latter being held within the organic molecule as if by a claw (Chelate is derived from the Greek word "chele" meaning 'claw'). Tetraclines form chelates with calcium and other polyvalent cations which interfere with antimicrobial activity of an antibiotic.

Three types of chelates are recognized in biological systems:

1. Chelates that serve to transport and to store metal ions: Amino acids, especially cysteine and histidine, are particularly effective metal binding agents and are of use in the transport and storage of mineral elements (Cu^{++}, Zn^{++}, Fe^{++}) throughout the animal body. Ethlenediamine tetraacetic acid (EDTA) may improve the availability of zinc and other minerals.

2. Chelates essential in metabolism: Many chelates exist in the animal body with metal ion in their strcuture e.g., haemoglobin, cytochrome enzymes and vitamin B_{12}. They have iron, cobalt, etc. that are very important to perform their metabolic functions.

3. Chelates which interfere with utilization of essential cations: Examples are phytic acid-zinc chelate, oxalic acid—calcium chelate, etc. These interfere with absorption of zinc and calcium.

Geophagia, or soil consumption is commonly observed in wildlife and has been suggested as an important means of meeting trace element requirements, including iron. (See page No. 251)

Balanced trace element nutrition helps to neutralize Oxidative Stress

High iron levels and insufficient amounts of zinc, copper and manganese in feedstuffs contribute to oxidative stress. Iron is a prooxidant, while zinc, manganese, copper or selenium has antioxidative properties. Balanced and bioavailable trace element supply will protect the animal from oxidative stress.

High iron levels in feedstuffs and water are common around the globe. Excessive amounts of iron are fed compared to the animal's requirement. Feeding excess iron affects the performance (cause retained placenta and udder oedema) and can cause oxidative damage to tissues. The iron requirement of an adult dairy cow is estimated to be about 100 mg/ day, depending on the DM intake and production. But intake may go up to 1840 to 2000 mg/day based on a work done in The Netherlands (Paul Perucchietti and Wilbert Litjens, 2010). Under normal circumstances, the harmful effects of iron are inhibited by complexing the mineral in larger molecules that are transported from sites susceptible to damage. Dietary imbalances, inflammation, environmental stresses or saturation of iron-binding sites are likely to negatively influence this process.

A diet deficient in zinc, manganese, copper or selenium can contribute to tissue oxidative damage. These are the active components of well-known antioxidant enzymes such as superoxide dismutase (SOD) and glutathione peroxidase (GSH-Px). Moreover, zinc is also associated with metallothionein, which can act as an antioxidant. It is shown that zinc can act as specific antioxidant protecting macromolecules against the negative effects of iron-induced oxidative stress. Vitamin E was only effective as an antioxidant at low iron dietary levels, but ineffective at high levels. Figure 4 shows the metabolism of prooxidants and antioxidants.

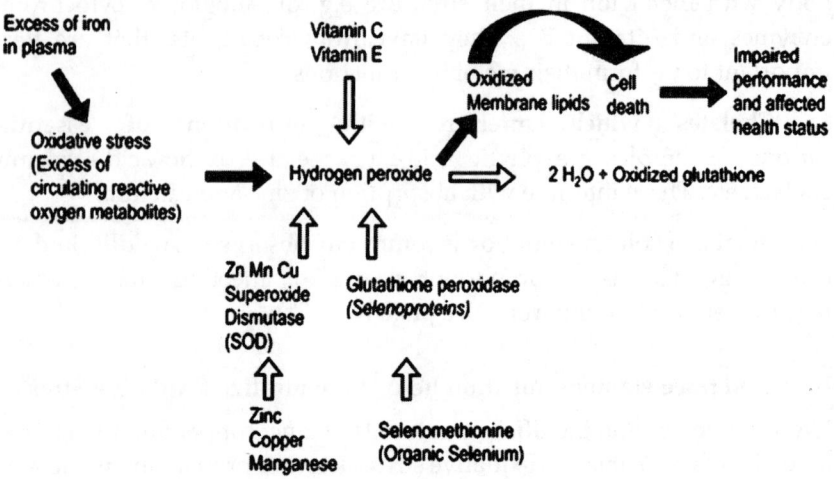

Figure 4   Balanced trace element nutrition neutralizes oxidative stress.
(Source: All About Feed – Vol. 1, No. 5, pp 28-29, 2010)

Chapter 12

The Vitamins

Introduction-Definition

Vitamins are chemical entities which are essential for maintaining the metabolic processes at a normal level in animals. Kazimierz Funk, a Polish scientist gave the name "Vitamine" in 1912, to the accessory food factor and later it was called 'Vitamin' since all vitamins were not vital amines. His pupil Drummond dropped the final 'e' from 'Vitamine'. Most of the vitamins are unrelated chemically but they are considered as a group because of certain advantages from a physiological and nutritional standpoint. Vitamins are defined as a group of complex organic compounds, chemically unrelated to each other, present in minute amounts in natural foodstuffs that are essential to normal metabolism and a lack of which in the diet causes deficiency diseases. However, under certain conditions and for specific species, vitamin C, choline (required in greater amounts), niacin and vitamin D would not always fit the classic definition of vitamin. The list of vitamins with their synonyms is presented in Table 1.

Synthesis of Vitamins

The vitamins are derived initially from the plants except vitamin B_{12}. Vitamins can not be synthesized by the animal and therefore must be obtained exclusively from the diet. Exceptions are vitamin D (synthesized on the surface of the skin by UV irradiation) and nicotinic acid (synthesized to some extent from tryptophan). Vitamin C is synthesized by all animals except human beings, guinea pigs. Choline can be synthesized in the liver and it apparently functions as a structural constituent. However, microorganisms are capable of synthesizing the water soluble vitamins, provitamin A (beta carotene) and menoquinones (vitamin K_2). Vitamin B_{12} can not be synthesized by either plants or animals, but is synthesized only by certain microorganisms.

Ruminal vitamin synthesis was confirmed through feeding experiments conducted by A.I. Virtanen in 1963 and R.R. Oltejen in 1969 in ruminants for at least one production cycle on purified diets free of B-complex vitamins.

Vitamins are of two types: Fat-soluble vitamins and water-soluble vitamins. Fat-soluble vitamins are vitamins A,D,E and K and water-soluble vitamins are B vitamins (thaimin, riboflavin, nicotinic acid, pyridoxine, pantothenic acid, biotin, folic acid, choline and vitamin B_{12}) and vitamin C. A comparison is made between fat-soluble and water-soluble vitamins in Table 2.

TABLE 1. Vitamins and their Synonyms.

Vitamin	Accepted name	Alternate names (some obsolete)
Vitamin A	Retinol	Vitamin A_1
		Antiinfective vitamin
	Retinal	Vitamin A aldehyde
	Retinoic acid	Vitamin A acid
Vitamin D	Ergocalciferol	Vitamin D_2
	Cholecalciferol	Vitamin D_3
		Antirachitic Vitamin
Vitamin E	D-alpha-Tocoferol	Antisterility Vitamin
Vitamin K	Phylloquinone	Vitamin K_1
		Antihaemorrhagic Vitamin
	Menaquinone	Vitamin K_2
	Menadione	Vitamin K_3
Vitamin B_1	Thiamin	Vitamin F
Vitamin B_2	Riboflavin	Vitamin G
Nicotinic acid	Nicotinic acid	Vitamin B_3, Vitamin pp
	Nicotinamide	
Vitamin B_6	Pyridoxine	Adermine
		Yeast eluate factor
Pantothenic acid	Pantothenic acid	Vitamin B_5, chick anti-dermatitis factor
Biotin	Biotin	Vitamin H
		Coenzyme R
		Egg white injury preventing factor
Folic acid	Pteroylmonoglutamic acid	Folacin
		Vitamin M
		Vitamin B_C, B_{10}, B_{11}
Vitamin B_{12}	Cyanocobalamin	APF
		APA factor
Choline	Choline	Vidin, Gossypine
Vitamin C	Ascorbic acid (or) L-Ascorbic acid	Antiscorbutic Vitamin

Vitamins: Dietary Essential and Metabolic Essential

Some vitamins are metabolic essential, but not dietary essential, for certain species, because they can be synthesized readily from other food or metabolic constituents, e.g. various B-vitamins are essential for normal

TABLE 2. A Comparison Chart between Fat-soluble and Water-soluble Vitamins

Fat-soluble vitamins	Water-soluble vitamins
1. **Solubility and occurrence in food** Soluble in fat and they occur in foods in association with fats	Soluble in water and present in food
2. **Chemical Nature** These consist only of carbon, hydrogen and oxygen.	Water-soluble vitamins (except pantothenic acid) are ring compounds, most of them being aromatic. Pantothenic acid is a straight-chain compound. They contain C, H, and O and N, S, cobalt or P. Vitamin B_{12} contain C, H, O, Co, N and P. Sulphur containing vitamins are thiamin and biotin. Each vitamin has its unique chemical properties on which the biological activities of the vitamin depend.
3. **Functions** A considerable uncertainty still surrounds *the chemical nature of the active metabolic forms* responsible for most of the known biological functions of the fat-soluble vitamins. However, *the role of vitamin D and vitamin A* in calcium absorption and metabolism and in vision, respectively, the chemical nature and mode of action of the active forms are known.	Water-soluble vitamins carry out functions in the form of coenzymes or prosthetic groups of enzymes, the only exception being vitamin C. Biological functions of a given vitamin can be related to the specific metabolic roles of its known coenzyme derivative. During absorption from the gut, B group of vitamin is converted to its coenzyme derivative. The coenzyme derivatives of B_1, B_2, niacin, B_6 and pantothenic acid contain high energy phosphate groups donated by ATP (Table 3) Vitamin C or ascorbic acid does not require conversion into a coenzyme derivative in order to function in metabolic reactions and it acts as a reducing agent.
4. **Synthesis** None of the fat soluble vitamins except vitamin K is synthesized to any appreciable extent by symbiotic microorganisms. Vitamin D can be synthesized in the skin upon exposure to sunlight.	Niacin can be synthesized from tryptophan except in cats. Vitamin C is synthesized in many animals except humans, guinea pigs. Ruminants can synthesize all B vitamins with inclusion of cobalt in the diet, with the aid of rumen microbes. Young ruminants need dietary supply of 'B' vitamins.

5. **Absorption**

These are absorbed from G.I. tract by passive diffusion through the lipid phase of the mucosal cell membrane. Consequently, if fat absorption is impaired, the absorption of A, D, E and K are also impaired

These are absorbed from the gut independent of fats. Most B vitamins (except B_{12}) are absorbed by passive diffusion but some may be absorbed by active process when the diet contains low levels of the vitamin. Thiamin, riboflavin and folic acid may be transported across the gastrointestinal wall by specific carrier mechanisms.

6. **Storage**

Fat-soluble vitamins are stored in the body in appreciable amounts. The polar bear has a very high vitamin A reserve in the liver. In times of dietary short supply the vitamin reserves are mobilized to make up for the deficit and the normal serum level of fat soluble vitamins is maintained for few days.

Water-soluble vitamins are not stored in the body except vitamin B_{12}, which is stored extensively in the liver and riboflavin also to some extent. Hence a constant supply of B vitamins (except B_{12}) and vitamin C in the diet are essential.

7. **Excretion**

These are excreted in the faeces via the bile

The portion of the absorbed vitamins in excess of immediate requirement is excreted in the urine.

8. **Toxicity**

Excess dietary intake cause serious problems because they are stored in the body. Hypervitaminosis A and D have been reported.

Water-soluble vitamins are relatively non toxic. Hypervitaminosis niacin and B_6 has been reported in man.

9. **Deficiency symptoms**

Deficiency of fat-soluble vitamins can sometimes be related to the function of the vitamin. For example, vitamin D is required for calcium metabolism and a deficiency results in bone abnormalities. Similarly vitamins A, E and K.

In case of water-soluble vitamins the signs of deficiency are much less specific and the signs are difficult to relate to function in most cases. Most B vitamin deficiencies result in dermatitis, rough hair coat, poor growth and reduced feed efficiency. Achromotricia and anaemia are also observed in certain cases.

ruminant metabolism (metabolic essential) but are not needed in the diet (not dietary essential) because of bacterial synthesis in the rumen. Vitamin B_{12} *is not dietary essential for* ruminants provided cobalt is present in the diet since bacteria can synthesize it in the rumen. *Vitamin C is not dietary essential* for many animals except humans, guinea pigs. While metabolic needs are similar in most of the animals, dietary needs for the vitamins differ widely among the species.

Chemical Structure of Vitamins

Many of the vitamins contain unsaturated carbon atoms, double bonds, or hydroxy or other chemical moieties that are highly susceptible to chemical reactions. When these chemical structures are chemically oxidized or reduced, vitamin activity in the feed is reduced or lost. The chemical structure of the vitamins is depicted in Fig. 1.

Vitamin A retinol has both free hydroxy group and five double bonds. The vitamin is made up of isoprene units with alternate double bonds, starting with one in the beta-ionone ring that is in conjugation with those in the side chain.

TABLE 3. B Vitamin Related Coenzymes and Enzyme Prosthetic Groups or Activated Carriers Important in Metabolism.

B Vitamin	Coenzyme or prosthetic group	Enzyme or other function
Thiamin	Thiamin pyrophosphate (TPP)	Oxidative decarboxylation
Riboflavin	FMN, FAD	Hydrogen carrier
Nicotinamide	NAD, NADP	Hydrogen carrier
Pyridoxine	Pyridoxal phosphate (PP)	Transaminases, Decarboxylases
Pantothenic acid	Coenzyme A (CoA) Acyl carrier Protein	Two carbon transfer Acyl transfer
Folic acid	Tetrahydrofolic acid (THFA)	One carbon transfer
Biotin	Biotin	Carbon dioxide transfer
Cyanocobalamin	Methylcobalamin	Isomerases, dehydrases

Ergocalciferol (Vitamin D_2) and cholecalciferol (vitamin D_3) do have double bonds. The vitamin E, as d-alpha-tocopherol, is an excellent natural antioxidant that protects carotene and other oxidizable materials in feed and in the body. The free phenolic hydroxy group in the molecule is responsible for the antioxidant activity. However, in the process of acting as an antioxidant it is destroyed.

The simplest from of vitamin K is the synthetic menadione (K_3), which is composed of the active nucleus (2-methyl-1, 4 naphthoquinone) and has no side chain. Phylloquinone (vitamin K_1 of plants) has a phytyl side chain composed of four isoprene units, the first of which contains a double bond.

Thiamin consists of a molecule of pyrimidine and a molecule of thiazole linked by a methylene bridge. It contains both nitrogen and sulphur atoms. Riboflavin consists of dimethylisoalloxazine nucleus combined with the alcohol of ribose as a side chain. Niacin is used as a generic descriptor of pyridine 3-carboxylic acid (nicotinic acid) and its amides

Vitamin A (Retinol) (all-trans form)

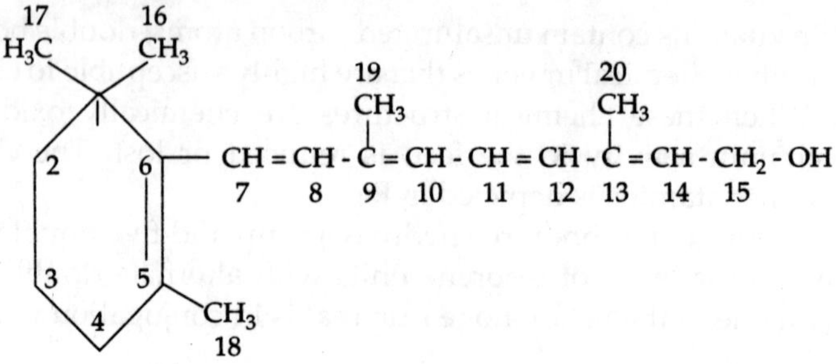

$$CH=CH-\underset{\underset{8}{|}}{\overset{\overset{19}{CH_3}}{C}}=CH-CH=CH-\underset{\underset{13}{|}}{\overset{\overset{20}{CH_3}}{C}}=CH-CH_2-OH$$

17 16
H_3C CH_3

2   6

3   5

4   CH_3
18

7   8   9   10   11   12   13   14   15

Vitamin D_2 (Ergocalciferol)

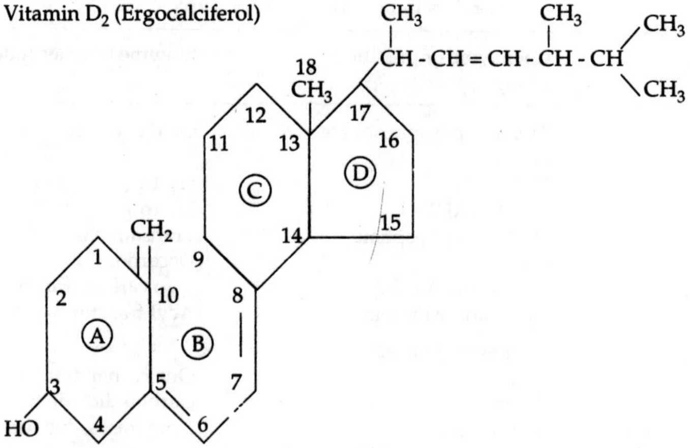

$$CH_3 \qquad CH_3 \qquad CH_3$$
$$CH-CH=CH-CH-CH$$
$$\qquad\qquad\qquad\qquad\qquad CH_3$$

18
CH_3

12   17

11   13   16

Ⓒ   Ⓓ

CH_2 14   15

1   9

2   10   8

Ⓐ   Ⓑ

3   5   7

HO   4   6

Vitamin D_3 (Cholecalciferol)

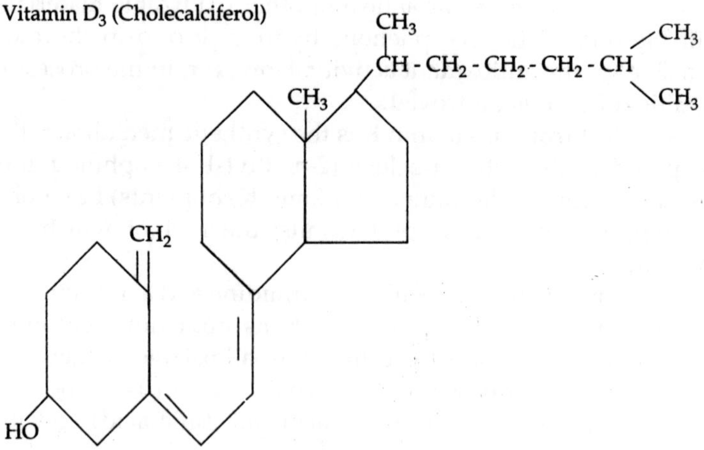

$$CH_3$$
$$CH-CH_2-CH_2-CH_2-CH$$
$$CH_3 \qquad\qquad\qquad\qquad\qquad CH_3$$

CH_2

HO

Alpha - Tocopherol

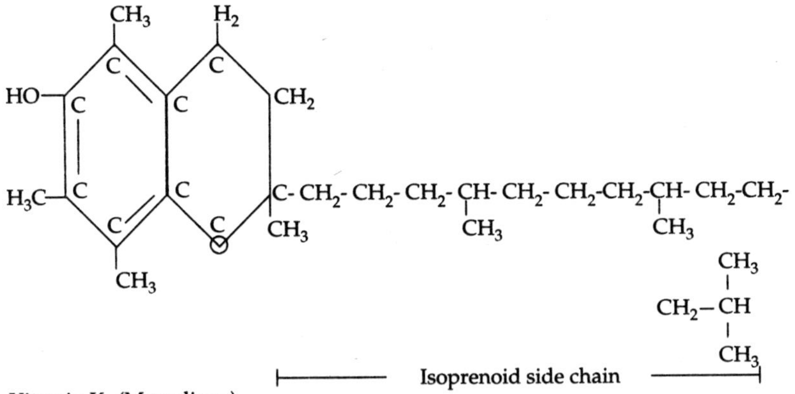

HO— ... C-CH$_2$-CH$_2$-CH$_2$-CH-CH$_2$-CH$_2$-CH$_2$-CH-CH$_2$-CH$_2$-
CH$_3$ CH$_3$ CH$_3$

CH$_3$
|
CH$_2$-CH
|
CH$_3$

├──────── Isoprenoid side chain ────────┤

Vitamin K$_3$ (Menadione)

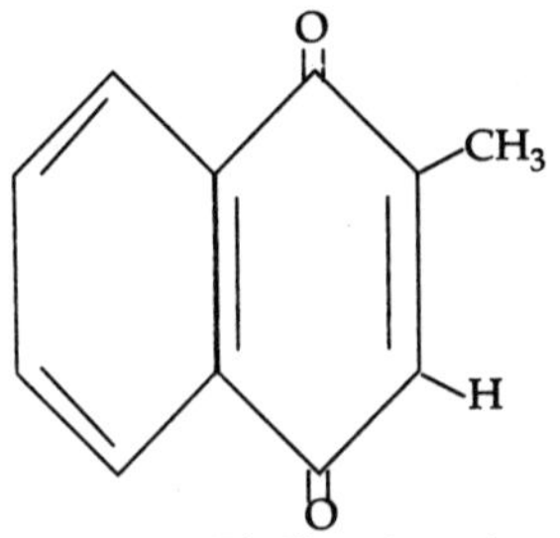

CH$_3$

H

Vitamin K$_1$ (Phylloquinone)

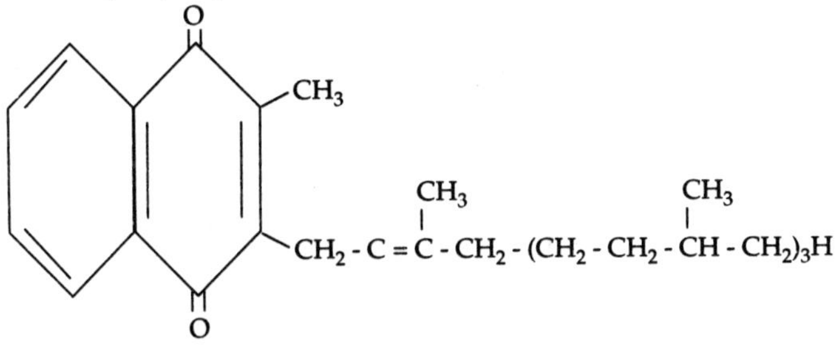

CH$_3$

CH$_3$ CH$_3$
| |
CH$_2$-C=C-CH$_2$-(CH$_2$-CH$_2$-CH-CH$_2$)$_3$H

Thiamin hydrochloride

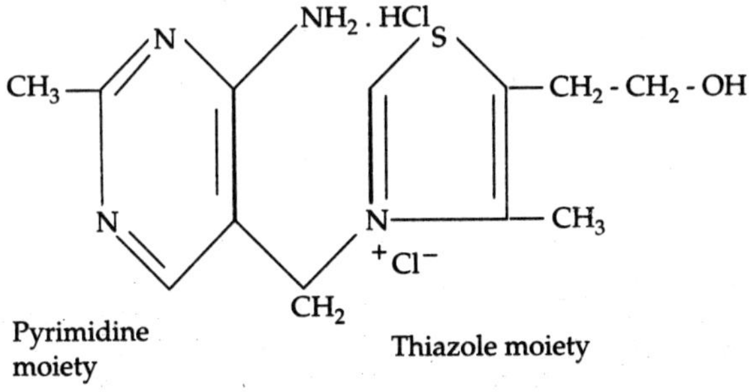

NH$_2$. HCl   S
CH$_3$—   CH$_2$-CH$_2$-OH

N   CH$_3$
$^+$Cl$^-$

CH$_2$

Pyrimidine
moiety   Thiazole moiety

Riboflovin (7, 8 dimethyl-10 (D, 1'- nibityl)- iso-olloeine)

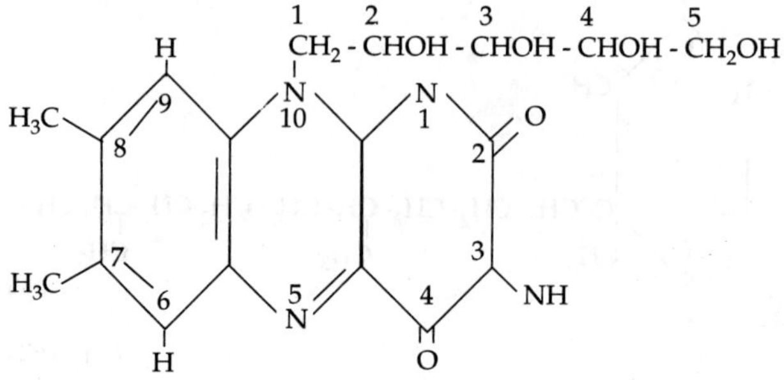

$$\overset{1}{C}H_2 - \overset{2}{C}HOH - \overset{3}{C}HOH - \overset{4}{C}HOH - \overset{5}{C}H_2OH$$

Nicotinic acid
(Pyridine - 3 carboxylic acid)

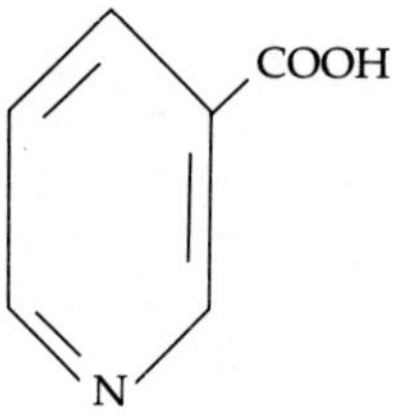

COOH

Niacinamide
(3-Pyridinecarboxylic acid amide)

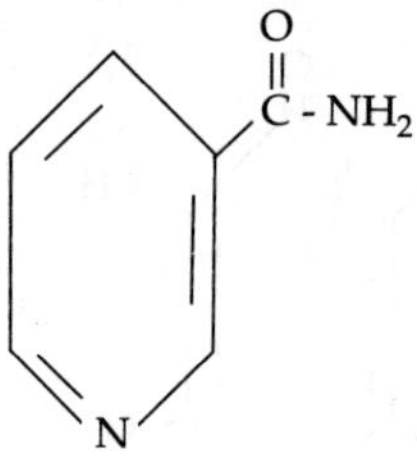

$$\overset{O}{\underset{||}{C}} - NH_2$$

Vitamin B_6

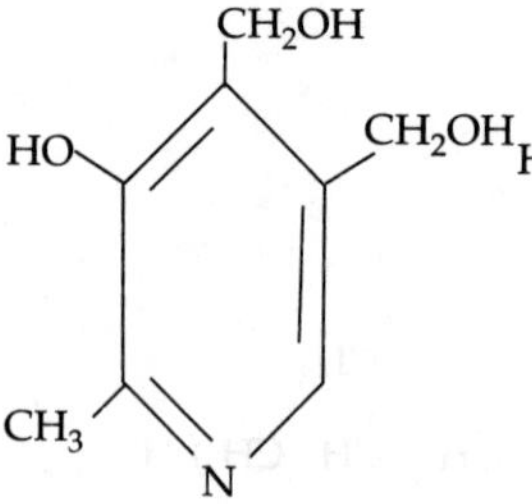

Pyridoxine

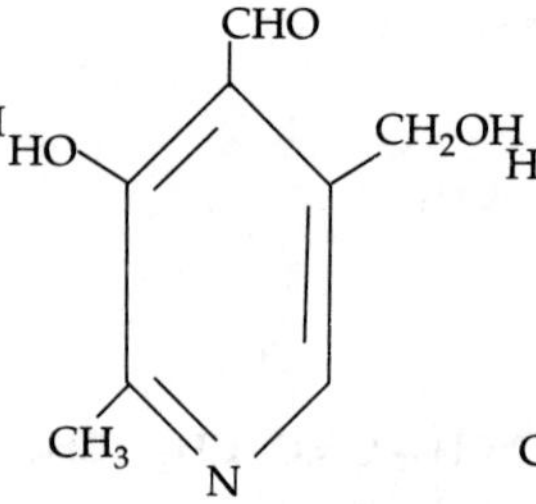

Pyridoxal

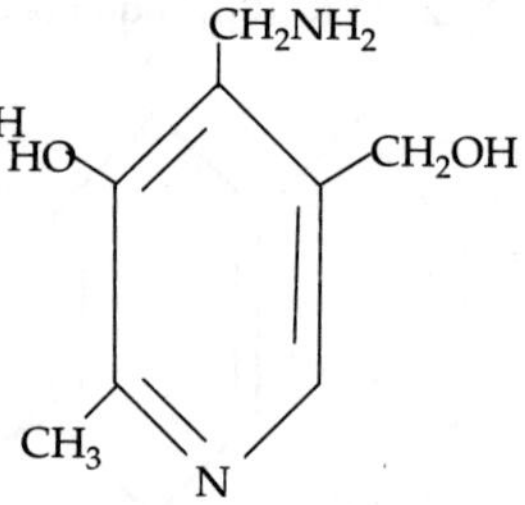

Pyridoxamine

Pantothenic acid

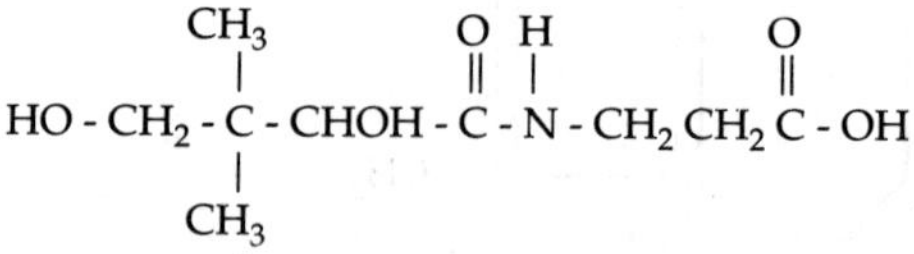

$$HO - CH_2 - \underset{\underset{CH_3}{|}}{\overset{\overset{CH_3}{|}}{C}} - CHOH - \overset{O}{\overset{||}{C}} - \overset{H}{\underset{|}{N}} - CH_2\ CH_2\ \overset{O}{\overset{||}{C}} - OH$$

Pantoic acid   β-alanine

d-Biotin

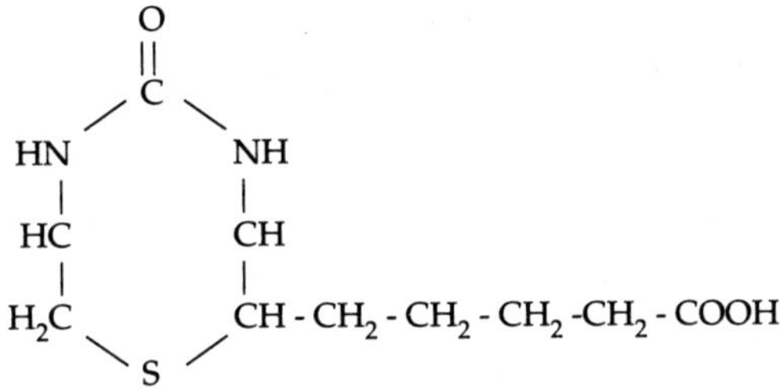

Folacin (Pteroylglutamic acid, Folic acid)

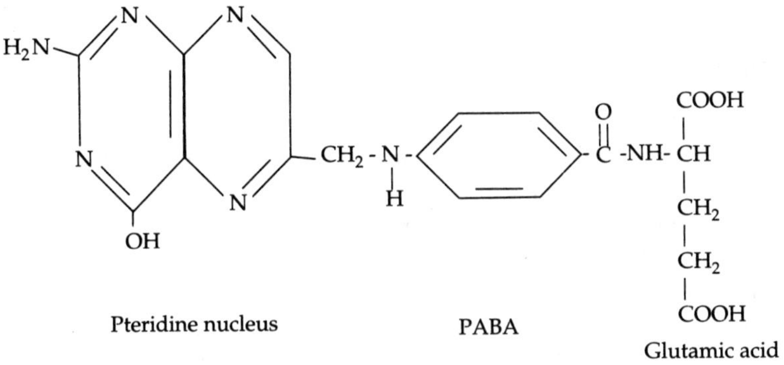

Pteridine nucleus   PABA   Glutamic acid

Choline

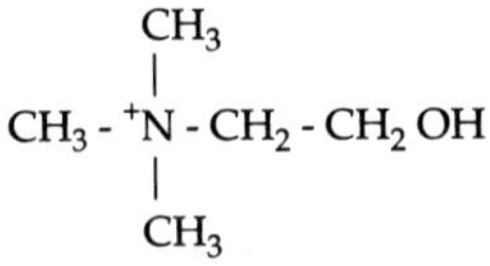

Vitamin C

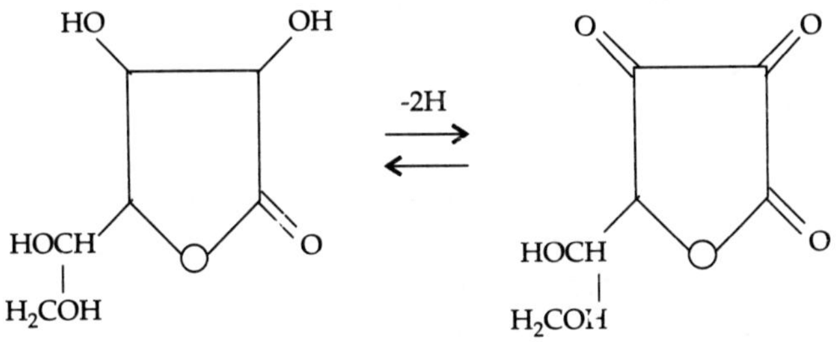

L-Ascorbic acid   Dehydroascorbic acid
(reduced form)   (oxidized form)

Figure 1. Chemical Structure of the Vitamins.

(nicotinamide or niacinamide) exhibiting the same qualitative biological activity of nicotinamide.

Vitamin B$_6$ is a relatively simple compound with three substituted pyridine derivatives that differ only in functional group in the 4-position; these are the alcohol (pyridoxine or piridoxol), the aldehyde pyridoxal, and the amine pyridoxamine. Pantothenic acid is an amide consisting of pantoic acid joined to beta-alanine. Biotin is a monocarboxylic acid with sulphur as a thioether linkage.

Folacin (pteroylglutamic acid) consists of glutamic acid, p-aminobenzoic acid and a pteridine nucleus. Vitamin B$_{12}$ is the heaviest compound of all the vitamins. Choline is a beta-hydroxyethyl-trimethylammonium hydroxide

Vitamin A

Introduction and Importance

It was discovered by McCollum and Davis and by Osborne and Mendel, independently, in 1913. *Vitamin A does not exist as such in plants*, but is present as *provitamins* in the form of *certain carotenoids* while vitamin A exists only in the animal kingdom. Vitamin A is an unsaturated 20 carbon cyclic alcohol containing *one beta-ionone* ring and is known as retinol. It also occurs as aldehyde (retinal) and acid (retinoic acid). The pure vitamin A is a nearly colourless liquid that is soluble in the fat and fat solvents and to only a very limited extent in water.

Carotenoids

Carotenoid pigments are synthesized only by plants and are conspicuously present in many blossoms, pollens, seeds, fruits, leaves, and roots. Many animals (e.g., insects, mollusks, crustacean, fish) concentrate and further metabolize the carotenoids they consume and become a rich food source.

Carotenoids may be divided into two main categories: *carotenes and xanthophylls*. Xanthophyllls are oxycarotenoids, because they have alcohol, keto, or ester groups on their terminal cyclohexenyl rings. The positioning and type of these groups determine the colour of xanthophylls. Carotene is a complex hydrocarbon containing no highly reactive functional groups such as alcohol, aldehydes, or acid. It contains *two beta ionone rings*. Theoretically one molecule of carotene yields two molecules of vitamin A. However, biologically the conversion is at best one molecule of carotene to one molecule of vitamin A. Lutein, zeaxanthin, canthaxanthine, astaxanthin, rhodoxanthin, cryptoxanthin, capsanthin are some examples.

TABLE 4. Carotenoids and their Relative Rat-biopotency.

Carotenoid	Relative rat-biopotency (all-trans forms)
Beta-carotene	100
Alpha-carotene	25
Gamma-carotene	14
Beta-zeacarotene	25
Cryptoxanthin (yellow maize)	29
Zeaxanthin	0
Lutein	0

Carotenes: Of the alpha-, beta-, and gamma-carotenes, β-carotene is the most biologically active form and this compound forms the main source of vitamin A in the diet of farm animals (Table 4).

Oxidative scission of β-carotene occurs in two stages (largely in the intestinal mucosa and also in the liver) catalysed by a dioxygenase and retinol reductase (NADPH or NADH as electron donor), respectively. The resultant retinol is seen in circulation. Anything that affects the integrity of the intestinal tract, such as a parasitism or a nutritional deficiency, can decrease carotene conversion to vitamin A. In certain situations, high nitrate levels in the forage or water also interfere with carotene conversion.

Buffaloes can convert carotene into vitamin A but cow can not and hence cow milk is yellow. Very little carotene appears in the blood or body tissues. Horses and cattle have considerable carotene in the blood since only a portion of the digested carotene is converted to vitamin A and the rest is stored in the liver and adipose tissue. It has been estimated that only about one-third of the dietary provitamins ingested by man is absorbed while the preformed vitamin A is almost completely absorbed. Beta-carotene has been found in cellular membranes including those of lysosomes where it functions as an antioxidant. Some animals such as cat can not utilize carotenoids. The pure carotenoids differ in their colour. Beta-carotene is red in colour, but in dilute solutions it is orange to yellow.

It has been suggested that some species may have dietary requirement for beta-carotene *per se*. For example, deficiency of beta-carotene in dairy cattle causes fertility disorders.

Green plant tissues contain 90% beta-carotene and 10% gamma-carotene and other forms. In general, beta-carotene is twice as potent as the other isomers, and the all-trans forms are 2 to 3 times as potent as the mono-cis forms. Also, the biopotency of any given carotenoid such as beta-carotene differs for various species of animals and with various dietary levels of intake (refer Table 5).

The conversion factors of vitamins from traditional unit to their metric units are presented in Table 6.

TABLE 5. Conversion of Beta-carotene to Vitamin A by Different Animals.

Animal	1 mg β-carotene to IU of vitamin A
Standard	1667
Cattle	400
Sheep	400-500
Swine	280
Horse	
Growth	555
Pregnancy	333
Poultry	1667
Dog	833
Rat	1667
Human	556

In cat and mink carotene is not utilized.

TABLE 6. Conversion Factors.

Element	Traditional Unit	Converted Equivalent
		One US Pharmacopeia (USP) unit
Vitamin A	1 international unit	0.3 µg retinol
	1 international unit	0.344 µg retinyl acetate
	1 international unit	0.55 µg retinyl palmitate
	1 international unit	0.6 µg β-carotene
	1 retinol equivalent*	1 µg retinol
	1 retinol equivalent	6 µg β-carotene
	1 retinol equivalent	12 µg other provitamin A carotenoids
	1 retinol equivalent	3.33 IU vitamin A activity from retinol
	1 retinol equivalent	10 IU vitamin A activity from β-carotene
	1 mg β-carotene	1667 IU of vitamin A
Vitamin D	1 international unit	25 ng cholecalciferol (vitamin D_3)
Vitamin E	1 international unit	1 mg all-rac-α- tocopheryl acetate
	1 international unit	0.74 mg RRR-α- tocopheryl acetate
	1 international unit	0.91 mg all-rac-α- tocopherol
	1 international unit	0.67 mg RRR-α- tocopherol
Thiamin	1 international unit	3 µg thiamin hydrochloride
Pantothenic acid	1 g of d-calcium pantothenate	0.92 g of pantothenic acid activity
Biotin	1 g of d-biotin	1 g of biotin activity

Note : These terms are now obsolete; the preferred expression is the molar concentration. RE* is the new nomenclature used to describe vitamin A activity in foods and feeds.

Synthetic antioxidants and vitamin E protect the integrity of vitamin A in the gut, thereby enhancing bioavailability. Mycotoxins have been reported to decrease the absorption of carotenoids.

Physiological Functions

1. Vision: The retina of the eye has two photoreceptor systems, the rods and the cones. In the retinal cells of the eye, vitamin A (all-trans-retinol) is oxidized to the aldehyde (all-trans-retinaldehyde) which is converted into the 11-cis isomer in the dark. This 11-cis-retinaldehyde combines with the protein opsin to form rhodopsin (visual purple) which is photoreceptor (present in the retinal rods) for vision at low light intensities. When light falls on the retina, the cis-retinaldehyde molecule is converted back into the all-trans form and is released from the opsin. This conversion results in the transmission of an impulse up the optic nerve. The role of retinol in the visual cycle is depicted here.

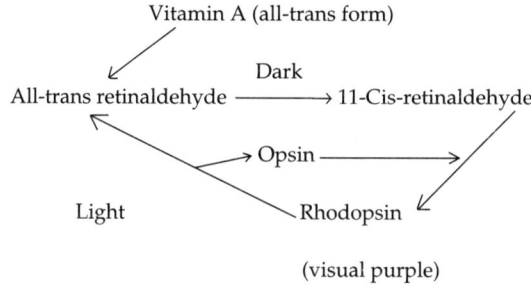

(visual purple)

2. Bone growth: Vitamin A is effective in controlling the activity of the osteoclasts and osteoblasts of the epithelial cartilage. In cattle, a blindness occurs as a result of narrowing of the bone canal through which optic nerve passes. Changes in the bone growth are reported to cause the rise in cerebrospinal fluid pressure.

3. Maintenance of mucus-secreting cells of the epithelia: It appears that the basal cells of epithelia have two pathways of cytodifferentiation depending on the presence or otherwise of vitamin A. Basal cells karatinize in the absence of vitamin A while they form columnar mucus secreting epithelium in the presence of vitamin A. Keratinization lowers the resistance of the epithelial tissues to the entrance of infective organisms. Thus vitamin A plays an important role in combating infection and it has been referred as the 'anti-infective vitamin'. Vitamin A is necessary to maintain the health and functional integrity of epithelial structures.

Deficiency Symptoms

1. Night blindness (Nictalopia): Deficiency of vitamin A first manifests as a slow, dark adaptation and progresses to total blindness.

2. Xerophthalmia (from the latin words for dry and eye): This is an advanced stage of vitamin A deficiency noted particularly in children, dogs, and rats. It is characterized by a dry condition of the cornea and conjunctiva, cloudiness and ulceration. It is not a common symptom in other species, although corneal changes occur.

In humans, this stage is called 'xerosis', the eye has a wrinkled and thickened appearance. Bitot spots or white foamy patches occur on the white portion of eyes, especially in children below 5 years. In untreated cases, keratinization may become irreversible leading to total blindness.

In poultry (mostly adult birds) it is known as **'Nutritional roup'** characterised by mucopurulent rhinitis and occulusion of respiratory tract, xerophthalmia and keratomalacia because of drying of tear glands. The discharge causes the lids to stick together. Breathing becomes rapid and difficult. Copious lacrimation is a more prominant eye symptom in cows and horses.

3.   Keratinization   of   epithelium: Normal   epithelium   (columnar epithelium) in various locations of the body became replaced by a stratified squamous, keratinizing epithelium (cornified cells). Epithelial cells from deficient animals fail to differentiate beyond the squamous type to the mucus-secreting cells and mesenchymal cells fail to differentiate beyond the blast stage. This effect has been noted in the respiratory, alimentary, reproductive and genitourinary tracts, as well as in the eye. So respiratory troubles such as cold and sinus infections and gastrointestinal disorders such as diarrhoea tend to be more severe in vitamin A deficiency since keratinization of epithelium lowers the resistance to infections.

The formation of kidney and bladder stones is favoured because the damaged epithelium interferes with the normal secretion and elimination of the urine and the sloughed keratinized cells may form foci for the formation of stones. In severe vitamin A deficiency, the blood level of uric acid increases from 5 mg to as high as 40 mg per 100 ml blood. Deposits of urates have been found on the heart, pericardium, liver and spleen of the affected birds.

4.   Reproductive   performance: There is a specific interference with reproduction   caused   by   the   altered   epithelium.   Reproductive performance is impaired in both the male and female. The male usually shows a decline in sexual activity, decreased number of spermatozoa with a marked decrease in motility, and the appearance of abnormal forms. In the female, estrus is disturbed. If the deficiency is severe, abortion or birth of dead, weak or abnormal offspring may occur. In avian species, egg production and hatchability of fertile eggs are markedly reduced.

5. Nervous lesions: Skeletal growth is retarded in young animals but nervous tissue and brain grow and hence there is pressure on nervous tissue. Increased cerebrospinal fluid pressure has been observed in vitamin A deficient chicken, cattle, etc. No lesions were observed in the cerebellum or cerebrum. A severe ataxia is the first symptom in the growing chick. This is different from the ataxia of vitamin E deficiency.

   6. *Retenoic acid for poultry:*   Retenoic acid carries out all of the functions of vitamin A except for vision and reproduction. When chicks were fed with vitamin A only in the form of retenoic acid, they grow and develop normally except that they became blind. Egg size and production were normal but the eggs contain no vitamin A. When such eggs were incubated they have malformed embryo at 72 hr incubation. Sight is restored in such hens within two days after providing them an adequate level of dietary retinol. Hatchability of the eggs also is restored immediately. This shows that feeding of retinoic acid affects only the production of retinene and storage of vitamin A in the egg.

Vitamin D

Ergosterol of plants and 7-dehydrocholesterol do not possess any vitamin D activity but on conversion to ergocalciferol (D_2) and cholecalciferol (D_3), respectively, by ultraviolet light they become active. McCollum in 1925 named the antirachitic factor as vitamin D (Rachitogenic means rickets - causing).

Sunlight and Vitamin D

By irradiation, the 7-dehydrocholesterol present in the skin is converted into vitamin D_3. U.V. light of 230 to 320 nm wavelength effects the conversion by imparting a definite quantity of energy to the sterol molecule and the light of wavelength between 290 and 315 nm is the most effective. Irradiation is less effective on dark pigmented skin. The conversion is greatly facilitated by a light complexion or a lack of melanin pigment. U.V. light also stimulates melanin formation. Ultraviolet radiation is greater in the tropics than in the temperate regions, more potent in summer than in winter, more potent at noon than in morning or evening and more potent at high altitude.

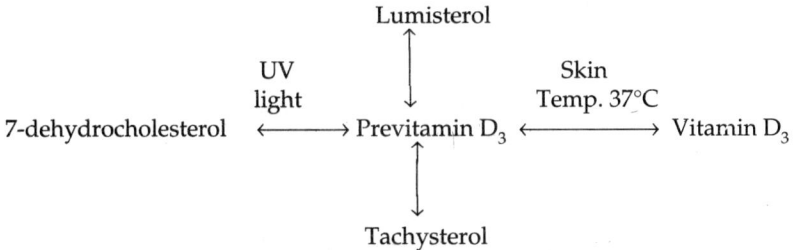

Ultraviolet light causes scissoring of the B ring of 7-dehydrocholesterol to form previtamin D_3 and this photochemical reaction is rapid. The rate at which this conversion proceeds depends on skin pigmentation, intensity of light and duration of exposure. The latter then undergoes a nonenzymatic, temperature-dependent isomerization to vitamin D_3. This reaction is slow and the overall rate of formation of vitamin D_3 is enhanced by the prompt uptake of the vitamin by the blood circulation.

A photochemical regulatory mechanism serves to prevent excessive accumulation of the vitamin and, hence, its toxicity to the skin during exposure to excessive sunlight by forming lumisterol and tachysterol.

On absorption in the lower half of the small intestine, vitamin D_3 reaches liver and it is converted to 25-hydroxy cholecalciferol in the liver. This in turn is converted in the kidney to 1, 25-dihydroxy cholecalciferol or Calcitriol.

- Vitamin D_3 + O_2 + NADPH

  $$\xrightarrow[\text{25-Hydroxylase}]{\text{Liver}} \text{25-hydroxy Vitamin } D_3 + NADP^+$$

- 25-Hydroxy vitamin D_3 + O_2 + NADPH

  $$\xrightarrow{\text{Kidney}} \text{1, 25-dihydroxy vitamin } D_3 + NADP^+$$

  Cytochrome P_{450}

  1-Hydroxylase

Functions

1. Active form of vitamin D (i.e., 1, 25-$(OH)_2$ D_3) stimulates the synthesis of calcium binding protein. The binding protein is necessary for efficient calcium absorption.
2. Vitamin D_3 is the third major hormone involved in the regulation of calcium metabolism and skeletal remodelling.
3. Vitamin D_3 stimulates both intestinal calcium and intestinal phosphorus transport. The mobilization of bone mineral (Ca and P) induced by parathyroid hormone is dependent upon the presence of vitamin D.

Vitamin D_2 and D_3 have the same potency for cattle, sheep and pigs but for poultry vitamin D_2 has only about 10% of the potency of vitamin D_3. Vitamin D_3 is much more effective than D_2 in the chick because of the fact that the chick catabolizes or breakdown vitamin D_2 much more rapidly than D_3. Thus, vitamin D requirements for avian species generally are expressed as International Chick Units. A 10-minute exposure to sun's radient energy would provide sufficient vitamin D to growing poultry.

$$1 \text{ ICU} = 0.025 \text{ } \mu\text{g of vitamin } D_3 = 25 \text{ ng.}$$

Deficiency Symptoms
1. The first symptom noted in fast growing animals and chicks is retarded growth and decreased feed consumption.
2. Rickets in young and osteomalacia in adults are not specific for vitamin D deficiency because of interrelationship among Ca, P and vitamin D.
3. Deficiency of vitamin D is rare in animals and humans that spend considerable time outside in the direct sunlight.
4. In humans, vitamin D deficiency has been reported due to failure of absorption of dietary vitamin D from the gut lumen and failure of the body to convert vitamin D to its biologically active form. Malabsorption of fat soluble vitamins occur in diseases associated with steatorrhoea and in conditions in which insufficient amounts of bile are secreted into the intestine. In severe liver and kidney diseases, the body may not be able to convert vitamin D to the biologically active form. Intestinal absorption of calcium and phosphorus is impaired and there is an increase in the loss of Ca and P in the urine.
5. Laying hens deprived of vitamin D for a period of 2 to 3 months laid thin shelled and soft shelled eggs. Egg production is decreased, hatchability is decreased. Penguin-like squat is observed. Parathyroid glands get enlarged. Vitamin D_3 is more than 30 times as efficient as vitamin D_2 for preventing rickets in poultry.

Evidence Suggesting that Vitamin D_3 Acts as a Hormone
1. Chemical structure resembles that of steroid hormones.
2. Very small quantities like nanograms are sufficient for full biological activity.
3. Synthesized by one organ (skin) by photoactivation and transported through blood in bound form to the target cells primarily in intestine and bone.
4. Mechanism of action is similar to steroid hormones. Enter into the cells and binds to cytosol receptors and nuclear receptors, facilitates transcription of mRNA from DNA, increases protein synthesis in target cells (e.g. calcium binding protein).
5. It is toxic in excessive amounts.
6. Ultraviolet light is less effective on dark pigmented skin to produce more D_3 and it also stimulates melanin formation. Thus melanin that is produced by UV light probably regulates the production of vitamin D_3.
7. It may appear confusing as to how 1, 25-$(OH)_2$ D_3 can serve as a hormone both for Ca and P since different signals are involved.

It must be kept in mind that the signal to raise plasma calcium comes by virtue of a stimulation of secretion of parathyroid hormone (PTH) by hypocalcaemia. Under these circumstances 1, 25-$(OH)_2$ D_3 increases in blood together with the increased levels of PTH.

PTH causes a phosphate diuresis (decreased P reabsorption from kidneys) which negates the 1, 25-$(OH)_2$ D_3 stimulation of intestinal phosphate absorption. On the other hand, calcium and phosphorus are mobilized from bone, additionally calcium absorption in intestine is increased by 1, 25-$(OH)_2$ D_3 and calcium is reabsorbed in the kidney under the influence of these two agents. Therefore, under the condition of a hypocalcaemic signal, plasma calcium will raise, whereas plasma phosphate will stay constant.

In case of hypophosphataemic signal, PTH secretion is suppressed and, therefore, 1, 25-$(OH)_2$ D_3 will have a minimal effect on mobilizing Ca and P from bone. On the otherhand it will stimulate both intestinal Ca and intestinal phosphate transport.

The absence of PTH would bring about a loss of some of this Ca in urine. On the otherhand, the low blood P causes the kidney to adjust its phosphate reabsorption mechanism to maximal affinity. As a result, the hypophosphataemic signal brings about an elevation of plasma P because of the intestinal effect of 1, 25-$(OH)_2$ D_3 and the change in reabsorption in the kidney.

Plasma Ca does not change since Ca mobilization from bone is minimum and furthermore Ca, which is absorbed from intestine in response to the increased 1, 25-$(OH)_2$ D_3 level, would in part be lost in urine. Thus 1, 25-$(OH)_2$ D_3 can act both as a Ca-regulating and P-regulating hormone.

Thus vitamin D_3 conforms to some of the conditions for defining it a hormone.

Vitamin E

In 1922 Evans Mattill and Bishop discovered it as a fat soluble factor. Later in 1936 it was isolated as alpha tocopherol. Eight naturally occurring forms of the vitamin are known in plant materials as the alcohols, tocopherols and tocotrienols. Alpha tocopherol is more active than beta, gamma and delta and the other four are alpha, beta, gamma and delta-tocotrienols. The word 'tocopherol' (greek word) denotes child bearing alcohol.

Functions

1. It is a natural antioxidant at the cellular level and play important role in biological oxidation-reduction reactions. The animal has two main methods of protecting itself against oxidative damage. Free

radicals that are formed during cellular metabolism are scavenged in the first instance by vitamin E and later glutathione peroxidase destroys any peroxides formed before they can damage the cells. Thus vitamin E and glutathione peroxidase complement one another. It protects carotenoids and vitamin A from oxidation both in the alimentery tract and in the cells.

2. Adequate dietary vitamin E appears to aid in the absorption and utilization of vitamin A, carotene and xanthophylls, and helps extend the storage of vitamin A in the liver. Excess vitamin E in relation to vitamin A tends to prevent proper storage of vitamin A and hastens depletion of vitamin A stores.

3. Vitamin E is also closely associated with sulphur amino acid metabolism, the synthesis of ubiquinone, phosphorylation reactions, and selenium and vitamin A metabolism.

4. Vitamin E also plays a significant role in the development and function of the immune system.

Deficiency Symptoms

1. Infertility is the classical manifestation of deficiency in female rats while in male rats, deficiency of vitamin E results in immotility of spermatozoa and degeneration of the germinal epithelium.

2. Nutritional muscular dystrophy (nutritional myopathy) is seen in chicks, pigs and lambs affecting primarily skeletal muscle and occasionally heart muscle. In pigs it is commonly known as mulberry heart disease.

3. Stiff lamb disease in suckling lambs and white muscle disease in calves are variable forms of nutritional myopathy. Enzootic disease of sheep and cattle may be due to deficiency of vitamin E or vitamin E and selenium.

4. Nutritional Encephalomalacia (cerebellum degenerating disease of chickens) or crazy chick disease: Haemorrhage, oedema and generation of the purkinje cells in the cerebellum are seen. The chick is unable to stand or walk.

5. Enlarged hock disorders in turkeys due to niacin and vitamin E deficiency.

6. Exudative diathesis (an edema caused by excessive capillary permeability), a haemorrhagic disease in chicks and turkeys.

7. Generally, vitamin E deficiency is characterized by increased haemolysis of RBCs.
   Both selenium and vitamin E appear to be involved in nutritional muscular dystrophy and in exudative diathesis but selenium does not seem to be important in nutritional encephalomalacia.

8. Vitamin E deficiency leads to 'yellow fat disease' or pansteatitis in cats. This occurs when high levels of PUFA are fed with low level of vitamin E leading to deposition of ceroid pigment in adipose tissue with fat cell necrosis and subsequent inflammation.

Vitamin K

Vitamin K was identified in 1935 by Henrik Dam and was designated as vitamin K for the Danish word Koagulation. Several naphthoquinone compounds with vitamin K activity are known. e.g. vitamins K_1, K_2 and K_3. Phylloquinone K_1 occurs naturally in green plants and oil seeds. Menaquinone K_2 is synthesized by bacteria especially the intestinal bacteria. Menadione K_3 does not occur naturally. It is a synthetic product. Presently K_1, K_2 and K_3 are renamed as phytylmenaquinone K_1, Multiprenylmenaquinone K_2, Menaquinone K_3. Much of the vitamin K_2 produced by the human intestinal microflora is subsequently absorbed from the gut. It does not appear to be stored in large quantities.

Functions

1. Vitamin K is required for synthesis of prothrombin and other clotting factors. If vitamin K supply is inadequate, the prothrombin molecule is deficient in gamma carboxyglutamic acid, responsible for calcium binding.
2. It has been found to be involved in electron transport and in bacteria, oxidative phosphorylation.

Deficiency Symptoms

Blood clotting time and prothrombin time are good indices of sufficiency of vitamin K. Ruminants consuming mouldy sweet clover develop vitamin K deficiency symptoms. The disease is referred as haemorrhagic sweet clover disease or bleeding disease. When sweet clover hay undergoes spoilage with certain moulds, the moulds convert the coumarin (that is present in clover) to dicoumarol, which is a potent vitamin K antagonist. Sulfaquinoxalene and warfarin are also vitamin K inhibitors. Vitamin K is synthesized by the microorganisms inhabiting in the GI tract of animals. However in hindgut fermentors it may not be useful to the animal unless coprophagy is practised. Partially fermented feed has large amounts of vitamin K. Putrefied fish meals has more menaquinone.

Poultry

The chicken does not have the type of microflora necessary to synthesize adequate amount of vitamin K. So it must receive adequate amounts from its diet. Poultry kept in confinement require synthetic source of vitamin K.

The deficient chicken may bleed to death from a very slight bruise or injury. Haemorrhages appear on the breast, legs, wings, surface of the abdominal cavity and intestines. An anaemia may develop and the bone marrow becomes hypoplastic.

Humans

Deficiency is restricted to newly born babies, especially premature infants and these infants need a supplementary source. While treating children for haemorrhagic diseases, anaphylactic reaction can occur after injection in sensitive individuals. Inadvertent overdosage can cause kernicterus in the new born — a severe form of infantile jaundice.

Antibiotics fed animals do not have microbes. Vitamin K synthesis is absent.

Thiamin

It was Eijkman (a Dutch Physician) and his coworkers who established the fact that there is a specific dietary factor essential for the prevention of 'beriberi' in man and 'polyneuritis' in pigeons. Eijkman (1897) observed polyneuritis in chicken that were fed on diets exclusively of polished rice and the symptoms disappeared when rice polishings were added to chicken diets. After absorption from the small intestine, thiamin is phosphorylated in the liver to thiamin pyrophosphate (TPP).

Functions

1. Thiamin pyrophosphate is necessary in a number of metabolic steps that remove carbon dioxide. These decarboxylations are particularly important to the ruminant in the glycolytic pathway in the central nervous system. Thiamin is essential for the utilization of carbohydrates to provide energy for body processes. TPP acts as a coenzyme for the oxidative decarboxylation of a-keto acids (pyruvic and a-ketoglutaric acid) and keto analogues of leucine, isoleucine and valine.
2. The requirement of the animal for thiamin is decreased as the level of fat in the diet is increased. This 'sparing action' of fat on thiamin need is related to the fact that the vitamin is needed in many more reactions in carbohydrate metabolism than in fat metabolism.
3. Transketolase reaction is a key reaction in the metabolism of pentose sugars in the pentose phosphate pathway. TPP is required.
4. Pyruvate dehydrogenase and oxoglutarate dehydrogenase also require TPP.

Deficiency Symptoms

The two major syndromes of thiamin deficiency involve the cardiovascular and nervous systems.

1. Thiamin deficiency inhibits carbohydrate metabolism and results in increased blood lactate, pyruvate and oxoglutarate level. Accumulation of these intermediates of carbohydrate metabolism cause peripheral neuritis. The conditions are known as **'beriberi'** in man and **'polyneuritis'** in birds. Chicken sits on its flexed legs and draws its head backward, assuming what is known as a 'star gazer' position. In foxes the deficiency is known as **chastek paralysis**.

2. Thiamin deficiency occurs in ruminants when ruminal synthesis decreases or when thiamin is hydrolysed by thiaminase in the rumen. These conditions are known as **polioencephalomalacia** (PEM) in USA and in Europe it is **'cerebrocortical necrosis'** (CCN). Symptoms are listlessness, circling, muscular incoordination, **opisthotonus** or **star gazing** (drawing the head back over the shoulder) and head pressing, progressing to blindness, convulsion and death. Thiaminase in prepared diets of monogastric animals and birds may also cause deficiency.

3. Bradycardia (a slowing of heart beat), enlargement of heart, oedema, gastrointestinal troubles such as lack of appetite, impaired digestion, etc. and nervous symptoms such as frequent convulsions, incoordination of gait, etc.

4. If diet lacks thiamin, highly acidic substrates of the oxidative phosphorylation reactions accumulate in the blood, conversion of pentose sugars to hexose sugars is impaired.

5. The affected cats often show ventroflexion of head.

Excess thiamin injection could cause anaphylactic shock.

Cause of Thiamin Deficiency

1. Thiaminases (enzymes that destroy thiamin) have been found in several ferns, raw fish and in a number of bacteria. Intraruminal thiaminases are also reported. Two types of thiaminases are known. Thiaminase I removes the thiazole ring and replaces it with cosubstrate and creates a thiamine analog that may act as thiamin antimetabolite. Thiaminase II destroys thiamin by splitting the molecule at the methylene bridge.

2. PEM has been induced by using large doses of amprolium, a coccidiostat and thiamin **antimetabolite**. Amprolium decreases thiamin phosphorylation and transport.

3. Sulphate (gypsum) content of feed and water. Sulphate appears to precipitate thiamin destruction in the rumen. The rumen converts the sulphate ion to sulphide through sulphite. The sulphite ion is known to destroy thiamin.
4. Thiamin deficiency is also caused by inactivation of thiamin by the preservative, sulphur dioxide.
5. High concentrate feeding with inadequate roughages may lead to decreased microbial synthesis of thiamin (in ruminants).

Riboflavin

Functions

1. Riboflavin is necessary for the formation of flavin mononucleotide (FMN) and flavin adenine dinucleotide (FAD). These are the compounds used by cells to transport hydrogen within metabolic cycles. FAD is contained in succinate dehydrogenase, which serves as a carrier in the electron-transport chain of two of the hydrogen atoms released in the TCA cycle to provide energy. Fumarate dehydrogenase and aldehyde oxidase also had FAD.
2. It is also a constituent of D-amino acid oxidase concerned in protein metabolism and purine metabolism and of xanthine oxidase which is concerned in the purine metabolism.
3. FMN containing enzymes are L-amino acid oxidase and cytochrome C reductase.

FAD and FMN are hydrolysed by phosphatases present in the intestinal brush border. Their absorption proceeds throughout the entire small intestine via an active but saturable transport system involving phosphorylation of free riboflavin.

The enzyme (flavokinase) is competitively inhibited by chlorpromazine, a compound in the phenothiazine category of antiemetic and antipsychotic drugs. Aflatoxin present in feedstuffs decreases riboflavin utilization. Ethanol inhibits enzymes required for conversion of FAD to riboflavin in the gut.

Deficiency Symptoms

1. Nervous symptoms caused either by degeneration of the myelin sheath covering the nerve or the nerve itself.
2. Inability to maintain the integrity of the epithelium.

Swine: Slow growth rate, diarrhoea, dermatitis, crooked and stiff legs, incoordination, nerve degeneration, corneal opacities and cataract formation.

Chicken: Exhibit a "curled-toe paralysis" which eventually develops into a total leg paralysis. The **"curled-toe paralysis"** is a very specific symptom and is caused by peripheral nerve degeneration. The toes curl inward and the chicken is soon forced to walk on its hock. Autopsy reveal that the sciatic and brachial nerve sheaths are four to five times of their normal size. Birds may otherwise appear normal. Dirrhoea is also common. In the hen, not only is the hatchability of fertile eggs decreased, but there is a high degree of embryonic anomalies and the embryo may show a **"clubbed" down condition**.

In very acute riboflavin deficiency, hens stop laying eggs altogether. The hen's liver becomes enlarged due to the deposition of fat. In more mild, chronic deficiency states, egg number may be reduced with a concomitant increase in egg size.

Humans: Deficiency causes inflammation of the tongue (glossitis). Deficiency also causes lesions of the lips, maceration with superficial ulcers on lips (cheilosis), and fissures at the angles of the mouth (angular stomatitis) and dermatitis, especially around the nose, eyes, ears and mouth. In humans, riboflavin deficiency has been found closely associated with pellagra or nicotinic acid deficiency.

Niacin or Nicotinic Acid

Nicotinic acid is the form of vitamin present in plants and nicotinamide is the metabolic form in animals. Nicotinic acid and nicotinamide (physiologically active form) are derivatives of pyridine. Elvehjem and his team discovered that nicotinic acid would cure black tongue in dogs in 1937. Nicotinamide is a component of two coenzymes-nicotinamide adenine dinucleotide (NAD) and nicotinamide adenine dinucleotide phosphate (NADP). Niacin is rapidly converted to nicotinamide after absorption and most of it is found in the form of NAD and NADP. Some amount of the vitamin is excreted unchanged in the urine while a fraction is excreted after methylation to N-methyl-nicotinamide. NAD and NADP are not interchangeable. Enzymes containing NAD and NADP are important links in a series of reactions associated with carbohydrate, protein and lipid metabolism. These enzymes are present in all living cells.

Tryptophan is the precursor for the vitamin and pyridoxine is required for the reaction. Cat and mink do not have the ability to convert tryptophan to niacin.

Niacin supplementation at 6 to 12g per day to ruminants during early lactation increased milk production, decreased incidence of ketosis (due to its effect on carbohydrate and fat metabolism), may enhance microbial protein synthesis and increase propionate production. (Maize diets are deficient in niacin and pantothenic acid).

Deficiency symptoms: Lesions of dermal epithelium and mucous membranes are general symptoms.

1. **Pellagra or blue tongue in man:** The term pellagra is derived from two Italian words (Pelle, agra) meaning rough skin, a typical characteristic of the disorder. The disease is common in populations eating a predominantly maize-based diet. Niacin is in bound form in maize and maize has low tryptophan. Pellagra is associated with tryptophan/niacin deficiency and not with excess ingestion of leucine. In Andhra Pradesh pellagra in sorghum eaters has been attributed to excess leucine-induced metabolic aberrations in tryptophan metabolism. The classical manifestations of pellagra are dermatitis, diarrhoea and dementia. Other symptoms include fiery red tongue, ulcers of the mouth, nausea, loss of appetite, etc. The skin may become thickened and scaly and show hyperkeratinization and uneven pigmentation. Erythema is also observed on such body parts exposed to light. Similar symptoms are also noticed in pig and chicken.

2. **Black tongue in dogs:** Symptoms include inflammation of the gums, inner surfaces of lips, cheeks, and inside of the mouth under the tongue. These tissues become necrotic and eroded, a foul odour is given off. The tongue becomes red, and dark bluish patches occur resulting in drooling of bloody saliva and halitosis. Bloody diarrhoea is also reported indicating involvement of whole G.I. tract. The dog stops eating and drinking, becomes very dehydrated and death follows.

3. Young chicks show **enlargement of the hock joint and bowing of the legs** similar to perosis. However, the tendon of Achilles rarely slips from its condyles. Other symptoms include inflammation of the mouth, diarrhoea and poor feathering.

4. **Pellagra in pigs:** Symptoms include severe diarrhoea, dermatitis and posterior paralysis.

Conversion of Tryptophan to Niacin

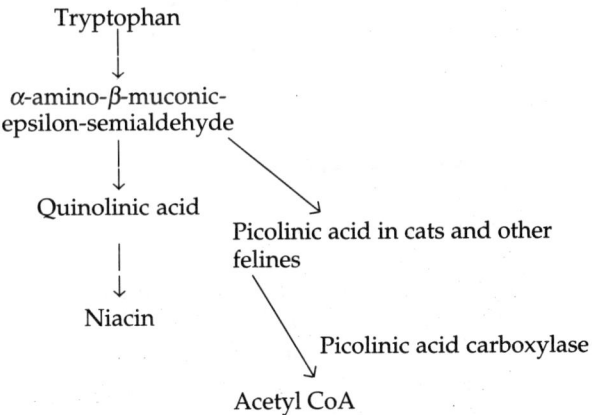

Ducks have a three- to four-fold higher level of picolinic acid carboxylase than chickens. So ducks may be less efficient than chickens in converting tryptophan to niacin. In nonruminant meat producing animals, 50 mg of tryptophan yields roughly 1 mg of nicotinic acid while in humans 60 mg yield 1 mg.

A recent report indicates that iron deficiency in chicks impairs the efficacy of tryptophan as a niacin precursor since iron is a cofactor for two enzymes required for conversion. Conversion of tryptophan to niacin is not available to cats, though the cat does possess all the necessary enzymes. This is due to the high level of activity (30 to 50 times higher than that in rats) of the enzyme picolinic acid carboxylase, which effectively diverts tryptophan conversion via an alternate pathway away from niacin.

Pyridoxine

Vitamin B_6 has three forms—pyridoxine, pyridoxal and pyridoxamine. The name pyridoxine was proposed by Gyorgy. It is present in plants as pyridoxine whereas animal products may also contain pyridoxal and pyridoxamine. This vitamin functions in several enzyme systems concerned with protein metabolism. Part of the B_6 absorbed from the gut is converted into pyridoxal phosphate (PP) while the remainder is excreted as pyridoxic acid in the urine. As phosphorylated pyridoxine, it serves as a coenzyme for enzymes which decarboxylate several amino acids and also serves as a coenzyme for transaminases. It is required for the complete metabolism of tryptophan. It is also concerned in fat metabolism. Linatine present in linseed is an antagonist of B_6.

Deficiency Symptoms

1. The requirement for B_6 is increased when high protein diets high in methionine and tryptophan are fed. In case of its deficiency, tryptophan metabolism would be incomplete. Abnormal metabolites-xanthurenic acid and kynurenic acid are formed and excreted in the urine.
2. Rats show a symmetrical dermatitis, acrodynia. It was called rat pellagra.
3. In swine and dogs microcytic, hypochromic anaemia, epileptic like fits or convulsions and slow growth are seen. Nerve degeneration and haemosiderosis (deposition of a dark-yellow iron pigment) are found on autopsy.
4. Chicks show excitability, aimless movement and spasmodic convulsions followed by exhaustion and often death. During these convulsions, the chicks run aimlessly with rapid 'jerking' motions. Compared to those of encephalomalacia, convulsions in pyridoxine

deficiency are of greater intensity during the seizure and result in complete exhaustion and often death.

5. Pyridoxine deficiency causes a marked rise in the iron and a fall in the copper content of the serum.

6. Deficiency is rare in humans.

Pantothenic Acid or Pantoyl-β-alanine

In 1933, R.J. Williams named this vitamin as pantothenic acid which means 'from everywhere'. It plays a basic biochemical role in the transfer of two-carbon units. It consists of dihydroxy dimethyl butyric acid or pantoic acid and β-alanine joined by an amide bond. The vitamin is absorbed intact from the gut since the bond is resistant to digestion. As a constituent of coenzyme A (coenzyme A contains the vitamin combined with ATP, pyrophosphate and β-mercaptoethylamine), pantothenic acid plays an essential role in the acetylation of choline and in many basic biochemical reactions. It also plays an essential role in fat and cholesterol synthesis. Another metabolically active form of pantothenic acid is acyl carrier protein (ACP) which is involved in the cytoplasmic synthesis of fatty acids. So coenzyme A and ACP are the coenzyme forms.

Deficiency Symptoms

1. Chicks exhibited retardation of growth and feather development. Dermatitis appears later, eyelids become granular and sticky scabs around the mouth develop.

2. In pigs the symptoms include scurvy skin, thin hair, brownish secretion around the eyes, gastrointestinal troubles, slow growth and a characteristic goose-stepping.

3. Deficiency of the vitamin result in a premature greying of the hair in rats, foxes and dogs.

4. Pantothenic acid deficiency is virtually unknown in humans. This no doubt is due to the wide distribution of it in plant and animal foods and its synthesis by intestinal bacteria. During world war soldiers had burning feet (neurological erythromyalgia), which was relieved by administration of pantothenate. A similar syndrome in pregnant women who are rice eaters has been documented.

Biotin

Kögl and Tönnis called this as "biotin" which was earlier referred as vitamin H. Biotin is necessary to prevent perosis in chicks and poults, and a fatty liver and kidney syndrome in chickens. Avidin of the egg white protein, which is a secretory product of the mucosa of the oviduct, is an **antimetabolite** to biotin. Streptavidin and dieldrin (a pesticide) are also antagonists. Administration of sulpha drugs and some intestinally active antibiotics result in a reduction of available biotin due to their effect on gut microflora biotin synthesis.

When raw egg white is fed avidin forms a stable complex with biotin preventing the absorption of biotin. About 20 (raw) egg whites per day have been estimated as the number needed to produce biotin deficiency in man.

It functions both in carbon dioxide fixation and decarboxylation. For example addition of CO_2 to pyruvate, adenine and guanine and in the decarboxylation of oxaloacetate and oxalo succinate. Similarly it is required in the formation of malonyl CoA from acetyl CoA + CO_2 in fat synthesis. The three important biotin-dependent enzymes are pyruvate carboxylase, acetyl coenzyme A carboxylase and propionyl coenzyme A carboxylase. PEPCK is another enzyme.

Deficiency Symptoms

1. Perosis in poultry is caused due to deficiency of biotin, manganese, choline and folic acid.
2. In poults, typical signs include broken flight feathers, bending of the metatarsus, and a dermatitis affecting the bottoms of the feet, the corners of the mouth, and the edges of the eyelids.
3. Egg hatchability is reduced in turkeys and chickens. Signs in embryos include 'parrot beak' chondrodystrophy, etc. (Stunted chick disease).
4. Pigs show spasticity of the hind legs, cracks in the feet, and dermatitis.
5. Rats exhibit a peculiar alopecia called spectacle eye because the skin around the eye loses its hair. Black rats may demonstrate achromotricia.
6. Biotin deficiency affects propionic acid metabolism in ruminants. Formation of methylmelonyl CoA from propionyl CoA is affected because of a decrease in propionyl CoA carboxylase activity (see p. 69).

Supplemental biotin has exerted beneficial effects on hoof health and integrity, milk production, protein yield, lactose yield and dry matter intake. Feeding high concentrate diets is common during the periparturient and early lactation periods. *In vitro* studies showed that biotin synthesis by rumen microbes reduced as the proportion of dietary concentrate increased. This indicates that biotin synthesis is lesser during this period, where the need of biotin is more. Low energy intake around calving causes the dairy cow to mobilize lipid from its adipose tissue, which can result in fatty liver infiltration. Feeding supplemental biotin at

20 g/d during the last 16 d postpartum and at 30 g/d from calving through 70 d postpartum elevated concentrations of biotin in plasma and milk compared with cows fed 0 mg/d of supplemental biotin (Rosendo et al., 2004). Supplemental biotin elevated plasma glucose and lowered NEFA. It is likely that metabolic responses to supplemental biotin are involved with hepatic gluconeogenesis.

Folic Acid (Pteroylmonoglutamic Acid)

Folic acid consists of glutamic acid, paraaminobenzoic acid (PABA) and a pteridine nucleus. The latter two are known as pteroic acid. Hence it is termed pteroylglutamic acid. Animal cells can not synthesize PABA, nor can they attach glutamic acid to pteroic acid. So folic acid must be supplied in the diet of nonruminant animals. Most of the folic acid taken up by the brush border is reduced to tetrahydrofolate (FH_4) or tetrahydrofolic acid. Tetrahydrofolic acid (THFA) is the coenzyme form and the main storage form is 5 methyl tetrahydrofolic acid. Its action is antagonised by aminopterin. It is indispensable in transfer of single-carbon units in various reactions, similar to that of pantothenic acid in the transfer of two-carbon units. These one-carbon units are generated primarily during amino acid metabolism.

Intestinal conjugase inhibitors may be present in certain beans and pulses, and these may impede folacin absorption.

Deficiency Symptoms

1. In young chicks, the chief signs are retarded growth, poor feather formation, feather depigmentation in coloured breeds, and mortality; macrocytic, hypochromic anaemia and perosis.
2. In turkey poults, growth rate is reduced, and a characteristic cervical paralysis develops in which the birds extend their necks and appear to gaze downwards.
3. Folate deficiency is very common in humans. A macrocytic, hyperchromic anaemia called megaloblastic anaemia is noticed in deficiency of folic acid and vitamin B_{12}. Leucopenia (a reduced number of white blood cells) also occurs.
4. Folic acid deficiency in pregnant women produce a child with a neural tube defect such as spina bifida.

Choline

Important Functions

Strecker in 1862 isolated this from hog bile and gave the name choline. Choline is a constituent of phospholipid lecithin. It is metabolic essential for building and maintaining cell structure. It plays an essential role in fat metabolism in the liver preventing abnormal accumulation of fat by promoting its transport as lecithins or by increasing the utilization of fatty acids in the liver itself. Hence it is designated as a lipotropic factor. Choline is necessary for the formation of acetyl choline. Acetyl choline makes possible the transmission of nerve impulses. Choline plays a nonspecific role as a source of "biologically labile methyl groups" and a specific one in the prevention of perosis.

Methionine can partially replace choline as a dietary essential since choline can be synthesized in the body by transmethylation process. It is prudent to supply choline in the diet to spare the methionine for its synthesis. In avians, however, methylation of phosphatidyl ethanolamine is limited such that excess methionine has minimal choline-sparing capacity. Moreover, excess levels of dietary protein markedly increase the bird's dietary need for choline, which is a reflection of the drain on the methyl pool resulting from increased uric acid excretion.

Choline therefore has two types of functions: functions of choline *per se* and functions as a methyl donor. The two principal methyl donors in animal metabolism are betaine, a metabolite of choline, and S-adenosyl-methionine (SAM), a metabolite of methionine. Choline is an essential nutrient for mammals when excess methionine and folate are not available in the diet.

Importance of Choline in Ruminants

Choline is rapidly and extensively degraded in the rumen of both cattle and sheep, both in its non-esterified form and as phospholipid. Only a minimal quantity reaches the lower digestive tract and can be absorbed. The choline methyl groups are metabolized to trimethylamine by rumen microorganism. Trimethylamine can accumulate in the rumen or be converted to methane, which is lost. The methanogenesis pathway is easily saturated by excess of substrates (trimethylamine, methylamine and methionine). Thus, less than 10% of choline escapes degradation by incorporation, as phosphatidylcholine into the structural membranes of ciliate protozoa.

In dairy ruminants, the dietary availability of choline is still low, but the output of methylated compounds in milk is high, and precursors from the tetrahydrofolate pathway are limiting, especially at the onset of lactation. Therefore choline may be a limiting nutrient for milk production in high-yielding dairy cows. Several studies have been conducted by R.A. Erdman and B.K. Sharma during 1988-94 and L. Pinotti and coworkers during 2000-02 on rumen protected choline (RPC) in dairy cows. The data do not provide precisely as to the amount of choline needed in dairy cow nutrition. The supplementation of unprotected choline ranged from 10 to 326g, while levels of RPC ranged between 2 and 50 g.

Deficiency Symptoms

1. Slow growth
2. Fatty liver
3. Perosis or slipped tendon in chicks

In ruminants, orally ingested choline is rapidly degraded in the rumen, but rumen microbes synthesise choline. Microbial choline synthesis may be inadequate to support a high level of milk production since higher milk yield has been reported in Holstein cows receiving 30 to 50 g choline per day via abomosal infusion.

Refined plant oils generally have been subjected to alkaline treatment and bleaching, and these processes almost totally remove the phospholipid bound choline.

Vitamin B_{12}

Discovery of Vitamin B_{12}

Its generic name is cyanocobalamin. The story of the discovery of this vitamin is a dramatic one made possible by the combined efforts of microbiologists, biochemists, nutrition scientists and physicians working in various laboratories. It was discovered in 1926 that humans suffering from pernicious anaemia would respond to the eating of large amounts of liver. It is named as antipernicious anaemia (APA) factor. The association of the unknown (unidentified) factor with animal protein sources was responsible for its designation as animal protein factor(APF). It was also referred to as the 'chick growth factor', 'cow manure factor', 'zoopherin'. Later around 1948 Merck group proposed the name vitamin B_{12}.

The tremendous task of working out the structure of B_{12} was completed by 1955. Thirteen different authors were involved in the task. This complex molecule has a cobalt atom in centre of a tetra-ring porphyrin structure. The large ring formed by the four reduced rings is called "corrin" because it is the core of the vitamin. Any compound with a corrin is called corrinoid. Vitamin B_{12} is stored in the liver in most animals. Levels of vitamin B_{12} in the blood is usually very low. It is a metabolic essential for all species. Plants do not synthesize or require vitamin B_{12}.

Vitamin B_{12} is synthesized by bacteria in the rumen (in ruminants) and in the large intestine (in ruminants and non-ruminants) when adequate cobalt is available. Restriction of roughage may decrease the synthesis in ruminants. So it is not dietary essential in ruminants with functional rumen. Intestinal synthesis of vitamin B_{12} is significant in other animals, but they meet their requirement only in such animals who practice coprophagy.

It is reported that several animals secrete intrinsic factor required for the absorption of vitamin B_{12} across the intestinal mucosa.

Functions

1. Vitamin B_{12} participates as a coenzyme in two reactions, the remethylation of homocysteine to methionine and the isomerization of L-methylmalonyl-Co A to succinyl-Co A. The former reaction is catalyzed by methionine synthase in the cytosol, and the latter is catalyzed by L-methylmalonyl Co A mutase in the mitochondria.
2. Vitamin B_{12} is concerned in the synthesis of labile methyl groups.
3. Synthesize methyl group from one-carbon precursors.
4. Concerned in the synthesis of nucleic acid, RNA and DNA. So it is essential for cell division.
5. Controls protein synthesis directly.
6. A ruminant animal may require more vitamin B_{12} than a monogastric animal of comparable size.

Deficiency Symptoms

Vitamin B_{12} deficiency is associated with anaemia, megaloblastosis, neuropathy, and neuroschychatric disorders. All these could theoretically be linked to the block in homocysteine remethylation or the resulting hyper-homocysteinemia. However, the block in the isomerization reaction and resulting build up of methylmalonic acid could also play a role.

1. Anaemia has not been noted as a symptom of deficiency in other animals except humans. Pernicious anaemia in humans is caused by vitamin B_{12} deficiency. This deficiency state may be caused by the failure of the absorption of B_{12}, usually due to a lack of intrinsic factor. Prior to absorption, cobalamine is bound to the intrinsic factor and some of it is bound to 'R' proteins derived from salivary glands and the stomach. The R proteins are largely degraded by pancreatic proteases in the gut lumen, but intrinsic factor is protease insensitive. In pancreatic insufficiency, cobalamine can not be released from the R proteins for subsequent binding by intrinsic factor. Intrinsic factor is a mucoprotein produced in the fundic region of the stomach and it facilitates the absorption of vitamin B_{12}. Hence, animals or humans lacking intrinsic factor or with pancreatic disorders are subject to B_{12} absorption problems. Pernicious anaemia is characterised by an arrest of erythrocyte

maturation in the bone marrow which result in a macrocytic hyperchromic anaemia. This is accompanied by leucopenia and progressive degeneration of the nervous system.

2. Swine show slow growth rate, incoordination of the hind legs and a wobbley gait.

3. In chicks, lower growth rate, kidney damage and bone abnormalities similar to perosis (if choline is inadequate) are seen. In hens, body weight and egg production are maintained despite a deficiency, but poor hatchability results.

4. In ruminants, B_{12} deficiency impairs the utilisation of propionate and causes an increase of methylmalonic acid in the urine. Vitamin B_{12} deficiency can be induced with the addition of high dietary levels of propionic acid (see p. 199).

5. In calves, cessation of growth, poor appetite and in some cases, incoordination in gait are observed.

6. Signs of folate deficiency almost always accompany B_{12} deficiency because vitamin B_{12} is required for folate metabolism.

7. Lack of either folate or vitamin B_{12} prevents proper transfer of methyl groups in the synthesis of thymidine. This, in turn, produces a defect in DNA synthesis.

Vitamin C (Ascorbic Acid)

Vitamin C is dietary essential to humans, guinea pigs, subhuman primates, bats, certain birds, certain fish and perhaps certain reptiles. All these species lack the enzyme L-gulunolactone oxidase which is required for vitamin C synthesis from 6 carbon sugars. Glycoascorbic acid acts as an **antimetabolite** for vitamin C. Vitamin C is precursor of oxalic acid.

Functions

1. It functions in the formation and maintenance of intercellular material having collagen or related substances as basal constituent in bones, in soft tissues.

2. It functions in hydroxylation reactions e.g. formation of hydroxyproline.

3. It occurs in two forms, L-ascorbic acid (reduced form) and L-dehydro-ascorbic acid (oxidized form). Both forms are biologically active. In conducive situations L-dehydroascorbic acid is further oxidized to diketo gulonic acid (an inactive compound) in an irreversible reaction.

4. Vitamin C is a fairly strong antioxidant and is used in the canning and freezing industry for the preservation of fruits and vegetables, especially when darkening is a problem.

Diets high in pectin, zinc, iron, or copper have been reported to decrease ascorbate absorption. It is absorbed from small intestine and is equalized with that in the tissues within 4h and the excess excreted. In humans excess ascorbic acid is excreted as ascorbic acid, diketogulonic acid, or oxalic acid, and very little appears in expired CO_2. However, in the guinea pig expired CO_2 is the major route of elimination of excess ascorbic acid.

Deficiency Symptoms

1. In 1753 James Lind described scurvy, a disease caused by deficiency of vitamin C. Symptoms include that the affected individuals have swollen, bleeding and ulcerated gums and loosening of teeth. Weak bones and fragility of the capillaries with resulting haemorrhages throughout the body are also found. Anaemia is associated with severe scurvy. The skin is dry, rough and covered with several reddish spots of varying sizes. The disease is more insidious in nature in the human infant, who at first fails to thrive, becomes irritable, and fails to grow. Costochondral beading of the ribs is also a frequent symptom. Baby often assumes a 'pithed-frog' position.

Antioxidant and Immunity Role of Vitamins

Antioxidant vitamins are carotenoids, vitamin E and vitamin C. These nutrients play important roles in animal health by inactivating harmful free radicals produced through normal cellular activity and from various stressors. Tissue defence mechanisms against free radical damage generally include vitamin C, vitamin E and β-carotene as the major vitamin antioxidant sources. In addition, several metalloenzymes which include glutathione peroxidase (selenium), catalase (iron) and superoxide dismutase (copper, zinc and manganese) are also critical in protecting the internal cellular constituents from oxidative damage.

Both *in vitro* and *in vivo* studies showed that these antioxidant vitamins generally enhance different aspects of cellular and noncellular immunity. A compromised immune system will result in reduced animal production efficiency through increased susceptibility to diseases, thereby leading to increased animal morbidity and mortality.

Carotenoids have been to have biological actions independent of vitamin A. Certain carotenoids, with antioxidant capacity but without vitamin A activity, can enhance many aspects of immune functions, act directly as antimutagens and anticarcinogens, protect against radiation damage, and block the damaging effects of photosentitizers e.g., canthaxanthin. Vitamin A and β-carotene have important roles in protecting animals against numerous infections including mastitis.

Polymorphonuclear neutrophils (PMN) are the major line of defence against bacteria in the mammary gland. β-carotene supplementation seems to exert a stabilizing effect on PMN and lymphocyte function during the period around dry off. Supplemental levels of vitamin E higher than recommended by the NRC (1989) have been beneficial in the control of mastitis.

Synthesis of B-vitamins in Ruminants

Unlike other B-complex vitamins, vitamin B_{12} (cyanocobalamin) is synthesized almost exclusively by bacteria and is therefore present only in foods that have been bacterially fermented or are derived from animals that have obtained this vitamin from their gastrointestinal microflora or their diet. As one atom of cobalt is part of the molecule of CBL, it is generally assumed that ruminant requirements for the vitamin equate with ruminal bacteria requirements for cobalt (McDowell, 2000).

Earlier research studies on B-vitamins led to the general dogma that dietary supply and ruminal synthesis are sufficient to meet dairy cow requirements (NRC, 2001). Although ruminal B-vitamin synthesis appears to be sufficient to prevent clinical deficiencies in most situations, supplementing dietary thiamin, biotin, niacin, and folic acid increased lactation performance. However, in other studies, lactation performance was not improved by supplemental folic acid, niacin, or biotin. Possible reasons for lack of consistent responses to B-vitamin supplementation are numerous, but a potentially important factor is variable amounts of ruminally synthesized B-vitamins. Data regarding amounts of B-vitamins flowing to the duodenum or ruminally synthesized in lactating dairy cows are limited.

E.C. Schwab et al., (2006; J Dairy Sci, 89:174-187) studied the effect of diets fed as total mixed rations (TMR) varying in forage (35 and 60%; silage and hay) and nonfibre (30 and 40%; soybean hulls, beet pulp and maize and barley processed grains) carbohydrates (NFC) contents on these parameters. No supplemental B-vitamins were fed. Dry matter and organic matter intakes were higher for cows fed the 35% forage diets and the 40% NFC diets.

When averaged across diets, ruminal apparent synthesis (AS) of individual B-vitamins as a percentage of B-vitamin intake was thiamin, 142; riboflavin, 228; total niacin, 120; total B_6, 39; folic acid, 137; and B_{12}, 24,276, clearly exemplifying the importance of ruminal synthesis for most B-vitamins. Negative AS values for biotin suggest minimal ruminal synthesis and/or appreciable ruminal degradation. Vitamin B_{12} AS was highest for 35% forage-30% NFC diets and was increased with increasing dietary sugars. Increasing dietary forage and NFC contents influenced B-vitamin intakes, duodenal flow, and AS. Dietary forage and NFC effects on AS could be due to changes in populations or functions of ruminal microbial species, their interrelationships, and subsequent effects on microbial B-vitamin metabolism.

Recent studies of C.L.Girard and his coworkers from Canada (J Dairy Sci, 2009, 92: 4524-4529) showed that dairy cows in early lactation could benefit from an increased supply of B_{12}, even when the dietary supply in cobalt is adequate. In primiparous cows, intramuscular injections of cyanocobalamin increased concentrations of the vitamin in milk and milk yields of solids, fat, and lactose compared with cows fed only supplementary folic acid. Intramuscular injections of cyanocobalamin also increased blood haemoglobin and decreased serum methylmalonic acid. In multiparous cows, oral or parenteral combined supplements of folic acid and B_{12} given in early lactation increased milk and milk component yields by improving efficiency of energy metabolism.

Calculation of apparent synthesis or destruction of vitamin B_{12} and its analogs in the rumen as well as their apparent intestinal disappearance in dairy cows showed that cyanocobalamin represented 38% of the total amounts of corrinoids produced in rumen. Approximately 11% of the average daily intake of cobalt was used for the synthesis of corrinoids, of which only 4% was incorporated into cyanocobalamin. Further, it is revealed that use of a dietary supplement of cyanocobalamin is not an efficient means to increase vitamin B_{12} supply to cows, because 80% of the supplement disappeared before reaching the duodenal cannula. But still cyanocobalamin seems to be the major form absorbed in the small intestine.

Factors Affecting Vitamin Requirements and Vitamin Utilization

1. *Physiological makeup and production function:* Vitamin needs of animals and humans depend greatly on their physiological makeup, age, health, nutritional status, and function, such as producing meat, milk, eggs, hair, or wool or developing a foetus. Productive animals require higher levels of vitamins compared to those maintaining body weight.

2. *Confinement rearing without access to pasture:* Confinement rearing of poultry and swine had a profound effect on vitamin nutrition (as well as mineral nutrition). Young, lush, green grasses or legumes are good vitamin sources. More available forms of vitamin A and E are present. Ample quantities of *b*-carotene and *a*-tocopherol are present in them. Confinement rearing of poultry in cages and swine on slatted floor has limited animal access to faeces (coprophagy) which is rich in many vitamins. Vitamin D has to be provided.

3. *Stress, disease, or adverse environmental conditions:* Intensified production increases stress and subclinical disease level conditions because of higher densities of animals in confined areas. Stress and disease conditions in animals may increase the basic requirement for certain vitamins. Diseases or parasites affecting the gastrointestinal tract will reduce intestinal absorption of vitamins, from both dietary sources and those synthesized by microorganisms. Micotoxins are known to cause digestive disturbances such as vomiting and diarrhoea as well as internal bleeding, and interfere with absorption of vitamins A, D, E and K and other vitamins e.g. biotin, folacin, etc. Coccidiosis increase vitamin K requirements due to reduced intake, reduction in absorption and increased requirement due to treatment.

4. *Vitamin antagonists:* Vitamin antagonists (antimetabolites) interfere with the activity of various vitamins. The antagonist could cleave the metabolite molecule and render it inactive. Some common antagonists are furnished here.

    a. Thiaminase (found in raw fish)   Thiamin antagonist
        Pyrrithiamine   ''
        Amprolium   ''

    b. Dicumarol   Vitamin K antagonist
        Sulfaquinoxaline   ''

    c. Avidin (raw egg white)   Biotin antimetabolite
        Streptavidin (Streptomyces moulds)   ''

    d. Oral contraceptives and drug   Antagonistic to B_6.
        therapy to control tuberculosis

    e. Rancid fats inactivate biotin
        and destroy vitamins A, D and E
        and possibly others

    f. Sulfonamides may increase
        requirements of biotin, folacin,
        vitamin K, etc.

    g. Isoniazid, cycloserine and penicillamine
        render pyridoxine inactive leading to
        peripheral neuritis.

5. *Levels of other nutrients in the diet:* Level of fat in the diet is important for the absorption of fat-soluble vitamins and possibly other vitamins. Fat-soluble vitamins may fail to be absorbed if digestion of fat is impaired.

6. *Interrelationships of vitamins with other nutrients:* Vitamin E and selenium, vitamin D with Ca and P, choline with methionine and niacin with tryptophan.

7. *Body vitamin reserves:*   Body storage of vitamins from previous intake will affect daily requirements of these nutrients. This is more true for fat-soluble vitamins and vitamin B_{12} than for other water-soluble vitamins.

Sources of Vitamins

Vitamin A: Carotenoids present in plants; yellow maize, carrots, greens are rich sources.

Long chain retinyl esters, largely palmitate esters in animal tissues. Fish liver oils, liver, egg yolk, butter, cream, whole milk are rich sources.

Vitamin D: It is not widely distributed in foods. The natural foods containing vitamin D are those of animal origin. e.g. egg-yolk, liver and salt water fish especially salmon, herring, sardines, etc. with higher content of body oils. Fish-liver oils (e.g. cod liver oil) are very rich in vitamin D and have been popular source of vitamin D for infant and child feeding.

Since most natural foods (milk, butter, cereals, etc.) contain little amount of vitamin D, it is a common practice to enrich (fortification) such foods especially when used in infant foods e.g. irradiated yeast, irradiated milk, etc.

Vitamin D sources for livestock are sun cured hay and roughages. The dead leaves of growing plants also contain vitamin D as ergocalciferol.

Vitamin E: Tocopherol is a plant product. It is also found in meat, fish, eggs, etc. of animal products. But there is no evidence suggesting its synthesis in any animal tissue. Cereals, wheat germ, oil seeds, green leaves are rich sources. Young green grass is a better source than mature fodder. The leaves contain 20-30 times as much vitamin E as the stems. Alfalfa meal is a rich source of tocopherol while maize grain has higher τ form. Milk has higher vitamin E during summer than during winter. Plant-source ingredients are richer in vitamin E bioactivity than animal-source ingredients.

Vitamin K: Green leafy vegetables are rich sources of phylloquinone. Liver, egg and fish meal are good animal sources and the amount is usually related to the diet. Menaquinones are synthesized by bacteria in the digestive tract of animals.

Thiamin: Widely distributed in both plant and animal tissues. Brans and rice polish are rich sources. Fermentation products such as brewers' yeast are rich sources. Animal products such as egg yolk, liver, kidney and pork are rich sources.

Riboflavin: It is one of the most widely distributed B complex vitamins. It can be synthesized by all green plants, yeast, fungi and most bacteria. Milk is a rich source. Eggs and meat are also high in riboflavin. Green leafy crops are also rich sources.

Niacin: Fairly widely distributed in both plant and animal tissues. It occurs naturally in foods in free, bound or coenzyme forms. About 40% of niacin in oil seeds and 85 to 90% of niacin in cereals is present as bound niacin. Leucine induces deficiency of niacin. Animal and fish byproducts and distillers' grain and yeast are good sources.

Pyridoxine: Widely distributed in feeds. In many sources this is chemically bound to protein. Groundnut meal, rice bran, wheat bran, cane molasses, liver and milk are rich sources. Bioavailability of B_6 in foods of plant origin is usually less than in those of animal origin. Whole grains and nuts are good sources.

Biotin: Widely distributed in foods. Liver, milk, yeast, oilseeds and vegetables are rich sources. A large portion of biotin requirement of humans and most animals comes from bacterial synthesis in the gut.

Pantothenic acid: It is synthesized in green plants and most microorganisms from pantoic acid and β-alanine. It is widely distributed. Outstanding sources are yeast, groundnuts, peas, liver and eggs. The vitamin occurs predominantly in bound form in food.

Folic acid: It is widely distributed in nature. Whole cereal grains, dark green leafy vegetables, nuts and oil seed meals are good dietary sources.

Choline: Green leafy materials, yeast, egg yolk and cereals are rich sources.

Vitamin B_{12}: Liver and kidney are excellent sources while meat and fish are moderate sources.

Vitamin C: Citrus fruits, tomatoes, green vegetables and potatoes are the principal sources. Raw milk is a good source, but most of it is lost during pasteurization.

Toxicity of Vitamins

There are reported cases of hypervitaminosis A, D, niacin and B_6. Let us know the toxicity symptoms.

Hypervitaminosis A: Results in reduced appetite and growth rate, inflammation of the membranes, bone abnormalities and increased spinal fluid pressure. Further, fatigue, lethargy, abdominal discomfort, bone and joint pain, headache and insomnia have also been observed in humans. Hypervitaminosis A may interfere with the absorption of other fat-soluble vitamins in diets that are marginal in these vitamins. Excessive vitamin A intake causes formation of new bone at the ventral aspect of the cervical vertebrae in a 3 year old cat (exostoses). It may be called as 'deformed cervical spondylosis'. Bony outgrowths may also be seen at joints of the foreleg.

Hypervitaminosis D: Results when a high dose of vitamin D is consumed over a long period. Initially it is exhibited as hypercalcaemia and subsequently the excess plasma ca^{++} is deposited not only in the bone tissue but also in soft tissues, more prominently the kidneys, myocardium, synovial membranes, the pancreas. Such calcification of the soft tissues may be lethal. Hypervitaminosis D is relatively uncommon in dogs and cats. It has been reported as a result of injudicious dietary supplementation, or of rodenticide (calciferol) poisoning.

Hypervitaminosis E: Symptoms observed in humans are nausea, muscle weakness, headache and blurred vision.

Hypervitaminosis niacin: Oral doses of 50 to 100 mg nicotinic acid are used as vasodilator in human patients. Hence, those with low BP should avoid excess of niacin. This high level causes marked flushing and 'tingling' sensation in fingers and toes. Excess nicotinic acid causes severe flushing, pruritis (itching), hyperhidrosis (sweating), nausea and abdominal cramps. Excessive doses may also aggravate asthma, activate peptic ulcer, impair glucose tolerance and damage the liver.

Hypervituminosis pyridoxine: Excess use can cause peripheral neuropathies characterised by muscular incoordination, clumsiness of hands and feet, tingling pains and, in rare cases, encephalopathy (a form of brain dysfunction).

Hypervitaminosis C: It is associated with an enhanced incidence of stone formation in the kidneys since urinary oxalate may arise from ascorbic acid. Excess vitamin C as sodium ascorbate may be dangerous to hypertensive patients.

Stress Factors that Promote Vitamin Destruction

Many vitamins are delicate substances that can suffer loss of activity due to unfavourable circumstances encountered during processing or storage of premixes and feeds.

Several factors can influence vitamin stability in premixes and in feeds during processing and storage, including temperature, humidity, conditioning time, reduction and oxidation (redox) reactions and light. Heat, pressure, humidity, friction and redox reaction vary drastically among the different ways, the feed can be processed. The level of stress on vitamins is high to very high in pelleting and extrusion of the feed.

Let us see how humidity is the root cause of all stability problems. Humidity is the primary factor that can decrease the stability of vitamins in premixes and feedstuffs. Water softens the matrix of vitamin A and thus the vitamin becomes more permeable to oxygen. Trace elements, acids, and bases are activated only by water. Humidity augments the negative effects exerted by choline chloride, trace elements, and other chemical reactions that are not found in dry feed. Thus, the water level is responsible for a higher reactivity of vitamins with other feed components. Elevated moisture content or incorrect storage of premixes and feedstuffs are the root of almost all stability problems.

Vitamins mixed and stored with minerals are subject to loss of potency. Hazards to vitamins from minerals are abrasion and direct destruction by certain trace elements, particularly copper. Some abrasion is inevitable in the mixing process but fortunately most minerals contain little moisture with the exception of salt, due to its hygroscopic nature. Therefore, packaging, careful transport, and storage become important. Few companies would willingly use very high levels of salt in a supplement containing fat-soluble vitamins.

Destruction of Vitamin A

Certain legumes, particularly soybeans and alfalfa contain an enzyme, lipoxygenase (proper heat treatment destroys lipoxygenase) which readily destroys the carotenes and xanthophylls and probably also destroys the vitamin A through a coupled oxidation with PUFA. Destruction of vitamin A in feeds takes place through oxidation, high temperature, etc., peroxidizing effects of rancidifying PUFA and catalytic effects of trace minerals.

Stabilization of Vitamin A

Vitamin A is stabilized by mechanical means wherein minute droplets of vitamin A are developed in a stable fat, gelatin, or wax, forming a small bead. This prevents most of the vitamin A from coming into contact with oxygen until it is digested in the intestinal tract of the animal. Synthetic antioxidants (ethoxyquin) are also used to markedly prolong the induction period which precedes active oxidation of vitamin A.

Destruction of Other Vitamins

* Vitamin D is destroyed by overtreatment with UV light and by peroxidation in the presence of rancidifing PUFA, especially when finely dispersed and in the presence of trace minerals.
* Dehydration and storage of alfalfa meal cause a loss of α-tocopherol. High temperature rapid drying of maize also cause loss of α-tocopherol.
* Some of the vitamins are destroyed by light. Riboflavin is stable to most factors involved in processing. However, it is very readily destroyed by either visible or ultraviolet light; vitamin B_6, vitamin C and folacin can also be destroyed by light. It is necessary, therefore, to protect premixes of feeds containing these vitamins from light and radiation.
* The most sensitive vitamins to irradiation are vitamins B_1, B_2, A and E. Niacin is relatively stable.
* Vitamin B_1 and niacin are extremely resistant to oxidation while vitamin C is highly susceptible to it.

Bioavailability of Vitamins

Most of the vitamins present in feedstuffs (refer Table 7) exist as precursor compounds or coenzymes that are often bound or complexed in some manner. Hence, digestive processes are required to either release or convert precursors or complexes to usable and absorbable chemical entities. Vitamin bioavailability in formulated diets for livestock and companion animals is dependent on two factors:
  (a) stability of free vitamins in vitamin and vitamin-mineral premixes as well as in diets and supplements.
  (b) utilization efficiency from plant- and animal-source feed ingredients.

Preparation of Vitamin Premixes

In preparing vitamin premixes, whether commercial or experimental, several precautions should be considered.

1. a. The carrier material should be uniform in texture and particle size. If it is a carbohydrate, it should not contain free aldehyde groups. That means dextrose and lactose should be avoided as carriers.
   b. Both thiamin and folacin have free amino groups that can react with free carboxyl groups to form Maillard linkages that cannot be

broken by digestive enzymes in the upper small intestine.

2. a. High potency vitamin premixes used for fortification of purified diets generally should not contain either choline or vitamin E activity.

   b. Pure choline chloride is extremely hygroscopic and pure DL-α-tocopheryl acetate (all-rac-α-tocopheryl acetate) is a liquid. As such, these substances are not suitable components of purified vitamin premixes. All-rac-α-tocopheryl acetate can be dissolved in ether or blended with fat, premixed with carbohydrate, screened, and then added directly to the diet.

   c. Commercial vitamin premixes generally use choline and vitamin E sources that are already premixed (i.e., diluted) and this makes them suitable as components of complete (feed grade) vitamin premix.

   The effect of the added choline chloride on the stability of Vitamins A, E and K_3 in premixes during storage in controlled conditions was studied over a period of one year. All vitamins were more stable in a premix containing no choline chloride than in a premix containing choline chloride.

3. a. Once prepared, vitamin premixes should be stored in a dark container that is as air-tight and oxygen-free as possible and kept in a cool, dry place. Avoiding heat, light, oxygen, and moisture will minimize loss of potency.

   b. Generally, the fat-soluble vitamins are less heat labile than the water-soluble vitamins, although the former can lose biopotency when subjected to high temperatures in the presence of oxygen. Among the water-soluble vitamins, thiamin, folacin, pantothenic and, and ascorbic acid are considered the most heat labile.

4. a. pH of the premix is also important. For maximal retention of vitamin A activity, premixes should be as moisture free as possible and have a pH above 5.

   b. Low pH causes isomerization of all-trans vitamin A to less potent cis forms and also results in deesterification of vitamin A esters to more labile retinol. The forms in which vitamins present in commercial supplements are presented in Table 7.

Rapid Vitamin Degradation in Premixes

A battle is raging in every bag of feed premix. Trace metals, fat and other nutrients ally themselves with oxygen and lay siege to the vitamins. Over time, the vitamins eventually lose the fight and their concentration in the feed is less than expected.

TABLE 7. Forms of Vitamins Present in Natural Food and Feedstuffs and in Commercial Preparations Meant for Supplementation.

Vitamin	Form available to the commercial foods & feeds	Form present in natural feedstuffs
Vitamin A	Vitamin A esters. Current commercial sources are generally "coated" esters of acetate or palmitate that contain a synthetic anti-oxidant in beadlet form. AD_3 beadlet form (cross linking). Crystalline β-carotene is absorbed from the gut more efficiently than that exist in foods and feeds.	Animal tissues, eggs and milk contain vitamin A while plant materials contain pro-vitamin A carotenoids.
Vitamin K	Water-soluble forms of menadione (K_3): Menadione sodium bisulfite (MSB); menadione dimethyl pyrimidinol bisulfite (MPB); menadione nicotinamide bisulfite (MNB)-most stable.	Green plants and oil seeds contain phylloquinone (K_1) and Fermented feed has menaquinone (K_2)
Vitamin D	D_3 beadlet form (cross linking), Mineral stable (MS) form	Ergosterol in plants, 7-dehydrocholesterol in animals
Vitamin E	Vitamin E alcohol, vitamin E acetate, dl-α-tocopheryl acetate gelatin beadlets	Alcohols, tocopherols and tocotrienols in plant materials. Of all the above α tocopherol is more active.
Thiamin	Crystalline thiamin is available as thiamin hydrochloride and thiamin mononitrate, latter being better. Stable up to 100°C and readily soluble in water.	Largely in phosphorylated forms, either as protein-phosphate complexes or as thiamin mono-/di- or triphosphates.
Riboflavin	Crystalline riboflavin. considered quite stable, although it is easily destroyed by UV light when in solution.	Primarily as nucleotide coenzymes, FAD and FMN.
Niacin	Nicotinic acid is a very stable compound when added to feed or premixes, being little affected by heat, light, oxygen, or moisture.	In plants it is present in the form of nicotinic acid. Much of the niacin activity exists as nicotinamide nucleotides in animals.

Pantothenic acid (PA)	Crystalline form as either D-or DL-calcium PA. Free flowing, nonhygroscopic D-Calcium pantothenate is available through complexing procedures	Most of the PA is contained in coenzyme A, acyl CoA synthetase, and acyl carrier protein.
Vitamin B_{12}	Crystalline cyanocobalamin is considered very stable when stored in feeds and premixes.	Plant foodstuffs are devoid of B_{12}. Microorganisms are the sole source of B_{12} in nature and this accounts for the B_{12} activity in animal and fermentation byproducts. In animal and fermentation based feedstuffs, B_{12} exists bound to protein in the methyl form (methylcobalamin) or the 5'-deoxyadenosyl form (adenosylcobalamin).
Choline	In its crystalline form, choline chloride (87% choline) is hygroscopic and is considered a stress agent to other vitamins in a vitamin-mineral premix. Choline bitartrate salt is also available.	Feed ingredients and crude unprocessed fat sources contain most of the choline as phospholipid-bound phosphatidyl choline.
Biotin	Crystalline D-biotin	Much of it exists in a bound form, ϵ-N-biotinyl-L-lysine (biocytin) which is a component of protein. Bioavailability of it varies and it is dependent on the digestibility of the proteins in which it is found.
Vitamin B_6	Crystalline pyridoxine hydrochloride.	Exists in food either in the free or the phosphorylated form. Plant products are rich in pyridoxine; some may have pyridoxine glucoside. Animal products contain primarily phosphorylated pyridoxal.
Folic acid	Crystalline folacin	Folacin exists largely as polyglutamates. A group of intestinal enzymes known as conjugases remove all but the last glutamate residue and this monoglutamyl form is thought to be absorbed into enterocyte.

Vitamin C	Crystalline L-ascorbic acid, 50% fat coated L-ascorbic acid, 97.5% ethylcellulose coated L-ascorbic acid, Ascorbyl phosphate (the most stable form).

Vitamin Degradation in Stored Feed

After four months of storage, vitamin losses have been found highest in premixes containing inorganic trace minerals. Potency of vitamins K, A, B_6 and thiamin mononitrates were most severely affected. Vitamin K potency dropped by up to 10% each month during the study. Vitamin premixes lost their potency only about half as fast as premixes containing both vitamins and trace minerals.

Premixes containing metal-specific amino acid complexes, which are an organic class of trace minerals, along with vitamins had only a slow loss in vitamin potency. The minerals in such premixes may be protected by organic compounds, preventing chemical degradation of the vitamins. However the cost of the organic trace minerals has been prohibitive for routine use or total replacement of inorganic trace minerals.

Feed industry recommends to limit storage of feed to a month or less. It is better to purchase vitamin and trace mineral supplements separately.

Effect of Processing on Bioavailability of Vitamins

* Any processing procedure that involves alkaline treatment generally leads to loss of B_1 activity.

* Coenzyme A contains peptide linkages and a free SH group. Hence, it seems possible that exposure of foods or feeds containing CoA to an acid or alkaline environment might decrease pantothenic acid bioavailability.

* Pyridoxal and pyridoxal phosphate have a free aldehyde group and so heat processing enhances Maillard-type reactions and decreases B_6 bioavailability.

* Heat processing, especially extrusion, can reduce vitamin A bioavailability.

* It is reported that only 1% of the β-carotene is absorbed from raw carrots, while mild cooking enhanced the absorption efficiency since mild cooking apparently releases carotenoids from protein-carotenoid complexes. Overcooking may reduce carotenoid bioavailability. This may be due to conversion of all-trans-β-carotene to the cis-β-carotene isomers during heating. β-carotene is also known to be rapidly destroyed by sunlight and air.

* Pelleting of feeds may have a beneficial effect on availability of vitamins such as niacin and biotin, which are often present in bound forms. Due the combined action of heat, pressure and moisture during pelleting, vitamins A, D_3, K_3, B_1 and C are most likely to show stability problems in pelleted feeds.

* Ascorbic acid in cooked cabbage is present in the bound form, ascorbinogen, a form that is absorbed very poorly by humans.

Chapter 13

Feed Additives and their Use in Livestock and Poultry Feeding

What are Feed Additives?

Feed additive is an ingredient or combination of ingredients added to the basic feed mix or parts thereof to fulfil the specific need. Usually used in microquantities and requires careful handling and mixing.

Any chemical incorporated in an animal feed for the purpose of improving rate of gain, feed efficiency, or preventing and controlling disease is feed additive.

A feed additive need not be a drug. A dose of a few mg/kg added to the feed of animals acts as a protection against untoward environmental influences.

A variety of feed additives are used in animal feeding. Some are approved to be used as implants or injectable form.

Types of Feed Additives

Feed additives are broadly classified into nutrient feed additives (e.g., amino acids, minerals and vitamins) and nonnutrient feed additives (e.g. antibiotics, arsenic and copper supplements, hormones, beta agonists, immunomodulators, coccidiostats, enzymes, probiotics, yeast culture and acidifiers, antioxidants, sequestrants, mycotoxin binders, anticaking agents, humectants, feed preservatives, flavouring agents, colouring agents, pellet binders, dietary buffers, methane inhibitors, roughage substitutes, propionate promoters, defaunating agents, ketosis and bloat controlling agents, surfactants, sweetening agents, tranquilizers, emulsifiers and stablilizers, bile acid, methyl donors, sweeteners, etc).

Five Categories of Feed Additives

European Union recognized 23 functions for feed additives (having added that of binding mycotoxins as recently as February 2009) indicating that each feed additive is recognized to explain its functionality. Accordingly, feed additives are organized in five categories:

Technological additives: This refers to products that influence the technological aspects of the feed while not directly affecting its nutritional value, although there may be indirect effects such as through improvements in the feed's handling or hygiene characteristics. Example, organic acid as preservative of feed.

Sensory additives: These improve the palatability and thereby voluntary intake of a diet by stimulating appetite, usually through the effect they have on the flavour or colour of the feed. Examples, vanilla extract, essential oils.

Nutritional, additives: They supply specific nutrients required by the animal for optimal growth. Examples vitamins, amino acids, trace minerals. This category of additives is simply the concentrated forms of nutrients supplied in the natural ingredients in the diet.

Zootechnical additives: The products in this case improve the nutrient status of the animal, not by providing specific nutrients but by enabling more efficient use of the nutrients present in the diet. Examples, enzymes and direct-fed microbials/probiotics (often referred to as pronutrients).

Coccidiostats and histomonostats: These are used to control intestinal health of poultry through direct effects on the parasitic organism concerned. They are not classified as antibiotics.

Advantages of use of Feed Additives

1. Increase feed quality and feed palatability:
    Emulsifiers, pelleting agents are used to meet the demands of feed manufacturers while antioxidants, fungistatic agents and fermentation inhibitors ensure proper shelflife of feed.
2. Improve animal performance:
    Feed additives are mixed with feeds in nontherapeutic quantities for the purpose of promoting animal growth, lowering feed consumption, protecting the animal against all sorts of harmful environmental influences (stresses).
3. Improve the final product:
    Addition of antioxidants to diets produce grades of meat in which the fat does not rancidify or does so more slowly. The use of additives such as enzymes also makes end products more homogenous and of better quality.
4. Economise the cost of animal protein:
    Low levels of additives, mainly of antibiotics or other growth promoters and related compounds in animal feed contribute to increased production of animal proteins for human consumption. Feeding antibiotics and other additives lower the cost of meat, milk and egg production.

Doubtful or Negative Aspects of Feeding Additives

Objections have been raised over the use of hormones and antibiotics which leave their residues in meat, milk and eggs. There is some concern that feeding of low concentration of antibiotics may favour the proliferation of antibiotic-resistant microorganisms, which could have serious consequences for disease control in humans or domestic animals. Continued monitoring of bacterial resistance in humans and animals has not provided clear-cut evidence to this concern.

It is difficult probably to envisage and develop intensive animal breeding without antibiotic feed additives. As animal concentrations increase in intensive farms, the use of antibiotic feed additives become even more indispensable.

1. Antibiotic Feed Additives: Antibiotics are a group of soluble organic substances produced from microorganisms, which in small concentration have the capacity of inhibiting the growth of other microorganisms and even of destroying them. The quantity of antibiotics to be added as an additive is much less than that used for therapeutic purpose.

Factors such as age of the animal, kind of production, nutritional status of the animal, level of hygiene in the farm, stress of the animals, etc. are to be considered before deciding the quantity.

Antibiotic feed additives are of two types: Ionophore antibiotics and non-ionophore antibiotics.

a) Non-ionophore antibiotics: e.g., chlortetracycline, oxytetracycline, zinc bacitracin, virginiamycin, flavomycin, bambermycin, avoparcin, tylosin, etc.

Mode of action: The antibiotics are drugs, not nutrients. Mode of action appears to be complex.

1.   A metabolic effect has been suggested in which the drug affects various enzyme systems such as some oxidative phosphorylation reactions. Intestinal alkaline phosphatase activity is high in germ-free animals, intermediate in specific pathogen free (SPF) animals, and lowest in conventional animals. Addition of certain additives (e.g. Bacitracin) to the diet increased intestinal alkaline phosphatase level. This enzyme is considered to be required in the transport of nutrients across the intestinal wall. It is probable that a decrease in bacterial load or specific interference with bacterial metabolism might have resulted in an increase of intestinal alkaline phosphatase with subsequent beneficial effects on nutrient absorption and improved animal performance.

2.   Some researchers suggested a nutrient-sparing effect which may be a result of

a) Stimulation of microorganisms in the gastrointestinal tract which favour nutrient synthesis. e.g. vitamins, amino acids.

b) Suppression of organisms which compete for critical nutrients (by their antimicrobial action).

c) Reduction in intestinal bacterial load may assist in a reduction of cellular proliferation in the intestinal wall. This leads to gut thinning. Improved nutrient absorption from the gastrointestinal tract as a result of thinner, healthier intestinal walls seen in antibiotic-fed animals. Intestines of young animals which have received antimicrobials appear especially healthy when examined under the microscope. These desirable features include undamaged finger-like villi projections and the absence of inflammatory cells or microcolonies of enterococci. Thinning of intestinal wall may reduce the metabolic energy cost of this most active tissue.

d) Antibiotics decrease the vitamin D requirements for normal bone calcification and lower manganese requirements for growth and prevention of perosis.

3. Inhibition of toxin-producing bacteria:
Antibiotics control the multiplication of toxin producing microorganisms. e.g., Antibiotics depress bacterial urease production leading to lower level of ammonia in the blood circulation. Ammonia toxicity increases the rate of destruction of mucosal cells resulting in increased thickening of intestinal walls and mucosal cell turnover. Prevention of this cellular loss could explain part of the growth response of antibiotic-fed animals.

4. "Disease level" theory:
Antibiotics suppress the subclinical level of infection (Bacterial load in the intestine is reduced) and increases feed efficiency and promotes growth. Growth promoting antibiotics cause lysis of gram-positive bacteria, while they produce discrete lesions in the cell walls of gram-negative species thereby weakening their cell wall.

Effect of feeding antibiotics: Both the ionophore and non-ionophore antibiotics have been used in nonruminants and preruminants, while only the ionophores have been successfully used in adult ruminants.

1. Ruminants

* Reduce incidence of diarrhoea in young calves.
* Check the subclinical infections and improves growth rate and feed efficiency. Most of the growth improvement occurs before the calves

are 8-10 weeks of age and beyond that age no beneficial effect has been reported.
* Reduce the incidence of liver abscesses in beef cattle fed high grain rations.

In India, inclusion of antibiotic feed additives in adult ruminant diets is not a common practice. It may be due to lack of sufficient feed resources and poor patronage for beef production. However, ionophores may be added to dietary regimen in organised male buffalo calf and lamb rearing programme to increase their production efficiency (See p. 347).

2. Swine: Growing-finishing Pigs

* Good effect is observed with animals given all vegetable protein diets than those receiving animal protein supplements.
* Increase in growth rate may vary between 10-20% and decrease in feed intake by about 2-5% depending upon degree of hygiene under which the pigs are reared. Higher the nutritive value of ration, the less would be the improvement in growth rate on antibiotic feeding. Feed efficiency is improved to the extent of 5-8%.
* The greatest beneficial effect is observed during the early growth period between weaning and 50 kg body weight. But antibiotic feeding has to be continued till the pigs reach the market weight. Runty pigs give better response.
* A mixture of two or more antibiotics is no more effective than the single effective antibiotic.
* The optimum level of most antibiotics lie within the range 1 to 50 mg/ kg. e.g., oxytetracycline, chlortetracycline, furazolidine, virginiamycin, avoparcin, bacitracin, flavomycin, avilamycin, tylosin, etc.

Sows: The benefits of antibiotic feeding in sows are shortened weaning to mating interval, increased litter size, improved quality of milk from lactating sows and increased weaning weight of 1 kg per piglet. Feeding of 40 mg of virginiamycin per kg feed to young gilts (sows) at their second oestrus showed improvement in their weight at first farrowing (4%), second farrowing (9%) and third farrowing (14%). It was also observed that weight losses in lactation were less.

Milk fat content is increased; total milk solids also increased with 50% increase being in the milk protein. Such changes in the sows' milk could be attributed to an effect of the feed additive on microbial activity in the animal's intestines, one result of which is an increased availability of amino acids for the sow. Most probably, less glucose was fermented by the gut flora in the small intestine. So more remained available for absorption and use as energy. Any unabsorbed glucose would pass into the large intestine where its fermentation yield volatile fatty acids that could enter the blood stream and be used by energy system.

3. Poultry

Antimicrobial feed additives are included in diets for the prevention and control of coccidiosis, etc. and to improve growth, efficiency of feed utilization and livability. As more low nutrient density ingredients are fed to contain costs, antibiotics can increase nutrient utilization, especially with several ingredients which are lower in digestibility. Direct-fed antimicrobials supplemented continuously at low levels can be beneficial for maintaining intestinal health. These are included in diets at relatively low concentrations (1 to 50 mg/kg), depending on the age and stage of development of poultry. Egg production is also frequently improved by dietary supplementation with antimicrobial agents. Antimicrobials do not stimulate growth of chicks kept in a germfree environment.

b. Ionophore Antibiotics

These are produced by several strains of streptomyces spp. e.g., monensin, lasalocid, salinomycin, lysocellin. The most studied single group of antimicrobial compounds used in animal feeds are the ionophores. These are small molecular weight molecules that bind ions of various minerals and modulate their movement across cell membranes.

All ionophore antibiotics possess the ability to facilitate the passage of inorganic cations like sodium, potassium and calcium across membranes by their capacity to form hydrophobic complexes with such ions. They are mainly active against Gram-positive organisms since the outer membranes of Gram-negative bacteria are relatively impermeable to hydrophobic complex of the molecular size of ionophores. Thus ionophores act by disrupting normal membrane physiology.

Monensin (Tradename: Rumensin):   Polyether ionophore antibiotic, it is produced by a strain of *Streptomyces cinnamonesis*. It is useful as an anticoccidial agent for broilers and lambs. It is also used in beef cattle rations. It is approved for feed efficiency but not for growth promotion in cattle.

Dose: 50 to 100 mg/head/day mixed in a minimum of 450 g of feed is the dose of monensin sodium to heifers above 182 kg body weight. It may be increased to 200 mg after 5 days. Survey of other findings revealed that monensin supplementation (25-33 mg/kg feed) gave 5.2% greater average daily gain, 4.03% less consumption and 8.7% better feed conversion ratio.

Effect of Monensin on Body Composition of Goats

Comparative slaughter data revealed a trend of higher protein in monensin-fed goats compared with controls (o vs 23 mg/kg dry matter). Magnitude of improvement tended to be greater with low, than high dietary protein treatments (8.3 vs 17.5% crude protein) suggesting a protein-sparing effect of monensin.

Effect of Ionophores on Rumen Fermentation

1. Increase the rumen propionate and decrease the acetate concentration and decrease the acetate: propionate ratio. 2. Decrease methane production. Monensin achieves this by affecting electrolyte transport across the cell walls of methanogenic and other bacteria while not disturbing propionate-producing bacteria. In this way more energy is conserved as propionate. 3. Ionophores depress the activity of some rumen enzymes like proteases, deaminases and urease which leads to improved efficiency of dietary protein utilization. 4. Monensin and lasalocid inhibit biohydrogenation resulting in the release of unsaturated fatty acids from the rumen which are deposited in the body tissues. 5. Lower calcium and potassium concentrations. 6. Decrease passage rate and this is associated with an increased amount of organic matter fermented in the rumen. This effect of rumen fermentation modification should increase the ME value per unit of feed intake. When ionophores which do not result in reduced feed intake are used, the effective ME value of the diet may be increased by approximately 10%.

Some of the changes in fermentation can be explained by the selective antimicrobial activities of the ionophores. Both monensin and lasalocid inhibit the growth of ruminal organisms which produce acetate, butyrate, lactate, formate and hydrogen as major end products. Other organisms such as those that produce succinate and propionate or utilize lactic acid tend to be resistant to the antimicrobial activities of these compounds and would be expected to grow more rapidly in the presence of the ionophore.

The production of increased levels of propionic acid in the rumen is related to improved animal performance. Fermentation changes which result in increased formation of propionate and decreased acetate formation can also be stoichiometrically related to decreased methane production. This is expected to provide more metabolizable energy to the animal. These activities coupled with the protein sparing effects of propionate and the ability of propionate to stimulate body protein synthesis are used to explain much of the growth-promoting activity associated with the use of ionophores.

Lasalocid (Trade name: Bovatec):   It is produced by fungi *Streptomyces lasoliensis* and is more potent than monensin. Lasalocid acts specifically against hydrogen producing bacteria and results in higher propionate production. Mechanism of action of lasalocid is similar to that of monensin.

Dose: 1 mg per kg body weight (or) similar to monensin.

Lysocellin: It is a divalent polyether antibiotic obtained from *Streptomyces cacaoci* Var. asoensis.

Benefits of Growth-promoting Antibiotics in Animal Feeds

* Seven per cent better daily weight gain in pigs across Europe and this means the time to reach slaughter weight is reduced.
* Antibiotic-fed animals have higher feed conversion ratio. A feed conversion saving of 0.14 and a reduction in protein content of the feed by 1.0% has been reported.
* Less quantity of manure with lower nitrogen and phosphorus content is produced.

Absorbable and Nonabsorbable Antibiotics

Antibiotics are absorbable and nonabsorbable depending on their absorption into the bloodstream. Tetracyclins, oxytetracyclins and chlortetracyclins are absorbable antibiotics. The concentration of tetracyclins (absorbable antibiotics) in the blood serum of poultry can be increased or "potentiated" by reducing the percentage of calcium in the ration and by substituting calcium sulfate and a soluble sodium phosphate for the commonly used calcium carbonate and calcium phosphate. "Potentiation" increases the concentration of an antibiotic in the blood and tissues of animals by adjusting the composition of the ration. More effective potentiation can be obtained through the use of certain sequestrants or chelating agents. Terephthalic acid in the feed increase the blood level of these antibiotics. But the commercial use has not been approved by the FDA.

Nonabsorbable antibiotics are zinc bacitracin, avoparcin, monensin, virginiamycin, halquinol. The growth-promoting effects of these antibiotics are primarily due to their beneficial effects on the microflora of the intestinal tract. These are **gut active agents**.

Examples of Commercial Preparations

1. TM-100 Feed Supplement (FS), Pfizer; Oxytetracycline
2. Aurofac 2A
   Aurofac 20   FS, Cyanamid; Chlortetracycline
3. Avotan 20, Feed Additive; Avoparcin
4. Bacitz FS; Zinc bacitracin

5. Flavomycin 40 Premix, Hoechst; Flavophospholipol
6. Stafac 20 FS, Pfizer; Virginiamycin
7. 3-care, Halquinol

Ban on the Antibiotic Growth Promoters

The worry is that as humans consume meat from animals that were fed antibiotics, these medications might enter the human body and build up a residue that will create intolerance to medication. Since the types of antibiotics given to agricultural animals are the same type as given to humans, some believe that bacteria may develop strains that are resistant to the medications, which would make the medications ineffective when needed by humans.

As a result of the "Swann Commission" in 1972 the use of tetracylins as well as penicillins was banned in Europe as feed additives. The fluroquinolones are found in milk when they were used in cows. The European Union has banned antibiotics used in human medicine from being added to animal feed to combat anti-microbial resistance. Consequently the WHO called for a ban on the practice of giving healthy animals antibiotics as growth promoters.

As per the European Union regulations (followed from September 1999) only monensin (monensin sodium), salinomycin (salinomycin sodium), bambermycin/flavomycin (flavophospholipol) and avilamycin are the 'final four' feed grade pharmaceutical antibiotics remaining on the approved list. The EU Agriculture Council and Parliament prohibited the use of these four substances in animal feed in July 2003 and came into effect from January 2006.

The Effects of these in-feed Antibiotics

Antibiotic growth promoters suppress the 'bad bugs' and allow the 'good bugs' which are essential to efficient digestion of feed, that is they work by modulating the gut flora.
* In the gut the 'bad bugs' compete with 'good bugs', reducing the conversion of feed into elements which can be absorbed through the gut wall.
* Bad bugs colonise the gut wall causing it to thicken as it fights the invasion. This reduces the food absorption.
* Bad bugs produce toxins which inflame the gut. This increases peristalsis leading to diarrhoea. In poultry, diarrhoea leads to 'wet litter' syndrome causing leg problems and breast blisters while in all species kept in sheds, the production of excess ammonia can lead to respiratory disease.

Potential Consequences of a Ban on Growth-promoting Antibiotics

* Seven to 10% more pig feeds are needed for the same output of meat because of poorer feed conversion. This leads to higher feed costs and thus higher cost of animal products.
* Higher doses of therapeutic antibiotics are needed to combat infectious diseases especially enteric diseases.
* Excretion of nitrogen, phosphorus and methane are increased and much more manure is produced all of which contribute environmental pollution.

It would be an environmental crime to ban the antimicrobial feed additives. Livestock industry, especially pigs and poultry, would become uncompetitive without the growth promoting benefits of antimicrobial feed additives.

Sulfa Drugs

During earlier days 5% flowers of sulfur was added to the feed to control coccidiosis in poultry. The SiO_2 formed in the intestinal tract was very destructive to the intestinal walls and fat soluble vitamins.

Then sulfa drugs were introduced. Sulfa drugs are also destructive to desirable intestinal flora which synthesize vitamins and decompose nondigested nutrients. Sulfanilamide reduces the synthesis of folic acid and cause anaemia in chicks.

Arsenicals

1. 3-nitro-4-hydroxy phenylarsonic acid (3-nitro)
2. P-amino phenylarsonic acid (arsanilic acid)

Arsenicals improve growth of broilers and such birds have bright red combs and wattles. Capillaries are enlarged and engorged through the dilator effect of arsenic. The amount of arsenic retained within the tissue is quite low, about the same as what is naturally found in some seafoods. Arsenicals must be removed from the feed 5 days before slaughter during which time practically all the chemical is excreted. Arsanilic acid is less toxic than 3-Nitro. Accumulation of arsenic in eggs and tissues is proportional to the amount in the ration and well below the allowable levels. Arsanilic acid is tolerated up to 0.1% in the diet of chicks and up to 0.02% in the diet of turkeys. Arsenicals should not be included in the rations for ducks and geese.

Examples of commercial preparations:

1. Nutrivet Feed supplement, Agvet, 3-nitro-4-hydroxy phenylarsonic acid 5%. (Dosage 1kg/ton poultry feed)

2. Roxarson Feed supplement, Merind, 3-nitro-4-hydroxy phenylarsonic acid. Dosage 50 g/ton poultry feed.

Copper supplements: These are routinely added to pig grower diets as growth promoters. Copper is believed to be an effective growth promotant with a mode of action at the intestinal level due to its bactericidal properties. A study in growing pigs revealed that a combination of copper sulfate and betaine resulted in an improvement of 15% in feed efficiency compared to a control diet containing betaine only.

Antibiotics, copper sulfate and 3-nitro-4-hydroxyphenylarsonic acid caused growth stimulation in swine (8-13%) and all inhibited *in vitro* deaminases of the intestinal microorganisms. Copper level, 250 mg/kg diet produces soft fat. In EU countries, level is limited to a maximum of 35 mg/kg. This soft fat is due to an increase in the ratio of oleic to stearic acid, possibly caused by a stimulation of the desaturase enzymes and also to a change in the structure of the triglycerides. Copper sulphate is added at 0.01% of the diet in fattening pigs to improve rate of gain and feed efficiency between weaning and slaughter. Sheep are particularly susceptible to copper poisoning. It causes partial defaunation in ruminants.

Hormones

The active principles secreted by the endocrine glands into the blood for transportation to target organs and tissues are known as hormones. These are of endogenous origin. These are broadly of two types.

1. Anabolic hormones: e.g. Somatotropin, Thyroxine, Androgens

Somatotropin stimulates growth of endochondrial bones and epiphysis of long bones while in protein metabolism it aids nitrogen retention and overall protein synthesis. Thyroxin also stimulates growth of long bones as well as protein synthesis. Testosterone is a potent androgen and at low dose testosterone increases the epiphyseal diameter, promotes muscle growth by augmenting nitrogen retention.

2. Catabolic hormones: e.g. Oestrogens, Glucocorticoids

Oestrogens inhibit skeletal growth although in ruminants it increases nitrogen retention. Glucocorticoids decrease growth of epiphysis and also aid in degrading protein and amino acids and thereby inhibit protein synthesis in extrahepatic tissues.

Exogenous Hormones and their Effect

Some oestrogenic activity is present in some clovers, soybean, sesbania, etc; some are synthesized chemically. These are exogenous sources of hormones. These are administered orally as feed additives, s/c implants or parenteral injections.

A. Hormones as Carcass Modifiers

In two comparisons of males and females, it was found that ewes were significantly fatter at the same empty body weight. It has been documented that intact males produce less fat and more lean from a given feed than either the females or the castrate males. When comparisons were made between steers and bulls, bulls contained less subcutaneous fat and intermuscular fat than steers.

Anabolic agents enhance nitrogen retention in the body and particularly in the muscle, by way of significantly decreasing blood and urinary urea and urinary nitrogen (i.e., controlling partition of nutrients absorbed) and result in the production of leaner carcasses. Androgens are mainly used in females and castrated males while oestrogens are used in males. Combination of oestrogens and androgens gave higher average daily gain than when a single agent was used. The mode of action of androgens and oestrogens in increasing nitrogen retention and average daily gain is different.

Anabolic Steroids

These are banned in European Union since 1989, because of health problems they might cause. e.g. Oestradiol, Trenbolone acetate (TBA) + Oestradiol, Zeranol (Ralgro) + TBA. Oestradiol—17 β is a natural oestrogen produced by ovaries and testes.

Zeranol: Non-steroid anabolic agent with estrogenic properties. It is a chemical derivative of resorcyclic acid lactone, a product of fermentation. It is a chemical derivative of Fusarium mould toxin produced by *Gibberella zeae*, zeralenone (fermentation estrogenic substance, FES). Zeranol implants (steers and lambs) increase apparent absorption of Ca, P, Mg and Zn. These increases in apparent absorption were accompanied by increased retention of Ca, Mg and Zn.

TBA: It is a synthetic anabolic agent with androgenic properties similar to testosterone in promoting growth rate but with no side effect (aggressive behaviour). TBA interferes with catabolic action of glucocorticoids on muscle protein thereby enhancing the rate of protein synthesis; 82% increase in daily carcass protein.

TBA + estradiol (E2) implant: Daily gain increase of 16% and feed efficiency increase of 13% are observed.

Hormone implants are legal and routinely used in USA.

B. Growth and Feed Efficiency

Implanting of calves not kept for breeding is a sound management programme and is cost effective.

Diethylstilbesterol (DES):   Increase rate of gain and feed efficiency.

Dose: Lambs 2 to 5 mg/day; Steers 10 mg/day. Steers 15 to 30 mg implant. Larger implants (60 to 120 mg) show undesirable side effects. Mammary development in steers and wethers, pelvic changes in cattle, vaginal and rectal prolapse, difficult urination and changes in the organs of the urogenital system.

Many widely used natural foods, including soybeans, contain higher oestrogenic activity than found in animal tissues.

It has been reported that traces of oestrogenic activity remained in meat of cockrels (caponettes)/animals implanted with DES. These traces are harmful. Hence DES has been banned since 1979. This was based on its known carcinogenicity as well as lack of an acceptable analytical method for the compound in meat.

Hexesterol is synthetic oestrogen. Melengesterol is synthetic progesterone.

Zeranol (Ralgro):   Implanted (12 mg pellet) subcutaneously on the backside of the ear. It stimulates pituitary gland to secrete increased amounts of somatotropin growth hormone. It is approved for growth promotion in cattle in an implantable form.

Trenbolone acetate (TBA):   It is very effective growth promoter especially in ruminants. Implanting steers with TBA and oestradiol-17 β made their growth rate comparable to that of bulls but, rather surprisingly, their carcass composition was still essentially that of steer.

Synovex plus: This implant contains 20 mg of oestradiol and 200 mg of TBA which is a 1:10 ratio of the drugs. Implanted steers gained more rapidly and converted more efficiently than unimplanted animals. Re-implanted cattle gained more rapidly than cattle implanted only once and they also tended to convert more efficiently. Implanting did increase the weight of saleable lean beef without increasing trimmable fat.

Synovex-S (Oestradiol benzoate, 20 mg and progesterone, 200 mg)
Synovex-H (Oestradiol benzoate and testosterone propionate)
Revelor-S (Trenbolone acetate and oestradiol)

Synovex-S and somavubove (R) (rbST) (look for greater details later in this section) act in an additive manner to improve growth and protein deposition in young growing steers.

C. Milk Production

Steroid hormones are orally active and they are not species specific. Somatotropin is a polypeptide and therefore not orally active and it is species specific. Hence the little, if any, somatotropin present in animal products get degraded in the gastrointestinal tract and thus has no influence on human health.

Bovine Growth Hormone (BGH)

Growth is under control of certain hormones secreted by the endocrine glands. The hormone which has the most general effect is secreted by the anterior pituitary and is called the growth hormone (GH). In 1954, at the International Symposium on the Hypophyseal Growth Hormone, it was proposed that the hormone be designated as somatotropin. Somatotropin and GH continue to be used interchangeably even to the present day. The secretion of this hormone is enhanced following feeding of protein.

Attributes of Somatotropin

* It stimulates various biosynthetic processes. It influences the biosynthesis of protein in muscle cells directly, and indirectly by supplying amino acids to the sites of biosynthesis as it facilitates the transportation of amino acids and their absorption into the muscle cells.
* The activity of somatotropins is mainfested in increased nitrogen retention in the body.
* It increases the growth of skeletal tissues as well.
* Growth hormone is homeorhetic because it manifests its actions by chronic influence on metabolism and involves partitioning of nutrients for selected processes such as growth, milk production.

Biotechnologically derived Somatotropin: Mass production of human GH (hGH) was started in 1979 using the recombinant DNA technology and this was used for treatment of GH deficiency syndromes in humans in Western Countries and was associated with some complications in contrast to insulin. In 1982, D.E. Bauman, Cornell University, USA reported increased milk production in cows with exogenous injections of bGH. Numerous studies have shown that BGH increases milk yield by 15-40% when administered to lactating dairy cows.

The availability of recombinant somatotropin (rST) and its effective use in both dairy cattle (bST) and growing pigs (pST) has provoked several studies in which the mechanism of action of the hormone has been investigated. These have confirmed the classical action reported in nonruminant species, with the protein mass of all the tissues increasing approximately equally, probably through increases in protein synthesis.

Growth hormone is a more powerful lactogenic stimulant than anabolic agent.

Exogenous Bovine Somatotropin (bST) Injections

A. Milk Production

A greater negative energy balance is often observed in cows during the first few weeks after beginning the administration of bST, but cows gradually increase their feed intake to obtain the required nutrients for body weight gain and increased milk production. BGH to increase milk yield was approved in the US in 1994 e.g. (Posilac from Monsanto company) while Canada, New Zealand, European Union banned its use. Indian Government has cleared the sale of BGH from August 1997, under prescriptions from veterinarians, only for use in buffaloes initially for one year based on the research findings of a 12-month trial conducted at NDRI, Karnal.

Long-term studies (Cornell University; published in 1986) with high-yielding cows treated with daily subcutaneous administration of bST (12-50 mg) prepared from the pituitary gland of cows or by DNA technology, gave increases in the milk yield in the range of 22 to 41%; milk composition showed little or no effect, and feed conversion was increased by 12-14%. However, at the higher levels of bST administration certain difficulties were encountered in subsequent reproductive performance. The increases in the milk yield were associated with increases in feed intake.

A continuous two-lactation study (published in 1993) with Friesian cows in their first lactation using a daily injection of 20.6 mg DNA-derived bST in the two lactations: The duration of the experiment was from 2 weeks postcalving to 42 weeks postcalving in one treatment and 2nd treatment starts from 10 weeks postcalving to 42 weeks postcalving and the 3rd treatment was control (without bST injection). The mean milk yields for each lactation were increased significantly by 17.8 to 18.7% and 13.5 to 16.2% for the cows under 1st and 2nd treatment, respectively. Although higher milk yields were recorded with administration of bST from week 2 of lactation, it was associated with some impairment of reproduction.

Production performance of dairy cattle (n=598) administered recombinantly derived bST (Somavubove)® daily from about 75 day postpartum until lactation end was studied. The results of the study (published in 1994) show that dosing of 4.3 to 13.2 mg/d enhanced the milk yield. Cows given 12.9 mg and above had reduced pregnancy and conception rates. Cows given bST should be managed well to meet the demands of their higher milk production level.

The availability of a slow-release device of bST has eliminated the necessity for daily injection. Lactating dairy cows injected 640 mg bST at 28 day intervals for a period of 112 days gave 11.8 to 15.2% higher milk yield over control animals.

B. Meat Production

Treatment of growing ruminants with exogenous GH increases nitrogen retention which is associated with an increase in the proportion of protein to fat and an increase in the fractional synthetic rate of muscle tissues. But this effect is mediated by age: adult animals being unaffected by exogenous GH or the duration of administration of GH. This is in agreement with the concept that there is a substantial influence of the developmental age on protein turnover and growth.

1. In beef cattle steroid implants and somatotropin produced additive increases in performance of finishing steers. Implanting estradiol benzoate + progesterone and trenbolone acetate increased gain and feed efficiency as did bST (80 or 160 mg/wk). Indicators of carcass fat decreased linearly with bST.

In growing lambs chronic administration of rST for 12 weeks led to a 3 kg increase in body weight which represented a 20% increase in rate of daily gain.

Importance of Conductive Environment

Heat stress reduces DM intake and milk yield and increases maintenance cost of the cow. Further, reproductive efficiency is also decreased. Hot or hot humid environmental conditions cause heat stress in dairy cattle. Although effects are more severe in hot climates, dairy cattle in areas with relatively moderate climates also are exposed to periods of heat stress. The high yielding cow has greater metabolic activity and produce more body heat than those with lower yields; thus greater milk yield may increase heat stress if the cause of that stress is not mitigated.

Decreased DM intake may help to maintain normal body temperature through reduced metabolic heat production. Use of bST increased milk yield and naturally such cows are subjected to heat stress as are other high-yielding cows if sufficient metabolic heat is not dissipated. Better housing environment in terms of cooling through shade, ventilation, spray of water and fans (if cost-effective) and strategies that improve DM intake are necessary to sustain the milk yield potential offered by bST administration.

Impact on Human and Animal Health

Extensive trials extending over several lactations have not revealed any adverse effects attributable to somatotropin administration. Indeed the cows previously subjected to long-term treatment with somatotropin are less likely to develop metabolic disorders associated with lipid mobilization after calving. However, recent reports showed fertility problems in multiparous cows.

Levels of somatotropin in milk produced by treated cows are exceedingly low and constitute no threat to the human consumer. Intact proteins which survive protease activity in the stomach and small intestine are not normally absorbed. Even if small amount of somatotropin were to be absorbed, species specificity would ensure that the absorbed hormone would not influence growth.

The availability of slow-release preparation of somatotropin has eliminated the need for daily injections.

Porcine Somatotropin (pST): Increase protein deposition and decrease lipid deposition; improve nitrogen retention; increase amino acid deposition. It alters the response of tissues to homeostatic signals and directs nutrients away from lipid deposition and towards muscle growth. Daily injections (3 mg) of PST improved growth performance and carcass characteristics of genetically lean or obese barrows and gilts, but the influence of genotype or gender was not expunged. A sustained release PST implant may also be used. Pigs treated with PST have less fat and more muscle.

Equine Somatotropin (eST)

The beneficial effects of eST in aged mares (n=7) in terms of body condition and enhanced immunocompetence compared with control mares (n=8) has been studied. The results of the trial of eST at a dose of 12 mg/d for 89 days showed lack of improvement in aerobic or exercise capacity of treated horses. This should dispel some of the concerns about eST having potentially powerful ergogenic effects in horses.

Studies in humans and animals have indicated that somatotropin has positive effects on bone density, immune function, wound healing and soft tissue repair. Since eST has been available for clinical trials, there has been much concern about its unauthorized use to increase growth rates of young horses and perhaps performance of racehorses.

Thyroprotein and Goitrogens

Thyroid-active materials are used to stimulate growth of body tissue and wool and milk secretion by creating mild hyperthyroidal state.

Thyroprotein (Iodinated casein): Thyroprotein has been available commercially since 1945 and is obtained by the iodination of casein. It increases the growth rate of pig and calves under some conditions. In dairy cows, feeding thyroprotein usually increases milk yields by 10-25% after they passed the peak milk production if concomitant increase in energy intake is maintained. The fat percent is also increased. But there is a sudden fall in production once it is discontinued.

Thyroprotein feeding is prohibited by the Purebred Cattle Association of USA. NRC has concluded that it is not advantageous to feed thyroprotein to dairy cows. In Britain it is used only for experimental purposes.

Dose: 15 mg/day in case of thyroprotein and 100 mg/d for thyroxin.

The following precautions should be observed while feeding thyroprotein.
1.   Should not be fed during the first 50-60 days of lactation.
2.   Should not be fed for more than 90 days.
3.   Should not be fed in hot weather as it increases rate of respiration and heart beat.
4.   When cows are fed thyroprotein 25% more TDN should be added. Otherwise they loose weight and run down in condition.
5.   While discontinuing thyroprotein feeding it should not be withdrawn abruptly from rations but gradually.

Goitrogens: These are antithyroid principles which depress the activity of thyroid gland and depress growth and often increase the rate of fattening. e.g. Thiourea and thiouracil fed to pigs and lambs at 2 mg/kg, BW. In poultry, thiouracil in combination with diethyl stilbesterol improves finish and market quality without depressing growth rate.

Thyroid-regulating substances seem to the have little practical importance in livestock feeding.

Phenethanolamine Repartitioning Agents: Phenethanolamines are often referred to as leanness-enhancing repartitioning agents because of their ability to redirect nutrients away from adipose tissue and toward muscle. In general, the effects of phenethanolamines are increased rate of weight gain, improved feed utilization efficiency, increased leanness, and increased dressing percentage. Several factors including dietary protein, age and weight of the animal and duration of treatment have been shown to influence the response to phenethanolamines. Higher dietary protein, older and heavier finishing stage have greater response.

The compounds most commonly studied are classified based on β-adrenergic receptor selectivity. These are β_1-selective phenethanolamines (e.g. ractopamine) and β_2-selective phenethanolamines (clenebuterol, cimaterol and L-644 and 969).

β-adrenergic Agonists (β-agonists)

These are structural analogues of the naturally occurring catecholamines, adrenaline (epinephrine) and noradrenaline. These are orally active. These are used to enhance the lean content and reduce the fat content of animals. Thus they increase feed efficiency and growth promotion.

Beta agonists react with special cell receptors and increase concentration of cyclic AMP which in turn results in reduced lipogenesis and increased lipolysis.

e.g. Clenbuterol, Cimaterol, Ractopamine, L-644, 969

Clenbuterol: It encourages lipolysis and these fatty acids in farm animals are reported to be utilized for protein synthesis. In lambs clenbuterol (2 mg/kg) increased live weight gain and protein content of the hind quarter with a corresponding reduction in fat content. In cattle clenbuterol (10 mg/day) had no effect on growth rate but affected carcass composition in a similar way, as in sheep. It has an effect on immune function in ewe lambs. It may inhibit humoral antibody response to infection.

Clenbuterol is also fed to pigs to prevent them from accumulating fat. It is banned as an additive in China because its residues are noticed in the flesh of pigs and is poisonous to humans if ingested.

Cimaterol: Dose: 4 mg/day in cattle. It markedly stimulate skeletal muscle hypertrophy in mammals. It did not affect dry matter intake (DMI), but improved feed efficiency (FE) and average daily gain (ADG).

Ractopamine: Elanco Animal Health, USA has come out with 'Paylean' brand of ractopamine as ractopamine hydrochloride. This is approved by USDA/FDA for use to increase weight gain, feed efficiency and carcass leanness in finishing pigs from 68 kg to 108 kg. It requires no withdrawal period. Formerly a repartitioning agent, now it is termed as 'leanness enhancer'.

Ractopamine (Paylean): Inclusion of this at 5 ppm rate in the last month of finishing is used as a management tool to increase growth rate and to obtain higher slaughter weight. Ractopamine stimulates the so-called beta-receptors in the body responsible for apportioning nutrients into lean and fat tissue. It repartitions nutrients away from the normal accumulation of fat before marketing and towards more muscle. China banned it.

Immunization Procedures

The anabolic steroids, although highly effective in enhancing lean tissue growth, failed to achieve public and political acceptance within the European Community. This fostered research into the more subtle technique of immunization, which utilizes the animal's immune response to alter endocrine pathways that control body growth and lean tissue deposition. So immunization procedures are an attempt to arrive at more acceptable approaches to controlling lean tissue deposition than hormone implants and injections or orally active β-agonists.

Somatostatin immunization: Somatostatin is a growth hormone-inhibiting peptide. The inhibition or neutralization (active immunization) of somatostatin has been considered as an approach to stimulate growth rate nowadays.

Adipocyte immunization: The existing normal physiological relationship between adipose tissue, muscle and the immune system may provide opportunities to the control of lean tissue deposition. Flint and his coworkers at Hannah Research Institute have carried out experiments on reducing carcass fat and enhancing lean tissue deposition in sheep and pigs by passive immunization with antibodies to their adipocyte plasma membranes.

Growth Hormone stimulation: Growth hormone-releasing factor (GHRF) is the main endogenous stimulator of somatotropin secretion. Hence as an alternative to direct administration of growth hormone (GH), stimulation of endogenous GH secretion, using GHRF is also highly effective in increasing lean and reducing fat of animals.

Within the general theme of enhancing the GH response, it is now thought that binding proteins for GH and the insulin-like growth factors (IGFs) attenuate the expression of the GH response and this had led to speculation that immunomodulation of the binding proteins may enhance the anabolic action of GH.

It has been demonstrated that monoclonal antibodies to GH potentiate the activity of endogenous GH. This opens up possibilities for the synthesis of specific peptides which simulate the GH epitopes that bind the monoclonal antibody. These could then be used to enhance the activity of endogenous GH via active immunization (Buttery, 1993). Antibodies to hormone antibodies, otherwise known as antiidiotypic antibodies, also hold promise in that their production for GH and other growth promoters, such as β-agonists, shows that they can mimic the GH effect. Their ability to target specific elements of the GH response and their protracted half life make them a much more attractive proposition for practical application than GH itself.

Immunomodulators: These are compounds obtained from organisms or synthesized chemically which are capable of enhancing the defence mechanism of animals, including fish and shrimps. The use of the immune response potentially has a lot to offer the animal production industry as a method of growth promotion and manipulation of carcass composition.

These are classified as:

1. Natural immunomodulators
2. Synthetic immunomodulators

Potent immunomodulators: Cell wall preparations, Vitamin C, Vitamin E, Levamisole, quaternary ammonium compounds (QAC).

1. They act as a barrier to infection against specific and non-specific pathogens.
2. They enhance the microbe killing activity of the macrophage, lymphocytes and natural killer cells.
3. Some activate the complement system also and enhance the phagocytosis of the cells, resulting in the development of the resistance and protection from various infections.

Glucans are one of the most important structural elements of fungal cell walls, *Saccharomyces cerevisiae*. Macrogard is the commercial name of one of the glucans marketed by a Norwegian company. Selenium along with vitamin E develop resistance against disease. Chitin is an immunomodulator. It is a polysaccharide obtained from crustacean shells, insect exoskeletons and cell walls of certain fungi.

Saccharomyces cerevisiae yeast cell wall (YCW)

Yeast cell wall is composed of complex polymers of β-(1-3/(1,6) glucan, mannan-oligosaccharide (MOS) and chitin. As shown in Figure 1, MOS is located on the surface of the cell wall. Yeast glucans are major cell wall components often present as the inner wall layer and associated with other cell wall components such as chitin.

Typically commercial YCW are composed of 30 to 60% polysaccharides (15 to 30% of β-1, 3/1, 6-glucan and 15 to 30% of mannan sugar polymer), 15 to 30% proteins, 5 to 20% lipids, and no more than 5% of chitin. Most of the protein is linked to the mannan oligosaccharides (MOS) and is referred to as the mannoprotein complex. The β-1, 3/1, 6-glucans present in YCW should be recognized as an immune modulator substance in animals and humans.

MOS is able to play important roles in binding mycotoxins and improving the micro-environment of the animal digestive tract. See page nos 375 and 384.

Growth Promoters for Fattening Ruminants

There is a considerable interest for the use of growth promoters to improve animal production efficiency which can be achieved in two main ways.

o

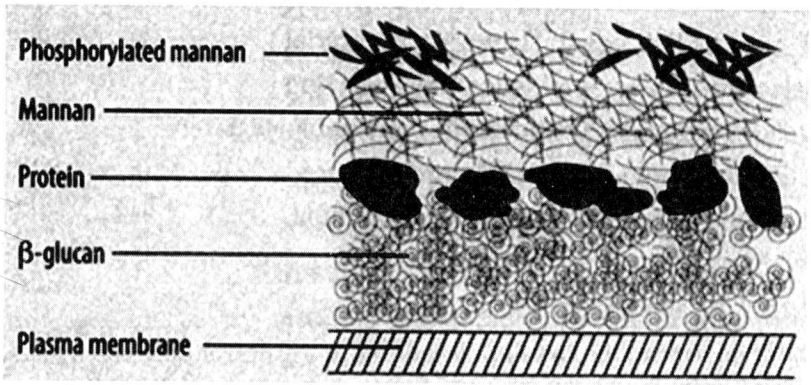

Figure 1 Structure of Yeast cell wall
(Source: AllAboutFeed, Yeast Special, March 2013, page 18)

1. Altering ruminal digestion with ionophore antibiotics (monensin (Rumensin), lasalocid (Bovatec), narasin, salinomycin) or nonionophore antibiotics (avoparcin; it is banned since Dec. 1996 in EU, Flavomycin/bambermycin and avilamycin) may favourably modify the quantity and quality of nutrients entering the body. In the EU, the recommended doses for fattening cattle are 20-60 mg/kg feed (optimum 30) for monensin.

2. It is possible to manipulate metabolic processes and utilization of absorbed nutrients with hormonal anabolic agents. The major anabolic agents used are testosterone (androgen produced in the testes), trenbolone acetate (TBA, synthetic androgen) and oestradial-17 *b* (oestrogen produced by ovaries and testes). Zeranol (Ralgro) is a non-steroid-anabolic agent with oestrogen-like activity produced by *Gibberella zeae*. Androgens are mainly used in females and wethers and oestrogens in males. In the EU, these products are forbidden since January 1989, because of health problems they might cause. Most common doses were 20 mg E-17 *b* + 140 mg TBA in veal calves, steers and bulls, and 180 or 300 mg TBA in heifers.

Ionophores improve average daily gain and feed conversion efficiency of growing kids by 10 percentage units. Ionophores suppress coccidiosis. Ionophores and nonionophore antibiotics induce modifications of rumen fermentation, increasing propionate/acetate ratio. Review of literature on partitioning of absorbed nutrients with anabolic steroids and consequences on growth performance showed average increase in daily gain by 13%, but results are very heterogeneous.

Coccidiostats: Amprolium, clopidol, lasalocid sodium, monensin sodium, salinomycin, robenidine, maduramicin, 3,5-dinitro-o-tolumide (DOT), diclazuril, narasin.

Use of Hormones in Animal Production and Food Safety

Phytoestrogens

Phytoestrogens are a diverse group of naturally occurring non-steroidal plant compounds. Soya proteins contain phytoestrogens and the phytoestrogens have been shown to help prevent heart disease and slow osteoporosis, just as oestrogen replacement therapy does, but apparently without increasing the risk of breast or uterine cancer. Researchers see no harm in suggesting that menopausal women include Soya in their diets to reduce the discomfort of menopause due to hot flushes, night sweats, etc.

Phytoestrogens of soya are isoflavones. The isoflavone genistein is similar to the body's natural estrogen but is much less potent in its effects. Many edible plants contain phytoestrogens and current research focusses on a group of compounds belonging to the isoflavone class, concentrations of which are particularly high in the soybean.

A number of epidemiological studies have found that people living in countries where the diet includes a lot of soybean products, such as Japan and China, tend to have less breast cancer, osteoporosis and cardiovascular disease. There have even been some animal studies which suggest that exposure to phytoestrogens early in life may help prevent cancer in adulthood.

The phytoestrogens are far weaker than oestrogens made by the human body. Soybean-based infant formulas can contain such large amounts of phytoestrogens and these have been on the market for 30 years in Western countries and so far they have not been linked to any health problems. To determine how much of these phytoestrogens were actually getting into the bloodstream, blood samples have been collected from three groups of healthy four-month old boys.

Group	Blood levels (ng/ml) of biologically active phytoestrogens	
	Genistein	Diadzein
Infants on cow's milk	3.2	2.1
Infants on human breast milk	2.8	1.4
Infants on soya-based formula	684	295

Hormone use in Animal Production

Several hormone implants *viz* oestradiol, zeranol, trenbolone and testosterone are used for economic animal production. Use of hormones in animal production has drawn much attention over the years, particularly in the European Union (EU) where anabolic steroids and growth hormone use has long been banned and it has also banned meat imported from countries, such as the United States (US), where growth hormone is used to achieve improved efficiency and leaner carcasses.

The data given in Tables 1, 2 and 3 from the Hormone Working Party of the Animal Health Register, London help put hormone safety into perspective. The US estimates that the EU ban on US beef costs the beef industry at least $ 100 million per year. It has gone to the World Trade Organization (WTO) to represent the case of ban and the dispute has been solved by labelling the product with the country of origin (i.e., "This beef is of US origin"). Doing so would allow US Beef into the EU marketplace and put the decision of which beef to eat back in the hands of EU consumers, where it should be.

TABLE 1. Comparative Estrogen Intakes from Food Sources.

Food	Weight of portion (g)	Estrogen intake (ng)
Unimplanted steer meat[a]	500	6.1
Estradiol-implanted steer meat[a]	500	11.4
Zeranol-implanted steer meat[c]	500	7*
Cow meat [ab]	500	75(7.2-540)*
Hen's egg	50-60	1,750*
Cabbage	100	2,400*
Peas	100	400*
Wheat germ	10	200*
Soybean oil	10 ml	20,000*
Milk	500 ml	75*

ng = nanograms; Steer means castrated bull
a = Assuming 25% fat, 75% muscle
b = Estrone only
c = Muscle tissue only
* = Estradiol equivalents

Many consumers are concerned over the long-range effects of the hormones fed to animals that might be residual in meat, eggs, milk, or other products. However, there is no evidence of any human health problem from the use of any natural or synthetic hormones fed to livestock.

TABLE 2. Comparative Androgen Intakes.

Food	Weight of portion (g)	Androgen intake (ng)
Unimplanted bull meat	500	1, 560
Steer or female implanted with Trenbolone[a]	500	135-150
Heifer implanted with testosterone	500	35

TABLE 3. Natural Production of Hormones in Humans *.

Sector of Production	Estrogen production (ng per 24 hours)	% increase from eating 500 g implan- ted steak	Androgen production (ng per 24 hours)	% increase from eating 500 g implan- ted steak.
Male child (pre-puberty)	41,000	0.0013	65,000	0.005
Adult man	136,000	0.0004	6,500,000	0.00005
Female Child (pre-puberty)	54,000	0.001	32,000	0.01
Non pregnant Woman	540,000	0.0001	320,000	0.001
Pregnant Woman	20,000,000	0.000003	320,000	0.001

Calculation based on the hormonal content of the steaks and availability of this material to be absorbed via the oral route.

* *Source:* The Hormone Working Party of Animal Health Register, The Association of the British Pharmaceutical Industry, London, England.

The data in Tables show the relative amounts of estrogen produced by people and the estrogen in beef from a steer that has been implanted with hormones and one that has not. In fact, a person will obtain thousands of times the amount of estrogen from a gram of soyabean oil than from a gram of beef from an implanted steer.

Feed Enzyme Additives

Maize and soybean meal are the most preferred feeds for poultry, swine, etc. High cost of these ingredients spurred the pursuit of alternate ingredients such as wheat, oats, barley, etc. and sunflower seed meal, rapeseed meal, etc. These alternate feedstuffs have deleterious factors hindering the utilization of nutrients. Feed enzyme additives act as biocatalysts to assist the digestion process and support utilization of nutrients that otherwise go unused.

The predominant non-starch polysaccharides (NSPs) in cereal grains are cellulose, arabinoxylans and mixed-linked betaglucans. Beta glucans are water soluble gel-forming polysaccharides present in the endosperm of barley and other grains of graminae crops. They cause sticky droppings and greater litter moisture; reduced nutrient utilization and growth rate in chicks; lead to dirty eggs. Depending on this the grains such as barley, rye and wheat are grouped under high viscosity grains while maize and sorghum are grouped under low viscosity grains.

The cellulolytic or hemicellulolytic enzymes degrade gel-forming viscous and structural polysaccharides. e.g. Beta glucanase, xylanase, mannanase, pectinase, betagalactosidase, 1-4-β-galactanase.

Feed enzymes such as β-glucanases and xylanases have enabled barley or wheat in poultry diets up to 50 or 60%. A combination of endo-1-4β-galactanase and β-galactosidase could be used to improve the ME of soybean meal. Feed enzyme complexes containing arabinases, xylanases and pectinases (pectin esterase, pectin lyase and polygalacturonase) breakdown the arabinoxylans and pectins present in sunflower seed meal, rapeseed meal, lupin seed meal, etc. and release the protein and other nutrients. This enzyme complex can convert sunflower meal into soybean meal in terms of nutritional value.

A multi-enzyme preparation with cellulolytic and proteolytic activity (cellulases, β-glucanases and protease) can degrade the structural polysaccharides and proteins. Phytase enzyme helps to increase the utilization of phytin phosphorus by swine, poultry, etc. Enzymes which can withstand high temperature (95°C) employed during pelleting are available now. Feed enzyme additives combine both economic and ecological benefits.

Protected Enzymes for Ruminants

Exogenous enzymes such as cellulases and hemicellulases are protected from rumen degradation by attaching a carbohydrate moiety to the protein of the enzyme. Extracellular enzymes produced by certain fungi are protected from the rumen degradation in this manner.

"Fibrozyme", (Alltech) is the first feed-grade enzyme that is rumen stable. It significantly increases dry matter digestibility, VFA production and carbohydrate utilization in cows fed diets containing high amounts of fibre. **Glycosylation process protects the fibrozyme enzyme in the rumen**, and also during pelleting. Feeds containing fibrozyme can be pelleted with only a slight loss in enzyme activity.

Enzymes that assist piglets of 3 weeks age are protease, xylanase, pectinase, hemicellulase.

Commercial Feed Enzymes

1. Avizyme series 1000,1300,2000
   Finfeeds Limited, Avizyme 1500 for corn soy based feeds
2. Natugrain (endo-xylanase, β-glucanase)
   Natuphos (phytase)
   Vevozyme (alpha-amylase) (BASF)
3. Kemzyme, (Kemin Europa)
4. Grindazym (Danisco ingredients)
   Flavodan: Feed flavourings.

Probiotics, Yeast Culture and Acidifiers

Over the last several years considerable attention has been given to the use of probiotics, yeast cultures, and acidifiers in pig, and poultry feeds primarily. Much of this interest has been generated because of increased public awareness and objection to the use of antibiotics as growth promotant feed additives.

Probiotics: Parker coined the term 'probiotic' in 1974 and defined it as "organisms and substances which contribute to intestinal microbial balance". The term probiotic means " for life" and has a contrast with the term antibiotic means "against life". Probiotics are advocated as an alternative to antibiotics for growth promotion. Probiotics are live cultures of non-pathogenic organisms which are administered orally. Later Fuller (1989) redefined probiotics as live microbial feed supplements which beneficially affect the host animal by improving its intestinal microbial balance. Probiotic products are available in the form of oral pastes, water dispersible powders or liquids or directly fed feed additives and include microbial cells, microbial cultures and microbial metabolites. Most probiotics get destroyed by up to 80% in the presence of antibiotics or when mixed with antimycoplasma drugs in the feed.

The term **'pronutrients'** is used in place of probiotics. The US Food and Drug Administration used the term **direct fed microbials** (DFM; p. 378) instead of probiotic and the manufacturers were directed to write DFM on their products (also see p. 376 for prebiotics).

Some firms developed 'thermo-positive process' to formulate microbial cultures and microbial viability is assured in the pelleted feeds. e.g. *'Primalac'* DFM. Some probiotics supply viable bacterial spores of selected Bacillus strain which are heat resistant. The recovery rate of organisms after pelleting is 95%. Microgranulated probiotic is available facilitating reduced dust and improved flowability, homogenous mixing even at very low inclusion levels with improved stability during storage and pelleting e.g. Paciflor Microgranulated.

Microorganisms used as probiotics: Some important are *Lactobacillus acidophillus, L. bifidus, L. bulgaricus, L. casei, L. fermentum, L. lactis, L. plantarum, L. ruminis, L. salivaricus. Bifidobacterium bifidum, Aspergillus oryzae, Torulopsis, Streptococcus faecium, S. thermophilus, Saccharomyces cerevisiae.*

Lactobacillus acidophillus produce lactic acid and the enzyme amylase. *Lactobacillus casei* compliments the growth of *L. acidophilus. Bifidobacterium bifidum* is found commonly in mother's milk and the intestine of humans and animals. *Aspergillus oryzae* produce enzyme cellulase. *Torulopsis* is the mother culture of yeast. The enzyme lipase is exhibited by Torulopsis.

Characteristics of a Good Probiotic

1. The culture should exert a positive effect on the host. It should be gram positive, acid resistant, bile resistant and contain a minimum 30×10^9 CFU (colony forming unit) per gram.
2. The culture should possess high survival rate and multiply faster in the digestive tract. It should be strain specific.
3. The culture microorganisms should neither be pathogenic nor toxic to the host.
4. The adhesive capability of microorganisms must be firm and faster.
5. Be durable enough to withstand the duress of commercial manufacturing, processing and distribution so that the product can be delivered alive to the intestine.

Mode of action may be competitive with the harmful enteric microorganisms, stimulatory for increasing growth rate and thus the productivity and nutrient sparing or the combined effects. e.g. The main metabolites of Lactobacilli are lactic acid and H_2O_2. The former is responsible for preventing the growth of coliform organisms by reducing the pH while the latter has bactericidal effect. Finally, an acid environment is conducive to increased enzymatic activity within the digestive system. Probiotics at the specific concentration stimulate the immune system.

Pigs and Probiotics: Probiotics have shown the greatest potential in very young and growing pigs. Probiotics prevent and control the incidence of diarrhoea in pigs. Feeding probiotics (*L. acidophilus* and *S. faecium*) improved weight gain and feed efficiency. Grower pigs receiving the probiotic in their feed showed either equal or superior daily gain, feed intake and feed efficiency compared to pigs fed the antibiotic.

Sows consuming diets supplemented with probiotic bacteria weaned larger, heavier litters. The probiotic species *Bacillus subtilis* reduce the number of *E. coli* in sows and thus reduce the incidence of *E. coli* scours in piglets.

Poultry and Probiotics: The role of the intestinal microflora in health and digestion of poultry is more extensively understood than in mammalian species. There is a delicate balance between beneficial and pathogenic bacteria. A low pH (4 to 5) favours Lactobacillus sp. and a high pH (6 to 7) is optimal for *E. coli.* It was reported that Lactobacilli can be found in crop epithelial tissue as early as day one of life. The crop of fowl normally contains a microbial population in which Lactobacilli predominate.

These microbes attach to the crop epithelium and colonize the surface. Attached bacteria are able to inoculate newly ingested food. Lactic acid-producing bacteria moving with digesta to the intestine serve to influence that microbial community. The result ensures dominance of lactic acid species for the suppression of *E. coli.*

Shortly after hatching, the chick or poult has a nearly sterile digestive tract with a pH range of between 5.5 and 6.0. In addition, the young bird lacks sufficient gastric acid secretion to maintain the ideal acidic pH. It was reported that the poults were born with high numbers of coliforms. So supplementation of a lactobacillus product in the water or feed along with an acidifying agent would be effective in controlling the coliform proliferation.

In addition to the production of lactic acid, the inhibitory effects of lactobacillus on other bacteria species have been attributed to hydrogen peroxide formation and production of an inhibitory substance termed "acidolin". Lactobacillus probiotic and zinc bacitracin had similar effects in stimulating weight gain and feed efficiency of broilers. The probiotic caused a distinct change in microbial flora of the caeca and small intestine in that by nine days of age, enterococci had essentially disappeared.

Yeast Culture

Yeast culture is known to contain compounds formerly referred to as UGFs which positively affect animal performance. The term **'nutrilite'** coined by Hungate (1966) better describes the unidentified growth factors (UGFs) contained in yeast cultures. Hungate observed that rumen bacterial concentrations increased when fermentation products such as yeast cultures were added to the diet. He concluded that the stimulatory effect was due to metabolites in the fermentation products which served as nutrients for the bacteria. Byproducts of fermentation include dried brewers yeast, dried distillers solubles, dried bacterial press cakes.

Yeast Cultures Vs Yeast Blends

True Yeast cultures composed of the entire culture-the yeast cells capable of fermentation and the media on which they were grown. So when it is dried, the product composed of live yeast and the growth media is rich in nutrilites. Yeast culture products do not contain many live yeast.

Yeast blends are marketed as yeast culture even though these products are only blends of active dry yeast and a diluent. Various diluents such as distillers dried solubles, wheat middlings, hominy feed or rice hulls are frequently used and may be augmented with saccharins, sucrose and traces of mineral salts.

Yeast is a relatively fragile living organism that is easily killed by heat, humidity and rough handling. Hence yeast cells are destroyed by pelletising the feed and storage conditions. Yeast packaged in a vacuum or inert gas has a much greater stability than yeast packaged in air. Significant losses of viable yeast cells can also occur over time for yeast products held at 35°C in paper bags. The rate of deterioration is time and temperature dependent under normal conditions. Yeast cells in products blended with minerals deteriorate more rapidly due to the action of the mineral salts.

Live Yeast Culture as a Feed Additive

The feeding of live yeast culture, *Saccharomyces cerevisiae* has attracted the attention of Animal Nutritionsts to improve the microbiological balance of the host animal and thereby extract the nutrients to the maximum extent and get them deposited in end products (milk, meat and eggs) for human use which simultaneously reduce environmental pollution. Live yeast species are highly probiotic.

Yeast, *Saccharomyces cerevisiae* is not a natural component of the ruminal microbial population. It is important to differentiate between *live cell* yeast *products* and yeast culture *products*. **A live yeast culture** is the living yeast cell and the medium upon which it was grown. *Saccharomyces cerevisiae*, a facultative anaerobe, has been shown to grow well when introduced in the rumen along with the medium upon which it is grown (Dawsen, 1987). More recent papers, however, indicate that live cells of *S. cerevisiae* do not grow in the rumen but show some degree of rumen viability (Dawsen *et al.* 1990) and influence the course of rumen fermentation and the population of microorganisms in the rumen.

There is much evidence to refute yeast growth in the rumen. Rumen temperature of 39°C alone is sufficient to prevent yeast survival in the rumen. Normal rumen pH (6.2 to 6.8) is too high for yeast (4.5 optimal) to survive any length of time in the rumen due to the impairment of the yeast cell wall and ensuing autolysis. In addition, yeast is unable to attach to either the rumen fibre mat or the rumen wall and flow from the rumen as fluid leaves. Yeast cells in the fresh brewers yeast slurry remained metabolically active at 39°C for about six hours.

Data from several studies do indicate the potential for yeast to produce nutrilites before being killed, digested or washed from the rumen. Yeast was used at less than 1% of dry matter in cattle diets in the 1950's and one report says an increase of 1.1 kg milk yield/day with inclusion of 50 g of an active yeast/day.

Examples of commercial preparations

1. YEA-SACC [1026], Alltech; Dose: 1 kg/ton of broiler feed; 400-600 g/ton of layer feed; 2.5-5.0 g/pet animal/day.
2. Lacto-Sacc (Microencapsulated Lactobacillus, Streptococcus, enzymes and yea-sacc [1026]), Vetcare/Alltech, Inc.
3. Nutri-Sacc for dairy cows (contains bypass protein, niacin, selenium and yea-sacc[1026]) Dose : calves 100 g/head/day; cows 200 g/head/day.
    Products with probiotics and other nutrients are used as nonantibiotic growth promoters.
4. Levucell (SC) for ruminants, Levucell (SB) for monogastrics, Lallemand.
    Alltech's Yea-Sacc[1026] has become the only yeast culture to gain EU approval as a performance-enhancing yeast additive for dairy cows, fattening cattle and calves. Alltech developed Yea-Sacc[1026] from a naturally occurring strain, *Saccharomyces cerevisiae* yeast.

Effects of Live Yeast Culture

1. Effect on the animal physiology: Reduces the temperature in heat stressed animals. The greatest benefit occur during the hotter months. Fungal cultures (*Aspergillus orizae, Armillaria heimii, etc.*) (3 to 5 g/d) in the diet decreased body temperatures and respiration rates in hot, but not in cool weather. The mechanism of action exerted by fungal cultures on body temperature and respiration rate is unclear.

2. Effect on the rumen: *Saccharomyces cerevisiae* could act by production of growth stimulating factors in the rumen, stabilisation of rumen pH, and reduction of lactic acid production in the rumen. It increases the bacterial population in the rumen.

	Control (C)	C + yeast culture
Cellulolytic bacteria/ml rumen liquor (RL)	1.82×10^7	3.16×10^7
Total bacteria/ml (RL)	6.41×10^8	13.4×10^8

The probiotic activity might be due to the metabolites (probably some unidentified growth factors) in the yeast culture. The increased population of cellulolytic bacteria and total bacteria increases the rate of forage degradation which eventually enhances feed intake and the supply of microbial protein from the rumen (Fig. 2).

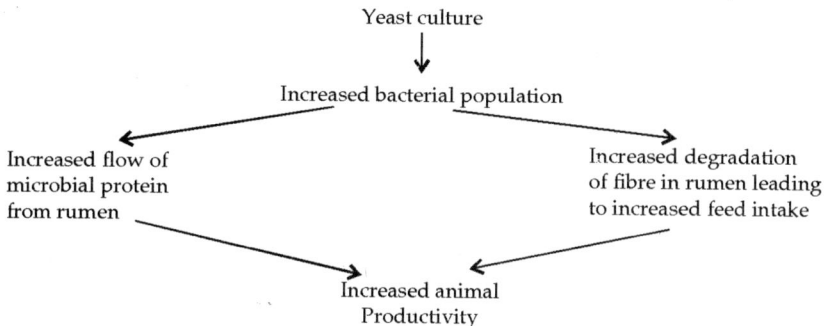

Figure 2. Action of Yeast Culture in Ruminants.

Regarding the possible mechanism of action of live yeast culture in elevating pH of the rumen, it has been suggested that protons (hydrogen ions) may be absorbed by yeast (Williams, 1988). Another possibility could be the removal by yeast of certain non-volatile fatty acids, perhaps even their transformation to VFA with higher PKa values. Removal of simple sugars from the rumen environment as they are actively transported across the yeast cell wall, reduce the negative associate effects of rapidly fermentable carbohydrates.

3. Effect on milk production: The results of several lactation studies revealed that the response ranged from a 6.8% decrease to a 17.4% increase in milk yield, the average response being an increase in the milk yield of 7.8%. Responses are greater in early lactation. Responses increase as the ratio of concentrate to forage in the ration increases. Total butterfat and milk protein production were increased in all the studies (i.e. the protein and energy output in the form of milk was increased). The effect of yeast culture may also be modified by more subtle variations in the diet. Inclusion of yeast in the diet of cows fed a 60% concentrate and 40% straw responded with an 18% increase in milk yield; but this decreased to 14% when the straw was replaced by hay.

Sources of additional nutrients for increased yield and butter fat: The increases in both yield and butterfat on yeast culture diets can only be achieved by an increase in nutrients supplied to the mammary gland. The additional nutrients must be supplied by the diet, since there is no reason to suggest that yeast culture stimulates mobilization of body reserves.

1. The nutrients can be supplied directly by a stimulation of appetite probably due to increased total number of bacteria and especially

cellulolytic bacteria and the consequent increased rate of cellulose digestion and intake of feed.

2. Alternatively, the nutrients can be indirectly produced: By an increase in the metabolizable energy content of the diet through a reduction in methane production or by changes in the composition of the digesta absorbed from the rumen or in that which leaves the rumen, passes into the abomasum and into the duodenum.

Live Yeast Culture for Ruminants

Dr. C.J. Newbold and his coworkers conducted several experiments on the live yeast culture as a feed additive in ruminants to explore its potential as an aid to manipulate the rumen fermentation. The addition of yeast culture to diets containing 40 to 80% oat straw increased *in situ* NDF digestibility in steers. Ruminal molar proportion of acetate was decreased while propionate was increased by yeast addition. Ruminal protozoa numbers were higher in steers fed yeast culture. Buffalo calves fed live yeast culture had lower ruminal concentrations of lactate than control calves up to six hour postfeeding on high concentrate diet. Protozoa numbers were not significantly affected by treatment, but total bacteria and cellulolytic bacteria were higher in ruminal fluid of calves fed yeast culture. *In situ* DM disappearance and ruminal acetate: propionate ratio were increased by yeast culture addition.

White rot fungi decompose lignin or lignocellulose with minimal degradation of hemicellulose and cellulose. Zadrazil (1976) showed that yeasts are always found in cultures of white rot fungi and yeasts can act as secondary microorganisms of lignin and lignocellulosic degradation by utilising the simple metabolic products so formed. The potential synergism between yeast (*S. cerevisiae*) and fungi (*Armillaria heimii*) had the best potential for increasing forage digestibility.

Live Yeast Culture for Horses

Inclusion of Yea-sacc (8 g/head/day) significantly increased neutral detergent fibre, hemicellulose and nitrogen digestibility of diets given to yearling horses. It was concluded that dietary supplementation with yeast culture increased hindgut fermentation, and thus increase the nutritive value of equine feeds resulting in a doubling of the percentage of digested nitrogen that was retained within body tissues.

Plasma amino acid profiles of the foals (10 weeks of age onwards) were significantly altered by yeast culture supplementation (10 g/day) within a week, with several amino acids exhibiting sustained increases. These observations reinforce the link between yeast culture supplementation and increased nitrogen utilization and increased weight gain.

Live Yeast Culture for Swine

Saccharomyces cerevisiae I – 1079 (Levucell SB®) is a specific live yeast strain designed for swine. It has been reported to increase performance and feed efficiency in sows and weaned pigs. Growing pigs fed a lactic acid bacteria plus yeast culture combination (Lacto-sacc; Alltech, Inc.) were heavier at 56 days (4.8 kg) and converted feed 9.6% more efficiently than pigs in the control group. VFA, the end products of bacterial fermentation, could contribute between 0.15 to 0.28 of the maintenance requirement of the pig. It is therefore possible that some of the responses in terms of growth and feed efficiency that have been reported in pigs may be due to effects of yeast culture on hindgut fermentation by a mechanism similar to that occurring in the rumen.

Live Yeast Culture for Poultry

Yeast culture is considered a probiotic by many when that culture supplies live yeast cells. However it is better known for its ability to enhance feed utilization. Hence live yeast culture plus lactic acid-producing bacteria (*L. acidophilus* and *S. faecium*) was supplemented in broilers (1 kg/ton) and the results showed that weight gain and feed conversion were improved. Lacto-sacc (Alltech, Inc) has also been shown effective in diets fed to pullets and layers.

Combined use of lactobacillus and yeast culture in the feed and water has been shown to be effective in reducing morbidity and mortality and improving growth performance and production characteristics.

Mannan Oligosaccharides (MOS)

Now evidence is accumulating that some of the positive effects of yeasts in monogastrics might be associated with the yeast cell wall (see Figure 1).

MOS, a complex carbohydrate extracted from yeast cell wall, improves the health and performance of monogastric animals. MOS blocks attachment of pathogenic bacteria to the animal's intestine and prevents colonisation that can result in disease. In addition, MOS may stimulate the animal's immune system, thereby further reducing the risk of disease. MOS increased the release of cytokines, which coordinate activity among different cells of the immune system. MOS also enhanced interleukin-2 concentration. The immune function requires interleukin-2 for T-cell proliferation and differentiation.

Studies in broilers showed that MOS, (in comparison with antibiotic growth promoters: virginiamycin and bacitracin), conferred intestinal health benefits by improving its morphological development (increased villi height and goblet cell number per villus) and microbial ecology.

Research findings strongly favour dietary supplementation of live yeast culture as a stress reliever during the hot season of the year and of intensive rearing of livestock and as a prebiotic to increase the rate of fibre degradation and thus increase feed intake and eventually animal productivity.

Fructo Oligosaccharides (FOS)

Short chain fructo oligosaccharides encourage the growth of beneficial bacteria in the gut such as Lactobacillus spp., Bifidobacterium spp. and Bacteroides spp. Feeding FOS helps proliferation of these probiotic bacteria which inhibit growth of more harmful bacteria and reduction of flatulence (since FOS are not digested by host intestinal enzymes) in animals. So these (FOS, MOS) are termed as *'prebiotics'*.

Prebiotics in Pet Food

Prebiotics were first defined by Gibson and Roberfroid in 1995. A prebiotic is a non-digestible food ingredient that beneficially affects the host by selectively stimulating the growth and/or activity of one or a limited number of bacteria in the colon and thus improves host health (Gibson et al., 1996). Prebiotics are normally simple sugars, oligosaccharides of between 3 to 6 fructose units in length or may also comprise soluble fibres, with longer monosaccharide chain lengths. Examples of prebiotics which are commonly used in the companion animal feed industry include inulin, MOS, FOS or oligofructose. Prebiotics are substrates for probiotic bacteria such as Bifidobacteria spp.

In companion animals, prebiotics improve gut microbial ecology and enhance stool quality. They are known to improve the efficiency of nitrogen utilization in the intestine resulting in less wastage through ammonia recycling and a more complete digestion of nutrients in the large intestine. This also helps to ward off the production of undesirable odours.

Due to the potential synergy between probiotics and prebiotics, foods containing a combination of these ingredients are often referred to as synbiotics. Intas Pharmaceuticals Ltd., India formulated a comprehensive microfloral rejuvenator: Ecolas Probioc enriched with prebiotic and growth stimulants, a fortified synbiotic.

Silver Nanoparticles as a Potential Antimicrobial Additive Alternative to Antibiotics

Nanoparticles

Most scientific data is reported in terms of metric measurements as mentioned here below. In general, particles are considered to be nanoparticles if one of their dimensions is less than 100 nanometers (nm) across. See the illustration

exa	peta	tera	giga	mega	kilo	10	milli	micro	nano	pico	femto	atto
10^{18}	10^{15}	10^{12}	10^{9}	10^{6}	10^{3}	10^{1}	10^{-3}	10^{-6}	10^{-9}	10^{-12}	10^{-15}	10^{-18}

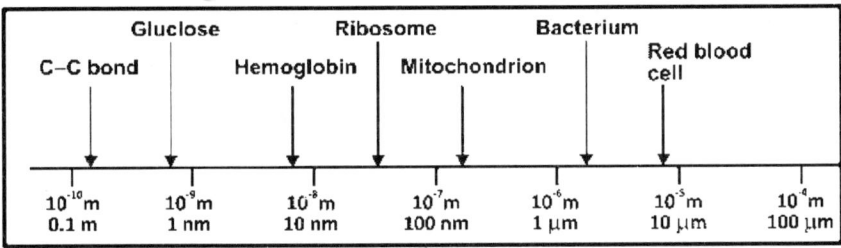

Figure 3 Objects ranging in size from nanometer molecules to the micrometer: The DNA double helix has a diameter of about 2 nm; eight-cell-stage human embryo three days after fertilization, about 200 μm. Source: Kamlesh Pawar (2011) Nanoparticles and their toxicity, *Pashudhan*, 37, 10, October 2011, pp2-4.

The birth of this nanotechnology is usually attributed to physicist Richard Feynman's 1959 talk, "There's Plenty of Room at the Bottom", suggesting the possibility of manipulating things at atomic level. There are two reasons for differences in a material's nanoscale behaviour. (1). Nanoparticles have a much great surface area per unit volume. (2). The smaller the particles get, the greater the changes in the particles magnetic, optical and electrical properties. Due to these unique features, it gives nanotechnology as a separate category in the science.

Nanotechnology enables development and production of novel silver-based composite materials (Egger et al., 2009). A silver-silica-containing polystyrene material was manufactured and the material exhibited very good antimicrobial activity against a wide range of microorganisms. The small size of nanoparticles of metallic silver (below 200 nm) in solid or colloidal state allows for a higher microbiological effect than silver salts. Besides, metallic silver is potentially less toxic and it would be deactivated at a slower rate by gastric HC1 than silver salts. NRC (1980) set the maximum tolerable level of silver for poultry and swine at 100 μg/kg feed. Research workers from Spain (Fondevila et al., 2009, AFST, 150, 259-269) reported that low doses of metallic silver nanoparticles could improve intake and growth of weaned piglets. The low concentration of silver included in weaned pigs' diets (20-40 mg Ag/kg), especially when compared with the currently used doses for other metals (250-350 mg Cu/kg or 2500-3000 mg Zn/kg) suggests a minimum environmental challenge of this metal.

Direct-fed Microbials (DFM)

Direct-fed microbials, particularly bacteria and yeast can replace antibiotics in livestock and poultry feed. The FDA defines direct-fed microbials as "a source of live (viable) naturally-occurring micro-organisms". One major difference between antibiotics and direct-fed microbials is that direct-fed microbials are living organisms. Advancements in stabilizing and packaging of bacteria and yeast have resulted in direct-fed microbial products that have shelf-lives that are acceptable to feed manufacturers. However, these advances can not protect direct-fed microorganisms during feed processing.

Direct-fed microbials include *Lactobacillus, Streptococcus, Bacillus* and yeast (*Saccharomyces cerevisiae*). These microorganisms vary considerably in their ability to withstand various environmental conditions.

Lactobacillus are delicate microorganisms that are unable to withstand environmental extremes, such as the heat and pressure of pelleting. Bacillus are very stable microorganisms that can survive pelleting due to their ability to form spores that are resistant to changes in temperature, pressure, and moisture. Yeast and Streptococcus fall somewhere between Lactobacillus and Bacillus in their ability to survive pelleting. The ability of yeast to grow in the rumen is limited, but is able to remain alive and metabolically active in the rumen and postruminally.

Direct-fed Microbials (DFM) for Calves

Calves are born with nearly sterile gastrointestinal tract. During the first two weeks of the calf's life, it is especially easy for toxin-producing coliform bacteria like *E. coli* to colonise the gut. This irritates the intestinal tract, resulting in a 'hyper-secretion' of fluids that leads to scours. Certain types of DFM oral pastes and feed supplements are designed to prevent or reduce *E. coli* scours in calves.

DFM are a type of 'probiotic' additive, usually composed of living or biologically active spore forming microorganisms. The rationale for their use in the calf is that feeding live, non-pathogenic bacteria may displace and suppress intestinal pathogens. DFMs may be of little benefit under good rearing conditions and husbandry practices. Stress such as extreme weather or transportation, would more likely enhance the potential benefit of feeding a DFM to calves.

Bacterial DFM for Dairy Cows

As we challenge dairy animals to produce higher levels of milk, we need to continue to find ways to moderate rumen pH, enhance rumen energetic efficiency, and promote efficient digestion and absorption of nutrients from the intestine. Bacterial DFM include species of *Lactobacillus, Bacillus,*

Bifidobacterirum, Streptococcus, Enterococcus, and *Propionibacterium.* Bacterial DFM may reduce fluctuations in rumen pH throughout the day. *Megasphaeri elsdenii* and propionibacteria ferment rumen lactate to form propionate. By doing this, rumen pH is controlled and energetic efficiency in the rumen is improved. In addition, additional propionate can increase gluconeogenesis, drive milk production, and possibly reduce subclinical ketosis.

A number of production studies with bacterial DFM in dairy and beef cattle have shown positive response in milk production and milk production efficiency, and promote efficient digestion and absorption of nutrients from the intestine. Lactobacillus bacteria are naturally in the intestine and if these organisms can be supplemented as bacterial DFM and survive passage through the rumen, they may enhance intestinal function. Research needs to prove that they can indeed survive the rumen and function in the intestine. More studies need to be conducted.

Acidifiers

Organic acids usually are added only as preservatives, but they do positively influence performance when included at higher quantities. Liquid acidifiers are

1. Formic acid 6-8 kg/ton and 2. Propionic acid 8-10 kg per ton.

Organic acids in powder form are 1. Fumaric acid 12-15 kg/ton and 2. Citric acid 20-25 kg/ton.

The optimal dose depends on the age of the pig and the environment in which it is being grown as well as on the acid-binding capacity of the dietary ingredients (see appendix no. 3).

The organic acids are capable of providing equivalent performance benefits to those obtained from growth-promoting antibiotics. One recent German study had compared 14-25 kg pigs on a 40 ppm growth promoter or on a 1% propionic-formic acid mixture (BASF's Lupromix product) and found daily gain improvements of 13% and 10% respectively. Feed conversion rates actually were better with the acids. Propionic and formic acid (50 : 50) mixture reduced the potential of *E. coli* bacteria for adhering to the gut wall, the adhesion of these organisms being essential before they can give rise to diarrhoea. Acidifying the feed always reduces the number of piglets with diarrhoea after weaning.

Certain feed plants installed corrosion resistant stainless steel pumps, pipes and nozzles to allow formic acid to be used more readily as a preservative and acidifier. At pH 6.6-6.8 in the small intestine, the formic acid becomes totally dissociated so that only the formate anion is active. This anion exerts a positive influence on the microflora of the digestive tract which improves the utilization of feed nutrients.

Now it is reported that there is synergy between formic acid and phytase to improve the growth performance and feed conversion rates of young pigs in the 22-47 kg weight range.

In diets for laying hens, the feed additive calcium formate (1.3%), which is converted to formic acid in the crop, offers potential benefits beyond reducing *E. coli* and *Salmonella* populations. They include mould inhibition effect and general preservative effects, improved consistency of droppings, resulting in fewer dirty eggs, better calcium absorption and egg shell quality.

Feed additive calcium formate is chemically stable in storage, safe in food and the environment without destructive effects for other feed supplements, such as vitamins and yolk pigments. Calcium formate additive is non-corrosive, odour-free and non-caustic. It is a relatively safe acidifier for use in feed manufacturing process. It is approved by European commission (EC) for use as a food and feed preservative.

Organic Acids as Alternative Hydrogen Sink

Fumaric acid as a feed supplement has the potential to decrease methane production as well as increase glucogenesis (fumarate - succinate - propionate; of course, fumaric acid not converted quantitatively to propionate) and hence milk yield, but the quantity fed has to be restricted because of a risk of acidosis and a consequent decrease in fibre breakdown and feed intake. To avoid the downside on ruminal pH fumaric acid salts such as sodium fumarate may be tried. But what about its effect on osmotic load due to large addition of sodium?

Dr. R. John Wallace, head of the microbial biochemistry group at the Rowett Research Institute in Aberdeen, Scotland and one of the world's leading ruminant nutritionists in association with C.J. Newbold and coworkers (Wood et al., 2009 AFST 152, 2009, 62-71) tried feeding of encapsulated fumaric acid at 100g / kg diet to growing lambs. The results indicated a decrease of methane production by 76%, and improved live weight gain and feed efficiency in the lambs. The encapsulation of fumaric acid seems to provide the optimal conditions to the ruminal microbiota by enabling the slow release of fumaric acid.

As consumer preference tends towards all-natural products, the use of probiotics, live yeast culture, or acidifying agents as a natural way to enhance production of milk, meat and eggs is a viable concept and the farmers who use this knowledge of application of natural additives in rearing their livestock and poultry will be the successful producers of the future.

Acidifiers May Reduce the Effects of Ascites in Poultry

Growing broiler chicken at a quicker rate than their predecessors has resulted in skeletal and metabolic problems. High growth rates have led to higher incidences of diseases such as ascites (scientifically known as pulmonary hypertension syndrome), cellulites (caused by *E. coli* and is characterized by infected scratches on the surface of the skin), sudden death syndrome and disorders such as tibial dyschondroplasia (TD). Ascites represents a spectrum of physiological and metabolic changes leading to the excess accumulation of fluid in the abdominal cavity. These changes occur in response to a number of dietary, environmental and genetic factors. Feed restriction and diet acidification are to be followed, after duly identifying the underlying causes of ascites.

Feed Additive Comprising Organic Acids, their Salts and Surfactants for Effective Moisture Management of Feedstuffs

Moisture is a nightmare for the feed manufacturer or the farmer, because moisture is the largest promoter of various degradation mechanisms in feed. Moisture favours both chemical and microbial degradation mechanisms, which act in perfect synergy adversely affecting their nutritional and storage characteristics. Moisture is not the culprit by itself, but it is the water activity. The numerical amount of moisture is not the guiding factor, but its water activity. Moisture does not contribute to degradation mechanisms as long as its water activity is controlled. The longer storage life of certain liquid and gel food products is a classic example. Moisture managed raw materials and feeds have been proven to be stored for a longer period than normal without any complications. Diet acidification contributes to environmental hygiene due to its antimicrobial effect and prevented feed from microbial and fungal deterioration.

Antioxidants

Oxidation of feed fat causes rancidity spoiling the taste and flavour of the feeds through a process known as lipid peroxidation or autooxidation (see p. 37). These rancid fat containing diets impart undesirable off flavour to the feeds, the milk and milk products. Oxidation also causes much loss to carotenes, vitamin A and vitamin D. The use of antioxidants limits this oxidative spoilage.

Antioxidants prevent fat oxidation and so help avoid rancidity. The addition of antioxidants mops up the free radicals. Primary antioxidants are capable of interrupting and terminating the free radical propagation step. Secondary antioxidants are chemicals that can prevent free radical formation. Primary antioxidants are natural and synthetic. Natural ones are vitamin E (alpha tocopherol), rosemary extract, carotenoids, flavenoids, sulfides and thiocyanates. In biological systems the alpha-tocopherol is most active. Alpha-tocopherol is natural with good consumer acceptance, high heat stability, good process carry-through, low volatility and excellent solubility in fats. However, it increases the cost of the diet. Rosemary extract is also natural with good consumer appeal. It is effective in stabilizing unsaturated oils such as fish and vegetable oils. Negative points are poor carry-through in extrusion processing, higher cost, only regulatory approval is as a flavour or spice and there is a high level of variability amongst suppliers of rosemary extract.

The most common synthetic antioxidants are ethoxyquin, tertbutyl hydroxyquinone (TBHQ), propyl gallate, butylated hydroxyanisole (BHA) and butylated hydroxytoluene (BHT). BHT and BHA tend to be more effective in preventing oxidation of animal fats than of vegetable oils while ethoxyquin is most effective in protecting both animal fats and vegetable oils. Ethoxyquin is a key antioxidant used in shrimp feed. Ethoxyquin levels in feed should be well within the prescribed limits so that the minimum residue limits (MRL) in shrimp do not exceed 0.2 ppm. TBHQ lacks broad global regulatory approval. Propyl gallate can form coloured complexes with copper and iron ions. It has poor process carry-through and poor oil solubility. Ethoxyquin, though very effective antioxidant, has a negative consumer perception. In 1997, the FDA requested a voluntary reduction of ethoxyquin in dog food from 150 ppm to 75 ppm. Since then its usage has steadily decreased. BHA and BHT are susceptible to losses due to steam distillation. Gum guaiac is an antioxidant used in lard, as well as in liquid fats and dehydrated fats and foods.

The main secondary antioxidants are metal chelators (citrates and phosphates) and reducing agents (ascorbates and sulfites). Increased usage of omega fatty acids, which are highly unsaturated fatty acids, has led to feeds more difficult to stabilize. Antioxidants should be added as early as possible since the oxidation process is an irreversible process. There is a growing demand for natural products.

Sequestrants: Certain metals such as copper and iron are active catalysts of oxidation (pro-oxidants) and therefore need to be immobilised. Sequestrants are the compounds added to do this. Sequestrants or sequestering compounds are also referred to as metal scavengers since they combine with trace metals such as iron and copper and remove them from solution. So these compounds should have affinity to the metal ions e.g. calcium salt of EDTA, polyphosphates and citric acid.

Mycotoxin binders: Mycotoxins are diverse group of chemicals that are harmful to animals and humans and have the greatest impact on human and animal health. The three major mycotoxin producing fungi are *Aspergillus, Fusarium* and *Penicillium* and the toxins are aflatoxins, zearalenone, trichothecenes, fumonisins, ochratoxin A, etc. (refer chapter 17).

Mycotoxins are stable compounds and, are not easily removed from finished feeds. Basic hygiene and good management of grain and other feeds, use of mould inhibitors are the initial steps often used as a preventive measure. But once mycotoxins are suspected in the feed addition of mycotoxin binder is the only solution.

Mycotoxin binding agents include activated charcoal, yeast cell wall products, synthetic zeolites and mined mineral clays such as aluminosilicates, sodium bentonite. Effectiveness of these compounds depend upon the adsorptive capacity, their molecular structure, their purity and the characteristics of the targeted mycotoxin.

Mineral clays bind to mycotoxins through electrical charges (e.g. aflatoxins) and thereby prevent their absorption in the intestine. All mycotoxins do not have electrical charges. Thus mineral clays only bind a narrow spectrum of toxins and offer little or no protection against toxins such as zearalenone or trichotecenes.

Some Examples

a. Zeolites (sodium zeolite A) and aluminosilicates have strong affinity to aflatoxins and form a stable complex.

1. Hydrated sodium calcium aluminosilicate (HSCAS) and nutrients with antioxidant capabilities (Se, methionine and vitamin E).
2. HSCAS and virginiamycin

Commercial preparations: UTPP-5 (Ultimate Toxin prevention programme), Vetcare, India-contains organic acids and treated aluminosilicates.

b. Mycosorb (**Mannan oligosaccharides**, Alltech Inc.), developed by esterifying yeast cell wall glucomannans (functional carbohydrates) can specifically adsorb aflatoxins, ochratoxin and fusariotoxins. It is used at lower inclusion rate; About 50 g is as effective as 4 kg of clay.

c. Dietary supplementation of activated carbon reduces the toxic effects of many insecticides, pesticides and other toxins by adsorption and elimination in the faeces. However it has no effect in reducing the DDT (dichloro-diphenyl trichloroethane) and dieldrin in milk or body tissue.

Anticaking agents: In the preparation of mash type feeds, problem of cake or lump formation is observed. This can be considerably minimised by using certain anticaking agents. Anticaking agents not only retard

384 Principles of Animal Nutrition and Feed Technology

caking due to humidity but also cause the mash feeds to flow much easier. These are anhydrous substances that can pick up moisture without themselves becoming wet. They are added to dry mixes to prevent the particles clumping together and so keep the product free flowing. They are either anhydrous salts or substances that hold water by surface adhesion yet themselves remain free flowing. e.g. salts of long chain fatty acids (calcium stearate).

Cal. phosphate, ferrous ammonium citrate, yellow prussiate of soda, potassium and sodium ferrocyanide, magnesium oxide, kaolin, attapulgite clay, ball clay, sodium aluminium silicate, hydrated sodium calcium aluminosilicate (HSCAS), calcium aluminium silicate. HSCAS is used at 0.5% level.

Humectants: These are the substances which are required to keep the product moist, as for example, bread and cakes. Anticaking agents immobilise moisture that was picked up.

Firming and crisping agents: These are substances that preserve the texture of vegetable tissues and by maintaining the water pressure inside them, keep them turgid. They prevent loss of water from the tissues.

Preservatives: The aim of preservatives is to prevent microbial spoilage. e.g. nisin, benzoic acid, methyl-4-hydroxybenzoate, ethyl-4-hydroxybenzoate, propyl-4-hydroxybenzoate, sodium nitrate, sodium nitrite, propionic acid, sorbic acid and sulphur dioxide.

Antifungal agents: sodium propionate, sodium benzoate, nystatin (antifungal antibiotic).

Deodourising Agents

Odour of litter in poultry and other species is more than a nuisance to farmers/breeders. Urea/uric acid is present in urine and stools of all animals. Urease enzyme hydrolyzes the urea to ammonia. The level of ammonia should be less than 25 ppm in farmhouses. Yucca shidigera extract blocks the action of urease enzyme. Lower doses are sufficient for ruminants while high doses are required for swine. Ammonia concentration in the shed was decreased when yucca shidigera was added to the diet while growth rate was increased. Feeding oligasaccharides to pigs reduce objectionable smells. Tea based polyphenol is applied as a feed additive. It stops bacteria producing ammonia and other malodorous compounds.

Flavouring Agents

Flavours are used to improve palatability and thus food appeal. Palatability and feed conversion ratio are interdependent. Types of flavours are spices and sweeteners. Taste and odour are important properties of a food or feed by which they are recognized and enjoyed. The four basic taste qualities are salt, sour, sweet and bitter. Commercial flavouring agents only try to influence sweetness. Flavouring compounds are nonvolatile water soluble substances which have little or no taste of their own, but modify or potentiate the flavour of a product. e.g. esters, alcohols, terpenes, etc.

Flavour in Poultry Feed

Chicken possess a sense of taste but a very limited ability to smell. Yet poultry accept or reject feed according to their preference. Flavour helps to improve rudimentary taste perceptions, aids in rudimentary salivary secretion, helps to regulate water intake and helps to overcome stress. Hence flavours increase feed intake, improve feed efficiency and reduce mortality. e.g. monosodium glutamate (MSG) at 0.2%.

Flavours can be used in conjunction with antioxidants in high fat dairy feeds to mask the rancid taste.

Flavours are sometimes useful as a top dressing for feeds that are supplemented with high concentrations of niacin.

Meat flavours, cheese flavours, mint, onion and garlic flavours are used in feeds for pets at less than 0.1%.

Yeast products are also used at 0.25% in combination with MSG for the improvement of dry dog food.

Capsicum, red pepper, MSG, fennel, fenugreek seed, ginger are examples of spice and seasoning.

Food colours: They make the food more attractive and pleasing. e.g. acid fuchsine, amaranth, brilliant blue. brilliant black, eosin, indigo carmine, sudan red, azolutin, erythrosine, β-carotene, canxanthin, bixin (obtained from annatto seed), crocation (saffron), beetroot red, chlorophyll, anthocyanins.

Pigments

Colour of an egg yolk or egg shell may due carotenoids or porphyrins. Pale yolk is not deficient in vitamin A (vitamin A is colourless). Yolk colour is improved by the addition of either dried alfalfa leaf meal at 2-3% (if yellow maize is not part of the ration) or synthetic carotenoid pigments. Most yellow and red pigments synthesized in vegetable materials are a closely related group of chemical compounds known as carotenoids (see also p. 157). Green leafy materials are excellent sources of xanthophyll. Alfalfa has 5 major carotenoids: lutein (xanthophyll), cryptoxanthin, zeaxanthin, violaxanthin and neoxanthin. These produce yellow pigmentation of the skin and fat of chickens also. Under normal feeding practices, 70% of the yellow colour of egg yolk is due to xanthophyll, and most of the remainder is due to zeaxanthin.

Alfalfa caroteniods and xanthophylls are absorbed, as well as those of corn or corn gluten meal. Alfalfa is a low energy source while yellow corn gluten meal is a high energy source. The biological availability of xanthophylls from various feed sources is variable-corn gluten meal 47 to 89%, dehydrated alfalfa 37 to 65%.

Canthaxanthin and beta-apo-8'-carotenal are synthetic carotenoids. The latter is an intermediate compound produced by the body during the stepwise degradation of β-carotene to vitamin A. Dose 2-8g/ton of feed. Xanthophylls are not stable compounds and can be lost from poultry feeds by oxidation. Antioxidant is added to protect xanthophylls against oxidation.

Annato contains bixin and xanthophyll. Bixin produces red yolks while canthaxanthin produces orange-coloured yolks. *Carophyll* is an example of commercial preparation from Roche Scientific Company.

Carotenoids in Avian Immunity

Carotenoids consist of a class of lipid-soluble polyunsaturated hydrocarbons (carotenes) and oxygenated derivatives (xanthophylls). These are produced by plants, algae and microorganisms. While vertebrates can't synthesize carotenoids endogenously, many species ingest carotenoids in their diets, and are capable of digesting and absorbing these compounds. Carotenoids have a variety of biological functions, including light absorbing properties (providing the basis for pigmentation), antioxidant capabilities, and immunomodulatory functions.

Pellet Binders

Calcium lignosulphonate, sodium lignosulphonate are byproducts from wood pulp manufacture. These are widely used as pellet binders in animal feeds. Lignin is the most widely used feed binder in the world today advantages being improved pellet quality, more control over the additions of fat and moisture, greater pelleting efficiency, improved press capacity and die life, lower power consumption, lower production costs, less fines returns and feed rejections and less dust in the mill.

In rabbits lignosulfonates cause ulceration of colon and consequent mortality. Hence it is not used in pelleting of diets for rabbits. Sodium bentonite at 2.5% is used.

Sepiolite is an effective pellet binder in swine diets especially when diets contained 4% added fat. The others are molasses 5-10%, calcium aluminates 0.6-1%, and guar meal 2.5-5%.

Buffers: Feeding high grain (low fibre) diets to meet the energy requirements of high yielding (over 35 kg milk/day) cows to minimize the energy crisis during early lactation leads to changes in rumen pH and rumen fermentation pattern. Buffers are used to correct these changes. e.g. sodium bicarbonate 200 g/cow/day or 1.5% of grain ration, sodium sesquicarbonate, magnesium oxide, calcium carbonate, sodium bentonite. Salt level of the ration may be reduced to half normal.

Magnesium oxide: Magnesium plays a major role in the synthesis of milk fat in the udder. Dietary requirement is 0.23% of DM intake.

Sodium bentonite: It prevents milk fat depression when fed at 5% of the grain ration. However bentonite may absorb other minerals in the rumen and thus reduce their availability to the microbes and to the animal. It also increases rate of passage.

Sodium bicarbonate for poultry: It has been proved to potentiate ionophore coccidiostats and is being used commercially to improve weight gain, feed conversion, livability and processing yields under stressful conditions such as built-up litter and/or coccidia challenge.

For broiler chickens: 1.8 to 2.7 kg/ton continuously in feed. For Layers: 1 to 1.8 kg/ton. Benefits in layers include improved egg shell quality and better litter condition.

During heat stress the dose is 3.6 to 4.5 kg/ton. It increases water intake and improves survivability and performance of broilers more than 4 weeks of age and adult poultry. Part of the sodium bicarbonate may be given via water. It is known that sodium bicarbonate through water is slightly more potent than through the feed.

Pigs: Adding dietary buffers (1% $NaHCO_3$ or $KHCO_3$) to finishing diets may reduce severity of gastric ulcers.

Methane inhibitors: Methane production could be inhibited by fatty acids and related compounds, particularly unsaturated fatty acids. Other methane inhibitors are chloroform, carbon tetrachloride, chloral hydrate, bromochloromethane (BCM), sulphites and nitrites, amichloral (very potent) and halogenated methane analogues. Rumen microbes require 22 days for adaptation for the latter.

Roughage substitutes: In Western countries and other places where high concentrate diets are used for ruminants in huge mechanized feedlots the possibility of using roughage substitutes is examined. Polyethylene cubes sold as Rufftabs produced beneficial responses in gain and feed conversion in beef cattle fed high concentrate rations.

Propionate production promoters: Ionophores affect principally gram positive bacteria, *Ruminococcus albus, R. flavefaciens.* e.g. monensin, lasalocid.

Defaunating agents: Examples are copper sulphate, sodium lauryl diethoxy sulphate, sodium lauryl sulphate, oil rich in PUFAs and dioctyl sodium sulphosuccinate.

Ketosis controlling agents: Examples are sodium propionate, propylene glycol.

Bloat controlling compounds: Examples are poloxalene (Bloat guard), a non-ionic surfactant 10-20 g/day.

Microbial growth factors (for ruminants): These include niacin, thiamin, branched chain fatty acids (isobutyric acid, 2-methyl butyric acid and isovaleric acid) and straight chain fatty acid (n-valeric acid).

Surfactants: These act like antibiotics or arsenicals by selective inhibitory effects on intestinal microorganisms. Surface-active agents possess the property of stimulating the growth of chicks. e.g. alkyl benzene sulfonate, lauryl ethelene oxide condensate, ethmiod C-15.

Tween 80 (Poly oxyethylene sorbitan monoolate) is a surfactant and appears to have some effect on protozoa, gram negative bacteria and non cellulocytic bacteria. Tween 80 was added along with enzyme as a surfactant, to facilitate the action of enzyme.

Non-ionic surfactant (NIS) is well known as an effective surfactant that stimulates the release of enzymes from a range of aerobic microbes. When NIS was included at a concentration of 0.5g in the 1L of anaerobic growth medium, this material increased the growth rate of rumen bacteria and fungi, and the rate of cereal grain and rice straw digestion, and polysaccharide-degrading enzymes activities. S.S. Lee and group of workers from South Korea (Animal Feed Science and Technology 115 (2004) 37-50) found increased enzyme activities of protease, amylase, carboxymethyl cellulose and xylanase in the rumen contents, concentration of VFA and NH_3-N in rumen fluid and growth rate of rumen anaerobic microorganisms upon administration of NIS solution into the rumen. Hence NIS might be of use as an alternative feed additive to stimulate multiple enzyme activity and microbial growth in the rumen.

Role of Surfactant During the Pelleting Process

Recent studies indicated that the incorporation of food-grade surfactants into the mash feed can enhance the overall conditioning of the feed during pelleting. The surfactant reduces the surface tension of the water, thus allowing a much faster permeation of the feed particles during the conditioning process. Since moisture serves as the conduit for heat transfer into the feed particles, faster rate of moisture permeation facilitates faster heat transfer to the feed in the pelleting conditioner.

Biopreservative

Nisin is a natural antimicrobial peptide produced by strains of *Lactococcus lactis* subsp., lactis that effectively inhibits Gram-positive and Gram-negative bacteria and also the outgrowth of spores of Bacilli and Clostridia. Nisin has been used as a biopreservative and a potential agent in pharmaceutical, veterinary and health care products.

Sweetening agents: Molasses, dextrin, sugars are added to improve palatability.

Tranquilizers: Bring about weight gains in farm animals by controlling stress. Energy otherwise spent in restlessness and irritability is conserved for body gain.

Examples for Sheep: Hydroxyzine hydrochloride 1-2 mgs/day
Triflomephazine
Reserpine 5-10 micrograms/day

Emulsifiers: A substance which aids in the formation of a stable mixture of two otherwise immisible substances (e.g. fat and water) is called an emulsifier. It should have one group with an affinity for water and another with an affinity for fat. e.g. lecithin, glycerides esterified with acetic acid, lactic acid, citric acid, glyceryl monostearate, propylene glycol monostearate.

Stabilizer: Any substance that helps to maintain an emulsion when it has been formed is called a stabilizer. e.g. alginic acid or its sodium/calcium salt, tragacanth, acacia, karaya gum, etc.

Bile acid: Mixed bile acid for shrimp feed and broiler chicken feed are available and are claimed as natural growth promoter. This increases fat utilisation, improves absorption of fat soluble vitamins, growth rates and feed efficiency.

Nutritional Emulsiflers

The ability to digest lipids is not fully developed in young animals. But several studies have demonstrated that the supplementation of **bile salts, lipase or phospholipids** to young animals improves the digestibility of fats. Bile salts are excreted by the gall bladder; they enhance fat digestion by reducing the size of the large fat globule since the efficacy of lipase (released in the small intestine) increases with decreasing fat particle size. Furthermore, bile salts enhance the formation of a micelar phase in the small intestine which enhances fatty acid digestibility in dry diets.

Natural growth promoters: These include acidifiers, probiotics, prebiotics, synbiotics, feed enzymes, phytogenics, and immune stimulants.

Nutricines

Nutricines are components of food which are considered for their beneficial effect upon health rather than their direct contribution to nutrition. Nutricines provide the crucial link between health and nutrition. Nutricines play important roles in delaying the onset of diseases, controlling microbial spoilage of food, improving the digestion of food and helping the absorption of nutrients from the gastrointestinal tract. Examples include antioxidants, nondigestible carbohydrates (NDC), natural acids, enzymes, lecithins.

Nutraceuticals

The term nutraceutical was coined from the words 'nutrition' and 'pharmaceutical' in 1989 by Stephen DeFelice, founder and chairman of the Foundation for Innovation in Medicine, Cranford, New Jersy, USA. A nutraceutical can be defined as a food or part of a food that provides medical or health benefits, including the prevention and/or treatment of a disease. Nutraceuticals may range from isolated nutrients (antioxidants, minerals, amino acids, fatty acids and vitamins), herbal products, dietary supplements and special diets to genetically engineered 'designer' foods and processed products such as cereals, soups and beverages.

Essential Oils (EO)

Essential oils are a secondary metabolite present in spices, tree leaves and bulbs of some plants. Essential oils are described as follows: volatile aromatic compounds with an oily appearance extracted from plant materials typically by steam distillation; alcohol, ester or aldehyde derivatives of phenylproponoids and terpenoids. EO compounds available include thymol (thyme and oregano), eugenol (clove), pinene (Juniper), limonene (dill), cinnamaldehyde (cinnamon), capsaicin (hot peppers), terpinene (tea tree), allicin (garlic), anethol (anise), peppermint oil, eucalyptus oil. They have antimicrobial activity and have been shown to modify rumen microbial fermentation. From an extensive review of the literature primarily related to *in vitro* work, Calsamiglia et al. (2007) concluded that EO inhibited deamination and methanogenesis. However, the impact of dietary EO supplementation on ruminant animal performance has been equivocal.

Oils that contain phenolic structures have stronger antimicrobial properties than oils without phenolic structures. Essential oils are extremely potent substances, they can lead to feed intake reduction, micro-flora disturbance in the gastrointestinal tract and accumulation in animal tissues and products. Most essential oils are generally recognized as safe (GRAS) but they must be used cautiously because they can be toxic (allergens) and potent sensitizers and their odour/taste may contribute to feed refusal. They are also very volatile and will evaporate rapidly, leading to large variation in concentration in the finished products.

Essential oils can act in synergy with organic acids for their growth promoting effect and prevention of specific intestinal diseases. It has been demonstrated that when both organic acids and essential oils are protected in a special matrix, the quantity required to achieve maximum performance in poultry can be reduced drastically. The active ingredients can be delivered into the intestine, directly where the bulk of gastrointestinal bacteria are located.

Methyl Donors

Methionine, betaine and choline are sources of methyl groups (see fig. 4 for details). Activated methionine, S-adenosyl-methionine is the primary methyl donor. But betaine is cheaper than methionine and choline is cheaper than betaine. However, choline is not a methyl donor, because its methyl groups are not metabolically available for methylation. Choline has to be converted to betaine to fulfill this function and this conversion is not highly efficient. Thus choline is not as efficient a methyl donor as betaine. Commercial preparations of betaine are 'Betafin' and 'Finnstim' from 'Finnsugar Bioproducts' of Finland as betaine anhydrous extracted from sugar beets. Nowadays, it is available as betaine hydrochloride from synthetic production.

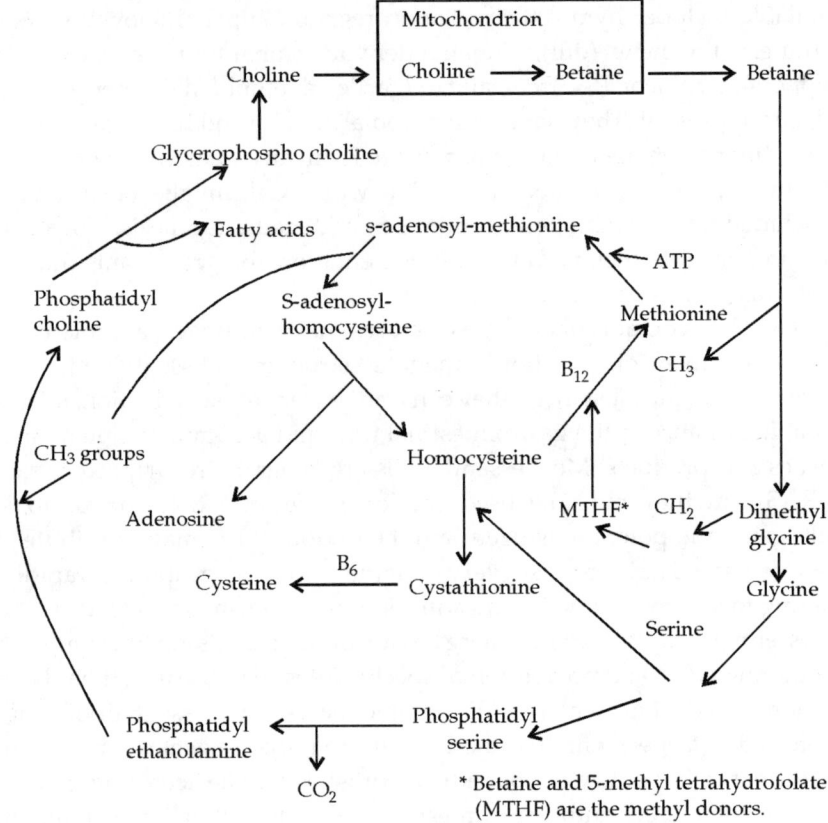

Figure 4. Methyl Donors: Biochemical Interrelationship.

It is wise to supplement betaine/choline in formulating diets for poultry, swine, fish, pet animals, dairy cattle, etc. to spare the essential amino acid, methionine and also important vitamins, such as vitamin B_{12} and folic acid as potential methyl donors.

5-Methyl tetra-   cobalamin-dependent methionine synthase
hydrofolic + homocysteine   ⟶ Tetrahydro- + Methionine
acid   folic acid

Feed Additives for Transition Cows and Buffaloes

Transition period is the period 2-4 weeks prior to calving through 2-4 weeks after calving. Depression of feed intake pre-calving and slow intake increase post-calving is observed during this period. During the transition from pregnancy to lactation, the dairy animal is under enormous stress both physically and metabolically. Further some cows showed a relatively high frequency of inflammations, mostly subclinical; they impair performance and welfare of dairy cows. Hence feed additives such as propionate production promoters, propionate enhancers (flumarate, malate), ketosis controlling agents, methyl donors, rumen inert fats or rumen bypass fat, rumen bypass protein, biotin, niacin, vitamin B_{12}, pantothenic acid, riboflavin are included in their diets. Propionate is converted to glucose in the liver of ruminants by a series of enzymatic reactions which require biotin, vitamin B_{12}, niacin, pantothenic acid and riboflavin. Apart from proper feeding management during the dry period, addition of PUFA such as omega-3 and conjugated linoleic acid (CLA) in diet can contribute to modulation of the inflammatory process and attenuation of the systemic inflammatory response.

Feed Additive Sweeteners: A number of lab and field trials with sweeteners have demonstrated increased feed intake in young animals, especially pigs. In many cases, sweeteners also improved feed conversion.

Natural Sugars: Natural sugars such as sucrose, dextrose, fructose and lactose are the first feed sweeteners. Sucrose (cane or beet sugar) is included up to 2% in certain young animal diets as a highly palatable energy source. However, the 2% dose of sucrose proved far from adequate to sweeten a finished feed and this led to the search for cheaper alternatives.

Alternatives to sucrose: Modern alternatives to sucrose include blends of 'high intensity' sweeteners (HISs). High intensity sweeteners are of two types:

1. High intensity sweeteners that have short term effects e.g. aspartame, cyclamate, saccharin, moneline, alitame.
2. High intensity sweeteners that have long lasting effects or potentiators e.g. thaumatine, neohesperidin dihydrochalcone (NHDC).

In feeds for young animals it is often necessary to prolong saccharin's initial sweet taste as well as to 'mask' its characteristic unpalatable metallic aftertaste. These are the functions of the second HISs, called a 'potentiator' or 'enhancer', which normally is incorporated at a concentration of ppm (parts per million) in the finished feed. That is how 'blends' of high intensity sweeteners are used in feeds. e.g. Saccharin-NHDC blend. This blend has a synergistic sweetness effect. Saccharin is added at levels up to 150 ppm in the finished feed and the potentiator, NHDC is added at 1 ppm to enhance, extend and modify the sweetening effect of saccharin.

Sweetener power of some of the high intensity sweeteners is presented in Table 4. It has been reported that sweetener effectiveness is inversely proportional to the feed raw materials quality. This means that as the quality of raw materials in the diet increases, there is a corresponding decrease in the efficiency of the sweetener. Nevertheless, in most cases of least cost ration formulation, palatability of the diet can be improved by means of a sweetener.

TABLE 4. Sweetener 'Power' of HISs in Relation to Sucrose.

Sweetener	Sweetener power where surcrose equals 1
Cyclamate	30
Aspartame	180
Saccharine	300
Moneline	1500–2000
Alitame	2000
Thaumatine	1000–2000
Neohesperidine dihydrochalcone	1500–1800

Dosage of the sweetener: There is no single dose of a sweetener for all feeds or even for particular types of feed products, such as piglet creep or weaning feeds. The dosage has to be optimised based on the type of feed raw materials, feed intake or other measures of animal performance.

Particle size of the sweetener: The sweetener manufacturer must make sure that the particle size of the sweetener is uniform and its distribution throughout the sweetener premix is homogenous. One brand of commercial sweetener (SUCRAM) has particle size into the range of 8-121 μm, with a median size of 57 μm and a mode of 48 μm. A high particle-per-gram helps to ensure that a greater number of finished feed pellets will have an effective concentration of sweetener. Thus the micro particles provide a uniform degree of sweetness throughout the feed and optimise the effect of sweet taste potentiators. Also, they provide improved masking of the bitter and metallic aftertaste of saccharin and medicinal products.

Sweeteners are of great help to increase feed palatability, especially in young animals. But the nutritionist should use the sweeteners with care to improve feed intake and animal performance because of availability of a huge variety of feed raw materials.

Palatants: Aromas, flavours, sweeteners and/or their combinations to improve the palatability of feeds.

Amino acids and Amino acid anologues: Methionine is the most limiting amino acid in lactating cows. Structural manipulation of amino acids is one of the potential methods for rumen bypass of amino acids by making them resistant to rumen degradation. An ideal analogue would have to survive rumen degradation, absorb from the small intestine and must have biological potency at the cellular level for metabolism. Many analogues of methionine have been tried effectively in ruminant diets by *encapsulation*, (rumen bypass methionine) e.g. methionine hydroxy analogue Ca (MHA), N-Hydroxymethyl-L- methionine Ca (HMM-Ca), L-Stearyl-L-methionine, α-hydroxy-τ-methyl mercapto butyrate Ca-(HMB-Ca).

HMB-Ca is not completely protected from rumen degradation. The most consistent response of these amino acids is to increase milk fat percentage or milk yield or both. Rumen-stable methionine is used in lactation feeds. 25 to 35 grams daily or 0.2 to 0.25% of the grain mixture is used during early lactation per day for high producing cows.

Commercial Preparations

1. dl-methionine; Hydroxy methyl thiobutanoic acid (HMB) or methionine hydroxy analogue free acid MHA-FA (Alimet liquid)
2. MHA, Methocare
3. Methomin, (Methionine + Cu, Co, Zn)
4. G-Promin (HMB, Lys, choline chloride and chelated trace minerals)
5. Mepron (Rumen protected methionine), Degussa.
6. Smartamine (Rumen protected methionine), Rhone Poulene Animal Nutrition.

L-Lysine HCL 98.5% (Feed grade), DL-Methionine 99.0% (Feed grade) are imported since they are not manufactured in India. These are available in dry and liquid form. L-Threonine and L-Tryptophan are also available.

Carnitine: Lysine and methionine are carnitine precursors. L-carnitine significantly increased the cholesterol in egg yolks and had some positive effects on hatchability (3 to 4%) when fed to broiler breeders. The U.S. FDA stated that L-carnitine can be added to swine diets at levels not exceeding 0.1% and finfish feed at 0.25%. e.g. Lonza-L-carnitine.

β-carotene: It is precursor of vitamin A with an activity of 400 IU of vitamin A per milligram. It has been reported that beta carotene has been linked to bovine fertility.

Niacin: It helps the animals to do better and visibly better. It prevents ketosis in dairy cows. Dose is 12 gms/day. Feeding niacin daily in early stages of ketosis decreases fat mobilization and increases blood glucose levels, usually correcting ketotic condition within a week.

Encapsulated Nutrients

Balchem's Animal Nutrition and Health Division (Balchem Corporation, USA) produces several encapsulated products with its patented proprietary encapsulated technology. Encapsulation protects nutrients and other sensitive compounds, and allows them to become available when and where they are of the most benefit to the animal. Without protective encapsulation, many compounds experience losses in activity due to feed processing and storage or prematurely in the rumen, long before they can be absorbed in the small intestine and used. It released products such as rumen-protected lysine, rumen-protected choline and rumen-protected niacin. Product encapsulated-urea makes nitrogen available in the rumen in proper proportion to carbohydrates for the production of microbial protein. Encapsulated vitamin C product protects vitamin C from typical losses during feed processing and storage and deliver vitamin C in a highly bioavailable manner, in ruminants, nonruminants and in aquatic species.

Meat and Bone Meal (MBM): It is manufactured by the rendering plants designed and supplied by Firms such as Alfa level FME of Denmark and Flo-Dry Eng. Ltd of New Zealand. The process is in compliance with the EU regulations. The high temperature drying and sterilization guarantees that the MBM is free from *E. coli, Salmonella, Clostridia* and at the same time retaining the nutritional value. MBM is a vital ingredient in the manufacture of high quality compounded feeds for livestock and poultry. Allanasons Ltd. (Mumbai) manufactures a sterilised meat and bone meal.

Product specifications : Protein,   min 45%

Fat,   min 4%

Moisture,   max 8%

Sand and Silica,   max 1%

Mesh size   6 mm

Dicalcium phosphate: It can be prepared from two sources, bones and rock phosphate. Bone based DCP is a byproduct of gelatine/ossein industry. Rock phosphate has tricalcium phosphate and fluorine. Food and pharmaceutical grades of DCP are manufactured by the defluorination of rock phosphate. Brindavan phosphate private Ltd. (Bangalore) prepares it from rock phosphate.

Product Specifications (On DMB):

Moisture	, max	7%
Ca	, min	23%
P	, min	18%
AIA	, max	1%
Fluorine	, max	0.1%

Mineral Mixture

Dicalcium phosphate (DCP)-Animal Feed Grade (BIS:5470-1969; as per the latest amendment Jan. 2000):

- Highly bioavailable phosphorus source for Poultry and Livestock
- Guaranteed 18% P
- Fluorine maximum: 0.1%
- Free from pathogenic bacteria
- Free from undesirable odour, harmful nonsterilised putrefied animal protein, dead animal cells, etc.
- Does not contain less bioavailable salts of phosphorus like calcium metaphosphate/tricalcium phosphate/defluorinated phosphate.

Minmix, Pfizer Ltd. is a fortified Mineral Feed Supplement for cattle and buffaloes.

Dosage specifications are

a) 1 kg per 100 kg of concentrate mixture.
b) 28 g per animal per day (which does not receive concentrate mixture) for adult cattle and buffaloes.
c) 5 to 15 g daily for calves, sheep and goats.

Chromium Supplement

Chromium improves glucose metabolism in swine. It is available as chromium picolinate, chromium nicotinate. It increased muscle and decreased lipid deposition when fed to pigs of 20 to 105 kg body weight at 200 ppb. Greater longissimus muscle area, greater absorption and retention of nitrogen have been obtained in chromium fed pigs.

Sows fed diets with supplemental chromium picolinate from 40 kg through two parities had larger litters than sows that had never received supplemental chromium. Sows received supplemental chromium had lower insulin: glucagon ratio in mid gestation, indicating greater efficiency of insulin action. It has been reported that chromium nicotinate is better than chromium picolinate.

Part II

Evaluation of Feedstuffs and Feed Technology

Part II

Chapter 14

Common Feeds and Fodders for Livestock and Poultry Feeding: Their Classification, Composition and Nutritive Value

Introduction

Feeds for livestock and poultry feeding composed of naturally occurring products from food crops and field crops and of many of the byproducts of the milling, oil seed processing, sugar industry, starch manufacturing, vegetable and fruit processing, dairy, meat, fish, prawn, etc. processing and other food processing industries. This shows that there are various types of feedstuffs available for the livestock and poultry feeding.

Though strictly speaking no two feedstuffs are alike in the composition and characteristic, substitution of one feedstuff is made with another depending upon the market price and availability in a particular region/ season in practical feeding. Therefore, it is necessary to know the categories of the feeds within which substitutions are justified for the feeds with similar nutritional properties.

The Advantages of Feed Classification Are

1. Feeds with similar nutritive characteristics are grouped together;
2. Such grouping helps in the selection of feedstuffs for formulation of rations, and
3. This also helps in the substitution of one feed with another feed from the same group.

Classification of Feeds Based Upon Use

This was proposed by Crampton and Harris (1969) and utilized by the National Research Council (NRC) of USA. This is known as NRC classification of feeds. Feeds are classified into eight groups/classes on the basis of their physical and chemical characteristics. The same is also referred to as international feed classes. These are dry forage and roughage, succulent forage and pasture, silage, energy feed, protein supplement, mineral supplement, vitamin supplement and additives.

Classification of Feeds in General

Feedstuffs can be grouped into different classes on the basis of bulkiness (bulk density) and chemical composition. Feedstuffs are classified into roughages and concentrates based on the crude fibre content, which is primarily responsible for bulk density of the feeds. Roughages are classified into succulent (those which contain more than 80% moisture) and non-succulent; leguminous and non-leguminous; green and dry. Roughages can also be grouped based on their nutritive value (on DMB) into maintenance type, productive type and nonmaintenance type.

1. Maintenance type of roughages have about 3-5% digestible crude protein (DCP). e.g. non-legumes: cereal fodders and grasses and their hay.
2. Productive type of roughages have more than 5% DCP e.g. legume fodders and their hay.
3. Nonmaintenance type of roughages have below 3% DCP. e.g. straws and stovers.

Concentrate feedstuffs are further classified into 3 groups based on energy and digestible protein: Carbonaceous-rich in energy and low in DCP (cereal grains), proteinous-very rich in DCP (oil seed meals and cakes, animal protein supplements) and products with energy and protein in intermediary position (brans, husks, chunies, etc.).

Broadly feeds and fodders can be classified into roughages, concentrates and additives (nutritive and non-nutritive).

Forages and roughages: The term 'roughage' is usually used to designate feeds that are high in fibre and low in net energy. Technically forages mean hay, straw, silage and pasture while roughages include rice husk, groundnut (peanut) shells. However, the terms forage and roughage are used interchangeably. Products containing more than 18% crude fibre or more than 35% cell wall in their dry state are classified as forages and roughages. Feedstuffs with less than 18% CF or less than 35% cell wall are called as concentrates.

Hay: Hay is the product obtained by drying in the sun or in the shade, tender stemmed leafy plant material in such a way that they contain not more than 12-14% moisture.

Straw: Straw is the byproduct of any cereal, millet or legume crop leftover after harvesting, threshing and removal of the grains or pulses. Straws form the main feed of cattle and buffaloes (see page 498).

Fodder: Aerial parts with ears, with husks or heads are called fodder.

Stover: Aerial parts without ears, without husks or heads are called stover. While harvesting maize, jowar, ragi, etc. commonly the earheads are removed and the remaining dried portion can be classed as stover.

Sugarcane Plant Byproducts in Animal Feeding

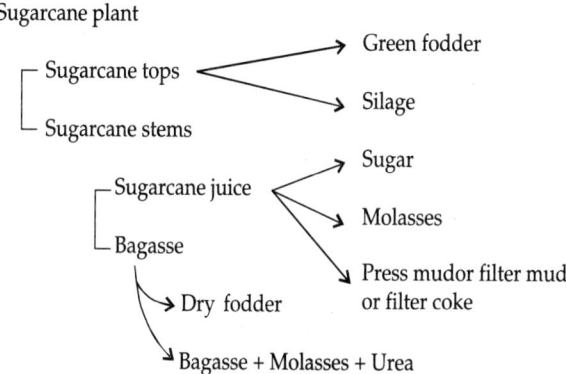

Sugarcane plant

┌ Sugarcane tops → Green fodder
│ → Silage
└ Sugarcane stems

┌ Sugarcane juice → Sugar
│ → Molasses
└ Bagasse → Press mudor filter mud or filter coke
   → Dry fodder
   → Bagasse + Molasses + Urea

Bagasse: It is the fibrous material leftover in sugar factories after extraction of all the juice from sugarcane.

Hull: Outer covering of beans, peas e.g. cottonseed.

Husk: Dry outer covering of grains, grams e.g. rice husk, gram husk.

Shells: Hard outer covering of nuts. e.g. groundnut shells.

Hulls, husks and shells are high in crude fibre. They are light and bulky feeds containing very little protein.

Corn cobs: After removal of corn grains, the corn cobs can be fed to ruminants.

Succulent Forage or Roughage (Pasturage, Range Plants and Soiling Crops) See Appendix I for scientific names.

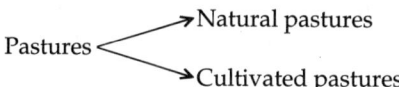

Pastures < → Natural pastures
          → Cultivated pastures

Some Examples

Pasture grasses: Cenchrus ciliaris, Cenchrus setigerus, Heteropogon contortus

Pasture legumes: Stylosanthes hamata, Stylosanthes scabra, **Siratro,** Butterfly pea *(Clitoria ternatea).*

Natural pastures: Natural postures are grasslands where grasses of several different species grow wild as natural vegetation. They occur in forest regions and uncultivable wastelands.

Cultivated pastures: Cultivated pastures are grasslands which are regularly cultivated and maintained in condition by means of periodical weeding and manuring. Cultivated pastures may be allowed to be grazed as such by livestock or may be cut green and fed as soilage.

Soilage: Pasture whether natural or cultivated when cut and fed green to an animal in its own stall is known as soilage.

Soiling or zero grazing: The method of feeding of an animal with soilage is known as 'soiling' or 'zero' grazing.

Soiling crops: The grasses or crops which act to provide the fodder are known as 'soiling crops'. These crops are nothing but fodder grasses or other crops raised by farmers for feeding livestock.

Advantages of 'Zero Grazing' or Soiling

1. The energy spent on walking in search of fodder is saved in 'soiling'. This is especially more important in the case of dairy cattle.
2. The quantity of fodder required by the animal can be accurately rationed and fed which is not practicable while pasturing (grazing).
3. Soiling is preferable and economical if green fodder is scarce.

Fodder Crops

1. Kharif fodders	:	Sorghum, Maize, Bajra, Teosinte, Sunnhemp, Cowpea
2. Rabi fodders	:	Oats, Lucerne, Berseem,
3. Improved legumes	:	Berseem, lucerne, Kudzu vine
4. Fodder grasses	:	Napier, Guinea, Rhodes, Para, Anjan, Sudan.
5. Fodder trees	:	Babul, Subabul, Sesbania, Glyricidia.

Energy Feeds: These are concentrate feedstuffs with less than 20% protein and less than 18% crude fibre or less than 35% cell walls on dry matter basis. In case of certain brans, chunies some samples may contain over 18% CF and more than 20% CP and still they are classified as energy feeds. e.g. Cereal grains, mill byproducts, fruits, nuts and roots. Many of the fruits and some roots are excellent sources of vitamins and minerals for humans.

Energy Supplements: Examples

Cereals: Bajra, sorghum, maize, wheat, barley, ragi.

Cereal byproducts: Rice bran and polish, wheat bran, maize bran.

Legumes/pulses: Horse gram, black gram, Bengal gram, red gram (not strictly as energy supplements)

Byproducts of pulses: chunies, husk.

Roots and tubers: A root crop consists of the fleshy subterranean (underground) parts of a harvested plant, grown primarily for its sugar content. e.g., turnips, sugarbeet, carrots, swedes, etc. Tubers are short, thickened, fleshy stems usually formed underground such as potatoes, cassava, sweetpotatoes, etc. Tubers differ from the root crops in containing either starch or fructan instead of sucrose as the main storage carbohydrate.

Protein Supplements: These are concentrate feedstuffs which contain 20% or more protein and less than 18% CF or less than 35% cell walls on DMB.

Examples

Plant origin: Oil cakes and meals: Groundnut cake/meal, soybean meal, gingelly cake/sesame cake/til cake, cotton seed cake, coconut cake, mustard seed cake, rape seed meal and canola meal, sunflower cake, safflower cake, linseed meal

Animal origin: Meat meal/meat scraps, blood meal, liver residue meal

Marine/aquatic origin: Fishmeal

Avian origin: Feather meal, hydroyzed feather meal

Methods of extraction of oil from the seeds: Cakes and meals are the products leftover after extraction of oil from the seeds.

1. Hydraulic pressure method or Ghani pressed: Oil seeds are pressed under high pressure. The cake obtained by this method contains 8% fat.
2. The expeller process: This is a continuous process in which the seeds are fed into a revolving screw of diminishing circumference, the oil being collected and carried off in small channels. The cake obtained by this method contains 6% fat. The heat developed during the process due to the friction denatures the protein. This denaturing of protein helps in reducing the solubility of protein in the rumen and thus protects the protein degradation in the rumen.
3. Solvent extraction process: Seeds are crushed and placed loosely in a large container and a solvent like ether, benzene or petrol is allowed to percolate. Extracted material is heated with steam to remove the solvent. This meal contains less than 1% fat.

Soybean meal is produced by the solvent extraction method. Heat treatment is necessary to inactivate trypsin inhibitor, haemagglutinins, saponins, etc. which affect monogastric animals.

Rapeseed meal contains glucosinolates which are hydrolysed by endogenous myrosinase during the crushing of seeds. Low glucosinolate varieties of rapeseed have been developed in Canada and are registered as canola. Meals from such varieties can be added in the diet of pigs at higher levels than those containing high glucosinolate (see page 547 for more information).

Cakes Versus Meals

Meals differ from cakes in having higher protein and lower fat content. Meals are derived from solvent extraction process where the oil extraction is much more complete than in expeller process. The byproduct obtained in the expeller process of oil extraction is called as cake.

INTERNATIONAL FEED VOCABULARY

Nowadays feedstuffs have been described as per the International Feed Vocabulary (IFV) to minimize the identification difficulties by assigning descriptive name to every feed. IFV is widely used in North America and South America, parts of Europe, the Middle East, Australia and Southeast Asia.

IFV is designed to give a comprehensive name to each feed as concisely as possible. Feed descriptions are selected to specify qualities among feeds that relate to differences in nutritive values. Each international feed description (feed name) is coined by using descriptions from one or more of six facets. These include the following:

1. Origin: comprises scientific names (genus, species, variety), common names (generic, breed or kind).
2. Part: The actual part of the parent material feed given to animals as affected by process.
3. Processes and treatments: a system of operations to which the part has been subjected.
4. Stage of maturity.
5. Cutting (primarily applicable to forages).
6. Grade (official grades with guarantees).

A complete international feed description consists of all description applicable to a specific feed.

1. Origin

The origin of the parent material of plants may be specific (sorghum, maize, etc.) or non-specific (cereals, grasses, legumes, etc.).

2. Part

This facet of feed description represents the actual part of the parent material. Today, due to extensive fractionation of plant seeds and reconstitution of many parts into new processed foods many byproducts are available for animal feeding e.g. bran, germ, maize cob. Also, there are many byproducts from meat, fish and prawn industry for human consumption.

3. Processes and treatments

Various processes are used in the preparation of animal feeds and some of these may significantly alter their nutritive value. Heat may damage some nutrients; conversely it may make other nutrients more available. Treatments like grinding, pelleting and heat treatments affect the nutritive value. Some of processes and treatments like drying, expeller, solvent extraction process, etc. also affect the chemical composition.

4. Stage of maturity

Stage of maturity is an important factor that influences the nutritive value of forages, silages and some animal products. In case of perennial fodders the actual growing time of plant is used as stage of maturity.

Early Vegetative	:	Stage at which the plant is vegetative and before the stem elongates.
Late vegetative	:	Stage at which stems are beginning to elongate just before blooming; first bud to first flower.
Early bloom	:	Stage between initiation of bloom and stage in which 1/10 of the plants are in bloom; some grass heads are in anthesis.
Mid-bloom	:	Stage in which 1/10 to 2/3 of the plants are in bloom; most grass heads are in anthesis.
Full-bloom	:	Stage in which 2/3 or more of the plants are in bloom.
Late-bloom	:	Stage in which blossoms begin to dry and fall, and seeds begin to form.
Milk stage	:	Seeds well formed, soft and immature
Dough stage	:	Seeds with dough like consistency

| Mature | : | Stage at which plants are harvested for seeds |
| Past ripe | : | Stage that follows maturity; some seeds have been cast and plants have begun to wither. |

5. Cutting

Many forages like berseem and lucerne are cut and harvested a number of times and need description.

6. Grades

Some commercial feed and feed ingredients have been given official grades on the basis of their composition and other quality characteristics. The Bureau of Indian Standards has given specifications in which 'minimum' and 'maximum' per cent of feed nutrients have been described.

The International Network of Feed Information Centres (INFIC) identified eight classes of foods (Harris et al., 1968, 1980).

International Feed Classes

Code	Class description (on dry matter basis)
1.	Dry Forages and Roughages
2.	Pasture, range plants and forage fed green
3.	Silages
4.	Energy Feeds or Basal feeds
5.	Protein supplements
6.	Mineral supplements
7.	Vitamin supplements
8.	Additives

Chemical Composition and Nutritive Value of Common Feeds and Fodders

Average chemical composition of common feedstuffs along with their nutritive value is presented in Table 1, 2, 3 and 4. Chemical composition of rice straw (Table 5), BIS specifications for certain concentrates (Table 6) and feedstuffs with their nutritive value at a glance (Table 7) are delineated for a quick grasp.

International Feed Number

All international feed descriptions are listed in the Feed Description File (Harris et al., 1980). Each new entry in this file is assigned a current number for its identification. It consists of 5 digits. This number is the link

TABLE 1. Average Chemical Composition (%) of Common Feedstuffs (on as fed basis)

	DM	CP	EE	CF	NFE	Ash	Ca	P
Roughages: Green fodder								
Non-leguminous green fodder	25	2.2	0.8	8	12.2	1.8	0.11	0.05
Leguminous green fodder	20	4	0.8	5	7.7	2.5	0.4	0.08
Hays (on DMB)								
Indigenous grasses	88	5	1	35	47	12	0.3	0.2
Improved pasture grasses	88	7	1.5	30	51.5	10	0.35	0.25
Legumes	88	15	2	30	41	12	1.5	0.25
Straws (on DMB) Cereals	90	3.8	1	35	48.7	11.5	0.34	0.17
Legumes	90	6.0	1	39	43.5	10.5	1.0	0.12
Concentrates (on DMB) **Cereal grains**	90	10.2	2.7	4	79.8	3.3	0.04	0.35
Legume seeds	90	23.3	2.3	6.8	63.6	4.0	0.16	0.41
Brans	90	12.5	3.5	13	64.0	7.0	0.1	1.0
Oilseed cakes (sesame and GNC)	90	48.5	9.5	6	27.7	8.3	0.5	1.0

between the international feed description in different languages, the international feed name and country feed names, and the chemical and biological data in the data bank.

The numbers are particularly useful as tags when calculations involve various feeds. The feed class number usually precedes the international feed number when feed tables and reports are prepared.

International feed name is a complete international feed description. It consists of all description applicable to that feed. The first digit is the class followed by other characteristic features.

Examples:

Rice straw	1-03-925
Rice hulls	1-08-925
Para grass (fresh)	2-03-525
Maize silage	3-02-818
Rice grain	4-03-939
Groundnut cake	5-03-648
Fenugreek seeds	8-01-856

TABLE 2. Chemical Composition of Common Feedstuffs (on DMB)

Feedstuff (1)	DM (2)	CP (3)	EE (4)	CF (5)	NFE (6)	Ash (7)	Ca (8)	P (9)
Cereal Straws							0.5-0.6;	0.12-0.14
Rice straw	90	3	1	32	49	15		
Wheat straw	90	3	1	38	46	12		
Oat straw	90	4	1	36	52	6		
Ragi straw	90	3	1	36	52	8		
Jowar straw	90	5	1	34	50	10		
Legumes Straw							1.0-1.4;	0.08-0.15
Gram straw	90	6	0.5	45	36	13		
Groundnut straw/ haulms	90	8	1	41	42	8		
Hays								
Indigenous grasses	88	5	1	35	47	12	0.3	0.2
Improved grasses (Cenchrus spp.)	88	7	1.5	30	51.5	10	0.35	0.25
Legumes (Cowpea, Lucerne, Berseem)	88	15	2	30	41	12	1.5	0.25
Green fodders (on as fed basis)								
Non-leguminous							0.07-0.09;	0.04-0.05
Maize	25	2	0.6	8	13	1.4		
Oat	25	3	0.8	6	14	1.2		
Jowar	25	1.5	1	9	12	1.5		
Napier bajra hybrid	25	2	0.5	10	11	1.5		
Guinea grass	25	1.5	0.5	8	14	1.0		
Dub grass	35	3.5	1	8	17.5	5.0		
Sugarcane tops	35	2.5	1	8	21	2.5		
Leguminous							0.3-0.5;	0.05-0.10
Cowpea	20	4.5	1	5	5.5	4		
Lucerne	20	4.5	1	5	5.5	4		
Berseem	15	3	0.5	4	8.5	4		
Cereal grains								
Maize	90	11	2.5	2	82.5	2	0.04	0.35
Oat	90	9	1.5	5	80.0	4.5		
Legume seed								
Cowpea	90	25	2	5	64	4	0.16	0.41
Brans								
Deoiled rice bran (DORB)	90	12	2.0	13	68.0	5	0.08	1.5
Wheat bran	90	13	2.5	13	64.5	7	0.1-0.3	0.8-1.2
Oil cakes								
Gingelly cake/ Til cake/ Sesame cake	90	45	10	5	29	11	0.5	1.0
Groundnut cake (GNC)	90	52	8	7	27.5	5.5		
Coconut cake	90	24	10	13	45	8		
Cottonseed cake	90	23	9	24	37	7		
Mustard cake	90	36	11	10	33	10		
Linseed cake	90	31	6	10	43	10		

TABLE 3. Nutritive Value of Common Roughages (Average Values) (on as fed basis).

Feedstuff	DM	DCP	TDN	Ca	P
	←		%		→
Dry roughages					
Cereal straws	90	0	44	0.5-0.6	0.12-0.14
(Rice, Wheat)					
Legume straws					
Groundnut straw	90	8	53	1.0-1.4	0.08-0.15
Cereal hays					
Jowar hay	88	3	51	0.3	0.2
Legume hays	88	10	60	1.5	0.25
Green roughages					
Cereal fodders					
(Maize, Jowar, Bajra)	20	1	13	0.07-0.09	0.04-0.05
Green grasses	25	1.0	16	0.11	0.05
(Hybrid napier					
Para, Guinea)					
Sugarcane tops	25	0.7	10		
Legume fodders					
(Berseem, Lucerne					
Cowpea)	15	3	12	0.3-0.5	0.05-0.10

TABLE 4. Nutritive Value of Common Concentrate Feedstuffs (on as fed basis).

Feedstuff	CP	DCP	TDN	Ca	P
	←		%		→
Maize	9.0	7.4	84.9	0.04	0.35
Jowar	9.0	8.0	75.0		
Wheat	13.2	10.2	79.2		
Deoiled rice bran	12.0	6.0	60.0	0.08	1.5
Wheat bran	14.0	10.0	68.0	0.1-0.3	0.8-1.2
Gram husk	6.0	0.5	55.0		
Chuni (mixture of					
broken gram and husk)	10-12	6-8	60.0		
Tapioca tippi/waste	4.0	2.0	64.0		
Molasses	4.8	1.0	54.0		
Groundnut cake (exp)	45.0	42.0	71.0	0.2	0.7
Groundnut cake (extr)	52.0	46.0	70.0		
Gingelly cake/					
Til cake/sesame					
cake (extr)	47.8	38.0	78.0	2-3	0.8
Sunflower cake (extr)	33.0	23.0	71.0		
Cottonseed cake					
(extr, decorticated	39.0	32.8	72.5		
and delinted)					
Cottonseed cake					
(undecorticated)	39.0	18.0	70.0		
Coconut cake (extr)	24.0	19.0	81.0		
Mustard/rapeseed					

[Table Contd.]

[Table Contd.]

cake (extr)	36.0	27.0	74.0	0.6	1.0
Soybean meal (extr)	45.8	42.0	78.0		
Fish meal	50.0	45.0	65.0		
Meat meal	50.0	45.0	70.0	8-10	4-5
Bone meal	-	-	-	29.0	12.6
Calcite	-	-	-	36.0	-
Dicalcium phosphate	-	-	-	21.0	18.5

TABLE 5. Chemical Composition of Rice Straw *.

Constituent	Range	Mean
	% DM	
Crude protein	2.2 to 7.6	4.0
Ether extract	2.0 to 4.0	2.0
Crude fibre	29 to 45	33.0
Total ash	10 to 21	18.0
Nitrogen free extract	30 to 50	43.0
Neutral detergent fibre	74 to 80	77.0
Acid detergent fibre	50 to 58	55.0
Hemicellulose	19 to 25	22.0
Cellulose	45 to 52	50.0
Lignin	4 to 6	5.0
Silica	5.0 to 14.0	13.0
Macro minerals		
Calcium	0.27 to 0.67	0.37
Magnesium	0.10 to 0.33	0.19
Phosphorus	0.02 to 0.54	0.14
Potassium	0.25 to 2.40	1.50
Sodium	0.14 to 0.30	0.20
Sulphur	0.01 to 0.07	0.04
Micro minerals	mg/kg	
Copper	3.0	
Iron	449.0	
Manganese	276.0	
Zinc	58.0	

* Data based on several references

TABLE 6. BIS Specifications for Certain Concentrate Ingredients (on % DMB).

Feedstuff	Moisture	CP		EE	CF	AIA
	Max	Min	%	Min	Max	Max
Groundnut cake (GNC)						
GNC (exp) grade 1	8	48		7	8	2.0
grade 2	8	43		6	12	2.5
GNC(extr) grade 1	8	51		-	7	2.5
grade 2	8	47		-	10	2.5

[Table Contd.]

[Table Contd.]

Cottonseed cake (CSC)					
Decorticated CSC					
„ grade 1	8	40	7	12	2.0
„ grade 2	8	35	6	15	2.5
Undecorticated CSC					
„ grade 1	8	24	7	22	2.0
„ grade 2	8	20	5	26	2.5
Rapeseed cake type 1	10	37	5	8	1.5
„ type 2	10	35	8	8	2.0
Coconut cake grade 1	11	22	6.5	12	1.5
„ grade 2	11	18	11	10	1.5
Linseed cake (LC)					
LC expeller grade HF	8	29	8	10	1.5
„ „ LF	8	31	5	10	1.2
LC (extr) sp. grade	10	33	1	9	2.5
LC(extr) grade A	10	29	1.5	11	2.5
Maize gluten grade 1	10	45	4	3	0.5
„ grade 2	10	23	3	8	0.5
Wheat bran	12.5	13	-	12	0.25
Rice polish	10	11	15	4	1.5
Calf starter meal	10	23-26	4	7	2.5
Calf growth meal	10	22-25	4	10	3.5

The minimum specified limit for molasses, the Brix value is 85 for grade 1 and 80 for grade 2 and 3 (ISI, 1958).

Availability of Feeds and Fodders and their Importance for Livestock and Poultry Production

India is blessed with the most fabulous livestock wealth in the world (Table 8). All this livestock and poultry have to be supported with only 2.4% of the world's geographical area and 4% of world's fresh water resources.

In recent times human nutritionists have highlighted the important role of animal protein in human health since a balanced diet supports an efficient immune system and promotes resistance to parasites and infectious diseases even in adults. Meat protein appears superior for stature development (Waterlow, 1998), while milk proteins have a greater effect on prenatal development and size of the newborn child (Moore, 2002).

Purchasing power often limits the amount of meat and milk consumed by the people. As disposable income increases, people tend to consume more of these commodities. The progress, prosperity and accelerated growth in economy spur the demand for animal products.

TABLE 7. Feeds and their Nutritive Value at a Glance.

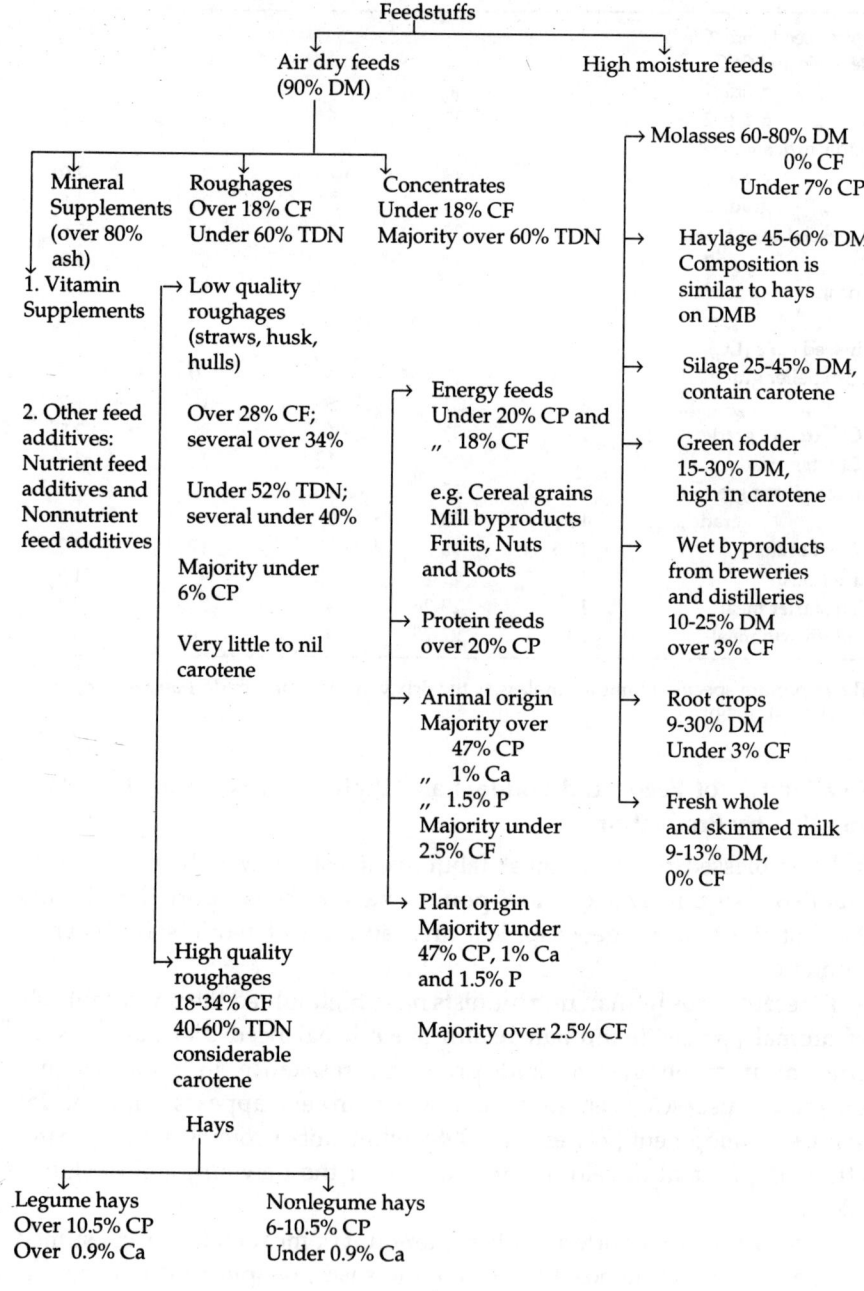

Feedstuffs

Air dry feeds
(90% DM)

High moisture feeds

→ Molasses 60-80% DM
0% CF
Under 7% CP

Mineral
Supplements
(over 80%
ash)

Roughages
Over 18% CF
Under 60% TDN

Concentrates
Under 18% CF
Majority over 60% TDN

→ Haylage 45-60% DM
Composition is
similar to hays
on DMB

1. Vitamin
Supplements

→ Low quality
roughages
(straws, husk,
hulls)

→ Silage 25-45% DM,
contain carotene

→ Energy feeds
Under 20% CP and
„ 18% CF

2. Other feed
additives:
Nutrient feed
additives and
Nonnutrient
feed additives

Over 28% CF;
several over 34%

Under 52% TDN;
several under 40%

→ Green fodder
15-30% DM,
high in carotene

e.g. Cereal grains
Mill byproducts
Fruits, Nuts
and Roots

→ Wet byproducts
from breweries
and distilleries
10-25% DM
over 3% CF

Majority under
6% CP

→ Protein feeds
over 20% CP

Very little to nil
carotene

→ Animal origin
Majority over
47% CP
„   1% Ca
„   1.5% P
Majority under
2.5% CF

→ Root crops
9-30% DM
Under 3% CF

↳ Fresh whole
and skimmed milk
9-13% DM,
0% CF

↳ Plant origin
Majority under
47% CP, 1% Ca
and 1.5% P

↳ High quality
roughages
18-34% CF
40-60% TDN
considerable
carotene

Majority over 2.5% CF

Hays

Legume hays
Over 10.5% CP
Over 0.9% Ca

Nonlegume hays
6-10.5% CP
Under 0.9% Ca

TABLE 8 Indian Livestock population in the year 2012 (in Million Numbers) and growth pattern

Species	2007	2012	% Change
Cattle	199.08	190.90	−4.10
Buffaloes	105.34	108.70	3.19
Yaks	0.083	0.077	−7.64
Mithuns	0.264	0.298	12.88
Total bovines	304.76	299.98	−1.57
Sheep	71.56	65.07	−9.07
Goats	140.54	135.17	−3.82
Horse & ponies	0.612	0.625	2.12
Camels	0.517	0.400	−22.36
Pigs	11.133	10.294	−7.54
Mules	0.137	0.196	43.07
Donkeys	0.438	0.319	−27.17
Total livestock	529.696	512.057	−3.33
Poultry	648.829	729.209	12.39
Dogs	19.08	11.67	−38.85
Rabbits	0.424	0.592	39.55

Source: 19th Livestock Census 2012 (15th October 2012 as the reference date); Animal Husbandry Statistics Division, Department of Animal Husbandry, Dairying & Fisheries, Ministry of Agriculture; elephant population increased from 1000 to 22000 during 2007 and 2012.

Feed Supply Position

Feed is an important input for milk and meat production from livestock and egg and meat production from poultry. The cost of feed constitutes 50 to 75% of production cost of livestock products. While milk production in the country is increasing, the feed and fodder resources are depleting due to increased population, urbanization and pressure on land for cereal and cash crops and for industrial and infrastructural projects. This led to qualitative and quantitative insufficiency of feeds and fodders, which is one of the main impediments for orderly development of livestock industry in India.

As early as in 1970s, National Commission on Agriculture (1976) estimated the requirements of feed and fodder vis-à-vis availability to feed the country's livestock and poultry on scientific lines. It was reported that green fodder, concentrates and dry fodder were in short supply to the tune of 38%, 44% and 40%, respectively. Scientists at National Institute of Animal Nutrition and Physiology (NIANP), Bangalore prepared a database on availability and requirements of feeds and fodder. The deficit with regard to dry fodder, green fodder and concentrates had been shown to the tune of 11, 28 and 35%, respectively (NIANP Disc, 2005).

As per the 19th livestock census (2012) India has a total livestock population of 512.05 million (Table 8).

As per the estimate of Planning Commission with the current fodder availability and requirement, in the year 2015 there will be a deficit of 63% green fodder and 23% dry fodder. With the trend in livestock growth, by 2025 there will be a shortfall of 32.6, 24.7 and 46.7 % of dry fodder, green fodder and concentrates, respectively (Ravi Kiran et al., 2012). Hence, there is a need to look for alternate feed resources, relentlessly, to sustain livestock productivity for food and nutritional security of the populace. Byproducts from agricultural, forestry, food processing industries and bio-energy sectors fulfill the need of additional concentrate feeds while those from agro-forestry systems provide the roughage component for the herbivores.

Further, the agricultural crop production in India is dominated by cereal grain production to meet the requirements of food grains for ever increasing human population. It is therefore difficult to use cereal grains for livestock farming in developing countries like India. Hence, there is a need to develop grain saving feeding system (Swaminathan, 1998) to spare cereal grains for human consumption and make the livestock farming more remunerative for farmers of low-income group.

There is a gradual shift in the cropping pattern from cereals to more remunerative fruit and horticultural crops. This results in generation of huge quantity of fruit and vegetable residues from the respective processing industries (See Table 9). These include dried apple pomace, grape pomace, dried mango peels and mangoseed kernel, citrus fruit byproducts (citrus pulp from orange, mandarin orange and lemon), tomato pomace, jack fruit residue, banana fruit byproducts, pineapple fruit residue, areca sheath, vegetable wastes from cabbage, cauliflower, carrot and turnip.

The imbalance existing between the animal numbers and the available feed resources associated with frequent exposure to drought or dry spells of 4-5 months in a year with virtually no green forage for grazing led to more dependence on crop residues, agro-industrial byproducts (AIBP) and non-conventional feed resources (NCFR) for feeding of ruminant livestock. To bridge the gap between availability and requirement of nutrients, efficient utilization of the available feedstuffs is of paramount importance. Refer chapter 17 on Feed Technology for details.

Nonforage fibre sources (NFFS)

High - fibre byproducts are generated by several food industries, and the supplies of these nonforage fibre sources (NFFS) are increasing (Table 9). NFFSs have small mean particle size and are typically low in lignin and

TABLE 9 Examples of Nonforage fibre sources (>30% NDF)*

S. No.	Product	Description / derivation
1	Brans	Consists of the fibrous components of cereal grains, but also contains portions of the germ. Most often derived from maize, wheat, rice, oats, or barley
2	Wheat middlings	A byproduct of the flour milling industry. Contains residual portions of wheat endosperm, bran, and germ.
3	Maize gluten feed	A byproduct of maize wet milling. Gluten feed consists of maize bran and others remaining after starch extraction.
4	Brewers spent grains	A byproduct of beer brewing. Primarily consists of residue from malt and grain remaining after the mashing and lautering processes.
5	Distillers grains	A byproduct of dry milling that can be derived from maize, sorghum, or any cereal grain. After production of alcohol through fermentation and mash distillation, the remaining solid residue is known as distillers grains. Often, solubles remaining after distillation of ethanol are added back to the grains, producing distillers grains with solubles.
6	Cull beans	Beans that are discoloured, shrunken, or broken; may be composed of a single type of bean or a mixture of beans including stems.
7	Hulls	The outermost seed coat of cottonseed, soybean, almond, peanut, red bean, etc.
8	Sugar beet pulp	A byproduct of sugar production. After extraction of sucrose from sliced beets, the remaining solid residue is beet pulp.
9	Fruit / vegetable pomace	The solid portion of the fruit or vegetable (especially the skin) that remains after it is pressed to remove the liquid. The common examples are apple, tomato, grape, and olive pomace
10	Cotton seed and cottonseed cake/meal	Whole linted cottonseed (the cotton seed after removal of the recoverable cotton fibre); the residue after oil extraction is cottonseed meal.
11	Palm kernel cake/meal	The residue remaining after extraction of oil from palm kernel fruit.
12	Coconut cake/meal	The residue remaining after extraction of oil from copra

*B.J.Bradford and C.R.Mullins, 2012; Journal of Dairy Science, 95: 4735-4746.

high in digestible fibre, so replacing forages with these nonforage fibre sources will decrease the physical effectiveness of NDF. This can improve energy supplied by the diet, especially if ruminal distension is restricting dry matter intake (Straws and stovers restrict the DMI due to their low digestibility). Thus they are quite useful in formulating high-energy diets for lactating dairy cows. It is imperative to bear in mind that adequate physically effective fibre (peNDF) is required to maintain rumen health and milk fat yield. Bradford and Mullins (2012) reviewed the research and summarized, with judicious use, these NFFS represents an opportunity to improve the productivity and health of cattle in all stages of lactation while potentially controlling feed costs. Studies of K.Izumi et al. (2014) showed that normal rumen function could be maintained even when a low peNDF diet that contained red bean hulls was given to dairy cows because the ruminal mat was stratified and rumination activity was not reduced.

Seaweeds

Seaweeds have a long history of use as a livestock feed (Makkar et al., 2016; Animal Feed Science and Technology, 212, 1-17). Seaweeds are macroalgae and include brown algae, red algae and green algae. They have a highly variable composition, depending on the species, time of collection and habitat, and on external conditions. They contain considerable amount of water. They may contain NPN resulting in an overestimation of their protein content. Most essential amino acids are deficient in seaweeds except the sulphur containing amino acids. Seaweeds concentrate minerals from seawater and contain 10-20 times the minerals of land plants. They contain only small amounts of lipids (1-5%), but majority of those lids are polyunsaturated n-3 and n-6 fatty acids.

Animal experiments in ruminants, pigs, poultry and rabbits reveal that some seaweeds have potential to contribute to the protein and energy requirements of livestock; seaweeds could be used as prebiotic (taking advantage of number of bioactive compounds present in them) for enhancing production and health status of both monogastric and ruminant livestock. Seaweeds tend to accumulate heavy metals (arsenic), iodine and other minerals; hence feeding such seaweeds could deteriorate animal and human health.

Chapter 15

Evaluation of Feeds for Energy for Ruminants and Nonruminants

Evaluation of Feeds in General

In Principles of Animal Nutrition we study which substances are required by animals, how these substances are supplied in feeds and the manner in which they are utilized. Evaluation of feeds is concerned with the assessment of the quantities in which nutrients are supplied by feeds as well as the assessment of the quantities in which they are required by different classes of farm animals.

The potential value of a feed for supplying a particular nutrient can be determined by chemical analysis, but the actual value of the feed to the animal can be arrived at only after making allowance for the inevitable losses that occur during digestion, absorption and metabolism. The major losses occur through faeces in the first instance. Determination of digestibility of the feed has to be done. Evaluation of feeds by digestion experiments shall be studied in Applied Nutrition I (refer chapter 2 of 3 ed Applied Nutrition Livestock, ...;).

The major organic nutrients i.e. energy and protein are required by animals as materials for the construction of body tissues, the synthesis of milk and eggs and for work production. A unifying feature of these diverse functions is that they all involve a transfer of energy - from chemical energy to heat energy (when nutrients are oxidized) or when chemical energy is converted from one form to another (when body fat is synthesized from carbohydrate). The ability of a feed to supply energy is therefore of great importance in determining its nutritive value. In the evaluation of feeds for energy, the fate of feed energy in the animal body, the measurement of energy metabolism and the expression of the energy value of feeds are discussed.

Energy is not a chemically identifiable nutrient but is a property that is realized when nurients such as amino acids, carbohydrates and lipids are oxidized during metabolism. Energy may be defined as the capacity to do work.

Evaluation of Feeds for Energy

Forms of energy: The original source of energy, the sun, or solar energy is stored in plants in the form of carbohydrates, lipids and protein through photosynthesis. This stored chemical energy becomes available to man and animals. Thus this is the form of energy which has significance in nutrition. The other forms of energy include electrical energy, thermal energy, radiant energy, nuclear/atomic energy. The animal body also absorbs solar energy from sunshine as a source of heat to warm the body, but this can not be stored in chemical form for later use as plants are able to do.

In November 1958 the NRC committee on Animal Nutrition passed a resolution to start using the calorie system, along with TDN system, to describe the energy value of feedstuffs, rations and nutrient requirements of animals.

The joule has been selected by the International System of Units and the US National Bureau of Standards as the official unit for expressing energy.

Schemes for Describing the Energy Value of Feeds

According to the first law of thermodynamics all forms of energy can be quantitatively converted into heat energy. It is convenient to express heat energy in the body as heat units.

Basic Terms

Calorie (cal):   A calorie is the amount of heat required to raise the temperature of one gram of water to 15.5°C from 14.5°C. However, since the specific heat of water changes with temperature, a calorie may be defined more precisely as 4.184 international Joules.

Kilo calorie (Kcal):   A kilo calorie is the heat required to raise temperature of 1 kg of water by 1°C. A kilo calorie is equal to 1000 calories.

Mega calorie (Mcal):   A mega calorie is equivalent to 1000 Kcal or Therm. But Mcal is the preferred term.

British Thermal Unit (BTU):   A BTU is the amount of heat required to raise 1 lb of water by 1°F. One kilo calorie approximately equals 4 BTU.
1 Kilo calorie = 4.184 KJ
1 KJ   = 0.239 Kcal

The quantity of chemical energy present in a food is measured by converting it into heat energy, and determining the heat produced.

Gross energy (GE):   Gross energy is the amount of heat given off when a substance is completely burnt/oxidized (to its ultimate oxidation products, viz, CO_2, water and other gases) in a bomb calorimeter containing 25 to 30 atmospheres of oxygen. This is also called heat of combustion (Table 1).

Measurement of GE of Feedstuffs

Bomb Calorimeter

Bomb calorimeters are of two types: The ballistic bomb calorimeter and the adiabatic bomb calorimeter.

Ballistic bomb calorimeter: The ballistic bomb calorimeter is considerably simpler, and less expensive than the adiabatic calorimeter and, inevitably, lacks some of the accuracy of the latter instrument. In the ballistic bomb calorimeter the bomb assembly is very similar to that in the adiabatic version, but without water, can or outer jacket. A known weight of a sample is ignited electrically and burned in an excess of oxygen in the bomb and the maximum temperature rise of the bomb is measured with the thermocouple and galvanometer system. By comparing this rise with standard sample of known calorific value is burnt, the calorific value of the sample material can be determined. In this case, calibration constant is calculated by combusting benzoic acid in bomb calorimeter. Calorific value of the test sample is estimated by multiplying galvanometer deflection due to the sample with calibration constant.

Adiabatic bomb calorimeter: The under-lying principle of the bomb calorimeter is simply that the material (feedstuff, faeces or urine) under test is burned, in an excess of oxygen, inside the calorimeter bomb that is immersed in a known quantity of water. The heat liberated by the combustion of the test sample warms this water and can be calculated from the increase in temperature.

The calorimeter bomb is a hollow, thick-walled stainless steel cylinder of about 300 ml capacity and fitted with a screw-on lid. The material to be tested is usually dried, and a sample of it, of about 1.0 g to 1.5 g is formed into a pellet for ease of handling. A short length of cotton thread may be included in the pellet, the free ends of which are wrapped around the ignition fuse wire to aid the initial stage of combustion. The sample pellet is then put into the bomb's crucible and connected to the fuse wire and ignition terminals. The bomb is closed and filled with oxygen to the required extent; it is then placed in a can containing an accurately determined quantity of water (usually 2 litres). The can containing the bomb and water is placed inside an outer insulating jacket.

Once an initial thermal stability has been obtained the test sample in the bomb is ignited electrically and the heat liberated by the burning sample warms the bomb, water and can. This rise in temperature is precisely mimicked by that of the water in the outer jacket, until a new temperature equilibrium is attained. The 'water equivalent/bomb equivalent' is calculated with a substance of known heat of combustion/ calorific value/ gross energy value (benzoic acid calorific value = 6324 cal/g).

Water equivalent = weight of benzoic acid ÷ rise in temperature × calorific value

Microprocessor units are available which can be attached to the adiabatic bomb calorimeter and which can automatically monitor the rise in temperature following ignition of the sample and then calculate the calorific value with virtually no intervention on the part of the operator.

Calculation of gross energy value of feed sample

Weight of empty crucible = 7.71530 g

Weight of empty crucible + feed pellet = 8.09730 g

Weight of feed sample = 0.382 g

Initial temperature = 33.276°C

Final temperature = 33.868°C

Temperature rise = 0.592°C

$$\text{Gross energy} = \frac{T \times W - (C_1 + C_2 + C_3)}{\text{Weight of the sample}} = 0.592 \times 2629 - 20 \div 0.382 \times 0.95$$

= 4.234 Kcal/ g

T = Rise in temperature; W = Bomb equivalent; C_1 = Sulphuric acid correction (12 cal); C_2 = Nitric acid correction (0.7 cal); C_3 = wire correction (7.3 cal)

Metabolic body size: Metabolic body size is defined as the weight of the animal, in kg raised to the three fourths power ($W_{kg}^{0.75}$). This may be termed 'physiological' weight while body weight is the physical weight, i.e. gravitational weight. More about basal metabolism will be dealt in applied livestock feeding. (refer chapter 3 of Applied Nutrition Livestock, ...;).

Energy Terms used in the Conventional Partition of Biological Energy (Fig. 1)

Gross energy feed intake (GE$_i$): GE$_i$ is the gross energy of the feed consumed. GE$_i$ = dry weight of feed consumed multiplied by GE of feed per unit of dry weight.

GE Losses from the Animal Body

The gross energy present in a feedstuff can not be fully utilized by an animal. A portion of it is not digested and excreted in the faeces. A portion

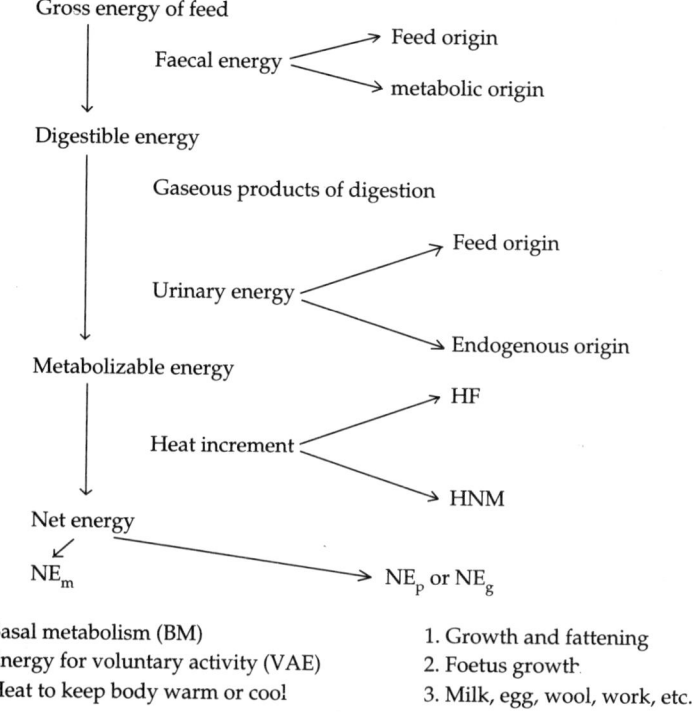

Figure 1. Conventional Scheme of Energy Utilization.

of it is lost in the form of combustible gases (methane chiefly) formed during fermentative digestion of nutrients in the gastrointestinal tract of the animal (Ruminants chiefly). A portion of it is lost in urine in the form of urea, uric acid and creatinine due to incomplete oxidation of proteins in the body. A portion of it is lost in the form of heat due to digestion and metabolism of nutrients.

Faecal energy (FE):   FE is the gross energy of the faeces. It consists of the energy content of the undigested feed and of metabolic fraction (digestive fluids and abraded mucosa) of the faeces. Faecal energy reflects undigested feed, microbial cell residue and metabolic energy from endogenous sources (FE_m). FE_m fraction is larger in producing animals since they consume more feed than comparable nonproducing animals. FE = dry weight of the faeces multiplied by GE of faeces per unit of dry weight.

Apparent digestible energy (DE): $DE = GE_i - FE$. The first loss of energy occurs in digestion is through faeces. By determining the GE of the faeces and subtracting this value from GE_i one obtains, the apparent DE. The value is labelled "apparent" because the faecal energy includes energy of undigested feed, microbial cell residues and metabolic products such as spent digestive fluids and abraded intestinal mucosa. The term 'true DE' is used to denote the value arrived at by subtracting the faecal energy of feed origin only from the GE_i. Faecal energy losses represent a substantial part of the GE_i. FE losses per unit of feed intake increase with level of feeding.

Ruminants	:	In case of roughages 40-50% of GE_i,
		In case of concentrates 20-30% of GE_i,
		Average 30-40%
Horses	:	35-40% of GE_i
Pigs	:	20% of GE_i

Gaseous products of digestion (GPD): GPD includes the combustible gases produced in the digestive tract by the fermentation of the ration. These include hydrogen, carbon dioxide, carbon monoxide, hydrogen sulphide, acetone, ethane and methane. Methane makes up the largest portion of the combustible gases produced and these reach significant proportions only in ruminants. Forbes and associates analyzed the data from 12 experimental periods in the respiration calorimeter with cattle receiving maize and lucerne, fed at levels ranging from one-half maintenance to twice maintenance and found 6.42 to 9.83% of GE was lost as methane energy. The values tended to be lower as the level of feed intake increased. Generally the energy lost as methane is of the order of 7% of GE.

In the nonruminants GPD is negligible. A substantial amount of cellulose fermentation occurs in the caecum and colon of the horse. The production of methane is less in the case of horse than in ruminants.

Determination of methane with respiration chamber is expensive and hence formulae have been developed for sheep (Swift *et al.*, 1948) and cattle (Pennsylvania workers).

Sheep E = 2.41 X + 9.80
Cattle E = 4.012 X + 17.68

Where E is methane in grams and X is digested carbohydrates in. hundreds of grams. Methane contains 13.34 Kcal per gram.

Urinary energy (UE): UE is the gross energy of the urine. It includes the energy content of the non-oxidized portion of the absorbed nitrogenous products, primarily urea in mammals and uric acid in birds and the energy contained in the endogenous fraction of the urine (UE_e). It is of the order of 2 to 3% of GE_i in pigs and 4 to 5% of GE_i in cattle. Under true energy distribution system, FE_m and UE_e are part of the maintenance requirement of the animal.

Metabolizable energy (ME): It is the portion of total energy ingested which is actually capable of transformation in the body.

Ruminants : $ME = GE_i - FE - GPD - UE$
Nonruminants $ME = GE_i - FE - UE$

Nitrogen corrected ME (ME_n): The ME value of a feed will vary according to whether amino acids it supplies are retained or are deaminated and their nitrogen excreted in the urine as urea/uric acid.

For this reason, ME values may be corrected to zero N balance (NB) by deducting for each 1 g of N retained or by adding for each 1 g of N catabolized. The values per gram are as follows:

Pigs   6.7 Kcal (28 KJ)
Poultry   8.1 Kcal (34 KJ) 34.4 KJ = 8.2216 Kcal
Ruminants   7.4 Kcal (31 KJ)
Ruminants $ME_n = GE_i - FE - GPD - UE \pm (NB \times 7.4)$

The urine loss of energy results from the excretion of incompletely oxidized nitrogenous compounds associated with protein metabolism, primarily urea, in mammals and uric acid in birds. The energy value of each gram of nitrogen excreted as urea is 23 kJ and as uric acid is 28 kJ. For this reason each gram of urinary nitrogen excreted by ruminants account for 31 kJ, in pigs 28 kJ and in poultry 34 kJ.

Heat increment (HI): It is the increase in heat production following consumption of food when the animal is in a thermoneutral environment. HI is due to heat of fermentation (HF) and heat of nutrient metabolism (HNM). Heat of fermentation is the heat produced in the digestive tract as a result of microbial action. HNM is the heat produced in intermediary metabolism of absorbed nutrients. This corresponds to the specific dynamic action/effect (SDE) or calorigenic effect or thermogenic action. Rubner coined the term SDE. The energy of HI is wasted except when the temperature of environment is below the critical temperature when it is used to keep the body warm.

Rubner's studies showed that protein caused a larger increase in heat production than either carbohydrates or fat. High protein feeds were considered 'hot' because of the size of the SDE.

The high heat increment of protein or amino acids when fed at a high level in the diet can be at least partially explained: Protein synthesis requires a large amount of energy; excretion of nitrogen products requires energy.

Research findings have suggested that heat increment can be lowered by decreasing dietary protein. For non-ruminant animals this can be accomplished by following ideal protein concept of protein feeding.

Net energy (NE): It is that energy which is available to the animal for useful purposes.

$$NE = ME - HI$$

NE includes the amount of energy used either for maintenance (NE_m) only or for maintenance plus production. NE_m is the fraction of total NE expended to keep the animal in energy equilibrium. Below the critical temperature some of the HI is also part of NE_m. NE_m for a producing animal is higher than that for a nonproducing animal of the same weight, because of changes in amounts of hormones produced and differences in voluntary activity. NE_m includes the energy required for basal metabolism, voluntary activity and to maintain body temperature.

Net energy for production (NE_p) or NE gain: NE_p is the fraction of net energy required for growth, fattening, milk, wool, work, egg, etc. production.

Basal metabolism is the minimum energy required by a non-producing animal at rest to carry on its essential processes of life, such as breathing, circulation of blood, maintenance of body temperature and repair of the daily wear and tear of body tissues.

Energy for voluntary activity (VAE) consists of the amount of energy needed in getting up, standing, moving about to obtain feed (grazing), water, etc. Heat to keep the body warm (HBW) is the additional heat needed to keep the animal's body warm when the environmental

TABLE 1. Gross Energy Values of Some Nutrients/Substances.

Nutrient/Substance	Kcal/gram
Carbohydrates	4.15
Fats	9.40
Proteins	5.65
Glucose	3.76
Sucrose	3.96
Starch	4.23
Acetic acid	3.49
Propionic acid	4.96
Butyric acid	5.35
Urea	2.53
Uric acid	2.74
Hippuric acid	5.65
Methane	13.34 (9.45 Kcal/L)

temperature is below critical temperature. Heat to keep body cool (HBC) is the extra energy expended by the animal when the body temperature is higher than that of the environment.

$$\text{Total heat production (HP)} = \text{HI} + \text{NE}_m$$
$$\text{NE}_g/\text{NE}_p \text{ or Energy retention} = \text{ME} - \text{HP}$$

Among pure nutrients fats have more than twice the energy value of carbohydrates. The primary determinant of the gross energy content of an organic substance is its **degree of oxidation,** as expressed in the ratio of carbon plus hydrogen to oxygen. For example, a carbohydrate has 50 : 50, a protein has 58 : 22, a fat has 89 : 11. Further proteins have additional oxidizable element, nitrogen and also sulphur.

There is enough oxygen present in the carbohydrate to take care of all the hydrogen present, and thus heat arises only from oxidation of the carbon. But in the case of fat, there is much less oxygen present, and combustion involves the oxidation of hydrogen as well as carbon. The burning of 1 g of hydrogen produces 34.5 Kcal heat while 1 g carbon gives 8 Kcal. Methane has a very high energy value because it consists solely of carbon and hydrogen. In protein, heat is produced from the oxidation of both carbon and hydrogen and nitrogen gives no heat at all because it is set free as such in its gaseous form.

Physiological fuel values (PFVs): These are the calorific values originally established by W.O. Atwater (1902) for use in human nutrition to calculate the portion of gross energy which is available for transformation in the body. This has a similar significance as metabolisable energy. These are derived by multiplying the gross energy values with their digestibility coefficients. In the case of protein, 1.25 Kcal per gram was subtracted from GE of protein as an allowance for the loss of energy through urine.

Nutrient	GE Kcal/g*	Digestibility coefficients		PFV Kcal/g	
Carbohydrate	4.15	×	98	=	4.0
Fat	9.40	×	95	=	9.0
Protein	(5.65-1.25)=4.4	×	92	=	4.0

*Whereas the energy value of carbohydrates or fats absorbed by animals equals their heats of combustion determined in the calorimeter, the energy value of absorbed protein is lower than its heat of combustion because of the energy lost in nitrogen-containing constituents excreted with the urine.

In the case of protein a subtraction of 5.3 kJ or 1.25 Kcal has to be made from the GE content of 1g of protein (23.7 kJ or 5.65 Kcal) for the energy lost in urine.

These values are not applicable to feeds of farm animals because the digestibility coefficients of carbohydrates, fats and proteins are very high and based on human diets; the factor 1.25 was obtained from studies with human beings eating mixed diet; this figure is too low to estimate the urine loss in the herbivores because of the relatively large amounts of hippuric acid excreted.

Total digestible nutrients (TDN): It is a measure of apparent digestible energy, but it is expressed in units of weight or per cent rather than energy *per se.* It is the most widely used expression of energy system in the 20th century. Digestibility coefficients are used to compute the TDN. Digestible EE is multiplied by 2.25 since its energy is 2.25 times of carbohydrates.

$$TDN = DCP + DCF + DNFE + (DEE \times 2.25)$$

Examples:

	Proximate Principle	%	Dig. Coe.	Digestible nutrient	TDN
1.	CP	20.11	75.0	15.08	
	CF	16.25	73.9	12.01	
	NFE	40.99	80.6	33.03	64.16%
	EE	3.34	53.9 (1.8×2.25)	4.04	
2.	CP	18.2	72	13.1	
	CF	25.0	63	15.8	80.2%
	NFE	27.5	59	16.2	
	EE	18.4	85	15.6	

Nutritive ratio (NR): It is the ratio of the digestible protein to the sum of digestible carbohydrates and fat, the latter being multiplied by 2.25. It is also called albuminoid ratio sometimes. It is computed in recognition of the fact that protein serves some special functions in the animal body, which can not be performed by the digestible nonprotein nutrients present in the TDN. Feeds richer in protein have narrow nutritive ratios (GNC = 1:0.7), while feeds poor in protein content have wide nutritive ratio. It is usual to consider that rations with wide nutritive ratio (1:9) are suitable for idle horses and cattle; a medium ratio (1:6) for early fattening, lactation, working animals, etc. and a narrow ratio (1:0.7) for young stock.

Example 1. Calculation of NR of groundnut cake (GNC):

DCP = 42   ;   DEE = 6
DCF = 1   ;   DNFE = 14.5

$$NR = \frac{DEE \times 2.25 + DNFE + DCF}{DCP} = \frac{TDN - DCP}{DCP}$$

$$= \frac{(6 \times 2.25) + 14.5 + 1}{42}$$

$$= \frac{29}{42}$$

$$= 0.70 \quad \text{A narrow nutritive ratio of } 1{:}0.7$$

Example 2: Calculation of NR of maize grain:

Maize has 82% TDN and 7% DCP.

$$NR = \frac{TDN - DCP}{DCP} = \frac{82 - 7}{7} = \frac{75}{7} = 10.7$$

A wide nutritive of 1:10.7. It means that for each kg of DCP, maize contains 10.7 kg digestible nonprotein nutrients.

Calorie Protein Ratio or Energy Protein Ratio

It is defined as the ME (Kcal) per kg divided by the percentage of crude protein in the ration. It is of paramount importance in poultry, swine as well as ruminants for efficient feed utilization.

Nutrient to Calorie Ratio

It is found logical to express nutrients in weight per unit of energy needed. Examples: g protein/1000 Kcal ME; available lysine/1000 Kcal ME; g Ca/1000 Kcal ME; mg riboflavin/1000 Kcal ME.

Nutritive Value Index (NVI)

The feeding value of roughage depends on its digestible nutrients as well as on its voluntary intake. Crampton and his coworkers in Canada evolved the term nutritive value index in 1960. NVI is obtained by multiplying the intake relative to some defined standard forage which is given a value of 100 and TDN value of the roughage. The consumption of standard forage is 80 g per kg metabolic body size. If the daily dry matter intake of a test roughage is 1.1 kg for a ram of 50 kg body weight, then the consumption of the roughage per kg metabolic body size is $1.1/50^{0.75} = 1.1/18 = 58.5$ g. The relative intake of the test roughage is $58.5 \times 100/80 = 73$ per cent. The TDN of the test roughage is 60 per cent. Then

$$NVI = \frac{73 \times 60}{100} = 43.8\%$$

True Metabolizable Energy Value of Feeds for Poultry

Chemical evaluation of feedstuffs must be backed up by biological methods and the three basic measures of the energy value of diets/rations and of feedstuffs are DE, ME and NE. For most animals DE is easiest to determine. With avain species, however, it is more convenient to determine the ME of a diet by treating the excreta (faeces and urine) as a single material representing the unutilized portion of the feed energy.

Different methods are used for measurement of ME of feedstuffs. Determining the ME value of a feed ingredient involves the feeding of two diets to two groups of chicks. One is a reference diet containing a high proportion of glucose (45.7%) and the other, test diet containing the ingredient (40%) to be studied, substituted for part of glucose. Both the diets have a premix of 54.3% which supplies other nutrients. The diets are fed for 15 days and collection of excreta are made during the last four days. Chromic oxide indicator method or total excreta collection method may be used to determine the ME of the diet.

The true ME (TME) value developed by Sibbald and coworkers is another method. Adult cockerels are starved for 34 hours and are force-fed a fixed amount of the test feed ingredient. Excreta are collected over the next 24 hour period. Excreta are also collected from a starved cockerel of similar body weight. Both the dried excreta and the test feed ingredient are assayed for gross energy. The energy voided by the starved cockerel is used as the correction for endogenous and metabolic energy ($UE_e + FE_m$). The energy of these endogenous losses is deducted from the energy of the excreta of the fed-birds. Thus TME value of test feed ingredient is estimated.

TME for poultry = Gross energy of the feed – Gross energy of the excreta of feed origin

Factors for Interconversion TDN to DE; DE to ME

In 1947, B.H. Schneider gave the formula: 1kg TDN = 4.38 Mcal DE. In 1957 Crampton and associates and R.W. Swift carried out studies with swine and sheep and cattle, respectively. Both digestible energy and total digestible nutrients were measured.

$$1 \text{ kg TDN} = 4.41 \text{ Mcal DE}$$

This value is somewhat variable according to species and type of ration, but this variation is small.

A factor 0.82 is used to calculate ME from the DE of the feedstuff/ration in ruminants. Ratio of ME to DE varies little from mean values of 0.82 for roughages, 0.85 for cereals and 0.79 for oilcakes and meals. NRC has adopted factor 0.82; ME = 0.82 DE. For pigs ME = 0.96 DE. But for fibrous feeds that give rise to methane in the hind gut of the pig, the factor is 0.90 rather than 0.96. 1 kg TDN = 3.616 Mcal ME.

Example 1: Calculation of Digestible Energy

Proximate principle	%	Av. calorific value /g	GE Kcal	Dig. Coe (%)	Digestible energy, Kcal
CP	10	5.65	56.5	75	42.5
EE	3	9.40	28.2	90	25.4
CF	10	4.15	41.5	50	20.8
NFE	65	4.15	269.8	90	242.8
Ash	2				
Water	10				
Total	100		396.0		331.5
Per gram			3.96		3.32

Example 2: Calculation of Metabolizable Energy of Feeds for Sheep

Feed	Dry matter eaten per day per head, kg	Intake Food per kg	Faeces	Urine	Methane	Metabolizable Energy, Mcal
Soybean hay	0.795	4.333	2.033 DE=2.3	0.196	0.208	1.896
Soybean straw	0.674	4.345	2.676 DE=1.669	0.042	0.229	1.398

Example 3: An Example of an Actual Energy Balance

Partitioning of the energy of grass within the animal

Dry matter intake	=	1.829 kg	
Gross energy intake	=	35.0 MJ	(1 MJ = 0.239 Mcal)
Faecal energy	=	13.5 MJ	
Urinary energy	=	1.2 MJ	
Methane energy	=	2.4 MJ	
Heat increment (HI)	=	7.0 MJ	

Nutritive value of feed

Digestible energy $= \dfrac{35.0 - 13.5}{1.829} = 11.8$ MJ / kg

ME $= \dfrac{35.0 - (13.5 + 1.2 + 2.4)}{1.829} = 9.8$ MJ / kg

$$NE = \frac{35.0 - (13.5 + 1.2 + 2.4 + 7.0)}{1.829} = 6.0 \text{ MJ} / \text{kg}$$

Net energy: H.B. Armsby (1921) coined this term and defined it as "the metabolizable energy minus the expenditure of energy by the body which results from the ingestion of food".

$$NE = ME - HI$$

Energy Value of Maize and Oats for Young Swine

	GE	DE	ME	ME_n	NE
		Mcal/kg, dry basis			
Maize	3.96	3.43	3.32	3.16	2.33
Oats	4.13	2.84	2.73	2.59	1.40

Note: The difference in DE values reflect the indigestibility of the fibre in oats and this high fibre level resulted in the low ME and NE values due to the greater GPD and heat increment losses.

Heat increment (HI) is subject to many variables. These include the nature of the ration (proportion of roughage), nature of the feedstuff (content of crude fibre), purpose for which it is fed (maintenance, lactation, etc). A value measured at the maintenance level in a warm environment is not a suitable measure of maintaining an animal in a cold climate because below the critical temperature some of the HI is part of the NE_m. A value measured at maintenance does not apply to productive functions. So specific NE values have been set up for maintenance (NE_m), growth (NE_g) and lactation (NE_l) in the NRC reports. Energy value of selected feeds is presented to illustrate these things.

Energy Value of Selected Feedstuffs (on DMB)

Feedstuff	GE	DE	ME	NE_m	NE_g	NE_l
	←			Mcal / kg		→
Alfalfa hay	3.89	2.51	2.03	1.35	0.49	1.25
Maize grain	4.41	4.01	3.43	2.28	1.48	2.42
Cottonseed meal	4.84	3.47	2.56	1.81	1.20	1.12

* FE and HI are considerably larger in roughages (35-41%) than for concentrates (6 to 28% of GE).

* The percentage of ME lost as HI for growing cattle (NE_g) for roughages is 71 to 76%; concentrates, it is 55 to 68%.

* HI losses were considerably less when the ME was utilized for maintenance (NE_m) or lactation (NE_l).

Formulae for true digestible, metabolizable and net energy are presented in the following. These apply to ruminants and need to be modified to nonruminants.

$$TDE = GE_i - (FE-FE_m) - GPD - HF$$
$$TME = GE_i - (FE-FE_m) - GPD - HF - (UE-UE_e)$$
$$TNE = GE_i - (FE-FE_m) - GPD - HF - (UE-UE_e) - HNM$$
$$TNE_m = BM + VAE + FE_m + UE_e$$

Efficiency of utilization of energy

Energy is utilized differently according to its source and the species and weight of the animal. Net energy considers the amount of energy used in digestion and deducts this from ME to leave the amount available for growth and maintenance of the animal. The main difference between the NE system and the DE and ME systems is that the NE system considers the amount of heat lost during digestion and subsequent deposition of nutrients in protein and adipose tissue. This point is illustrated in Table 2, which lists the DE, ME, and NE of several commonly used ingredients. When used in conjunction with digestible available amino acids and the ideal protein concept, a net energy system will allow the nutritionist to formulate diets that provide the animal with the energy and amino acids that it needs for efficient and predictable growth and carcass performance.

TABLE 2 Digestible, metabolizable and net energy values of selected ingredients for swine*

Feed ingredient	DE, kcal/kg	ME, kcal/kg	NE, kcal/kg	ME:DE	NE:ME
Maize	3390	3310	2650	0.98	0.80
Wheat	3310	3210	2510	0.97	0.78
Barley	3070	2970	2280	0.97	0.78
Wheat middlings	2650	2530	1830	0.95	0.72
Field peas	3320	3160	2320	0.95	0.73
Soybean meal (48%)	3520	3210	1940	0.91	0.60
Canola meal	2760	2530	1510	0.92	0.60
Tallow	7964	7914	7104	0.99	0.90

Source: Sauvant et al., 2004

DE and ME energy analysis systems overestimate the value of feeds high in fibre or protein and underestimate ingredients rich in starch and fats.

NE provides the closest estimate of the true energy available for maintenance and production purposes.

The efficiency of ME conversion to NE depends on the interaction of 3 factors:

1. The nature of the chemical compounds in which the ME is contained.

2. The purpose for which ME is used by the animal (maintenance or production)

3. The level or intensity of production.

* Structural carbohydrates like cellulose need more energy for their digestion and metabolism than any other nutrient.

* Proteins need less than cellulose, but still more than sugars and starch, while fats and oils generate the least heat increment.

* A feed high in fibre (e.g. alfalfa meal) or in protein (sunflower meal) will lose a greater proportion of its ME as heat than will a feed high in starch (maize) or in fat (full-fat soybean meal). This fact justifies the recommendation of feeding diets high in fibre during winter and rich in fat during summer.

* Less heat is generated and so the efficiency is higher (80%) when it is used for maintenance than when it is directed to growth (70%) or milk production 72%).

* The higher the intensity of production, the better the usage of ME.
* Separate NE values apply for maintenance, growth and lactation.

Example 4:　Calculation of net energy of a roughage for maintenance from metabolisable energy data.

Data :　Dry matter of feed　　　　　　=　　3.79 kg

Metabolizable energy　　　　=　　10508 Kcal

Heat production,
maintenance period　　　=　　9803 Kcal

Heat production,
fasting condition　　　　=　　7790 Kcal

Calculations:

Heat increment　(HI)　　　　　=　　2013 Kcal

$$NE = \frac{ME - HI}{DM \text{ of feed}} = \frac{10508 - 2013}{3.79}$$

$$= 2241 \ \text{Kcal/kg DM}$$

Example 5: Calculation of NE value of a feed for fattening cattle.

Ration	DM fed, kg	ME Mcal	Heat Production Mcal	Energy retained by the animal Mcal
Maintenance plus fattening	12.691	23.14	18.9	4.24
Maintenance plus slow growth	9.620	17.64	15.62	2.02
Difference	3.071	5.50	3.28	2.22

$$NE/kg\ DM\ =\ \frac{5.50 - 3.28}{3.071} = 0.723\ Mcal$$

$$= 723\ Kcal$$

Direct and Indirect Calorimetry

In order to study the extent to which the ME of the feed is utilized by the animal, it is necessary to measure either the animal's heat production (HP) or its energy retention (NE_p/NE_g)

$$NE = ME - HI\ ;\ HP = HI + NE_m$$
$$NE_p = ME - HP$$

NE
NE_g/NE_p NE_m

Heat production is due to oxidation of food constituents and oxidation of fat and protein liberated from body tissues. HP can be measured directly with the help of an animal calorimeter. This process is known as direct calorimetry. HP can also be estimated from the respiratory exchange of the animal using a respiration chamber. This approach is one of indirect calorimetry. Respiration chambers can also be used to estimate energy retention rather than heat production by calculating the carbon and nitrogen balance.

Direct calorimetry: The heat produced by an animal can be measured directly in a respiration calorimeter or animal calorimeter. Lavoisier was the first to recognize that animal heat is produced by oxidations in the body. Lavoisier and Laplace (1780) devised the first animal calorimeter to measure this heat, using a guinea pig as the subject. The animal was enclosed in a chamber surrounded by ice and the amount of ice melted in a given period of time was recorded as a measure of the amount of heat given off by the animal. More precise animal calorimeters were later developed replacing the ice with water (Adiabatic type). The latest type is known as the gradient-layer calorimeter and is so constructed that the average temperature gradient between the inner and outer spaces is proportionate to the total heat produced by the animal.

Respiration calorimeter combines the features of a respiration chamber and a calorimeter. The first accurate respiration calorimeter was constructed by Rubner in 1881 for dogs. Atwater and Rosa constructed one for human beings in 1897. It was equipped with a bed, desk, chair and a bycycle. Later Armsby built a respiration calorimeter for large animals. This calorimeter is preserved as an antique at Pennsylvania State University. In the respiration calorimeter it is possible to account for the intake of feed, water and oxygen and the outgo of solid, liquid and gaseous excreta and of the heat eliminated.

It is assumed that the quantity of heat lost from the animal is equal to the quantity produced. Heat is lost from the body principally by radiation, conduction and convection from the body surface (sensible heat loss) and by evaporation of water from the skin and lungs (evaporative heat loss).

The animal calorimeter/respiration calorimeter is an air tight chamber and has a special insulated construction which prevents the chamber from gaining or losing heat. The heat loss of the animal kept in the chamber is measured by the rise in temperature of the cold water flowing in various pipes (see the example 6). In the adiabatic type the rate of flow of the water and differences in the temperatures at the entry and exit are used for calculation of heat loss. In addition to metabolism trial, CO_2 and CH_4 are accounted. Daily energy balance of the animal can be calculated from the data of the respiration calorimeter.

The heat increment of the test feed is determined as the difference in the heat production of the animal at two levels of intake. Two levels are needed because a part of the animal's heat production is contributed by its basal metabolism and it is assumed that the basal metabolism remain the same. The increase in heat production at higher intake is attributed to the heat increment of the extra feed given to the animal.

It is also possible to make the lower level of intake zero, and to estimate the heat increment as the difference in heat production between the basal (or fasting) metabolism and that produced in the fed animal. Measurement of heat production by direct calorimetry is very expensive. Therefore indirect methods are used. That is respiration calorimeter has been replaced by respiration chamber.

Indirect Calorimetry by the Measurement of Respiratory Exchange (Respiratory Quotient)

The substances which are oxidized in the body, and whose energy is converted into heat, fall mainly into three classes: carbohydrates, fats and proteins. The overall reaction for the oxidation of a carbohydrate (glucose) is:

$$C_6 H_{12} O_6 + 6 O_2 \quad \rightarrow 6 CO_2 + 6 H_2O - \Delta H \text{ (675 Kcal per mole)}$$

and for the oxidation of fat (stearic acid) is:

$$CH_3(CH_2)_{16} COOH + 26 O_2 \quad \rightarrow 18 CO_2 + 18 H_2O - \Delta H \text{ (2711 Kcal per mole)}$$

one gram-molecule of oxygen occupies 22.4 litres at NTP. Thus in an animal obtaining all its energy by the oxidation of glucose, the utilization of one litre of oxygen would lead to production of $2820 \div 6 \times 22.4 = 20.98$ KJ (5.014 Kcal) of heat. This value is known as **thermal equivalent of oxygen** and is used in indirect calorimetry to estimate heat production from oxygen consumption. The thermal equivalents of oxygen vary with the nutrients and their mixtures. Animals oxidize a mixture of these nutrients. In order to apply the appropriate thermal equivalent when converting oxygen consumption to heat production it is necessary to know how much of the oxygen is used for each nutrient. The proportions are calculated from what is known as the respiratory quotient (RQ).

Respiratory quotient: This is the ratio between the volume of CO_2 produced by the animal and the volume of O_2 used. Under the same conditions of temperature and pressure, equal volumes of gases contain equal numbers of molecules. So the RQ can be calculated from the

TABLE 3. An Example of Calculation of Heat Production of a Calf from Respiratory Exchange and Urinary N Excretion (Blaxter *et al.*, 1955. J. Agric. Sci., Camb., 45, 10).

Oxygen consumed	392 L	
CO_2 produced	310.7 L	
Urinary N excreted	14.8 g	
Heat from protein metabolism.*		
Protein oxidized	14.8×6.25	92.5 g
Heat produced	92.5×4.3 Kcal	398.8 Kcal
Oxygen used	92.5×0.96	88.8 L
CO_2 produced	92.5×0.77	71.2 L
Heat from carbohydrate and fat metabolism		
Oxygen used	392 - 88.8	303.2 L
CO_2 produced	310.7 - 71.2	239.5 L
Non-protein RQ		0.79
Thermal equivalent of O_2 at RQ 0.79		4.789 Kcal/L
(From the table)		
Heat produced	303.2×4.789	1452 Kcal
Total heat produced	$398.8 + 1452 =$	1850.8 Kcal

*In the combustion of one gram of protein 0.96 litre of O_2 is used and 0.77 litre of CO_2 is produced.

molecules of CO_2 produced and O_2 used. So RQ for glucose is 6 CO_2 ÷ 6O_2 = 1 and that of the fat is 18 CO_2 ÷ 26 O_2 = 0.692. Similarly for protein (alanine) the reaction is (complete oxidation)

$$4\ CH_3\ CH(NH_2)\ COOH + 15\ O_2 \rightarrow 12\ CO_2 + 14\ H_2O + 2\ N_2 - \Delta H\ (388\ Kcal/mole)$$

and the RQ is 0.83. In the body, however, nitrogen is excreted as urea and small amounts of other incompletely oxidized compounds, such as hippuric acid, creatinine, allantoin, ammonium salts, uric acid, etc. Considering urea as the principal incompletely oxidized product, the reaction is

$$4\ CH_3\ CH\ (NH_2)\ COOH + 12\ O_2 \rightarrow 10\ CO_2 + 10\ H_2O +$$
$$2\ CO\ (NH_2)_2 - \Delta H\ (312\ Kcal/mole)$$

and the RQ is 0.83. If the RQ of an animal is known, the proportions of fat and carbohydrates oxidized can be determined from standard tables. Further, it gives an approximate idea of the kind of nutrient which is being burned in the body. The closer the quotient approaches unity, the larger the proportion of carbohydrates being used, while values lying close to 0.7 indicate the fat being used, RQs considerably higher than unity may be obtained when **carbohydrate is being converted into fat.** RQs of 1.4 and higher are reported in rapidly fattening hogs while RQs below 0.7 have been observed in fasting, particularly in hibernating animals, which may be the result of the **conversion of fat into carbohydrate.**

Example 6: Example of use of Direct calorimetry to obtain heat production per day of a human subject (Data from respiration calorimeter experiment)

Data:

Volume of water through heat exchange coil system	2000 L
Average temperature of water at inlet	18.5°C
Average temperature of water at outlet	19.1°C
Increase in weight of the absorber containing sulphuric acid	1256 g

Calculations:

Heat removed by exchange coil	=	2000 × 0.6°C
	=	1200 Kcal
Heat removed by evaporation (585 calories is heat eliminated by evaporation of 1g of water at 20°C, the temperature at which calorimeter was maintained)	=	1256 × 0.585
	=	735 Kcal

Total heat production per day   =   1200 + 735 = 1935 Kcal

Heat is produced not only when organic nutrients are oxidized but also when they are used for synthesis of tissue materials. It has been found, however, that the quantities of heat produced during these synthesis bear the same relation to the respiratory exchange as they do when the nutrients are completely oxidized.

Apparatus for Measuring Respiratory Exchange

The apparatus most commonly used for farm animals is a respiration chamber. The determination of gaseous exchange can also be carried out by the use of a face piece which provides for the analysis of the inspired and expired air. The animal is fitted with a face mask which is connected through a rubber tubing to the 'Douglas bag'. This bag is an air tight container used for collecting the exhaled air. The samples of inspired air and expired air are analysed for oxygen and carbon dioxide to calculate the heat production. The use of the chamber makes possible an accounting for the water lost as perspiration and for the intestinal gases produced as well as the pulmonary exchange.

Two types of chambers are devised; the closed-circuit type designed by Regnault and Reiset and the open-air current type developed by Pettenkofer. **The closed-circuit type** derived its name since the same air is continuously circulated, with provision for the removal of the waste products and the addition of oxygen. It consists of an airtight container for the animal together with vessels holding absorbents for carbon dioxide and water vapour. The oxygen of the circulating air is renewed through a meter. The output of CO_2 and water is determined by recording the increase in weight of the absorbing vessels. Any methane produced can be measured by sampling and analysing the air at the start and at the close of experiment. The main disadvantage of the closed-circuit chamber is that large quantities of absorbents are required. A cow needs 100 kg of soda lime to absorb CO_2 and 250 kg of silica gel to absorb water vapour per day (Example 7).

Example 7: Example of use of indirect calorimetry for obtaining hourly heat production (10 minute test with closed circuit apparatus; face mask type).

Data:

Decrease in weight of O_2 cylinder	= 3.293 g
Increase in weight of CO_2 adsorption unit	= 3.703 g

Calculations:

Vol of CO_2	= 3.703 × 0.5094	= 1.886 L
Vol of O_2	= 3.293 × 0.6998	= 2.304 L

$$R.Q = \frac{1.886}{2.304} = 0.819$$

Thermal equivalent of 1 litre O_2 at R.Q. 0.819 =   4.824 Kcal

Calories per 10 minutes = 4.824 × 2.304   =   11.11 Kcal

Total heat production per hour   =   66.66 Kcal

(1 g CO_2 = 0.5094 L ; 1g O_2 = 0.6998 L)

(only carbohydrate and fat metabolism is taken into account)

In the open-air current type, air is drawn through the chamber at a metered rate and sampled for analysis on entry and exit. Thus CO_2 production, CH_4 production and O_2 consumption can be estimated. Here accurate measures of gas flow and composition are required. With the availability of modern equipment based on infra-red analysis, **open-air current type chambers have largely replaced the closed-circuit.** Measurements of respiratory exchange have now been greatly enhanced by the development of automated systems.

In respiration calorimetry, heat production is estimated, and energy retention is calculated as the difference between ME intake and heat production.

Measurement of Energy Retention by the Carbon and Nitrogen Balance Technique

Here energy retention is estimated directly and heat production is calculated by difference.

The main forms in which energy is stored by the growing and fattening animal are protein and fat, since the carbohydrate (glycogen) reserves of the body are small and relatively constant. The quantities of protein and fat stored can be estimated by carrying out a carbon and nitrogen balance trial. The energy retained can then be calculated by multiplying the quantities of nutrients stored by their calorific values.

Determinations are made of the N and C in the feed, faeces and urine and of the carbon in the gaseous output. Prior to 1870, Henneberg began experiments with farm animals following the studies of Voit and associates with humans. Respiration chamber for large animals was built at the Mockern Experiment Station (Germany) under the direction of Gustav Kuhn and his successor, O. Kellner carried out many experiments which led him to present starch equivalents. An example of carbon and nitrogen balance is given below for a steer.

Calculation of Carbon and Nitrogen Balance

Amount		Nitrogen(g)		Carbon(g)	
		Intake	Outgo	Intake	Outgo
Feed :	6.988 kg hay	56.4	-	2831.7	-
	0.400 kg linseed meal	21.9	-	172.6	-
Excreta:					
	16.619 kg faeces	-	33.5	-	1428.7
	4.357 kg urine	-	32.4	-	124.2
	37 g brushings	-	1.3	-	8.0
	4.730 kg CO_2	-	-	-	1290.2
	142 g CH_4	-	-	-	106.6
	Total	78.3	67.2	3004.3	2957.7
	Gain in carbon	46.6 g;		Gain in nitrogen 11.1 g	

The calculation revealed that the animal gained 11.1 g nitrogen. Body protein contains 16.65% nitrogen, hence the gain of protein is $11.1 \times 100 \div 16.65 = 66.6$ g. But this protein is known to contain 52.54% carbon, hence the carbon used for this protein is $66.6 \times 52.54 \div 100 = 35$ g. The total gain of carbon was 46.6 and the amount of carbon available for fat formation is $46.6 - 35 = 11.6$ g. Since fat contains 76.5% carbon, the gain of fat is $11.6 \times 100 \div 76.5 = 15.2$ g. From the C and N balance data, it has been calculated that 66.6 g of protein and 15.2 g of fat are formed in the body. Energy retention can be calculated by multiplying them with their respective calorific values viz. $(66.6 \times 5.64) + (15.2 \times 9.39) = 518$ Kcal. If ME intake is known, subtraction of energy retention from ME gives heat production of the animal.

The advantage of the carbon and nitrogen balance technique is measurement of oxygen consumption or RQ not required.

With the advent of respiration chambers for measuring heat production directly, the carbon and nitrogen balance has assumed less importance in energy studies.

Comparative slaughter method/technique is also useful for measuring energy retention. The gain of energy by the animal in the form of protein and fat can directly be determined by slaughter of the animal and determining the gross energy of the carcass in the beginning and end of the trial.

To summarise, HP is measured with the help of animal calorimetry; HP is measured in indirect calorimetry with the help of respiration chamber (oxygen consumption of the animal multiplied by the thermal equivalent (4.852 Kcal per litre) of oxygen at RQ 0.82), carbon and nitrogen balance, comparative slaughter technique and by the Brouwer equation.

Brouwer (1965) equation

HP kJ $\quad$ = $\quad$ $16.18 \times O_2$ (L) $+ 5.02 \times CO_2$ (L) $- 2.17 \times CH_4$ (L) $-$
$\quad\quad\quad\quad\quad$ 5.99 x urine N(g)

HP $\quad\quad$ = $\quad$ Heat production, kJ
O_2 $\quad\quad$ = $\quad$ Oxygen consumption, L
CO_2 $\quad\quad$ = $\quad$ Carbon dioxide production, L
N $\quad\quad$ = $\quad$ Urinary nitrogen excretion, g

For poultry, N is 1.2 as poultry excreta N in the more oxidized from of uric acid, rather than urea.

This formula may be applied to ruminants, nonruminants and birds; however, nonruminants and birds produce little CH_4, so the CH_4 component may be left out.

Calculation of heat production - An example

Twelve mature female dry sheep (62.3±2.3kg body weight) (n = 4 per group) were used to determine gas exchange and C–N balances. Diet was a mix of 130 gram barley grain and 870 gram alfalfa hay/kg. They were fed at three levels, approximately 1, 1.5 and 2 x metabolizable energy for maintenance (MEm; 374 kJ/kg$^{0.75}$). Sheep were allocated in individual cages. After the adaptation period, a 5-day collection period was followed. During this period, gas exchange was measured for each treatment during 15 min/h per sheep and repeated each 3h during 24 h (8 measures/d with 4 sheep/h) using open-circuit respirometry attached to the sheep by a face mask. The calculations (Table 4) revealed that HP determined by the Brouwer equation (RQ method) was in agreement with the estimation by CN method. Both the methods gave no significant different values accounting for 407 and 410 kJ/kg$^{0.75}$ BW/d, as average for CN and RQ methods, respectively.

Starch Equivalents or Starch Values

O. Kellner, a German Scientist put forward his concept of starch equivalent in 1905 before Armsby suggested net energy values. Starch equivalent (SE) is essentially the same as net energy value of feeds. Armsby determined net energy values near maintenance while Kellner measured the values above maintenance using carbon and nitrogen balance methods. So Kellner's values were for body fat production. NE is expressed in terms of calories while the SE is expressed in terms of kg starch which is regarded to be a source of net energy to the animal. Kellner objected to the TDN because it did not measure the energy actually available to the animal, since it neglected metabolic processes in which energy escaped in the urine and also as wasted heat.

TABLE 4   Determination of heat production per day in female dry sheep under three ME intake levels* (Daily energy balance [kJ/kg$^{0.75}$ BW] and Carbon - Nitrogen balance [g/kg$^{0.75}$ BW]

Method of calculation	Low	Medium	High
Brouwer (1965) equation			
Gross energy intake	1219.5	1330.6	1461.1
Energy in faeces	704.3	662.7	617.6
Energy in urine	33.6	37.0	38.0
Energy in methane (39.54 kJ/L)	29.2	36.9	42.1
Metabolizable energy intake (MEI)	452.4	593.9	763.3
Heat production (HP)**	379.8	404.4	445.5
Retained Energy = MEI - HP	72.6	189.6	317.9
Carbon - Nitrogen balance			
Nitrogen intake	1.6	1.65	1.81
Nitrogen in faeces	0.88	0.79	0.76
Nitrogen in urine	0.63	0.69	0.71
Nitrogen retained	0.09	0.16	0.33
Carbon intake	26.75	31.12	33.78
Carbon in faeces	17.52	16.07	15.16
Carbon in urine	0.59	0.75	0.66
Carbon in carbon dioxide	6.59	10.00	11.06
Carbon in methane	0.53	0.67	0.76
Carbon retained	1.52	3.63	6.14
Retained energy of protein (RE$_{protein}$)	13.0	24.4	50.0
Retained energy of fat (RE$_{fat}$)	66.3	165.7	269.9
Retained Energy = REprotein + REfat	79.3	190.1	319.9
HP = MEI - RE	373.1	403.9	443.4

* C.Fernandez, M.C.Lopez and M.Lachica, 2012, Animal Feed Science and Technology, 178: 115-119;
** HP was calculated as kJ = 16.18 × O$_2$ (L) + 5.02 × CO$_2$ (L) – 2.17 × CH$_4$ (L) – 5.99xurine N (g) (Brouwer, 1965 equation); Protein has 0.16 N, 0.52 C and 23.86 kJ/g; fat has 0.767 C and 39.76 kJ/g; REprotein = N balance (g) x 6.25 x 23.86; REfat = (C balance [g] - N balance [g] × 6.25 × 0.52) × 1.304 × 39.76

Kellner added pure carbohydrate, protein and fat to a maintenance ration and thus determined the relative amounts of these pure digestible nutrients required to produce a unit of body fat. The SE of a feed is expressed as the amount of feed required to produce as much animal fat as produced by one unit of starch when fed over and above the maintenance requirement. The values were called 'Starch equivalents' or 'Starch values'. For example, maize grain has a SE of 81 kg which means that 100 kg of maize grain can produce as much animal fat as 81 kg of pure starch when fed in addition to maintenance ration. A series of factors were established for the fat producing powers of these nutrients.

Carbohydrates :	Starch	1.0
	Fibre	1.0
Proteins		0.94
Fat (roughages)		1.90
Fat (cereals)		2.10
Fat (oil cakes)		2.40

1 Kg TDN = 0.869 Kg SE

When Kellner tested feedstuffs instead of pure nutrients, he found that the fat producing power was less than calculated from their content of digestible nutrients and the discrepancy was larger with those feeds high in fibre.

Kellner, therefore, instituted two types of correction factors:

1. The Werticeit or Value number for concentrates: The digestible nutrients are multiplied by a 'Value number' or Golden number. This ranges from 95 to 100.
2. The fibre correction for roughages: For every 1% CF present in the original feed, 0.58 units of SE are deducted in case of ordinary (long form) dry roughages, 0.29 units of SE are deducted in case of chaffed dry roughages, 0.29 to 0.58 units are deducted in case of green fodders with 4 to 16 or more % CF.

Calculation of SE of Feedstuffs

Example 1: Calculate the Starch Equivalent of barley for the following data (value no. of barley is 98). 100 kg barely contains 7.6 kg DCP, 1.2 kg DEE, 60.9 kg DNFE and 2.5 kg DCF.

Solution:

Nutrient	% Factor		SE
DCP	7.6 × 0.94	=	7.14
DEE	1.2 × 2.10	=	2.52
DNFE	60.9 × 1.00	=	60.90
DCF	2.5 × 1.00	=	2.50
			73.06

Calculated SE = 73.06
Value No. of barley = 98

Corrected SE of barley $= 73.06 \times \dfrac{98}{100} = 71.60$

Example 2: Green Fodders Such as Berseem (CF=6.0%)

Nutrient	% Factor		SE
DCP	2×0.94	=	1.88
DEE	0.5×1.90	=	0.95
Dig. total carbohydrates	9.0×1.00	=	9.00
			11.84

Calculated SE = 11.84

The crude fibre content of berseem on green basis is 6%. Therefore it has to be multiplied by a factor 0.34 which comes to $6.0 \times 0.34 = 2.04$.

Corrected SE = 11.84 - 2.04 = 9.80

Example 3: Calculate the SE of Paddy Straw for the Data Given (CF% = 35%)

DCP	=	0.00,	DEE = 0.80,
DCF	=	24.50, and	DNFE = 17.80

Solution:

Multiply the digestible nutrients with the appropriate SE factors

DCP	0.00	×	0.94	=	0.00
DEE	0.80	×	1.90	=	1.50
DNFE	17.80	×	1.00	=	17.80
DCF	24.50	×	1.00	=	24.50
		Calculated SE			43.80

Correction:

Deduct 0.58 units of SE for every 1% of original CF content

		$43.80 - (35 \times 0.58)$
	=	43.80 - 20.30
Corrected SE of P.S	=	23.50

Starch Equivalent Values of Some Feedstuffs

Feedstuff	SE per 100 kg
Maize grain	81.5 kg
Wheat	71.3
Oats	59.7
Wheat bran	45.0
Timothy hay	29.1
Oat straw	17.0

Chapter 16

Evaluation of Feeds for Protein for Ruminants and Nonruminants

It has already been studied that proteins are made up of indispensable (essential) and dispensable (nonessential) amino acids. The animal must receive sufficient quantities of both the types of amino acids to meet its metabolic demands and this ensures the use of feed with maximum efficiency. Simple stomached animals such as pigs and poultry obtain the amino acids from the breakdown of feed proteins during digestion and absorption while in case of ruminants the situation is more complex involving degradation and synthesis of protein in the rumen.

Measures of Protein Quality

It is generally accepted that usefulness of feeds as sources of protein depends primarily on two factors, the total concentration of the protein (N × 6.25) and the distribution of the amino acids making up the proteins. Protein quality is the kind and quantity of essential amino acids and non-specific amino nitrogen that arrive at the individual cell which determines the protein value of a feedstuff whether for ruminants or for nonruminants. Different approaches to the evaluation of protein sources are necessary for nonruminants and ruminants because considerable degradation of feed proteins and microbial synthesis of protein occurs in the rumen.

Evaluation of Protein of Feeds: Common Methods

1. Crude protein : Johann Kjeldahl of Denmark developed the method of nitrogen estimation in 1883. In calculating the protein content, it has been assumed that all N is present as protein and all food proteins contain 16% N. But both these assumptions are unsound. About 95% of N of most mature seeds is present as true protein, while leaves and stems contain 80 to 90 and 60%, respectively as true protein. The remaining occurs as amides, amino acids, glycosides, alkaloids, ammonium salts and compound lipids. Similarly different food proteins have different N contents and therefore different factors

TABLE 1. Factors for Converting N to CP.

Food protein	N (g/kg)	Conversion factor
Cottonseed	189	5.30
Soyabean	175	5.71
Barley	172	5.83
Oats	172	5.83
Wheat	172	5.83
Maize	160	6.25
Egg	160	6.25
Meat	160	6.25
Milk	157	6.38

(Table 1) should be used in the conversion of N to CP for individual foods.

2. *True protein:* Stutzer's reagent (alkaline copper sulphate) is used to precipitate the true protein and determination of its N by the Kjeldahl method and multiply with 6.25 gives the true protein content of the feed.

3. *Digestible crude protein (DCP):* Digestion of protein appears inevitably to be a prerequisite to its utilization. It is assumed that the difference between the quantities of N in food and faeces represents the quantity absorbed in utilisable form by the body and that all the nitrogen which appears in the faeces is of dietary origin. In view of rumen degradation of N compounds and fate of ruminal ammonia and the presence of N of metabolic origin in the faeces these assumptions are obviously untenable.

Digestible crude protein is a measure that has been widely used to evaluate the protein for ruminants inspite of its drawbacks. The digestibility figures routinely calculated are apparently digestible protein, which are generally lower than the true values. But since the loss of metabolic faecal nitrogen (see page No. 450) is inevitable, the apparent digestibility values are considered to be a more realistic measure of nutritive value. DCP is not employed with nonruminants because proteins can have the same digestibility and yet still differ in their value to the animal. That is, the proteins are said to differ in protein quality.

Measures of Protein Quality for Monogastric Animals

Estimation of CP and DCP are not enough since the efficiency of the absorbed protein varies considerably from one source to another and hence biological methods have been devised. These include weight gain methods, N balance experiments and body N retention method.

I Weight Gain Methods

i. Protein efficiency ratio (PER): It is defined as the weight gain per unit weight of protein consumed. Osborne, Mendel and Ferry in 1919 developed this method. This was carried out with rats to compare specific proteins or protein sources. A nitrogen free, otherwise adequate basal diet is used to which the protein sources to be compared are included for different groups of young animals and records for growth and feed consumption are maintained.

$$PER = \frac{Gain\ in\ weight}{Protein\ intake}$$

PER of some food materials:

Whole Wheat flour	:	1.2
Peanut flour and		
Cottonseed flour	:	2.0
Soyabean flour	:	2.4
Skimmilk powder	:	2.8
Meat, milk and egg	:	2.6 to 3.8

Limitations: It is a tedious method. This method can not assess the digestibility of protein. It cannot measure how much of the protein fed is used for maintenance and how much for tissue formation. Further, the weight gain may be due to bone or fat formation and so the protein content of the gain may be variable.

ii. Net protein retention (NPR): It is a modification of the PER method. It makes an allowance for maintenance. It is claimed to give more accurate results than the PER method.

$$NPR = \frac{Weight\ gain\ of\ TPG - Weight\ loss\ of\ NPG}{Protein\ intake}$$

where TPG = Group fed on test protein.
    NPG = Group fed on non-protein (protein free) diet.

iii. Gross protein value (GPV): It refers to a measurement with chicks fed a depletion diet containing 8% protein for 2 weeks, after which they are divided into three groups. The live weight gain of chicks receiving a basal diet containing 80 g CP/kg are compared with those of chicks receiving the basal diet plus 30 g CP/kg of a test protein, and of others receiving the basal diet plus 30 g CP/kg of casein.

$$GPV = \frac{g\ increased\ weight\ gain\ /\ g\ test\ protein}{g\ increased\ weight\ gain\ /\ g\ casein}$$

The extra live weight gain per unit of supplementary test protein, stated as a proportion of the extra live weight gain per unit of supplementary casein, is the gross protein value of the test protein.

II Nitrogen Balance Experiments

i. Biological value (BV): Karl Thomas has first used the term BV in the year 1909. It is defined as the proportion of the nitrogen absorbed which is retained by the animal.

$$\% \; BV = \frac{N \; intake - (FN + UN)}{NI - FN} \times 100$$

This is called apparent BV. It measures the BV of protein for growth purpose only. A more useful measure is one that takes account of maintenance as well. Karl Thomas method was modified by Mitchell (1924). This is called the Thomas-Mitchell formula.

Crampton and Harris (1968) called it as true BV.

$$\% \; BV = \frac{NI - (FN - MFN) - (UN - EUN)}{NI - (FN - MFN)} \times 100$$

Where   NI = Nitrogen intake

FN = Total faecal nitrogen

MFN or FN_m = Metabolic faecal nitrogen. It consists of 'spent' digestive enzymes, abraded mucosa and bacterial N (Look for more details in chapter 3 of Applied Nutrition).

UN = Total urinary nitrogen

EUN or UN_e = Endogenous urinary nitrogen. It is analogous to the energy equivalent of basal metabolism. The EUN refers to the nitrogen resulting from normal catabolism of nitrogen constituents in the body that are regularly voided in the urine (Look for more details in chapter 3 of Applied Nutrition Livestock, ...;).

In excluding the MFN and EUN from the losses, the Thomas-Mitchell method provides a measure of the efficiency of the absorbed protein for the combined functions of growth (formation of new tissues) and maintenance (replacement of existing proteins). The values for the metabolic and endogenous nitrogen can be arrived at by the Titus extrapolation method and from basal metabolism, respectively, without using nitrogen free diet procedure. Reported average values for MFN per unit of DM consumed and for EUN per unit of metabolic body size may also be used.

Determination of BV: Conditions to be fulfilled

1. Protein under test should form greater part of the dietary protein of the experimental animal.

2. Protein intake must be sufficient to allow adequate N retention, but should not be in excess of that required for maximum retention. TBV data for individual feeds will change according to the rations in which they are used. In order to compare the TBV for different feeds TBV must be determined at the same protein levels of intake and such rations are adjusted to 10% CP.

3. Sufficient non-nitrogenous nutrients must be given to prevent catabolism of protein to provide energy.

4. The diet must also contain other nutrients.

Factors that influence the effective TBV of a protein include age and class of the animal and amino acid composition of the protein. Proteins with all the essential amino acids in right amount and proportion have higher BV. Animal proteins have higher BV compared to plant proteins. Deficiency or excess of any one of the amino acids lowers the BV.

BV of some food materials:	Average/Range
Whole wheat	67
Whole corn	60 (49-61)
Soybean meal	62-65
Peas	63-76
Fish meal	74-89
Microbial protein	78
Whole egg	94
Milk	85-95

Nitrogen balance index: It is applicable to studies of BV for maintenance and some growth. A linear relationship exists between N intake and N balance in the region of negative and low-positive balance. This is represented by the following equation.

$Y = bx - a$ where y = N balance mg N per basal
  x = N absorbed KJ
  a = N loss at zero intake mg N/basal KJ.

b = the N balance index, represents that fraction of the absorbed N which is retained in the body. This is equal to the BV for maintenance.

Calculation of BV of a Protein for Maintenance and Growth of the Rat : An Example

Food consumed/day	6.0 g
% N in food	1.043
NI/day	62.6 mg
UN/day	32.8 mg
EUN/day	22.0 mg
FN/day	20.9 mg
MFN/day	10.7 mg

$$BV = \frac{62.6 - (20.9 - 10.7) - (32.8 - 22.0)}{62.6 - (20.9 - 10.7)} \times 100$$

$$= 79$$

Since farm animals are fed for productive purposes, BVs for the combined function of maintenance and production are ones of practical importance.

ii. Net protein utilization (NPU): The usefulness of a protein to an animal will depend upon its digestibility as well as its BV. NPU is the product of these two values and is the proportion of N intake which is retained. The product of NPU and the percentage CP is the net protein value (NPV) of the feed and is a measure of protein actually utilizable by the animal.

iii. Protein replacement value (PRV): Murlin (1938) devised this measurement to overcome the limitations of the Thomas - Mitchell biological value. Replacement value of food protein is a measure of the retention of the total nitrogen intake rather than the digestible nitrogen. It compares the extent to which a test protein will give the same N balance as an equal amount of standard protein.

$$PRV = 100 - \left(\frac{NB_1 - NB_2}{NI} \times 100 \right)$$

Where NB_1 is the N balance of animals fed standard protein, NB_2 is the N balance of animals fed the test protein and NI as N intake.

Example: Assume a comparison between two rations with whole egg is the protein in the I ration and soybean meal is the protein in the II ration. Two N balance experiments are conducted keeping the daily N intake at 50 mg. The N balances are + 20 and + 16 grams. Soybean protein failed to equal egg protein by (20-16) 100/50 = 8% and so soybean protein has an egg replacement value of 92%.

Weight gain methods are less accurate than nitrogen balance methods. The use of young animals and standard conditions, however, has given high correlations between the growth and nitrogen balance methods.

III. Body Nitrogen Retention Method

Miller and Bender (1955) devised this method. This is based on a comparison of the body N content resulting from a test protein with that resulting over the same period on a nitrogen-free diet. The value is computed as follows.

$$\text{Body N retention} = \frac{\begin{array}{l}\text{Body N content} \quad - \quad \text{Body N content with} \\ \text{with test protein} \qquad\quad \text{N-free diet}\end{array}}{\text{NI}}$$

The formula measures efficiency for growth. At the close of the experiment animals are killed, the body water determined and the N calculated from body water or actual analysis of the carcasses for nitrogen.

The efficiency of utilization of dietary protein may be estimated from the difference between nitrogen intake and excretion, or from the increase of body proteins. Comparison of balance trials with comparative slaughter data showed that balance determinations usually overestimate nitrogen retention, particularly with large animals. Further, retentions are often recorded with little or no change in body weight. These discrepancies are generally considered to be due to errors inherent in the conduct of metabolism trials.

Biological methods require a regular supply of standard young animals (rats, chicks, etc.) and are expensive and require considerable technical resources. Hence alternative methods were developed.

IV. Estimation of Protein Quality from Amino Acid Composition

To overcome the economical limitations of biological methods, chemical methods have been proposed. A comparison of the quantitative distribution of the essential amino acids in a feed with the relative amounts needed by the body per unit of feed provides a method of estimating protein quality.

i. Chemical score: R.J. Black and H.H. Mitchell (1946) devised this. In this concept the quality of a protein is decided by that constituent indispensable amino acid which is in greatest deficit when compared with a standard. The standard generally used is egg protein, but now many workers use a defined amino acid mixture recommended by FAO. For example, amino acid levels in % egg protein (standard) and % wheat protein (test protein) are given. Then amino acid deficiencies are calculated. The amino acid present in the greatest deficit is considered as the limiting amino acid and the complement of its percentage deficit is the chemical score for that protein. Between egg protein and wheat protein, calculation revealed lysine was the most limiting amino acid (-63% deficit) and hence chemical score for wheat is 100-63 = 37.

TABLE 2. Calculation of Mitchell's Chemical Score for wheat as an index of protein*

Name of Amino acid	% in egg protein	% in wheat protein	% deficiency in wheat
Arginine	6.4	4.2	– 34
Histidine	2.1	2.1	0
Lysine	7.2	2.7	– 63
Tryptophane	1.5	1.2	– 20
Phenylalanine	6.3	5.7	– 10
Methionine	4.1	2.5	– 39
Threonine	4.9	3.3	– 33
Leucine	9.2	6.8	– 26
Isoleucine	8.0	3.6	– 55
Valine	7.3	4.5	– 38

*Chemical score for wheat is 100–63=37 (based on amino acid in greatest deficit)

Chemical score appears to be a useful measurement for separating proteins into categories of usefulness. With protein that is deficient in several amino acids, correction of one deficiency still leaves a combination that is biologically imperfect.

ii. The essential amino acid index (EAAI):   B.L. Oser (1951) devised this measure based on the contribution the protein makes to all essential amino acids rather than to the one in greatest deficit. It may be defined as the geometric mean of the ten egg ratios found by comparing the content of ten EAAs in a feed protein with that found in whole egg protein. Algebraically the index is expressed as

$$EAAI = 10 \sqrt{\frac{100a}{a_e} \times \frac{100b}{b_e} \times \frac{100c}{c_e} \times \dots \dots \frac{100j}{j_e}}$$

Where a, b, c, ...j = % concentrations of the indispensable amino acids in a feed protein

$a_e, b_e, c_e \dots \dots j_e$ = % concentrations of the same amino acids in egg protein.

For computation it is convenient to express the equation in logarithmic form:

$$\log EAA\ index = \frac{1}{10} \sqrt{\log \frac{100a}{a_e} + \log \frac{100b}{b_e} + \dots \dots \log \frac{100j}{j_e}}$$

Antilog of the above gives the EAAI of that test protein.

It has the disadvantage that proteins of very different amino acid composition may have the same or a very similar index.

Both the chemical score and EAAI are based upon gross amino acid composition. A more logical approach, hence, would be to use figures for the amino acids available to the animal. The principal reason for the reduction of amino acid availability is heat damage occuring during processing or storage of feedstuffs due to maillard reaction (Fig. 1).

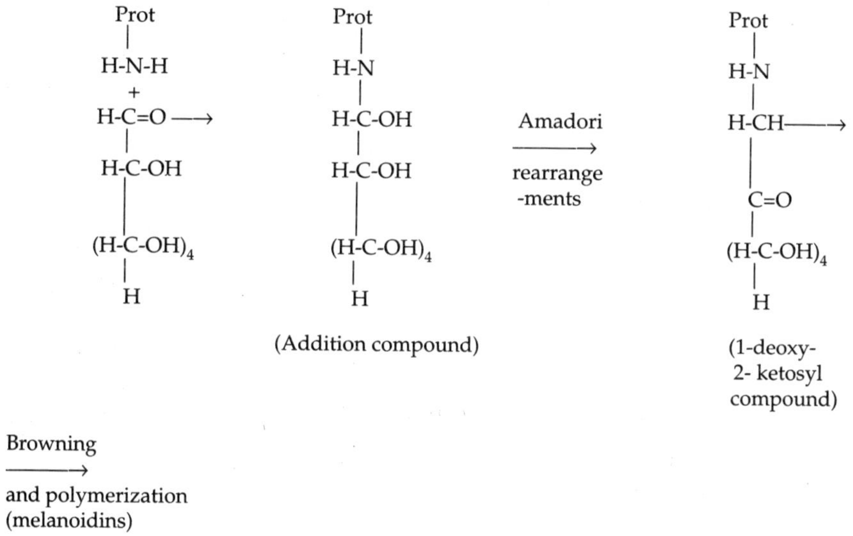

Prot
|
H-N-H
+
H-C=O $\longrightarrow$
|
H-C-OH
|
(H-C-OH)$_4$
|
H

Prot
|
H-N
|
H-C-OH
|
H-C-OH
|
(H-C-OH)$_4$
|
H

(Addition compound)

Amadori
$\longrightarrow$
rearrange
-ments

Prot
|
H-N
|
H-CH $\longrightarrow$
|
C=O
|
(H-C-OH)$_4$
|
H

(1-deoxy-
2- ketosyl
compound)

Browning
$\longrightarrow$
and polymerization
(melanoidins)

Figure 1. Maillard Reaction.

The reaction between sugars and amines is known as Maillard reaction (after the French chemist who studied it). Louis Camille Maillard (1878-1936) observed the reaction in 1912. The brown colour is caused by the formation of melanoidins. Maillard reaction is one of the nonenzymatic browning reactions. The reaction is also termed as "Sugar-amine reaction".

In this reaction, free amino groups of the peptide chain, most usually the ε amino group from lysine, react with the aldehyde group of reducing sugars such as glucose or lactose to yield an amino-sugar complex that is no longer available to the animal. As a result of the complexing, trypsin can no longer cleave the peptide bond and lysine is not available.

Amino Acid Availability

The bioavailability of amino acids is defined as the proportion of the total dietary amino acids not combined with compounds, which interfere with digestion, absorption or utilization for the purpose of maintenance or growth of new tissue (ARC, 1981). Defined as such, availability is an abstract concept that cannot be really measured but only estimated.

V. Estimation of the Availability of Amino Acids

i.   Biological Assay of Available Amino Acids: The available amino acid content of a food protein may be assayed by measuring the live weight gain, feed conversion efficiency or N retention of animals given the intact protein as a supplement to a diet deficient only in the amino acid under investigation. Chick is the usual experimental animal and the response to the test material is compared with responses obtained with supplements of pure amino acids.

The method has been used successfully for lysine, methionine and cystine. Disadvantages are time consuming, needs technical expertise, require regular supply of animals and the major problem is constructing diets deficient in specific amino acids but adequate in other respects.

ii.   Microbiological   methods: Certain   microorganisms   such   as *Streptococcus zymogenes,* a bacterium and *Tetrahymena pyriformis,* a protozoan have amino group requirements similar to those of higher animals. Hence these microorganisms have been used for evaluation of feed proteins. The methods are based on measuring the growth of the microorganisms in culture media which include the protein under test.

Streptococcus zymogens is used mainly for the determination of available methionine while *Tetrahymena pyriformis* is used for lysine.

iii. Chemical methods: It would be ideal if simple chemical procedures could be used to determine the availability of amino acids, provided the results correlated well with those of accepted biological methods.

a.   FDNB-reactive lysine method: One of the most promising chemical methods used is to test the availability of lysine, the amino acid most likely to be limiting in diets high in cereal grains. The method is based on the idea that the lysine that is unbound has free epsilon (ε)-amino group, and that is the available lysine. The free ε-amino groups of the lysine in the protein will react with the chemical called fluro-2,4-dinitrobenzene (FDNB) to produce a coloured derivative (DNP-lysine), the depth of the colour indicating the availability of the lysine. This method was originally proposed by Dr. K.J. Carpenter.

$$
\begin{array}{ccc}
\text{NH}_2 & & \text{NH}_2 \\
| & & | \\
\end{array}
$$

Lysine $CH_2\text{-}CH_2\text{-}CH_2\text{-}CH_2\text{-}CH\text{-}COOH$

The free ε-amino group reacts with FDNB and a coloured derivative, ε-dinitrophenyl (DNP) lysine is produced. Greater the depth of the colour higher the available lysine.

b. Dye-binding method: Dye binding methods have been used for protein in foods such as cereals and milk. These methods have been used for measuring total basic amino acids and reactive lysine. The latter requires blocking the ε-amino group to prevent its reaction with the dye. The dye 'orange G' has been used along with 2, 4, 6-trinitrobenzene sulphonic acid and propionic anhydride as blocking agents. It has proved effective for estimating the lysine content of cereals but less so for fish and meat meals.

Amino acid digestibility: It is defined as the difference between the amount of amino acids in the diet and in ileal digesta or in faeces, divided by the amount in the diet. Amino acid digestibility should not be confused with amino acid availability.

Ileal Digestibility of Protein

Digestibility coefficients based on collection and analysis of digesta from the terminal ileum (last part of the small intestine) are generally considered to give a more accurate measure of the nitrogen absorbed than do those based on the more usual total faecal collection method. Bacteria of the large intestine in poultry, pig, dog and cat change the amino acid composition of undigested food residues. These bacteria both add and consume amino acids, so that the mixture of amino acids in the faeces contains both undigested food amino acids and amino acids of bacterial origin. This makes accurate determination of nutrient digestion from 'total tract' collections impossible. Ileal collection eliminates the large intestine as a source of errors, and the method is justified since absorption from the large intestine makes little or no contribution to the protein status of the animal. It has been reported that there is a higher correlation between daily liveweight gain in pigs and ileal rather than faecal digestibility (r=0.76 vs 0.34), particularly with unusual protein sources.

True digestibility of protein may be calculated by using N^{15}-labelled dietary protein or by using homoarginine. However, these most favoured techniques also show average differences of about 5% in the true digestibility values derived from them.

Bioavailability of protein sources and other nutrients should focus only on digestion up to the end of small intestine, which would exclude the effects of hindgut fermentation. This measurement requires ileally cannulated animals and caecectomised roosters.

Ileal Digestibility and Faecal Digestibility

T-cannula were fixed at the distal ileum to piglets weaned at 21 days of age. An experiment was conducted to determine the ileal and faecal digestibilities of three protein sources by incorporating them in starch based semi-purified experimental feeds.

Treatments:	1	2	3
Protein: sources:	soybean meal	Extruded soybeans + soybean meal (50:50 on CP basis)	Full-fat canola + soybean meal (50:50 on CP basis)

Crude protein and amino acid digestibilities in the first feed were determined by the direct method. The digestibilities in the experimental diets containing extruded soybean or full-fat canola were determined by difference. The faecal digestibilities of CP and amino acids in SBM, extruded soybeans and full-fat canola were higher than the corresponding ileal digestibilities. This difference may have been due to higher amino acid degradation in the faecal samples.

The digestibilities of protein and most of the amino acids were significantly higher in soybean meal than they were in extruded soybean and in full-fat canola. The lower digestibilities may have been due to the trypsin inhibitor in the extruded soybean and tannins and pectins in the full-fat canola. (Anim Feed Sci. Tech. 1995, 52:189)

Measures of Protein Quality used in Practice in the Feeding of Pigs and Poultry

Several methods have been proposed to assess the value of a dietary protein. The crude protein figure gives a measure of the total N content and is useful since the digestibility of protein in feeds commonly given to pigs and poultry is fairly constant. The quality of dietary protein is indicated by stating the contents of all the essential amino acids or of those most likely to be in deficit. Practical pig and poultry diets are based largely on cereals and assessment of such feeds as sources of protein for the animals is important to supplement the amino acid deficiencies of the cereals. So here the most useful measure of protein quality such as available lysine or methionine content of the feed (mostly available lysine content) is analysed as a routine procedure.

The most recent method for evaluating dietary protein for growing pigs is based on the concept of 'ideal protein'. This is a modification of the chemical score with the amino acid pattern of the particular tissue protein serving as the reference pattern (Table 3).

TABLE 3. Recommended Balance of Amino Acids (g/kg) in Ideal Protein
[ARC (1981) The Nutrient Requirement of pigs].

Lysine	70	Leucine	70
Meth + cystine[a]	35	Histidine	23
Threonine	42	Phenylalanine + tyrosine[b]	67
Tryptophan	10	Valine	49
Isoleucine	38	Nonessential amino acids	596

[a] At least half should be methionine
[b] At least half should be phenylalanine

If the main limiting amino acid was lysine at 50 g/kg CP, then the score would be $50 \div 70 = 0.70$, and the ideal protein content would be 700 g/kg CP. A diet with 170 g/kg of this protein would then supply $170 \times 0.7 = 119$ g ideal protein per kg.

Ideal Protein Concept

In 1940s the ideal protein concept was introduced in the name of reference protein for evaluating protein quality using BV, Chemical score, etc. Later researchers more importantly H.H. Mitchell and R.J. Block reported that amino acids composition of high quality protein had the same with amino acids composition of body protein and this was the amino acids requirements of growing animal. Almquist in 1947 stated, that the "requirement of any indispensable amino acid for any rate of growth has a fixed proportion to the others in the diet".

The concept of an "Ideal Protein" was originally proposed by Mitchell (1964) to try to match exactly the amino acid requirements of the animal for growth and maintenance thus avoiding under- and over-supplying amino acids.

In 1981 ARC reviewed the idea of ideal protein and published the first estimate of an ideal protein requirement for growing pigs. The ideal protein concept was corrected, modified and applied in feeding systems of USA, UK, Australia, New Zealand, etc. The benefit of an ideal protein concept in diet formulation is to set all EAA requirements on the basis of lysine. Lysine was chosen as the standard because it is particularly well studied and it is not used extensively for purposes other than protein synthesis. So ideal protein concept is a statement of EAA requirements in a proportional relationship to the requirement for lysine. Thus, the dietary percentage of lysine is set and the concentration of other EAAs is determined as a percentage of the lysine concentration according to the ideal amino acid balance. In the latest edition of Nutrient Requirement of

Swine (NRC 1998) the amino acid requirements relative to lysine are presented for various growth stages of pigs.

For poultry, evaluation of protein sources is based upon their contents of the three major limiting amino acids, lysine, methionine and tryptophan. It is generally assumed that diets adequate in these acids will automatically provide sufficient amounts of the other amino acids.

Measures of Protein Quality for Ruminants

"Feed the rumen microbes and they in turn feed the host animal". This is what that has been said on feeding of ruminants. The quality of dietary protein is not important in ruminants in case of low producing animals since all the essential amino acids are synthesized by the rumen microorganisms. However, protein quality is important for high producing animals and a small portion of 'bypass' protein is advocated to meet their requirement for higher growth and milk production. See Applied Nutrition for more information.

1. *Crude Protein:* Since CP contains variable amounts of nonprotein nitrogen (NPN) compounds, true protein had come into use, but this was unsatisfactory since no allowance was made for the nutritive value of NPN fraction (crude protein-true protein).

2. *Protein equivalent:* In an attempt to have NPN fraction half the nutritive value of true protein a concept of protein equivalent (PE) was introduced in 1925.

$$PE = \frac{\% \ DCP + \% \ DTP}{2}$$

This means the PE is the arithmatic mean of the percentage of DCP and DTP.

3. *DCP:* For many years there has been considerable dissatisfaction with the use of DCP for evaluating feed proteins. This is due to the extensive degradative and synthetic activities of the microorganisms of the rumen.

   Orskov (1982) reported that the nutritional relevance of DCP for ruminants had ceased to exist and the use of DCP was rejected because (i) dietary proteins are largely degraded in the rumen (ii) the extent to which degraded N is utilized by rumen microbes is related to the amount of energy fermented, and (iii) faecal excretion could be altered by manipulating the site of fermentation between the rumen and caecum.

   Because of its easy calculation, DCP is a measure widely used to evaluate proteins for ruminants. While it was accepted that dietary protein was largely degraded, Orskov (1970) reported that microbial protein alone could not sustain high productivity in young early-weaned ruminants or in lactating ruminants. Furthermore, it was soon found that the extent of degradation of dietary proteins varied greatly.

4. Biological value does not apply to ruminants because of the ability of the rumen microorganisms to synthesize amino acid from a variety of N compounds.

5. Several new systems have been proposed in lieu of DCP system. These are the **'metabolizable protein'** system used in the USA (Burroughs *et at.*, 1975), 'rumen degradable and undegradable protein' system in the UK (ARC, 1980), true protein digested in the small intestine (PDI) system in the France and a similar system in the Germany.

The fundamental principle underlying these new systems is that N requirements of a ruminant animal is most logically considered in two parts: a requirement for N by rumen microorganisms and a requirement for protein by host ruminant animal.

The protein value of a feedstuff may be assessed from the determined or estimated flow of protein or amino acids leaving the rumen or entering the small intestine. Intestinal supply of protein to the ruminant comprises dietary protein escaping microbial degradation in the forestomachs, microbial protein synthesized as a result of rumen fermentation, sloughed epithelial cells and secretions into the abomasum. Metabolizable protein is that part of the dietary protein and microbial protein which is absorbed by the host animal and is available for use at tissue level.

A variety of *in vivo* and *in vitro* methods have been employed to estimate either the total protein supply or individual components. ARC (1980) adopted microbial protein yield as 30 g N/kg digestible OM. It can be estimated using rumen cannulated animals with the help of markers such as **bacterial marker** (α, τ-diaminopimelic acid DAPA), protozoal marker (2, aminoethyl-phosphonic acid AEPA; phosphatidyl choline). Isotopes such as ^{35}S, ^{14}C, ^{32}P and stable ^{15}N are also used.

Protein flow to the small intestine can be determined with animals equipped with either simple or re-entrant cannulae to the abomasum or duodenum.

Rumen degradability (N/CP) of feedstuffs is estimated by *in sacco/in situ* technique (page no. 26 of Applied Nutrition Livestock, ...;) to know the rumen degradable protein (RDP) and undegradable dietary protein (UDP). This aspect shall be studied in applied livestock feeding (refer chapter 5 of Applied Nutrition). Depending on the nature of the dietary N, microbial N contribute from less than 50% to over 90% of non-ammonia N (NAN) reaching the duodenum.

Protein rationing

Effective management of nitrogen inputs to the dairy cow is important because of the high cost of proteinaceous feeds, the relationship between protein intake and several metabolic diseases, notably reproductive disorders (Butler, 1998) and the cost to the environment due to high nitrogen emissions.

Flaws in the protein rationing based on DCP requirements led to its replacement. Later AFRC (1992) called the protein rationing as UK Metabolizable Protein system. This is also not a fool proof system. (1) Degradability of protein is based on feed factors and animal factors. Rumen outflow rate is one important factor. The rumen retention time is largely a function of the level of feeding. High-yielding cows have a high level of feeding and short retention time, whereas mature beef cattle are likely to have a low level of feeding and longer retention time.

(2) Some dietary protein that is undegraded in the rumen will not be absorbed at all. This part of protein is determined as ADICP. Feeds with high concentrations of tannins contain ADICP and will have reduced protein digestibility, because of the formation of indigestible tannin-protein complexes in the gastrointestinal tract.

Better definition of nitrogen capture by rumen microbes is already possible and is incorporated into the system devised by Cornell University, USA. This is Cornell Net Carbohydrate and Protein System (CNCPS) (Sniffen et al., 1992). This is described later.

Characterization of Proteins in Feeds

Feedstuffs contain a wide array of proteins and nonprotein N (NPN) compounds. Proteins are present in cell walls and cell contents of all plant and animal tissues, where they provide a variety of functions (e.g., structural, storage, catalytic, transport, and contractile). NPN compounds are smaller molecules that include peptides, free AA, nucleic acids, amides and amines, nitrate, and ammonia.

The first goal in characterizing feed CP is to obtain reasonably accurate estimates of ruminally degraded protein (RDP) and ruminally undegraded protein (RUP). These two fractions of feed CP have separate and distinct functions in ruminant diets. Ruminally degraded CP is required for ruminal fermentation because it provides the mixture of peptides, free AA, and ammonia required for microbial growth, activity, and synthesis of microbial protein. In contrast, RUP provides a direct source of digestible AA to the animal.

Several methods have been evaluated to partition feed crude protein (CP) into rumen-degradable protein (RDP) and rumen-undegradable protein (RUP) and to estimate the intestinal digestibility of RUP. These methods include *in vivo, in situ* (using nylon or dacron polyester bags with a 40- to 60 µm pore size), and a variety of *in vitro* enzymatic methods [(ruminal *in vitro* methods that involve incubations with mixed ruminal microorganisms (i.e., ruminal digesta) and nonruminal *in vitro* methods that involve incubations with cell-free enzymes], *in vitro* chemical methods and *in vitro* multi-chemical methods.

Cornell Net Carbohydrate and Protein System (CNCPS)

The most widely used and sophisticated multi-chemical approach for quantifying N fractions in feedstuffs is the protein fractionation scheme used in the CNCPS. The CNCPS partitions CP into 5 fractions using 3 solvents and a protein-precipitating agent. The 5 fractions are: A (NPN; soluble in borate-phosphate buffer but not precipitated with tungstic acid), Bl (rapidly degraded true protein; soluble in borate-phosphate buffer and precipitated with tungstic acid), B2 (moderately degraded true protein and large peptides; calculated as the difference between total CP and the sum of the other 4 CP fractions), B3 (slowly degraded true protein; calculated as the difference between neutral detergent insoluble CP [NDICP] and acid detergent insoluble CP [ADICP]) and C (undegraded true protein; measured as ADICP).

The NDICP is derived by determining CP on the insoluble residue of an NDF extraction without the use of sodium sulfite. The ADICP is determined as the CP associated with the insoluble residue of an ADF extraction. Fraction A is assumed to be 100% degraded in the rumen and fraction C is assumed to be undegradable.

The multi-chemical approach for characterizing feed CP was chosen for the CNCPS for 2 reasons. **First**, the procedures for determining the chemical fractions (NPN, soluble true protein, NDICP, and ADICP) that are required for determining the CP fractions (A, B1, B2, B3, and C) can be performed under routine laboratory conditions. An ongoing goal of the CNCPS is for it to be a field-usable model with inputs that can be collected onfarm. **Second**, one of the original purposes of the CNCPS model was to be able to predict, as accurately as possible, microbial growth and ruminal fermentation. (See page no. 40 also)

Methods for Estimating RUP Digestibility

Methods employed to protect protein from rumen microbial degradation (See Applied Nutrition Livestock, ...; page no. 110) should increase the efficiency of protein utilization in the animal. That is rumen-undegraded protein should be digestible and absorable subsequently in the gastrointestinal tract.

Accurate estimate of the intestinal digestibility coefficients of the RUP for each feedstuff is fundamental to balancing diets for RUP. Several methods have been used to obtain estimates of RUP digestibility. These include *in vivo* procedures, *in vitro* techniques, nonruminant animal bioassays, the *in situ* mobile nylon bag technique, and the use of ADICP. The most widely reported approach is the mobile bag technique. This approach consists of placing small amounts of washed ruminally undegraded feed residues in bags, pre-incubating them in a pepsin/HCL solution for 1 to 3 h, and then inserting them into the duodenum of cannulated ruminants. The bags are recovered from the faeces, washed thoroughly to remove endogenous and other contaminating protein, and analyzed for protein content. Research has shown good correlation between estimates of RUP digestibility with this method and *in vivo*-derived estimates.

Precision-fed roosters are valid models for the evaluation of small intestinal digestibility of protein in ruminants in the absence of animals fitted with duodenal and ileal cannulae. The use of caecectomized birds removes most of the fermentative capacity of the avian gastrointestinal tract, thereby allowing the rooster to simulate more closely only the small intestinal portion of the bovine gastrointestinal tract.

Use of '**the precision-fed caecectomized rooster bioassay**' offers promise as a method for assessing the availability of amino acids reaching the small intestine of cattle. Rumen-undegraded residues are crop-intubated to 4 caecectomized roosters and total excreta are collected for 48 h. Rumen-undegraded residues and excreta are analysed for amino acids. Basal endogenous amino acid loss estimates are estimated from fasted birds and are used to calculate standardized digestibility of RUP-amino acids.

Chapter 17

Feed Technology

Definition

The subject of feed technology deals with processing of feeds, fodders and preparation of formula feeds for which the knowledge of nutritional requirements of various livestock and poultry, quality control of feed ingredients, feed plant management and the storage of feed ingredients and feeds are essential. Animal feed technology may also be defined as the application of physical, chemical, biochemical, biological and engineering techniques to increase the nutrient utilization of feeds and fodders in animal system for the development of livestock and poultry and feed industry.

Beginning of Feed Industry and Related Activities in the US

In the United States (US) early mills were built for grinding wheat and maize for human consumption rather than for livestock feed. Wheat and maize milling, meat, milk and oilseed processing industries were developed by then. The byproducts were considered to be of no economical value and were dumped into the nearby rivers or streams. When such practice was stopped because of the pollution, efforts were made to explore means of eliminating the cost of disposal. By then proximate analysis system has come. Chemical analyses of the byproducts revealed their protein, mineral and vitamin contents. Thus the byproducts of milling, etc. found place in feeds for livestock and poultry proving 'necessity is the mother of invention'.

In 1875 Mr. John Barwell initiated the production of a calf meal at Blatchford of Waukegan, Illinois. It is credited with being the oldest feed manufacturing firm in the USA in continuous operation though the ownership has changed hands. Ralston Purina company was founded in 1894 as the Robinson-Danforth commission company to manufacture horse and mule feed. Since then scores of other firms entered the feed business. Increased competition and declining profits in flour milling industry led many of them to take up feed manufacturing.

The growth of commercial feed industry has been closely tied to the introduction of new byproducts. The Association of American Feed

Control Officials (AAFCO) defined 38 ingredients in its official publication published in 1911 and 440 in 1969 and more than 540 ingredients in 1985 publication. American Feed Manufacturers Association (AFMA) was founded in 1909 in Wisconsin and its name was changed to American Feed Industry Association (AFIA) in 1985. AAFCO was established in 1909.

Linear programming, a mathematical procedure, was developed by George B. Dantzig in 1947. W.V. Waugh of USDA was the first to see the potential of this mathematical procedure and developed a least cost dairy feed in 1951. Later Robert F. Hutton of Pennsylvania State University played a leading role in introducing linear programming to feed industry.

In North America and Europe, computers are controlling more processes and providing better quality control and operating efficiency. Almost every function of feed manufacturing is computerized-formulation of feed, purchasing, process control, inventory, warehousing, billing or payroll. Totally computerized feed manufacturing plants became a reality in 1975. Pelleting process was placed under the control of computers in the 1970's and in the 1980's proven automated systems were used worldwide. Inflation and rising labour costs along with new technology encouraged automation.

Food and Drug Administration (FDA) was passed in 1906 in USA. In 1938 Food, Drug and Cosmetic Act was passed to control addition of poisonous or deleterious substances to any food except where required. The Delaney Amendment to the Pure Food, Drug and Cosmetic Act was passed in 1958. It sets a zero tolerance for any feed additive that is known to produce cancer in man or animal. The Kefauve-Harris amendment to the Federal Food, Drug and Cosmetic Act (1962) required all firms manufacturing or mixing medicated feeds to register each plant. Later in 1965 FDA issued first good manufacturing practices (GMP's) for medicated feeds and started inspecting feed mills.

Feed Production School (FPS) was established in 1950 and it appointed a committee in 1960 to work up definitions of feed terminology used by manufacturers. Terminology in the feed industry was set up in the following broad categories: 1. Feed ingredients 2. Finished feeds 3. Feed in (manufacturing process) 4. Processing terms. Definitions prepared by FPS definitions committee were modified by AFMA Production Council committee under the chairmanship of Gerald A. Karstins.

Feed Production School published the "Feed Production Handbook" with Dr. Harry B. Pfost, as Editor-in-chief. Subsequently, AFMA published Feed Manufacturing Technology in 1970 and 1976, and the 1985 edition was published by AFIA. Fourth edition has also been brought out 1990s. Dr. Pfost served as Technical Editor and was a major chapter contributor to 1st and 2nd editions. It has been acknowledged that no person has contributed more to the technology of feed manufacturing or has had more influence in moving the industry from the state-of-the-art to the state-of-the science than Harry Pfost, a Professor in the Department of Grain Science and Industry at Kansas State University, USA.

Some of the AAFCO Definitions are Presented Here

Complete feed: A nutritionally adequate feed for animals other than humans; by specific formula compounded to be fed as the sole ration and is capable of maintaining life and/or promoting production without any additional substance, except water, being consumed.

Concentrate: A feed used with another to improve the nutritive balance of the total and intended to be further diluted and mixed to produce a supplement or a complete feed.

Supplement: A feed used with another to improve the nutritive balance or performance of the total and intended to be (1) fed undiluted as a supplement to other feeds, (2) offered free-choice with other parts of the ration separately available or (3) further diluted and mixed to produce a complete feed.

Premix: A uniform mixture of one or more microingredients with diluent and/carrier. Premixes are used to facilitate uniform dispersion of the microingredients in a large mix.

Development of Feed Industry in India

Feed industry came into existence in India in 1961 with the establishment of a feed plant in Ludhiana, Punjab. Compound Livestock Feed Manufacturers Association (CLFMA) was formed on 8th June, 1967. The installed capacity of CLFMA members put together is around 6 million tonnes and capacity utilisation is about 50% (CLFMA, 1998). Compound feed also produced by other feed manufacturers (non-members of CLFMA) and farmers directly and this comes to around four million tonnes.

Subsequently on 2nd June 1969, CLFMA was registered under the Bombay Public Trust Act 1950 as Charitable Public Trust. The constitution was further amended at the extraordinary general body meeting of the association held on 25th March 2002 at Hyderabad to make CLFMA a broad based association to cover all sectors of the livestock industry such as hatcheries, breeding farms, poultry integrators, milk processors, meat processors, aqua processors and exporters, egg powder manufacturers, equipment/machine manufacturers/suppliers, marketing firms (for branded products) and others who are involved in livestock industry as primary members.

CLFMA vision

To actualize the full potential of Animal Agriculture Industry of India and to converge the efforts of all sectors of Animal Production under one platform to get necessary recognition from all quarters of society for our contribution to the national economy.

Activities of the CLFMA are

1. The Association came to be known as CLFMA OF INDIA and was broad based to cover all sectors of the livestock industry keeping in line the objective of promoting animal husbandry.
2. CLFMA OF INDIA is the sole representative, national body of the livestock industry and has around 220 members that include all sectors of the livestock industry.
3. CLFMA OF INDIA is recognized not only by livestock industry but also by Central and State Governments, various Government Departments, Agricultural Universities, Veterinary Colleges and national research institutes in the country such as ICAR, IVRI, and NDRI.
4. CLFMA is also known in the livestock sector outside the Indian Union. CLFMA of India is also a member of International Feed Industry Federation (IFIF).
5. CLFMA's views are solicited and reckoned by Central and State Governments while formulating policies governing not only animal feed industry but also the entire gamut of animal production.
6. It represents the problems (such as import and export of feed ingredients and feed additives; matters related to tax) of the feed industry to the government.
7. To promote the concept of nutritionally balanced livestock feed as an imperative requisite of Animal Husbandry development on scientific lines and thus to help the increased production and usage of nutritionally balanced compound livestock feed
8. To promote and to organize scientific research designed to advance the industry, it provided research grants and instituted awards to honour the nutritionists who contributed substantially to the present day knowledge.
9. To foster and encourage the exchange of information relating to the livestock industry, it organizes orientation courses at veterinary colleges for the benefit of students and faculty.
10. CLFMA regularly interfaces with Central and State Governments to facilitate formulation of constructive policies for bringing about overall animal husbandry growth in general and development of livestock industry in particular.

11. To collect, classify and circulate statistical and other information relating to the industry among the members or the public at large in order to highlight the progress and prospects for the growth and development of animal husbandry
12. To impart training to livestock farmers, animal feed mill personnel, veterinarians, scientists and students of animal nutrition and any scientific livestock production
13. CLFMA publishes magazine to disseminate scientific information among the stakeholders.

PROCESSING OF FEEDS AND FORAGES

The Primary Reasons for Processing Feeds

1. *To make more profit:* Feed efficiency can be routinely improved as much as 10% and occasionally by as much as 15 to 20% by changing the method of grain processing.
2. *To alter particle size:* Some feeds need to be reduced in size to increase their intake or digestibility. e.g. grinding. In some instances, particle size is increased by pelleting or cubing to overcome dust problem, to prevent selectivity and to improve handling efficiency.
3. *To change moisture content:* The moisture content of a feedstuff may need to be changed to make it safer to store (reduced to 10% level), more palatable, more digestible, or to prepare it for other processes (moisture level is increased).
4. *To change the density of feed:* Bulky feeds (low density feeds) reduce feed intake. These are sometimes prepared for the purpose of limiting energy intake. These are preferred in feeding of horses because they cause fewer digestive disturbances. Grains are flaked rather than ground or pelleted.
   Very bulky feeds are pelleted or cubed to increase energy density and feed consumption. Transportation cost is reduced and storage space required is less.
5. *To change palatability:* Feeds are processed to increase acceptability and feed intake. Molasses, flavours and fats are added. Processing may be used to decrease palatability and limit feed consumption. Ex: salt-feed mixtures.
6. *To increase nutrient content:* When used alone and in their natural state, few feedstuffs meet the nutrient requirements of the animals.
7. *To increase nutrient availability:* Starch (70-80% of DM) and protein appear to be less available in sorghum than in other grains but new processing techniques produced dramatic improvements in the feeding value of sorghum. This is attributed to gelatinization of the starch granules rendering them more digestible. Pelleting of feeds increases the utilization of phosphorus for chicken and pigs.

8. *To detoxify or remove undesirable factors:* Considerable control of gossypol (the yellow pigment of cotton seed that is toxic to simple-stomached animals) is possible by heating. Addition of iron salts rupture pigment gland and thus protect against egg discolouration. Heating soybeans destroys the factors that inhibit the digestive enzymes, trypsin and chymotrypsin. The toxicity of linseed meal can be removed by adding two or three parts of water to the meal and allowing it to stand for 12 to 18 hours at a temperature between 22 to 37°C.

9. *To improve keeping qualities:* High moisture grains may be preserved by either drying or chemical treatment (adding an organic acid), or they may be stored in oxygen limiting silos. Similarly green fodders are also conserved as silage.

10. *To lesson moulds, sa!monella, and other harmful substances:* Sometimes feeds are subjected to a certain process to ensure safety and avoid contamination, especially from moulds and salmonella. Proper harvesting, drying and storage are important factors in lessening aflatoxin contamination and toxin production. Propionic and acetic acids will inhibit mould growth. Hence, they are used increasingly in the preservation of high-moisture grains. Treatment with ammonia or ammonium hydroxide will detoxify feeds.

Particle size reduction procedures: These are cutting, crushing, shearing and impact grinding.

Cutting: It is reduction accomplished by pushing or forcing a thin sharp knife through the materials to be reduced. e.g. Chaffing of green fodder, straw, hay.

Crushing: It is accomplished by applying a compressive force to the particle to be reduced. Ball mills, percussion mills and jaw crushers are examples of mills using the crushing principle.

Shearing: It is a combination of cutting and crushing. Ensilage cutter or rotary type knife and stationary bar cutter use the shear principle.

Impact grinding: It is most commonly used for reducing particle size in the feed industry. Hammer mills, Jet mills, Centrifugal input mills use this principle.

Mills that are Commonly used in the Feed Industry

1. *Hammer Mills:* These mills use impact grinding principle to reduce the particle size of feeds. Hammer mills are used for grinding of both concentrates and forages. It has been used for farm, commercial and custom grinding for many years.

The hammer mill consists of a cylinder or rotor made up of several plates keyed to the main shaft or axle and these plates, near the edge, carry the hammers. Outside the rotating cylinder is a perforated steel screen. The holes in this screen may be as small as 1/32" or as large as 2 or more inches (figure 1).

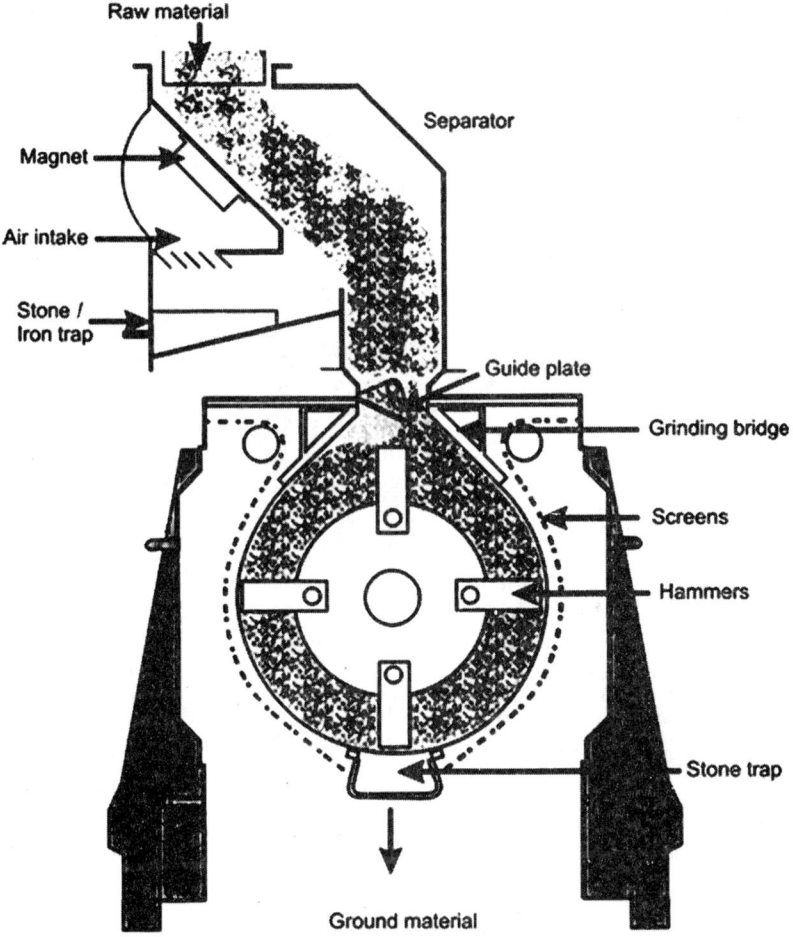

Figure 1 Cross-section of 'full-circle' hammer mill showing main features.

Hammer mills may be of the single, double or triple reduction type with either rigid or swinging hammers. The double or triple reduction types have knives or blunt discs on one side of the rotor to chop the longer stemmed materials such as maize fodder or alfalfa into small pieces before they come in contact with the hammers. This type of mill is usually fed from a central opening. So the material being reduced will come into contact with the knives and disks first.

It is assumed that most of the grinding occurs as the hammers strike the material in the air as it falls into the mill. The hammer tip may travel at a speed of 7000-25000 feet per minute. If the first impact of the hammers against the feed does not break it up so that it will drop through the screen, it rebounds and is again struck by the hammer tips. This process continues until all particles are reduced to a size that allow them to pass through the screen.

A fan or blower is usually used for product transport after grinding, the fan may be connected to the same shaft that drives the hammer mill or it may be driven seperatly. In either case the fan requires about 25-30% of the horse power (HP) of the mill and also cools the stock being reduced. See figure 2.

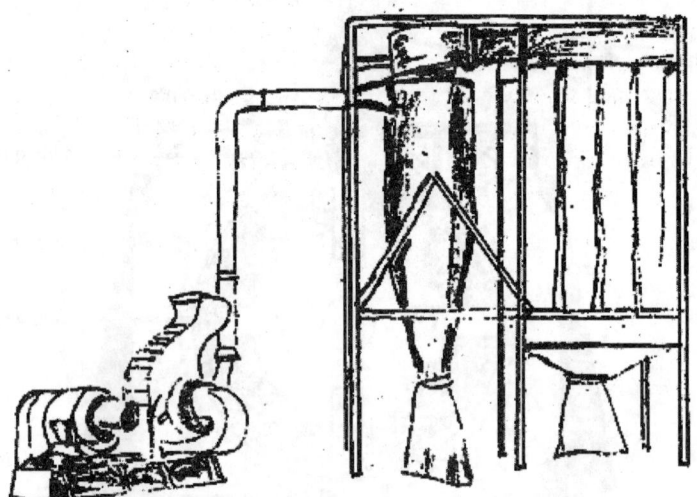

Figure 2   Hammer Mill: Pneumatic delivery - The blower carries the ground product from the mill and automatically delivers to cyclone collector. It is attached with a dust collector where fine dust particles are separated from air.

Mill Horse Power Requirements

Mill HP	Mill capacity (Lbs/hour)			Separate Fan	
	Fine grind	Medium grind	Coarse grind	H.P of the Fan	Capacity lbs
50	5,000	6,500	9,500	15-20	10,000-20,000
100	9,800	12,100	16,500	30-40	24,000-32,000

Factors that Affect the Performance of Hammer Mills

1. *Diameter and shape of screen openings:* Production and capacity increase as the screen openings are enlarged because the mill is doing less work per unit weight of material. Shape of the screen openings are mostly round.

2. *Screen area:* Production and efficiency were significantly lowered when one half of the screen area was blocked. Generally most hammer mills have 10-12 square inches of screen area per unit HP. Capacity varies directly with the percentage of open screen area.

3. *Moisture content:* It is reported that the power requirement in kilo watt hours (KWH) per tonne increases rapidly at higher moisture contents. Capacity in tonnes per hour is inversely related to the moisture. It is uneconomical to grind grains at moisture content higher than 12-14%.

4. *Peripheral speed (hammer tip speed):* It refers to the speed of the hammer tips and not the revolutions per minute of a mill. Most efficient peripheral speed is between 7000 to 9000 ft/mt and at this low speed mills produce more uniform grind. However, it is generally agreed that lower speed produce a coarser product and the product fineness is directly proportional to peripheral speed.

5. *Kind of feed:* Concentrates are easier to grind while roughages are difficult to grind. Cereal grains with higher starch contents are easier to grind.

6. *Location of feed intake:*
   (a) Central feeding: Feeding at the centre of the rotor.
   (b) Tangential feeding: Feeding tangential to the rotor.
      Central feeding is shown to decrease capacity up to 20% with a corresponding reduction in efficiency. In case of tangential feeding, the product is aided by incoming air and falls directly into the zone of greatest hammer velocity.
   In central feeding the material take a spiral path with almost the same peripheral speed as the hammers. The essential pulvarisation occurs at the screen because of the relative velocity and resulting impact.

7. *Hammer tip and screen clearance:* Product fineness is proportional to the clearance between the hammer tip and the screen. The optimum clearance has been shown to be 8 mm (0.31").

8. *Hammer width and design:* Hammer design is an important factor in the design of a hammer mill. The wear usually occurs at the tip of the hammer. Some hammers are manufactured so that they may be turned edge to edge and end to end. This arrangement allows for four

wear surfaces and is more economical than acquiring a new hammer when one edge wears out. See the illustration of conventional hammers and modern hammers. Modern hammers have more wear surfaces.

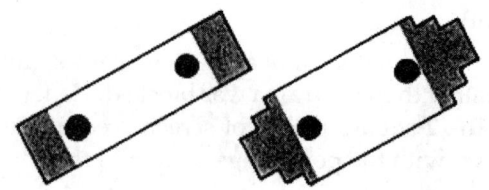

Hammers: Conventional hammers and Modern hammers

9. *Number of hammers:*   Number of hammers in a mill definitely affects production and fineness. It is desirable to have 15 hammers per 100 mm of rotor. Each hammer is of 3 mm thick.
10. *Feed rate:*   An increased rate of feed is associated with a coarser end product and also increases capacity. Therefore, feed rate is directly proportional to the applied power within the mechanical limitations of a given unit. The feed rate in most feed mills is controlled by an ammeter showing the current the motor is pulling. All motors have a rated amperage above which they should not be operated.
11. *Air flow through the mill:*   The amount of air flowing through the mill may affect the manner in which particles strike impact surfaces. The optimum value of about 4000 cu. metres/sq. metre area of screen surface is sufficient.

    Advantages of air flow are:

    a) it reduces the temperature of the material.
    b) it vacates the place and
    c) may help in changing the direction of ingredient.
12. *Mechanical conditions of the mill:*   Unworn screens and hammers with their sharper corners are more efficient.
13. *HP of the motor:*   Performance of the hammer mill is directly proportional to the HP of the motor.

2. Roller Mills

These are used in feed processing for the crimping or crushing of grains. Nowadays roller mills are preferred in Western countries for grinding of feeds for efficient grinding and uniform particle size.

The roller mill consists of two rolls rotating in opposite directions at the same speed or at different speeds. Rolls are usually corrugated or serrated. If the rolls are operated at the same speed, the reduction is mostly by crushing. If the rolls have a speed differential, cutting and shearing takes place. Roller mills may have one, two or three pairs of rolls in a strand.

Feed Mixing

The most important operation in a feed mill is mixing and this is the single operation that would be required in a plant to define it as a feed mill. The aim of mixing is to disperse the ingredients of a certain assortment (called formula) so that each small unit of the whole has the same proportion of each ingredient as in the original formula.

Feed Mixers are of Two Types

1. *Vertical batch mixer:* It is used in thousands of feed mills and farms. They may be single screw or double screw for elevating the material. However, single screw mixer is popular. These are relatively inexpensive and do a good job of mixing most ingredients. They are little slower than horizontal mixers and are not used in larger feed mills.

It consists of a vertical bin tapering to a point at the bottom. A tube containing a vertical screw conveyor elevates and mixes the material as the mixer is filled. The screw conveyor continuously elevates the product and distributes it over the top of the mixer. Repeated elevation of the product produces blending. Some mixers use two screw conveyors and few use other elevating devices. Normally screw is driven from the top but it can be driven from the bottom. These units range in capacity from 0.5 to 5 tonnes. See the illustration (Figure 3).

2. *Horizontal mixer:* This mixer is the one most commonly used in larger feed mills. This mixer has right and left hand augers which convey the material from one end of the mixer to the other while it is tumbled within the mixer. These mixers are equipped with openings at several places along the bottom to aid in more rapid discharge.

The mixer shaft is accurately machined and mounted on bearings and is fitted with ribbons/paddles which thoroughly agitate and blend the ingredients to produce homogenous mix. The ribbon assembly/paddle (Figure 4) is housed in a tub, the lower half of which is circular. Suitable speed reduction drive is provided to drive the mixer shaft at the designed speed to achieve proper mix with or without liquid additives.

Double paddle horizontal mixers: These have curved paddle blades which scoop, lift and tumble materials as they are conveyed to the centre of the mixer, where they are continuously over lapped and cross blended. In addition to the cross blending action, a turbulent upward and downward movement is secured which provides the intense type of action required to blend solids and liquid additives including molasses

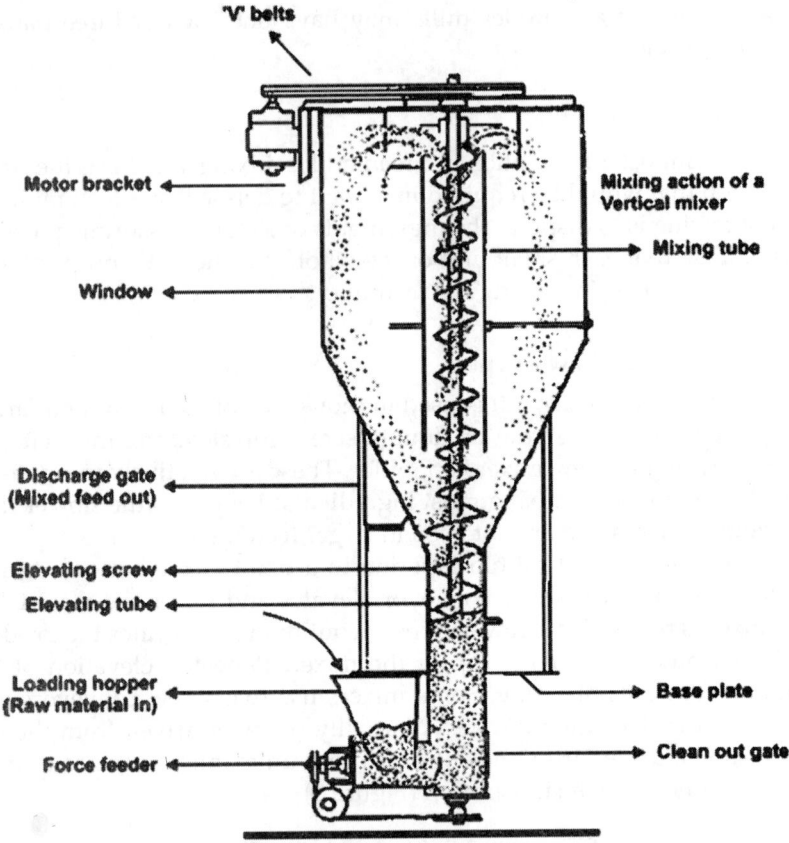

Figure 3   Vertical Mixer (Source: Feeds and Feeding by A.E. Cullison
2nd Edition 1979 Page 329)

blended with dry materials. These mixers have a side loading-cum-inspection platform.

Ribbon blenders: The principle of these blenders is the same as paddle mixers except that they have double worm type ribbons. The large one continuously conveys the material forward and the small one conveys it backwards. Material to be mixed is conveyed from end to end, top to bottom or side to side in the mixer. This continuous cross blending action tends to thoroughly mix the composition. The mixer is more suitable for blending powdery material of uniform fineness. In order to empty the mixer more rapidly than the product can be conveyed away with most elevators, a surge bin is usually provided. The mixed feed is dumped into the surge bin and another load can be mixed while the surge bin is emptying. See Figure 4 for illustrations of several designs in horizontal mixers.

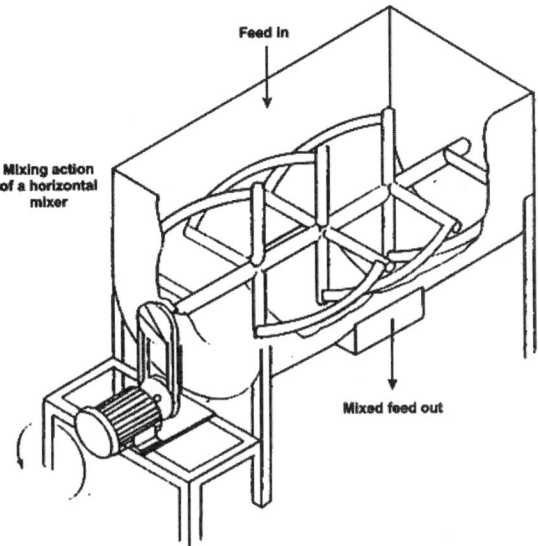

Figure 4 (a) Horizontal Mixer.

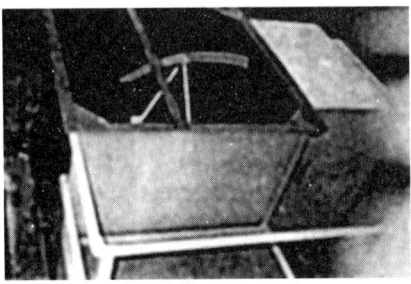

Figure 4 (b) Horizontal Paddle Mixer: 4
Curved paddle blades for Rapid Mixing by
Turbulent movement, Mixing high & low
density components and combination;
Wide range of applications.

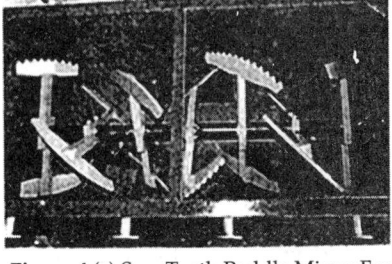

Figure 4 (c) Saw Teeth Paddle Mixer: For
rough & cellulose material mixing.

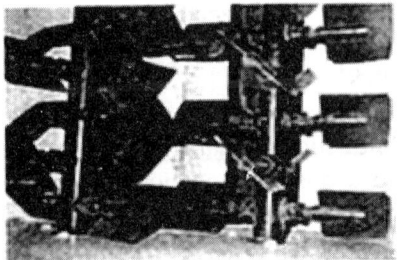

Figure 4 (d) Twin shaft Multi Paddle Mixer:
Fast Mixing Powders, Fibres or Solids with
liquids even of high viscosity & get thorough
blend in shortest time.

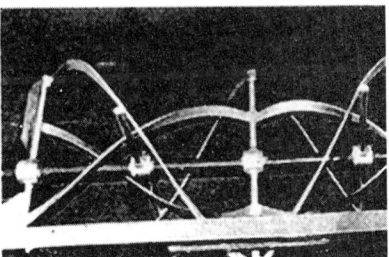

Figure 4 (e) Horizontal Ribbon Type
Mixer: Horizontal mixer with double
action ribbons embedded in the material;
Cross blending action of Ribbon gives
rapid and fine blend.

Merits and Demerits of the Mixers

	Attribute		Vertical mixer	Horizontal mixer
1.	Cost	:	Relatively inexpensive and do a good job of dry mixing.	Expensive and do a good job of dry and liquid mixing.
2.	Use	:	Used in thousands of feed mills and farms. Not used in larger feed mills.	Used in small mills as well as larger feed mills.
3.	Floor space	:	Require less floor space compared to floor mounted horizontal mixers	Require more floor space. Short leg mixers can be mounted to ceiling; However, these are not common.
4.	Time	:	Require 20 min. or more time per batch to obtain maximum mixing efficiency. These are slower.	Require 3-5 min. per batch and are faster than vertical mixers.
5.	Power requirements	:	Consumes less power.	Consumes more power.
6.	Discharge of mixed feed	:	Opening at one place for discharge of the mixed feed.	Openings at several places along the bottom to aid in more rapid discharge.
7.	Cleanout	:	Cleanout will be to a lesser extent.	Cleanout is generally 100% and is more efficient.
8.	Mixing efficiency	:	Require more time to obtain maximum mixing efficiency; Lower mixing efficiency.	Mixes feed at peak efficiency in 3-5 min. Mixing efficiency approaches 99%
9.	General cleaning of the mixer	:	There is only one small discharge gate	Hinged drop bottom doors are furnished for cleaning the internal ribbons and tub of horizontal mixer.
10.	Liquid addition	:	Liquids such as molasses, fats can't be effectively mixed.	Molasses, fats, etc. can be mixed effectively.

Principles of Mixing and Compounding of Feeds

The compounding of animal feed includes processing of raw materials of wide ranging physical, chemical and nutritional characteristics into a homogenous mixture suitable to obtain a desired nutritional response from the animals/birds. Certain feed ingredients such as cereals, oil seed cakes, soybean meal, meat meal, blood meal, fish meal undergo processing prior to their inclusion into a compounded feed.

Once the raw material is purchased, it is stored in the godowns in bags on wooden pallets placed away from the walls. The ingredients could also be stored in concrete or steel silos or in bins. The proper storage of raw materials is not only essential to prevent physical losses but it is also an important aspect of quality control (look for more details in chapter 17).

The feed compounding process consists of a) Grinding of ingredients, b) Mixing of ground materials, c) Further processing, if needed, d) Packaging.

Grinding of feed ingredients: Hammer mills and roller mills are used for grinding in feed industry though the former are popular in India. Expressing the particle size of ground feed is explained later (pp 484).

Mixing of ground ingredients: Importance of mixing has already been discussed elsewhere (pp. 475). Small quantities of animal feed can be adequately mixed manually using shovels. The ground raw materials should be layered one above one another, and then mixed and turned to form one heap. Mixing of the heap at least 3 to 4 times may produce an acceptable product. Microingredients such as vitamins, minerals, antibiotics, etc. are first mixed with diluents e.g. wheat bran and then it is added to ensure uniform mixing. Mechanical mixers such as vertical mixers, horizontal mixers are used for uniform mixing.

Factors that affect mixing: These include 1. Physical properties of ingredients and 2. Mixer designs.

1. *Physical properties of ingredients:* Feed mixing may require many combinations of solids and liquids. Physical properties of solids are particle size, shape, density, coefficient of friction, resilience and electrostatic charge. Physical properties of liquids are density and viscosity. Heating the liquids reduce the viscosity.

2. *Mixer designs:* Interior design of vertical and horizontal mixers.
   Particle segregation, during or after mixing has been attributed to differences in physical properties of materials and the design of the mixer. Particle size is more important. A decrease in particle size is necessary to attain a sufficient number of particles for dispersion into each portion of feed. Where very small amount of microingredients are added the required particle size is very small. The electrostatic properties, roughness of the mixer and cohesiveness are important factors that cause segregation when very small particles are mixed. Mixing time to achieve good distribution increase with very small particles.

Mixing equipment of different type with tumbling, stirring, smearing and impact actions have shown that the rate of mixing is dependent on the properties of the materials being mixed as well as type of equipment used. Differences in the performance of mixing equipment are reduced when the materials have nearly the same particle size and density.

Liquid addition: The addition of various liquids to feeds is a normal practice. These include molasses, vegetable and animal fats, fish solubles, phosphoric acid, choline chloride, etc. These are added to enhance palatability (e.g. molasses), energy (fats) and other nutrient content of the rations. However, addition of any liquid can complicate feed mixing operations. Special equipment for preheating and spraying of liquid are needed to avoid the agglomerate formation. Agglomerate formation can result in suboptimum microingredient distribution.

Liquids are preheated to reduce their viscosity. Molasses is preheated to 95 to 100°F while fat to 140 to 210°F. When liquids are added to the mixer they should be sprayed on over the entire length of the mixer. Before doing so, allow the dry feed ingredients to mix for a short time. This will allow the microingredients to be dispersed throughout the mixture. The maximum amount of molasses which can successfully be applied to feeds is governed by the viscosity of the molasses and by the absorptive quality of the ingredients.

Physical Properties of Feed Ingredients Important to the Daily Operation of Feed Plants

Physical properties of feed ingredients are important to the design as well as the daily operation of feed plants (Table 1). Some of them are discussed here.

1. Bulk density: It is the mass per unit volume of the material. The common units of bulk density are pounds per cubic foot (lb/ft^3) and kilograms per cubic meter (kg/m^3). It is good inventory practice to measure and record the bulk densities of materials as they are received at the plant.

Procedure:
1. Take a cubic foot test box.
2. Fill the box to heaping.
3. Lift it approximately 6 inches and drop it.
4. Repeat step 3.
5. Level the box with a straight edge.
6. Weigh the box and record the net weight of the material (deducting the known weight of the box from the gross weight).

This procedure is intended to duplicate the compaction of the material as it is stored. The density of a material varies significantly with particle

TABLE 1. Some Physical Properties of Dry Feed Ingredients.

Feed ingredient	Apparent density		Angle of repose (degrees)	Static coefficient of friction
	lb/ft³	kg/m³		
Animal Products				
Blood meal	38.5	617	45	1.7
Meat meal	37.0	593	45	0.9
Bone meal	50-60	801-961	40	1.7
Fish meal	30-40	480-641	45	0.9
Egg powder	16	256	-	-
Milk powder	20	320	50	0.4
Mineral feed				
Limestone	68	1089	38	1.0
Salt, coarse	45-50	721-801	30	1.4
Oyster shells, ground under 0.5 inch	53	849	40	0.9
Vitamins				
Riboflavin	37	593	-	-
Vitamin A, dry	48	769	-	-
Cereals, oilseeds and their byproducts				
Barley, whole	38-43	609-689	-	-
Brewers' dried grains	14-15	224-240	-	-
Brewers' grains, spent, dry	25-30	400-480	45	0.44
Maize, ground	34-36	545-577	35	0.8
Maize bran	13	208	30-45	0.5
Cottonseed cake	40-45	641-721	45	1.0
Cottonseed hulls	12	192	43	0.9
Maize distillers' dried grains	18-19	288-304	-	-
Oats, ground	20-25	320-400	40	0.4
Oat hulls, unground	8-9	128-144	45	1.0
Groundnut meal	29	464	-	-
Rice bran	20-41	320-336	45	0.4
Soybean meal	36-40	577-641	35	0.5
Wheat bran	11-16	176-256	30-45	0.4
Wheat ground	38	609	40	0.7
Bagasse	7-10	112-160	-	-
Hay, loose	5	80	45	0.8
Urea	34-42	545-673	30	1.0

size and compaction of the material. Factors that affect the compaction rate include the size, shape and moisture content of the feed material, size and shape of the storage bin, storage capacity and the material used for construction of the bin, seismic occurrences.

2. Coefficient of friction: In the movement of materials, the force of friction plays an important role. There are two different frictional forces that deal with the movement of materials: static and dynamic. The static frictional force is the force needed to start movement of a material. The dynamic frictional force is the force needed to stop the movement of a material.

It has been reported that the coefficient of friction increases slightly with an increase in moisture while it decreases slightly with an increase in temperature. The dynamic coefficient of friction is approximately 20% less than the static coefficient of friction. The coefficient of friction is variable depending on the surface of the bin/conveying area such as wood, plastic, metal.

3. Angle of repose: It can be simply defined as the maximum angle in degrees at which a pile of material retain its slope. It increases nearly linear as the moisture content of the material increases.

Microingredient Premixing

Microingredients

Microingredients are nutritional adducts or drugs that are added to the feed at very low levels. Dispersion of such low concentrations of active ingredients presents a challenge to the manufacturers of the compound feed. This challenge can be met by the premix-the dilution of an active component with a suitable carrier.

Physical characteristics of microingredients such as particle size, particle shape, specific weight, hygroscopicity, susceptibility to electrostatic charges, adhesiveness of the particles due to physical properties, such as rough surfaces or additions of adhesives such as oils influence mixing them with the other feed ingredients. Microingredients have a very small particle size and high density compared to other feed ingredients. A significant uptake of moisture by a microingredient can seriously hamper its ability to distribute and mix well. A hygroscopic ingredient can affect the chemical stability of any moisture sensitive component. This problem may be dealt with during formulations by complexation or through a coating that acts as a moisture barrier.

During intensive grinding to reduce particle size, a pure crystalline compound frequently develops a static charge and hence the individual particles repel one another which may affect its distribution in the premix and in the feed mixture. An antistatic agent such as an unsaturated vegetable oil is suggested.

Premix

Premixes are formulations of one or more microingredients, such as vitamins, minerals, or drugs mixed with diluent and/or carrier ingredient.

Diluent and carrier should be inert and inactive. Premixes are used to facilitate uniform mixing of the microingredients in the complete feed or concentrate mixture.

Diluent is an edible substance used to mix with and reduce the concentration of nutrients and/or additives to make them more acceptable to animals, safer to use and more capable of being mixed uniformly in feed. The mixing properties of the original ingredients are not drastically altered. Carrier is an edible material to which ingredients are added to facilitate uniform incorporation of the latter into feeds. The active principles are absorbed, impregnated or coated into the edible material in such a way as to physically carry the active ingredient. When a carrier is used with a microingredient the mixing properties are drastically altered.

Processing Methods of Grains:

A. Dry processing methods:

1) Grinding	2) Dry rolling	3) Popping
4) Extruding	5) Micronizing	6) Roasting

B. Wet processing methods:

1) Soaking	2) Steam rolling	3) Steam processing & Flaking
4) Pressure cooking	5) Exploding	6) Pelleting
7) Reconstitution		

Out of the above processing methods, grinding is the one commonly used for grains and other feeds. Soaking, extruding and pelleting of feed mixtures are also done in India.

A. Dry Processing Methods

1. Grinding: Grinding is a process of particle size reduction. It is the simplest and least expensive method for preparing grain for feeding livestock. It is a prerequisite for mixing, pelleting or extruding. The grinding may vary from fine to coarse, depending upon the mesh size of the screen used. It is usually accomplished by means of a hammer mill, which reduces the particle size of the grain by impact grinding. Medium-fine grinding is best. This can be distinguished by a gritty feeling as some of the feed is rubbed between the fingers. Very fine grinding makes feeds dusty, lowers palatability resulting in poor animal performance from lowered feed consumption or due to loss of fine material containing the essential nutrients. Further, the propionic acid content is increased, the ratio of acetate to propionate is altered and is narrowed resulting in reduced fat content of milk in milch animals. But in beef cattle the propionate helps in better fattening and increased growth rate.

Advantages of Grinding

1. Increases the particle numbers and thereby increase the surface area which facilitates the digestive enzymes to act resulting in increased digestibility.
2. Improves the feed utilization and thereby increase the performance of the animal.
3. Mixing different feed ingredients is aided by grinding since uniformity of particle size helps in uniform mixing.
4. Pelleting and extruding of feed will be easy, more effective and efficient.
5. Segregation of particles or ingredients or nutrients will be avoided.
6. Selective feeding by livestock will be minimized or avoided. So wastage in feeding will be minimum.
7. Palatability of ingredients will be improved.
8. Energy loss due to mastication will be decreased.
9. Feed passage time will be decreased. Feed consumption will be increased. But decreased feed passage time reduce the digestibility of fibre in ruminants since residence time in the rumen is less.

Expressing the particle size of ground feed: Ground feed is expressed in terms of modulus of uniformity and modulus of fineness. Equipment required is 'Rotap Sieve Shaker'.

Modulus of uniformity: It is expressed as a ratio of coarse, medium and fine particles in ground feed. The optimum ratio is 1:6:3.

Modulus of fineness: It varies from 1 to 7. It decreases with decrease in the particle size of the ground feed. It gives no indication of the proportion of coarse, medium and fine particles in the ground feed.

2. *Dry rolling:*   Rolled or cracked grain are usually prepared by passing the grain through a roller mill. The physical properties of dry rolled or cracked grain would be very similar to that of grains coarsely ground in a hammer mill. Depending upon the rate of flow and the tolerance set between the rollers, the grain can be rolled to a consistency that resemble finely ground grain. Wheat and barley are dry rolled for beef cattle rations.

3. *Popping or puffing:*   Popping is produced by the action of dry heat (700-800°F or 370-425°C) for 15 to 30 seconds causing a sudden expansion of the grain which rupture the endosperm and this results in rupture of starch granules and makes the starch more available to the rumen

microorganisms and/or to the animal. Popped grains will have less moisture (3%) and will be bulky. Popping increases palatability and feed consumption by 5-10%. Popping increases the digestibility. Popped grains are good molasses carrier.

4. Micronizing: It is similar to popping except that heat is furnished in the form of infra-red energy. Micro waves with 3×10^8 to 3×10^{11} cycles/ sec. that are emitted from the infra-red burners are used here. The grain is then rolled to produce a uniform dense product.

5. Extruding: Extrusion cooking has become an important part of the feed industry in the production of pet feeds, fish feeds, feed for laboratory animals, in the gelatinization of cereals for a variety of animal feed and in the cooking of soybean and pulses for control of growth inhibitors. This technology is also used for cooking meat, fish and feather meals for control of salmonella, the cooking of cereals/starch with urea for ruminants, etc.

Gelatinization of starch occurs in this process. Gelatinization is defined as the irreversible destruction of the crystalline order in a starch granule, so that the surface of every molecule is made accessible to solvents or reactants by a combination of moisture, heat, mechanical energy, pressure differential and/or by pH modification. It enhances the ability of starches to absorb large quantities of water leading to improved digestibility and improved feed conversion.

Extrusion cooking technology is becoming popular for manufacturing fish feeds since product densities can be readily controlled and so the feed is utilized by fish completely. These expanded feeds will hold their identity in water and will retain that identity in water without fragmentation for long periods of time. This helps top feeders (e.g. catfish) attain maximum feed conversion.

Density of expanded and gelatinized feed for catfish is 27 to 35 pounds per cubic feet and trout is 20 to 30 pounds per cubic feet.

6. Roasting: It is accomplished by passing the grain through flame resulting in heating to about 300°F (148.9°C) and some expansion of the grains which produces a palatable product. Moisture content of the grain is 5%. Roasting of whole soybeans inactivates enzymes or inhibitory factors, which improves the nutritive value for poultry and swine.

Wet Processing Methods

1. Soaking: Grains soaked for 12-24 hrs in water has long been used for livestock feeding. Sometimes concentrate mixture is also soaked before offering to swine. However, problems in handling and potential souring discouraged its large scale use.

Soaking of mustard cake, neemseed cake in water and offering of filtered product eliminates the toxic effects since the toxic factors are soluble in water.

2. Steam rolling: The grain is subjected to live steam for different periods of time depending upon the pressure used prior to rolling. In case of steam preconditioning at atmospheric pressure, grain is subjected to live steam for 8 to 20 min. and temperature and moisture content of grain are 210-215°F (100°C) and 16-20%, respectively. In case of pressure (20 to 60 psi.) preconditioning, grain is subjected for 50 sec. to 2 min. Temperature and moisture of the grain are 250 to 300°F (121 to 148.9°C) and 18-25% respectively. Pressure preconditioning of grains prior to rolling increases gelatinization of starch to 45-50%.

Steam rolled grains are usually less dusty than dry rolled grains.

3. Steam processing and flaking: The process is a modification of steam rolling to which rigid quality control standards are practiced.

After steam treatment, grain is passed through the roller mill. The tolerance set between the rollers depends upon the flatness of the flake desired. In order to produce a thin flake of grain, the capacity of the steam chamber should be approximately 1/3rd of that of the roller mill.

If the steam processed and flaked material is to be stored for more than one day, it must be dried.

4. Pressure cooking: Pressure cooked grain are similar to steam processed and flaked grain. Grains are cooked with live steam at 50 psi for 1.5 min in air tight pressure chambers. Temperature of 300°F is obtained. The temperature is reduced to below 200°F and the moisture to 20% by passing them through cooling and drying tower prior to flaking. Pressure cooked grains are difficult to flake to the same degree of flatness (as steam processed grain) due to the spongy nature of the pressure cooked grain. The pressure cooked grain should be flaked fairly thin. The capacity of roller mill to handle pressure cooked grain is about 4 times that of pressure cooker. Pressure cooked flakes are less brittle and don't break.

5. Exploding: It is accomplished by subjecting the grain to high pressure steam (to 250 psi) for about a very short time (20 sec.) followed by sudden decrease to atmospheric pressure. This results in rapid expansion of the grain kernels. Similar to popped grain, it produces a low density product.

6. Reconstitution: Reconstituted grain is mature grain (10% moisture) to which water is added to raise the moisture level to 25-30% and the wet product is stored in an oxygen-limiting silo for 14-21 days prior to feeding. Reconstitution of grain increases the solubility of the grain protein.

7. Pelleting: Pelleted feeds are agglomerated feeds formed by extruding individual ingredients or mixtures by compacting and forcing through die openings by any mechanical process.

The purpose of pelleting is to change dusty and unpalatable feed material into more palatable easy to handle larger particles by application of optimum amounts of heat, moisture and pressure. The normal size of pellets is 3.9 mm to 19 mm though the maximum used pellet diameter is 6.25 to 9.4 mm. The shape is mostly cylindrical. If smaller pellets are required, it is economical to produce 3.9 mm pellets and reduce it to the desired particle size by crumbling process.

Advantages of Pelleting

1. Increases the palatability of feed and thereby improves the feed intake.
2. Improves the feeding value of different feeds especially with roughages as compared to concentrates.
3. Increases the density of feed and thereby reduce the storage space required.
4. No segregation and selective feeding.
5. Reduces the wastage of feed by the animal.
6. Pelleted feed is in a free flowing form and can be handled mechanically thereby saving labour cost.
7. Heat labile inhibitors are destroyed; gelatinization of starch occurs.
8. Feeding pelleted feeds enhance the growth rate and milk production and reduce cost of the end product, meat/milk.

Roughage Processing Methods

Dry Processing Methods

1. Baling
2. Field chopped
3. Grinding
4. Pelleting
5. Cubing
6. Dehydration

Wet Processing Methods

1. Green Chopped
2. Soaking

Processing methods such as baling, field chopped, cubing are to be done to make handling easy, to reduce the cost of transportation and space required for storage.

Baling: It is one of the most common methods used to increase convenience of handling forage. The forage is cut and permitted to dry in the field. Dried forage is then baled with a stationary or field baler. It is very popular in developed countries.

Cubing: It is modification of wafer production. Density of long hay is 7 lb/cft while density of cubed hay and density of pelleted hay are 25-32 lb/cft and 40 lb/cft, respectively.

At the time of cubing the hay is broken rather than ground. So there is minimum of fine particles in the cube. Most of the cubing is done with excellent quality alfalfa hay. At the time of cubing water is sprayed on the hay to raise the moisture level to about 14%. If the hay contains more than 10% grass, a satisfactory cube is difficult to make. The cuber may be either a stationary or portable type. It is popular in developed countries.

Grinding: Grinding of roughages is a prerequisite for mixing and pelleting. These mechanical processes increase voluntary intake, nutritive value and facilitate preparation of complete feeds. Roughage should be ground to 1-2" (2.5-5 cm) long for roughage feeding alone or from 0.5 to 1.0" (1.3-2.5 cm) when it is to be incorporated in complete rations. The dust loss can largely be prevented by addition of 1% tallow or water to the material at the time of grinding. Addition of molasses to ground hay makes it highly palatable and increases feed intake.

The Effect of Grinding Roughages

1. Feeding of ground roughages reduces rumination and rumen retention time. Feed consumption is increased leading to better animal performance.
2. Fine grinding of roughage usually reduces digestibility of crude fibre due to faster rate of feed passage. Feeding finely ground feed to dairy animals result in a lower butter fat content in the milk due to lower rumen acetate production.

In view of the cost of equipment, ever increasing cost of energy for running the equipment and transportation of straw to the feed plant and back to the farm, this method appears to be not feasible at farm level and questionable at commercial scale.

Grinding of low quality roughage increase the dry matter digestibility compared to high quality one. It is recommended that straws/stovers be chopped or coarsely ground prior to feeding.

Pelleting of Roughages

Roughages are usually ground before they are pelleted, size of the pellets range from 12/64" to 48/64" (4.8 mm to 19.1 mm). Pelleted roughages weigh about 40 lb/cft as compared to 5-6 lb/cft for long hay.

Pelleting poor quality roughages will markedly increase the consumption of roughage. In pelletising complete feeds incorporation of concentrate mixture at 30% level appear to be the upper limit for optimising the feed intake; otherwise feed intake is decreased. Feeding pellets particularly with a higher concentrate content to ruminants may cause parakeratosis - a degeneration of the rumen papilla. That is pelleting of diets low in forage has an adverse effect.

Feeding of roughage pellets *ad libitum* as the only feed result in increased feed consumption and milk production and decreased milk fat production. This effect on milk fat can be reduced by using large pellet size and by making pellets from coarsely ground roughages.

Dehydration

Green forage such as alfalfa/lucerne can be preserved by dehydrating the forage at high temperature (600-1500°F) in a dehydrator for a short time (3-5 min.). It is usually done with the young growing and good quality forage. This method of forage preservation retains a maximum amount of dry matter and protein and there is no loss of leaves in the process. There is a loss of carotene (5-15%) during the process of artificial drying. Dehydrated alfalfa pellets (17% CP) are usually used as supplement to cattle rather than as primary source of roughage. These pellets are not palatable as compared to cubed or baled hay.

Bulk Density: Bulk density of roughages is very low as compared to concentrate ingredients like cereal grains and oil cakes. However, grinding of roughage increases the density significantly (Table 2) which ensures uniform mixing of ground roughage with other ingredients. The increase in bulk density due to pelleting of mash feed range from 29 to 135% depending on the level and type of roughage used in the complete diets.

In view of low density, most of the roughages are not free flowing, and may create problems in conveying system and other processing machines, thereby affecting production rate and in turn cost of processing.

TABLE 2. Effect of Processing on Bulk Density of Several Roughages.*

	Bulk density (kg/m₃)		
	Chopped	Ground[1]	Pelleted
Sorghum stover	81.5	133.3	333.4
Maize stover	59.3	102.6	344.5
Cotton straw	- -	129.6	311.1
Sunflower straw	—	166.7	319.1
Heteropogon grass	47.4	87.3	213.9
Sehima grass	44.4	83.5	207.2
Cotton seed hulls[2]	148.0	196.0	356.0
Groundnut hulls[2]	104.0	185.0	331.0
Maize cobs[2]	148.0	233.3	359.1
Sugarcane bagasse[2]	55.6	100.0	244.0

1.   Ground in a hammer mill (40 HP) through 8 mm sieve. 2. Unprocessed

* Raj Reddy and Narasa Reddy (1991), Department of Feed and Fodder Technology,
  College of Veterinary Science, Rajendra Nagar, Hyderabad.

Densification of Crop Residues, Grasses and Tree Leaves

High volume low value crop residues and grasses can be densified with
the help of baling machines to permit there economic transport to distant
places. Successful efforts have been made at the Indian Grassland and
Fodder Research Institute (IGFRI), Jhansi (U.P.), India to develop
techniques for making high density packages of these materials so that
their handling, transport, processing and storage (Table 3) become easy
and economical too. On an average, 15 sq. ft. of space will accommodate
about one tonne of concentrates when they are stacked up to a height of
10 ft.

TABLE 3. Space Required for Storing Various Feeds.

Feedstuff	Weight per cubic foot in pounds	Cubic feet per ton
Hay, loose	4.5	456
Hay, baled loose	10.0	200
Hay, baled tight	25.0	80
Hay, chopped	10.0	209
Straw, loose	4.0	512
Straw, baled	22.0	167
Barley	39.0	51
Corn, cracked	40.0	50
Oats	26.0	77
Wheat	48.0	42
Soybeans	50.0	40
Most concentrates	45.0	44

1. *IGFRI Manually operated Hay baler:* IGFRI, Jhansi developed a portable Hay baler which is simple in design, construction, operation and maintenance and cheap compared to indigenous power operated balers. Capacity is about 2.5 M.T. of grass can be baled per day by 3 persons. The bale on an average weighs 25 kg and have density ranging from 150 to 165 kg/m^3.

2. *IGFRI Forage Densifying Machine:* It is a reciprocating ram type machine developed to produce high density bales of wheat bhusa, chaffed stovers, rice straw, grasses and tree leaves for economic storage, handling and transport. Wheat bhusa was baled at 15-36% moisture by adding 10 to 15% molasses. The output capacity of the machine is about 2.0 MT per hour. Weight of the bales is adjustable from 15 to 25 kg.

Feed Mixing Plant

A feed mixing plant has the following machinery (See Figure 5).

1. *Hammer Mills:* These are versatile grinding machines for powdering most of the materials. The feed ingredient is fed into the grinding chamber of the mill where it is reduced in size by a mechanical army of hammers. The material reduced in size is drawn out through a sieve located at the base of the grinding chamber. The degree of fineness is determined solely by the size of the screen used. By changing the screen the degree of fineness can be varied to meet almost any requirement. The screen can be changed in less than one minute.

Hammer mills are of two types:

1. Pneumatic conveying   2. Gravity fall

1. *Pneumatic conveying:* In these mills the ground material is conveyed pneumatically to a cyclone collector where it is disengaged and collected in bags. The feeding and bagging therefore are at a convenient level above the ground. See figure 2.

Capacity/8 hrs.	Power
6-8 tons	7.5 HP

2. *Gravity fall:* In these mills the ground material directly falls from the bottom opening into a pit.

Capacity/8 hrs.	Power
6-8 tons	5 HP

Note: The capacity of the mills is based on grinding of maize on 5/16" hole screen. The capacity will vary for different materials depending on the structure of the material to be ground. The capacity will also be proportionately reduced for finer mash.

Mixers: Horizontal mixer: Horizontal paddle mixer, saw teeth paddle mixer, twin shaft multi paddle mixer, horizontal ribbon type mixer, etc. are available to facilitate mixing of solid and liquid feedstuffs.

Double Paddle Horizontal Mixers and Ribbon Blenders

	Capacity Batch/kg	Shift/8 hrs.	Power
1.	Double paddle horizontal mixer 250 - 300	8 - 10 tons	3 -5 HP
2.	Ribbon blenders 250 - 300	6 - 8 tons	5 - 7.5 HP

Note: Capacity is based on maximum mixing time of 5 min. for each batch and discharge and bagging time of 10-12 min. for one ton of mixed feeds.

ii. Vertical mixer:

Capacity

Batch/kg	Shift/8 hrs	Power
500	8 tons	3 HP

3. Conveying Systems

Bucket elevator: The inlet hopper is designed and positioned for uniform and accurate feed to buckets. Buckets are shaped to hold the material and elevate to the required height. The casting is done dead straight to provide easy and dust-proof-housing for the chain and buckets. The spacing of buckets is designed to attain high efficiency.

HP	Capacity/hour
1	1.5 to 2.5 tons
1.5	3 to 5 tons

The feed ingredients to be ground as well as the powdery materials of the formula are dumped into the grinder. The ground material is lifted by the bucket elevator for mixing process. A batch holding bin is placed above the mixer to hold one batch in readiness for instant feeding to the mixer no sooner it gets emptied.

4. *Magnetic Separator:* Magnets are used for arresting ferrous thrash from feed ingredients and final mixed feeds. Removing of the ferrous thrash is not only to free the feeds from dangerous ferrous articles, especially sharp nails and pieces, which can cause death of an invaluable animal, but also to prevent damage to costly machinery.

Magnets can be placed at various points, preferably at the point where the flow is comparatively thin and at slow speed. Plate magnet is kept in the feeding hopper of hammer mill and a grid magnet or drum magnet is kept at the mixed feed discharge chute to arrest the ferrous thrash.

5. *Pellet Mill:* Pelleting has become an important and necessary process in the densification of a variety of materials. However, pelleting increases the cost of machinery and involvement of high energy.

Capacity	Mill motor HP	Feeder motor HP
0.75 to 1 ton/hr	35 to 40	2
1.5 to 2 tons/hr	50 to 60	2
5 to 10 tons/hr	120 HP (at maximum production)	3

6. *Packaging:* Compound feeds, whether in meal or pellet form, are packed in bags or stored in bins. Bags may be filled directly from mixers, pellet coolers or holding bins and weighed before sealing. Bags may be of jute, cotton, paper or plastic and can be hand or machine stitched or tied with string. The BIS standard requires that the packing of balanced cattle feed should be in clean and sound plain or polyethylene lined jute or laminated paper bags. However, normally the polyethylene bags are not used because of risk of sweating and mould growth. Bags used for fertilizers, pesticides or other chemicals may not be reused for filling animal feeds.

Proportional Motor Size and Cost for Feed Milling (% of Total)

Unit/Operation	Feed Mill (2 ton/hr)	
	Motor size (%)	Unit cost (%)
Weighing	-	7
Elevators/Augers	3	7
Holding bins	-	5
Grinding	34	13
Mixing (horizontal)	10	12
Pelleting	43	17
Steam production	1	11
Pellet cooling	9	11
Bag-off weigh	-	7
Electrical control system	-	10
	100	100
	110 KW	

Approximate Cost of Processing and Packing of Feed per MT

1. Cost of grinding and mixing mash feed   Rs. 100 - 125
2. Cost of pelleting one MT of mash into
   3 mm diameter pellets   Rs. 300
3. Cost of packing in HDPE bags   Rs. 220
   (cost of one empty bag × 20 + misc. charges)

Feed Mill Design

The engineering and design of feed mills vary throughout the world considerably depending on the capacity of the mill, availability of feed ingredients, storage and logistics of feed, availability of labour force, etc. If labour is expensive a fully computerised mill may be the answer. Several differences can be noted in the general design of feed mills present in the United States and in the European Countries. In the US most of the ingredients are transported by bucket elevators to bins above ground level. Gravity flow is then used in many cases and that is why

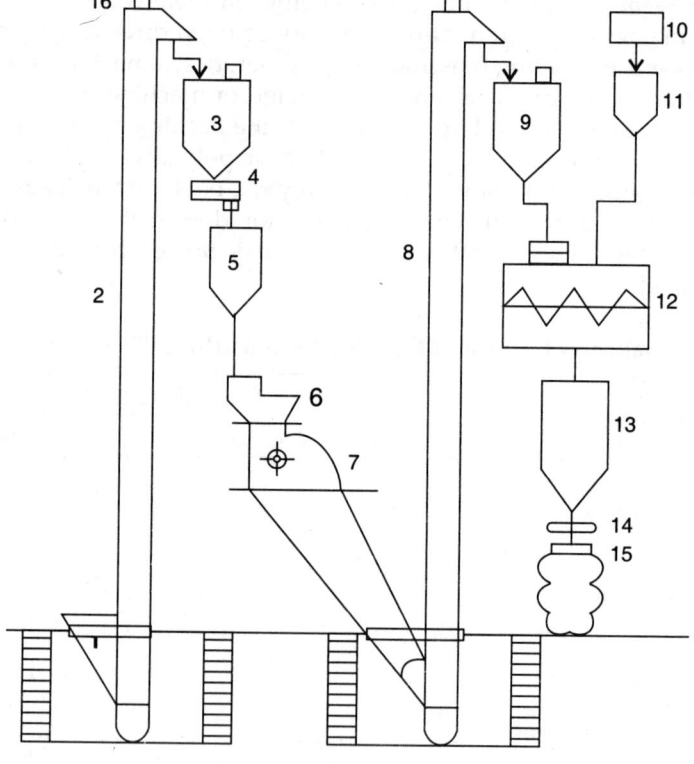

Figure 5. Symbolic Process Flow diagram: Feed Mill.

many mills in the US have rather high profiles. Horizontal conveyors are used in many European mills. Production systems in US mills are generally located below the bins while European mills have the processing systems located on a tower next to the bins and at the same level.

In most American systems, the ingredients are ground in the first phase of production. In many European mills, raw materials are first weighed together as a batch. Later the entire batch of feed goes through a separator where the material require grinding are diverted to pass through the hammer mill.

Legend

1. Intake hopper
2. Bucket elevator
3. Surge hopper (raw feed ingredients)
4. Separator
5. Surge hopper (feed ingredients for grinding)
6. Feeder and magnet
7. Hammer mill
8. Bucket elevator
9. Surge hopper (ground material for mixing)
10. Molasses service tank
11. Molasses dosing tank
12. Horizontal mixer
13. Surge hopper (finished mash feed)
14. Magnet
15. Feed packer (gunny bag)
16. Dust bag

An example of Soybean meal has been shown here how it is processed in a feed mixing plant.

Receipt of soybeans → cleaning (pass through less than 3.2 mm round-hole sieve to remove foreign materials in soybeans) → cracking (two sets of corrugated rolls) → dehulling → conditioning (71-76°C; 9-10% moisture) → flaking (0.25 → 0.3 mm thickness) → expanding/extruding of flakes (55-66°C; 7% moisture) → extraction (1 kg solvent to 1 kg flakes; time 30 minutes) → desolventiser toaster distillation → Soybean oil, and Soybean meal.

Soybean meal has poor flowability and has bridging characteristics. Addition of calcium carbonate, calcium bentonite or sodium bentonite at 0.25-0.5% level improves flowability. The soybean meal is hygroscopic. The moisture level at a given temperature and equilibrium relative humidity is its equilibrium moisture content (EMC). The EMC of soybeans and soybean meal by desorption (lose moisture) are higher than that by adsorption under the same set of conditions. The phenomenon is known as **hysteresis**. Jute bag storage has self-ventilating and cooling charcteristics.

The Maillard Reaction in Feed Manufacturing

The Maillard reaction (see p. 455) is an integral part of feed manufacturing. Its adverse effects are experienced via reduced nutrient availability from thermal processing and prolonged storage in both finished diets and ingredients. Before going into the Maillard reaction proper, let us know about the reason for brown colours.

Non-enzymatic Browning Reaction

Brown colours often develop during the processing, storage, and preparation of foods and food ingredients. Some reactions that produce brown colours are enzyme catalyzed. These reactions usually involve oxidation of food components. Other browning reactions are non-enzymatic. These include caramelization of sugars (Sugars in solution are quite stable to heat in the pH range of 3-7. Melting dry sugars or heating sugar solutions in the presence of acidic or basic catalysts, however, causes the sugars to caramelize. Caramelization results in brown colours and pleasing aromas.) and the Maillard reaction.

Several Factors Influence the Extent of Maillard Browning in a Food.

1. First, either an aldehyde or a ketone (reducing sugars are the most important in food systems) and an amine (protein is by far the most important) must be present. Under conditions of elevated temperature and humidity, any compound with a free amino group is vulnerable to the Maillard reaction, and this includes free amino acids, epsilon amino groups of protein-bound lysine, and free amino groups of thiamine, folacin, and gossypol. Lysine is the most susceptible amino acid in intact protein because it has a free amino group at the epsilon carbon unit that is readily available to react with reducing sugars. Free lysine is even more reactive because it has two free amino groups. See page No. 456.
2. The reaction rate is measurable at 37°C, as long as several days' reaction time are allowed; rapid at 100°C, and violent at 150°C.
3. The reaction is extremely slow in dry foods and in highly dilute solutions. Maximum rates of browning reactions occur in foods containing 10-15% moisture. This is because some water is necessary for the reactants to interact. In case of highly dilute solutions, the reactants would be relatively widely separated.
4. The Maillard reaction, may take place at room temperature, but its intensity increases as time, temperature, moisture, and alkalinity

(linear between pH 3 and 8). The initial reaction products have autocatalytic properties that further intensify the effects of heat treatment and storage.

Browning and Deterioration of Protein Quality

The Maillard reaction involves binding of amino groups to the carbonyl group of reducing sugars such as glucose or lactose. Although sugar losses are greater and more intense than amino acid losses, it is the deterioration of protein quality that is of most concern to nutritionists and farmers/producers. Browning is often confused with the intensity of the Maillard reaction. However, brown colouration and amino acid losses are two independent phenomena of the Maillard reaction that differ radically. During the initial stages of the Maillard reaction, products [early-Maillard reaction products of lysine include N- (1-deoxy-D-fructosyl) lysine and N- (1-deoxy-D-lactulosyl) lysine] remain colourless but amino acids have already become unavailable. Therefore, colour change is not a good indicator of protein quality damage, which occurs rather early. Formation of late-Maillard reaction products such as melanoides contributes browning colouration. It has been repeatedly demonstrated that thermal over-processing of high-protein materials reduces lysine bioavailability, depending on temperature levels and the duration of heat application.

Heat-sensitive Feed Ingredients

Creep feeds for piglets and calves are rich in milk products, which contain relatively high amounts of lactose and lysine. Creep diets may also contain other equally sensitive ingredients such as blood products, concentrated soybean proteins, fish meal, and wheat gluten that readily contribute to the Maillard reaction problem.

Pelleting of Feed and Destruction of Nutrients

During pelleting, feed is exposed to relatively high humidity and temperature levels. Usually two to six per cent moisture is added to the mash during conditioning at temperatures that can range from 50 to 90°C from several seconds to 20 or more minutes. Extremely high temperatures can also develop during pellet formation due to friction with the die walls as the conditioned mash is forced through die openings. More aggressive feed processing methods, such as expansion, extrusion, double pelleting, and prolonged mash conditioning, also increase the risk of greater nutrient destruction via the Maillard reaction.

Storage of Feed and Destruction of Nutrients

Storage of heat-senstive material in the form of finished diets or raw materials for prolonged periods of time can also initiate a second cycle of

Maillard reactons. This is of paramount importance in feed management during storage in silos and general feed storage godowns because the conditions of high temperature and relative humidity are extremely favourable for the Maillard reaction. A 10% moisture level in milk powder stored for 10 weeks at 30°C resulted in a 20% loss in lysine bioavailability.

Positive Side of Maillard Reaction

On the positive side, Maillard reaction products are responsible for the desirable cooked flavour of feed and foods. This may be a contributing factor associated with increased feed intakes usually observed with pelleted diets.

Improvement of Poor Quality Roughages

Characteristic Attributes of Straws

Straws are low density feeds characterised by large content of structural carbohydrates (cellulose and hemicellulose), low level of starch type carbohydrates, low nitrogen and minerals and varying amounts of lignin. Cellulose and hemicellulose are in complex form with lignin. Straws contain low levels of soluble carbohydrates (1-2%). The extent to which cellulose and hemicellulose are digested in the rumen depends to a great extent on the degree of their association with each other and lignin. It has been suggested that lignin acts as a physical barrier and impedes microbial breakdown of these materials. The usefulness of cellulose depends on the extent and rate at which it can be degraded by rumen microorganisms. High quality roughage is usually low in lignin and high in protein and is highly digestible. Low quality roughages are usually low in protein, high in lignin and are poorly digestible.

There is insufficient rumen degradable nitrogen (RDN) and other elements (S, P, Ca and Co) in the straw to supply the requirements of the rumen microbes for maximal fermentation of organic matter. Much of the small amount of N in the straw is probably in the insoluble acid detergent fibre (ADF) fraction and unavailable to the rumen microbes.

Since straws are deficient in nutrients required for rumen microbes, their colonisation gets delayed. Hence rate of degradation is slow and feed stays for more time in the rumen. With most poor quality roughages, animals may consume only about 60-80 $g/W_{kg}^{0.75}$/day, an amount hardly enough even to support maintenance requirement of an adult animal. So animals lose body weight. Therefore, it is imperative that these deficiencies are corrected before poor quality roughages are considered satisfactory ruminant feedstuffs.

Dry roughages	DCP%	TDN%
Paddy straw	0.2	45.9
Wheat straw	0.0	48.3
Ragi straw	0.2	50.0
Gram *bhusa*	2.2	51.0
Bajra *karbi*	0.8	48.0
Jowar *karbi*	1.0	51.0

Methods of Improving the Feeding Value of Poor Quality Roughages

A. Supplementation with Deficient Nutrients

The purpose of supplementing a poor quality roughage is to correct nutrient imbalances and thereby create optimum rumen conditions for efficient microbial fermentation.

1. Enrichment with urea and molasses
2. Ensiling with animal wastes such as faeces and urine
3. Supplementation with green fodders either leguminous or non-leguminous
4. Supplementation with legume straws (Sunnhemp, horsegram, cowpea and gram straws)
5. Supplementation with urea-molasses liquid supplements

B. Treatments: The main objective of treating a poor quality roughage is to increase its digestibility and or voluntary intake so as to increase the intake of digestible energy.

Methods of Improving the Nutritive Value of Poor Quality Roughages

Poor quality roughages

Physical methods	Chemical methods	Physico-chemical methods	Biological methods
1. Soaking	1. Alkali -NaOH,Ca(OH)$_2$ KOH, NH$_4$OH	Combination of physical and	Enzymes Rot fungi
2. Chopping	2. Ammonia	chemical treatments	Mushrooms
3. Grinding	Gaseous, Aqueous, Urea-ammonia	e.g. NaoH/ pelleting; NaOH/steam	
4. Pelleting	3. Acids		
5. Wafering	H$_2$SO$_4$, HNO$_3$		
6. Steam under pressure	4. Salts Na$_2$CO$_3$ NaCl		
7. Irradiation	5. Gases Chlorine SO$_2$		
	6. Oxidizing agents H$_2$O$_2$,O$_3$		

Physical Treatments

Soaking of wheat straw increased the dry matter intake and volatile fatty acid production but has no effect on the digestibility of nutrients. The paddy straw is rich in oxalate and the major portion of it is present in the form of soluble potassium and sodium oxalates and small fraction is present in the insoluble form of calcium oxalate. Soaking of paddy straw removes some of the oxalates and may improve the nutritive value of straw and improve Ca retention more importantly. Chopping of rice straw or maize stover increased the voluntary intake of these roughages.

Chaffing or Chopping of Fodder: Chaff Cutter

Animals are prone to eat only the leaves of plant material wasting the stem part. By chaffing the green fodder or dry fodder selective feeding and thus wastage of fodder can be avoided. Fodders are chopped uniformly into fine (0.5 cm) or coarse (1-2 cm) particles.

There are two types of Chaff cutters.

1. Hand operated:

    a)   Sickle type chaff cutter

    b)   Hand operated chaff cutter: This machine is made from sturdy angle iron frame with cast iron well-balanced wheel on which two knives are fixed. This wheel is enclosed by wire mesh cover from top to avoid accident. The main shaft has 3 ball bearings in the line in oil immersed gear box.

        Output: Hand drive: 75-100 kg/hr at 40 RPM

                   Power drive: 200-250 kg/hr at 100 RPM with 0.75 KW

        Output depends on quality and condition of fodder.

2. Power Operated:

Chaff-cutters working on 5 HP or 10 HP are useful for medium size to big Dairy Farms. The Chaff cutter is fabricated from heavy duty angle iron. The impellar is made from 1/2" M.S. (mild steel) plates with 3 straight knives. The impellar is fully enclosed and the sliced or chaffed material is thrown from the overhead spout. The knives can be accurately adjusted to give around 3/8" (9.4 mm) cut chaff. It has a gear box for forward and reverse motion so that any clogging of chaffed material is immediately released by reversing the motion. The feeding of fodder is done either by hands or by a belt conveyor. The machine can be made mobile on wheels for toeing it from one place to another.

Output: 1000 kg to 2000 kg/hr with 5 to 10 HP motor (output depends on quality and condition of fodder).

Advantages of Chopping of Roughages

1. It avoids wastage.
2. It facilitates feeding of roughages and concentrates together in the form of complete feed.
3. Chopping of green fodder facilitates good silage making.
4. It facilitates mixing with other ingredients of ration and checks the selective feeding.
5. It facilitates easy handling due to increased bulk density.
6. It improves digestion due to exposure of relatively larger surface area of roughages for microbial digestion.

Boiling under high pressure or steaming method: Among all the physical treatments, this method has greater effect on improvement of feeding quality of straw.

The basic and precise technology behind this process is to break the chemical bonds (ligno-cellulose/ligno-hemicellulose) through steaming at high pressure which in turn increases the digestibility of the final product. D.V. Rangnekar (1982) from BAIF, Ahmedabad proposed utilization of surplus steam in sugarcane industries for treatment of bagasse which could economise the process with effective improvement in the nutritive value of bagasse.

Chemical treatments: The aim of chemical treatment is to increase lignin solubility or decrease the bonds between lignin and other cell wall constituents, thereby making cellulose and hemicellulose more susceptible to (rumen) microbial attack. This increases the voluntary feed intake as well as the digestibility of straw. Several types of chemicals such as sulphuric acid (acid), sodium hydroxide, potassium hydroxide, calcium hydroxide, sodium carbonate or ammonium hydroxide (alkalies), hydrogen peroxide, sulphur dioxide, sodium chlorite or ozone (oxidizing agents) have been investigated for treatment of crop residues.

1. Treatment with NaOH: This process was first used on straw in Germany in 1919, during Ist world war when there was a critical shortage of livestock feed. Straw was treated with NaOH under high pressure and temperature. The product was called as 'fodder cellulose'. This process was very expensive and only relevant in emergency situations. It can be of two major types.

1.	Wet method:	This includes Beckmann method, modified Beckmann method or Torgrimsby method and dip method.
2.	Dry method.	

Beckmann's method: Proposed in 1921, it consists of treating chopped straw in 8-10 times its weight of 1.2 to 1.5% (W/V) solution of NaOH for atleast 4 hours. The treated straw was drained and washed with a large quantity of water until free from alkali [(i.e.) it should be neutral to litmus paper]. As NaOH is caustic and rapidly attacks animal tissues, it should be thoroughly washed with water.

The treatment dissolved 20-25% of DM from the straw and therefore, was lost.

Modified Beckmann method: An improvement over the Beckmann method, it uses less NaOH and less water; DM loss is reduced; there is no pollution problem because it is a closed system.

Dip treatment: This method was developed by Sundstol and coworkers (1981) in Norway and Tanzania. After draining the excess alkali solution, the straw is allowed to 'ripen' for 3-6 days as there is evidence to show that digestibility of treated straw increases during the 'ripening' process.

Dry method: With a view to eliminate the disadvantages of the Beckmann system, Wilson and Pigden (1964) evolved a dry process. The straw is sprayed or sprinkled with NaOH while being mixed. 4 to 6 kg of NaOH dissolved in 200 litres of water is adequate to wet 100 kg straw. The treated straw is moist and has pleasant odour. Intake of straw is increased by 30-40%. Digestibility is increased by 10-15 percentage units.

2. Treatment with calcium hydroxide: It is a cheaper, safer to use and easily available chemical; but its low solubility in water and being a weak base has deterred researchers in their studies with fibrous feeds. With spray treatment $Ca(OH)_2$ has consistently been inferior to NaOH, unless longer reaction time is allowed. Ensiling $Ca(OH)_2$ treated straw (4 kg $Ca(OH)_2$/100 kg straw), with enough water to give 50% moisture in freshly treated straw, for 90 to 150 days has resulted in higher fermentability of treated straw. Longer incubation period gave higher treatment effect.

Treatment with combination of calcium and sodium hydroxides: Combined treatment produced some what better gains than either of the hydroxide alone, and treatment with 4% NaOH produced significantly greater gains than with 4% $Ca(OH)_2$. Treatment of straw with $Ca(OH)_2$ will be effective when the treated straw does not constitute more than 70% of the diet, because the calcium content increases more than the normal requirement (1.5 to 2.0%). One approach could be to use lower concentration of $Ca(OH)_2$ either alone or in combination with urea or NaOH.

Due to high cost of the chemical, problems of pollution, corrosive nature of the chemical and addition of sodium to animal diets, NaOH treatment could not find popularity.

3. a. Treatment with anhydrous NH₃: Among the several alkalies/ oxidising agents suggested, ammonia treatment is by far the most appropriate for straw treatment. It serves as an alkali to improve the potential rate and extent of digestion of straw and it further serves as an essential nutrient (nitrogen) to rumen microbes to ensure efficient rumen fermentation. The stack method for ammonia treatment of straw was developed by Sundstol and coworkers in Norway during 1970-75. Stacks of straw were wrapped with polyethylene cover and injected with 3% of anhydrous ammonia. This method has become popular and was standardised under Indian conditions for wheat straw, cotton straw and paddy straw. The effect of ammonia treatment on the digestibility of straw is less than that of dip treatment with NaOH. When materials with a high sugar content (5% e.g. hays) are treated with anhydrous NH_3 at high temperature (70°C) a poisonous compound '4-methyl imidasol' can be formed which may cause hyperexcitability **(crazy cow or angry cow or bovine bonker)** in farm animals and may also be transferred into the milk of dairy cows. With straw, treated at environmental temperatures, the risk of this disturbance should be negligible.

b. Treatment with aqueous NH₃: Aqueous ammonia (20-35%) is also used commercially for treatment of straw. One advantage here is that at ammonia concentration of about 20% the solution can be transported and handled at normal temperature and pressure.

c. Ammoniation through urea hydrolysis: Anhydrous or aqueous ammonia are costly, not freely available and even if available transportation of equipment is difficult and need to be handled with much care. Fertilizer grade urea which is well known to the farmer can also be used to generate ammonia from urea hydrolysis. Urine has also been used as source of NH_3 for straw treatment. Ammonia treatment through urea hydrolysis is a promising alternative to several problem ridden chemical treatments because of simple technology and low cost involved in it.

The method developed by Jackson (Pantnagar, UP) and tested and modified at IVRI, Izatnagar, NDRI, Karnal and at several State Agricultural Universities in India, Bangladesh and Sri Lanka has clearly demonstrated that this treatment increases digestibility and intake of the straws leading to increased animal production. On-farm trials in India, Sri Lanka and Bangladesh have shown that urea-ammonia treated straw offers a great promise for the future of animal production in the Indian sub-continent. These studies have also stressed the necessity for a simple and economic treatment system for the rural farmer.

Optimum Conditions for Urea Hydrolysis

a. Level of urea: The basic principle is the breakdown of urea to its components of NH_3 and CO_2 by urease enzyme.

$$H_2N - \overset{\overset{\textstyle O}{\textstyle ||}}{C} - NH_2 + H_2O \xrightarrow{\text{Urease}} 2NH_3 + CO_2$$

Molecular weight	60	18	17	44
Weight produced	60	18	34	44

This indicates that adding 6.2% (wt/wt) of urea is equivalent to adding 3.5% ammonia, assuming 100% conversion. It was considered a dose of 3.0% NH_3 optimal and this corresponds to 5.3% urea (wt/wt) for treatment.

b. Moisture level: It was demonstrated that for sufficient ureolysis a minimum of 350 ml water/kg straw must be added.

c. Preservative effect of NH_3: It was reported that when the moisture content of straw is 300 g/kg DM or more, then a concentration of urea greater than 40 g/kg DM is required in order to achieve preservative effect of NH_3. NH_3 has a fungicidal effect.

d. Source and activity of urease: Urease enzyme is a natural contaminant of straw. Urea was extensively hydrolysed even in the absence of an exogenous source of urease. However addition of an urease source (soybean powder, 8.5%) reduced the treatment time from 21 days to less than 5 days. NDDB workers used watermelon seed powder as a source of urease.

e. Temperature: The optimum temperature for urease activity in soil is approximately 30°C, and urease activity tends to decrease at temperatures lower than 20°C. Ammoniation was accelerated at higher temperatures (14, 24 and 35°C) particularly at the higher moisture levels (250 Vs 375 g/kg wheat straw). Comparable IVOMD (*in vitro* OM digestibility) values were obtained after a treatment period of one to two weeks at 35°C and approximately six weeks at 24°C. The significant ($P < 0.01$) interaction found between temperature and treatment period and moisture level and treatment period indicates that the slow reaction at lower temperature and at lower moisture levels can partly be compensated for by longer treatment period. Low urease activity at 4°C indicate that this method may not be practical under field conditions in extremely cold regions.

Effect of Ammonia Treatment on Feeding Value of Wheat Straw

Ammoniation of straw improves the quantity of cellulose (hemicellulose) for microbial attack, because the small NH_3 molecules are able to penetrate the interfibroid spaces of the crystalline cellulose in order to break down the H-bridges. In contrast with NaOH, ammonia is too weakly alkaline to have an appreciable effect on (hemi) cellulose-lignin bonds.

The effect of wheat straw ammoniation using 5% urea as a source of ammonia at 40% added moisture level was evaluated by chemical analyses and *in sacco* polyester bag technique (Table 4). Ammonia treatment increased the soluble phenolics by 52% and decreased the total cell wall phenolics by about 12%. Treatment increased crude protein content by 300%, decreased neutral detergent fibre (NDF) and hemicellulose content by 8 and 20% respectively. About 54% of added N was retained in the ammoniated straw 66% of which was soluble in water. Ammoniation had changed the colour of straw from yellow to dark brown. The pH of treated straw measured after 24 h aeration was 8.86. Ammoniation has enhanced the rate of rumen degradability of wheat straw by more than 60% and potential degradability by 10% compared to those of untreated straw.

Ammoniation through urea hydrolysis has many advantages. It is relatively inexpensive, creates no known pollution problems, acts as

TABLE 4. Effect of Ammonia Treatment of Wheat Straw

Parameter	Untreated Straw	Treated Straw	Significance
Crude protein %	2.59	10.37	P < 0.01
Metabolisable energy (Mcal/kg dry feed)	1.62	1.99	-
Buffer soluble phenolics (absorbance/mg straw at 280 nm)	0.52	0.78	-
Total cell wall phenolics (absorbance/mg straw at 280 nm)	2.56	2.26	-
Rate of degradability in the rumen (%/h)	3.21	5.07	P < 0.001
Potential degradability in the rumen (%)	63.36	69.10	P < 0.01

preservative of high moisture material preventing mould attack, NPN is added to the straw and treated straw is pliable and palatable.

Biological Treatments

1. Enzyme treatement: Cellulase solution is sprayed on straw at 25 mg/ 100 kg straw.
2. Fermentation: Chopped straw is pretreated with 3-5% NaOH, and steamed at 120°C for 15 min; then fermented with bran type media cultured with cellulolytic microorganisms at 40-50°C for 2 days.
3. White-rot fungi, mushrooms and other microbes

The efficient utilization of lignocellulosic straws is limited because of metabolic block caused by lignin which occurs in a range of 3 to 13%. Some of the white-rot fungi like *Phanerochaete chrysosporium* degrade lignin to the extent of 65-75% while other fungi like *Ganoderma applanatum* and *Coriolus versicolor* degrade over 45% of lignin in the lignocellulosic materials. Preference is given to species which degrade only lignin but not hemicelluloses.

Indo-Dutch Project on Bioconversion of Crop Residues

Studies have been conducted on white-rot *Basidiomycetes,* often belonging to the non-toxic and edible mushrooms.

1. *Zadrazil process:* Straw was treated with Pleurotus sp. The process has enormous losses of organic matter. It is unfit for small level operations at farmer's level.

2. *Karnal process:* It is essentially a biological treatment of ligno-cellulosics in a solid substrate fermentation (SSF) system under non-sterile conditions which causes a promising improvement in the enhancement of quality of straw. It is a two stage technique wherein cereal straws are pretreated with 4% urea and 40% moisture and ensiled for 30 days in the first stage and followed by second stage in which the urea treated material is mixed thoroughly with 1% single superphosphate, 0.1% calcium oxide and then moisturise to 60-65% before inoculation with 3% *Coprinus fimetarius* (alkalitolerant strain) culture grown on millets. The solid substrate fermentation was terminated at mycelial stage of growth of C. fimetarius.

The use of urea in the first stage has many advantages. Besides, breaking the ligno-carbohydrate bonds in the treated straw, ammonia also helps in creating conducive environment (high pH), increases CP content from 3-4% to 12-14% and acts as a chemical sterilent in preventing the growth of unwanted organisms.

In the second stage, the fungus traps the excess free ammonia in the urea-treated straw and synthesize amino acids. Thus there was substantial increase in the amino acid content of fungal treated straw. Considerable dry matter losses were there. However, dry matter losses were reduced from 35% to 7% by applying certain modifications.

Complete Feed Manufacturing Machine

Low productivity of Indian livestock is a matter of concern, and one of the contributing factors is the insufficient and poor quality feed resources. To bridge the gap between availability and requirement of nutrients to feed the most fabulous livestock wealth (Indian cattle, buffaloes, sheep and goats constitute to 14, 58, 6 and 16% of the world population, respectively), there is an urgent need to optimize the use of our limited feed resources through effective feed management.

Blending the coarsely ground (8mm) crop residues, AIBPs, NCFRs in the form of complete feeds / Total mixed rations (TMR) helps developing low-cost feed, avoids refusal of unpalatable portion or selective feeding, improves utilization of supplemental urea or uric acid of poultry droppings resulting in efficient feed resource use [Reddy, D.V. (2008) Sixth regional conference of Animal Nutrition Society of India held at Tirupati on 15th October, 2008; pp. 22-27].

The complete feed manufacturing unit consists of chopper cum grinder and paddle type mixer. The chopper cum grinder had a motor with specially designed impact type beaters and blower fan. It had 2 inlets one for crop residues (straws and stovers in long form) and the other for other feed ingredients (sunflower heads, maize cobs etc. which are small in size can be fed along with concentrates). It has a separate gear box used to drive the intake mechanism. The gear box had forward, reverse and neutral gear operated by a lever. The reverse gear is used in case of roller jamming rising due to bigger than acceptable column of stalk entering the intake mechanism. The chopper cum grinder operates on 15 hp motor while the gear box operates on ½ hp geared motor drive. At the bottom of the chopping/grinding chamber is a screen of 8mm diameter. Once the material reaches the size of the hole of the sieve, it will pass through the sieve and reach the mixer via blower. Hardcase Engineering Works Pvt. Ltd., Secunderabad fabricated the machine with technical support from Dept of Feed and Fodder Technology, CVSc, Hyderabad, (then Andhra Pradesh), Telangana State.

The mixer is paddle type, capable of mixing the roughages, grains, oil cakes, microingredients and molasses. It can accommodate 250kg concentrate or 100 kg complete feed. The mixer is provided on the top with large hopper with lid to add micro nutrients and also with a bottom-perforated tray to add molasses. The mixer works on 3 hp motor. To operate the motors, a motor control centre is essential.

The roughages and concentrates as per the feed formula after weighing are fed to the machine for the necessary particle size reduction. Micronutrients can be added directly to the mixer in the form of a premix. Molasses heated to 70°C has to be added as the process of mixing continues. Mix all ingredients for 7-10 min and collect the complete feed into gunny bags.

Densified Feed Blocks

Densification of such complete feeds (compressed feed blocks) reduces the volume of feed which makes its handling, storage and transportation easy. For the production of 'feed blocks', the mixture of roughage and concentrate is compressed in a machine. Dr. Amar Singh and his team of scientists from IARI, New Delhi developed a prototype of 'block making machine', which has been patented as well. M/s Poshak feeds India Pvt. Ltd., Karnal, Haryana has come up commercially to manufacture complete feed blocks for medium and high yielding dairy animals.

Expander-extruder Processing of Complete Feeds

The nutritive value of the complete feeds could be further improved by expander extruder technology. This is a system which combines the features of expanding (application of moisture, pressure and temperature to gelatinize the starch portion) and extruding (pressing the feed through constrictions under pressure). The feed material is conditioned to 16-17% moisture by adding sufficient quantity of water and then fed to the machine. The Expander-extruder is a single continuous barrel with about 5.25 inches internal diameter and of approximately 2.56 meter working length.

The feed material enters into the barrel and is pushed in forward direction. The feed material is subjected to steam and pressure leading to rise in temperature to about 100°C, as the material is extruded through the 16 mm die holes present at the other end of the barrel. The pellets coming out of die holes are cooled and collected into sacks. This process increases the bulk density, ensures detoxification of antinutritional factors and destruction of microbes.

Expander extruder processing is simple to operate with less maintenance cost and high production efficiency. Further, it ensures complete gelatinization of the feed material comprising roughage and concentrate when compared to conventional pellet mill. Dr. G.V.N. Reddy and his team of scientists standardized the technology at CVSc, Hyderabad as part of the TOE on Feed Technology and Quality Assurance (NATP) ending 2003.

Chapter 18

Storage of Feeds and Feed Ingredients

Storage loss: Storage loss is measured as reduction in weight. But this loss may be qualitative as well in terms of nutritional and germinative. The storage loss can be prevented or reduced by better management at preharvest stage, during harvesting, threshing and shelling and drying and by applying sound storage practices.

Factors that Affect Food Value and Deterioration during Storage

1. Physical factors: These are moisture of grain, temperature and relative humidity (RH) of air, grain size and shape and storage period. Clean sound and unbroken grains will have higher weight and longer storage life compared to immature, broken, germ-eaten and shrivelled grains because of increased susceptibility to insect pests, fungus and moisture. A temperature of 28 to 30°C and 65-80% RH favour microbial and insect growth.

2. Biological factors: These are insects, fungi and rodents. Major storage insect pests are granary weevil, lesser grain borer, saw-toothed grain beetle, flat grain beetle, grain moth, rice weevil, meal moth, red flour beetle.

The fungus development occurs in the stored feed ingredients due to inadequate drying, high humidity and wetting.

Rodents not only consume food but also spoil with their excretions (faecal pellets and urine) and hair. Further they destroy containers by gnawing holes that results in leakage and wastage of grain.

3. Mechanical factors and chemical factors: Damage to the grains during harvesting, transportation and mechanical handling and conveying expose the nutrients and may result in rapid spoilage during storage; pesticide residues affect the food value because of their adverse effect on the health of the consumer.

4. Engineering factors: Structures-bag or bulk storage.

Design of storage structures: A good storage structure provides for effective fumigation, proper ventilation, protection from rodents, birds, rain water leakage, fire and floor moisture seepage and ease of loading/ unloading. Concrete walls for the storage of feeds and feed ingredients must be watertight. The roof, walls, doors, windows and floor must be leakproof. The floor must not transmit water vapour from the soil. Doors and windows should be sealable in order to permit control of ventilation. Buildings must have devices to protect against the entry of rats and mice and birds; gaps between roof and walls should be sealed with sheet metal or close netting; pipes, shafts, ducts, etc. should be fitted with wide metal guards outside and netting inside.

Factors that influence deteriorative changes during storage: These are moisture, temperature, oxygen supply and condition of the product. Moisture and temperature are the principal factors for safe storage.

1. Moisture: The maximum moisture content at which grain can be stored safely depends on the kind of grain, the locality in which it is stored, the method of condition and the length of storage period. The maximum moisture content for safe storage in the U.S. are as follows: corn, oats and sorghum, 13%; soybeans 11.0%. The lower the temperature, higher the level of permissible moisture for storage. For grains stored as seed stock or for long time storage up to 5 years the moisture levels should be 2% lower.

The difference between one kind of grain and another (in moisture level for safe storage) is attributable to the different equilibrium relative humidities of different grains at the same moisture content. Since the relative humidity of air is common to all grains stored, the moisture content of grains is to be different for safe storage. See equilibrium moisture content and grain quality later in this chapter; Page No. 526.

Moisture content of grain is also an important factor in the activity of insects and moulds. At low moisture contents (below 9%) most of the destructive insects become inactive. e.g. rice and maize weevils. Flour beetles on the other hand can produce progeny in flours or in grain dust that are extremely dry. During larval development and growth, an insect produces metabolic water and heat. It has been reported that when the density of *Sitophilus oryzae* (weevil) rose from 15 adults to 2100 in a closed container of wheat the moisture content increased from 15 to 35%.

Mould growth can readily develop in stored materials if the moisture content in any one area rises above 13%. Thus insect activity is usually beneficial to mould growth. The increase in moisture content and tempera-ture due to growth of insects frequently is followed by rapid growth of moulds. Insects may also be carriers of mould in their intestinal flora.

2. Temperature:

a. Temperature of environment: All foods and other biologicals keep better under refrigeration. It is based on the fundamental fact that the speed of the most chemical reactions increase with increasing temperature. Reaction is rapid at higher moisture levels. Temperature below 15°C retard insect reproduction. Temperature between 21-43°C speed up the life processes of all microorganisms.

	Insect species	Mould species
Weevils	*Sitophilus oryzae*	*Aspergillus flavus*
Beetles		
Grain beetle	*Oryzeaphilus*	*Aspergillus flavus*
	surinamensis	*Aspergillus ochraceus*
Flour beetle	*Tribolium castaneum*	Penicillium spp.

b. Temperature of stored grain: If the temperature of the storage area is lower there is less likelihood of spoilage of stored feeds and feed ingredients. Low temperature offset the effects of high moisture with respect to the hazard of mould growth and insect development.

The interaction of moisture content, moulds and insects can rapidly lead to spoilage of stored feed raw materials. Insect infestation enhances the moisture content of stored feeds due to their metabolism and can result in temperature increase up to 42°C. Increased moisture and temperature are conducive for the growth of moulds and can produce temperatures as high as 65°C.

In materials with 11-15% moisture both insects and moulds become active and heating occurs. A small local rise of temperature referred to as 'hot spot' will accelerate the metabolism of insects and speed up the rate of population increase. This follows the growth of moulds.

3. Oxygen supply: Grains are living entity and they respire continuously during storage. Aerobic respiration of grain and of microorganisms associated with grain involves consumption of O_2 and liberation of CO_2 and production of water molecules. In closed storage bins the concentration of CO_2 increases and the concentration of O_2 decreases and so the rate of respiration tends to decrease due to limited oxygen supply.

Ample supply of O_2 supports respiration and if the rate of respiration is high enough the heat produced in the process will exceed the heat lost and spontaneous heating will occur.

The factors controlling grain respiration are moisture, temperature, aeration and condition of grains including maturity, harvest methods and handling techniques.

4. Condition of the feed: As mentioned already, respiratory activity and tendency of the grain to deteriorate in storage are considerably influenced by the 'condition' or soundness of the product.

Unsound grain (grain with broken seed coat) usually be expected to harbour greater number of mould spores and bacteria than sound grain. Respiratory activity in a mass of grains is believed to be largely that of microorganisms rather than the grain itself. Hence unsound grain might be expected to exhibit more rapid respiration than the sound grain. Hence storage of grains containing higher percentage of damaged kernels or showing other evidence of unsoundness is much more likely to heat in storage than in sound grain of the same moisture content.

Free Water and Bound Water

Mould growth can occur in damaged grain even at lower moisture level because of the more readily available nutrients in damaged grains. The increased deterioration in unsound grain compared to sound grain lies in the possible relation between the bound and free water ratio in sound and damaged grains to the rates of mould growth and respiration. As the grain undergoes deterioration part of moisture that is held firmly in close physical union with proteinous and other constituents of the grain may be released gradually and thus increase the free water content of the grain without changing its total moisture content.

Relative humidity of the air surrounding the grain depends more closely upon the free moisture than upon the total moisture of the grain. Higher the free moisture, greater the relative humidity.

Electrical conductivity of unsound grain is usually higher than that of sound grain of the same moisture content.

Mycotoxins in Animal Feeds and their Management
Mycotoxins and Mycotoxicoses

Mycotoxins are a diverse group of chemicals that are harmful to animals and humans and have the greatest impact on human and animal health. They are secreted by fungi growing under favourable conditions in the field even before harvesting the crop, during transport and in the storage place. The severity of mycotoxin contamination is determined by major environmental factors such as excessive moisture in the field and in storage place, temperature extremes, humidity, variations in harvesting practices and insect infestations. Global climate change has also contributed to an increased frequency of mycotoxin contamination of grains. Drought, excessive rainfall and flooding can also promote mould growth. Mycotoxicoses are diseases caused by the ingestion of foods or feeds contaminated with mycotoxins. In addition to being acutely toxic, some mycotoxins are now linked with the incidence of certain types of cancer, and it is this aspect which has evoked concern over feed safety.

Fungi in stored feeds: The three major mycotoxin producing fungi are *Aspergillus, Fusarium* and *Penicillium*.

Favourable Conditions for Growth of the Fungi

Fungi	Temperature	R.H.	Moisture
Asperigillus flavus *A. nomius* *Fusarium graminearum*	Range 12-41°C Optimum 25-32°C	86-87%	More than 10-12%
F. Sporotrichioides	Below 21°C	High humidity	22-25%

The mycotoxins and the causative fungi are presented in Table 1.

Consequences of Consumption of Mouldy Feed in Farm Animals and Humans

In farm animals consumption of mycotoxin feed reduces growth efficiency, lowers feed consumption and reproductive rates, impairs resistance to infectious diseases, reduces efficacy of vaccination, induces pathologic damage to the liver and other organs, etc.

Aflatoxins: Aflatoxins are a group of closely related, highly toxic, mutagenic and carcinogenic compounds. Aflatoxins affect liver functions and lead to unthriftiness. Aflatoxins can lower resistance to disease and interfere with vaccination and acquired immunity in livestock. Aflatoxins may also cause rectal prolapse.

Zearalenone: Zearalenone is best known for its role in the oestrogenic syndrome in swine. In the pre-pubertal gilt, the vulva become swollen and this may progress to vaginal or rectal prolapse. In pregnant animals, abortions and still births are also reported. Young male pigs undergo symptoms of "feminization", such as enlarged nipples and testes atrophy. Dairy cows have decreased fertility, prolonged oestrus and swelling of vulva. Turkeys develop greatly enlarged vents within four days.

Trichothecenes: Trichothecenes are a group of more than 150 structurally related compounds that inhibit eucaryotic protein synthesis causing human and animal health impairment. The main sources of trichothecenes in the food/feed supply are contaminated cereal grains. The toxic effects in animals include gastrointestinal disturbances such as

TABLE 1. Mycotoxins and the Causative Fungi.

Mycotoxin	Fungal species
Aflatoxin B$_1$ (AFB$_1$), AFB$_2$ and cyclopiazonic acid	*Aspergillus flavus*
AFB$_1$, AFB$_2$, AFG$_1$ and AFG$_2$	*A. Parasiticus and A. nomius*
Fusaral mycotoxins	
A. Zearalenone	*Fusarium culmorum* *F. graminearum* *F. sporotrichioides*
B. Trichothecenes	

Type A: T-2 toxin
       HT-2 toxin
       neosolaniol
       Diacetoxyscirpenol (DAS)
	F. sporotrichioides
	 F. poae
	
	 F. sporotrichioides
	 F. poae
	 F. graminearum

Type B: Deoxynivalenol (DON) or
       vomitoxin,
       nivalenol, fusarenon - x
	F. culmorum
	 F. graminearum
	 F. sporotrichioides

C. Fumonisins	
FB$_1$, FB$_2$ and FB$_3$ are the major toxins, while FB$_4$, FA$_1$ and FA$_2$ are produced in small amounts	*formerly (F. monoliforme) Fusarium verticillioides; F. priliferatum*
Ochratoxins (Nephrotoxin) Ochratoxin A	*formerly (Aspergillus ochraceus) A. alutaceus* *Penicillium viridicatum* *P. verrucosum* *P. cyclopium*
Tremorgens and Rubratoxin	*Penicillium sp* *Aspergillus sp*
Patulin **Phomopsins** **Sporidesmins** **Ergopeptine alkaloids** **(ergovaline)** **Lolitrem alkaloids**	*Penicillium expansum* *Phomopsis* *leptostromiformis* *Pithomyces chartarum* *Acremonium coenophialum* *Acremonium lolii*

vomiting, diarrhoea and inflammation. In addition, trichothecenes are potent immunosuppressive agents that affect immune cells and modify immune responses as a consequence of other tissue damage.

Feeds containing more than 1 ppm of deoxynivalenol (DON) may reduce the feed intake and weight gain in swine. Vomiting also has been reported giving it the term vomitoxin. Deoxynivalenol has been found worldwide, especially in temperate zones. Swine ate less toxin-containing feed while dairy cattle seem to be less susceptible. Chicken suffered no detectable ill effects from rations containing up to 18 ppm of deoxynivalenol and the toxin was not detected in the flesh or eggs.

Unthriftiness, decreased feed consumption, slow growth, lowered milk production, sterility, gastrointestinal haemorrhages and death can occur when cattle consume rations containing T-2 and diacetoxyscirpenol (DAS).

Effects of T-2 on swine include infertility accompanied with some lesions in the uteri and ovaries. Drastic and sudden decrease in egg production in laying hens has been reported due to T-2 toxin in ppm range. Lesions on the beak and in the mouth, also have been reported in turkeys and chickens.

Fumonisins: These have long been associated with occasional outbreaks of blind staggers (equine leucoencephalomalacia) in horses. It is characerized by facial paralysis, nervousness, lameness, ataxia and inability to eat or drink. Fumonisins have also been shown to be carcinogenic to rats and have been reported to be associated with pulmonary edema in swine and esophageal cancer in humans. Fumonisins reduced feed intake and weight gains in chickens. Cattle, however, seem to be less susceptible than either swine or horses. Fumonisins increased the free sphingosine levels which means that the sphingolipid biosynthesis is inhibited. Monoliformin is a cardiotoxic mycotoxin.

Ochratoxin A: It can damage the kidneys and limit growth rates. Ochratoxins cause renal tubular failure in swine, rats and mice and pale swollen kidneys are observed. It has also been reported to kill young pigs if their feed is heavily contaminated.

Some moulds and bacteria can destroy nutrients in feeds. For example, the *Pseudomonas* species of bacteria and *Aspergillus* species of moulds can separate glutamic acid from pteroic acid in the vitamin, folic acid. Thus they can destroy the vitamin and cause folic acid deficiency.

Indirect exposure of humans to aflatoxins can occur by consumption of foods derived from animals that consume contaminated feeds. In addition, handling contaminated feed can also result in uptake of mycotoxins through the skin and by inhalation.

Metabolism of Mycotoxins

1. Most of the toxins are detoxified in the liver and kidney and hence do not appear in meat, aflatoxin B_1's appearance as aflatoxin M_1 in milk being the notable exception. Dairy cows consuming rations contaminated with aflatoxin B_1 excrete its toxic metabolite aflatoxin M_1 in milk in dose related concentration. AFM_1 excretion in milk reached its maximum and stabilized after 6 to 9d from the start of feeding toxin-contaminated feed and excretion rate from feed to milk was between 0.4-0.6% to 1.7%. So the complete feed for dairy cattle should contain a maximum of 0.5µg/L (20 ppb) (Table-2). One publication reported the ratios of the levels of aflatoxin B_1 in the feed to that in milk as about 300:1 and other as a range of 29 to 989. After complete withdrawal of AFB_1 contaminated ration, AFM_1 excretion in milk of cows dropped to a negligible level (0 < 0.01µg/L) within 4 to 5d. Hens fed aflatoxin-contaminated feed laid aflatoxin-contaminated eggs. A four to five days time is required to see the effect. However, ochratoxin A binds to plasma proteins and accumulate in the kidneys and, to a lesser extent, in the liver.

2. Even when mycotoxins are metabolized, their breakdown does not always result in a less toxic residue. Zearalenone in feed is well absorbed from the pig's intestinal tract and rapidly converted into α-zearalenone (primarily) and β-zearalenone. α-zearalenone is more active than zearalenone itself having a higher affinity for oestrogen receptors. This process is known as bioactivation. Pigs are most susceptible to zearalenone toxicity.

3. Cyclopiazonic acid (CPA) is widely reported to occur in maize, cheese, peanuts and sunflower seeds. Cyclopiazonic acid has been reported to markedly distribute to the skeletal tissue in rats and poultry on oral feeding of it. Dorner and coworkers reported in 1994 that CPA was found in milk and eggs after oral administration of CPA to lactating ewes and laying hens. These findings indicate potential source of human exposure via ingestion of contaminated animal meat and byproducts.

Safe Level of Aflatoxin in Poultry Feed-Indian Data

Aflatoxin was one of the subjects discussed at the 38th meeting of the Animal Feeds Sectional Committee (AFDC) of Bureau of Indian Standards (BIS) held on 7.4.1989. A limit of 20 parts per billion (ppb) was laid down for poultry feeds and for duck feeds, the maximum limit was 3 ppb. It was contested later at the symposium on "Aflatoxin and Aflatoxicosis" conducted by the Compound Livestock Feed Manufacturers' Association

(CLFMA) of India on 7.10.1989. It was generally accepted that chicken can tolerate far higher levels (say up to 400 ppb) than originally assumed to be toxic, provided farm conditions are appropriate, nutritional care is efficient and total farm management is perfect.

Research results of Central Avian Research institute (CARI), Izatnagar indicated up to 150 ppb as safe level for chicks, 400 ppb for broilers, 900 ppb for layers in commercial egg production. For breeding stock the maximal level of aflotoxin should be less as hatchability is affected at 300 ppb (Table 2) and fertility is affected at 750 ppb although the male reproduction is affected at 20,000 ppb.

It is not uncommon to import feedstuffs such as maize grain, soyabeans etc., to meet the domestic needs of poultry industry now-a-days. Maize samples collected in Karnataka (Janardhana et al. 1999) were analysed for mycotoxins and were found to have contaminated with aflatoxin (17.7%), ergosterol (15.2%), zearalenone (9.6%), T-2 toxin (4.5%), ochratoxin (1.5%) and deoxynivalenol (1%). In the present scenario of increased international trading of feedstuffs and blending those feedstuffs in feed formulations, the chance of feeds containing mixtures of different mycotoxins only increase. This can result in toxicological synergies that increase the severity of mycotoxicoses (Speijers and Speijers, 2004).

How to Salvage the Mycotoxin Contaminated Feedstuffs?

It is estimated that mycotoxins affect as much as 25% of the world's food crops each year. Mycotoxin production in the field is hard to control. However recent research indicates promising prospects for the development of plant genotypes devoid of or resistant to infection by toxigenic fungi. Several pre- and post-harvest approaches are to be followed to reduce or eliminate mycotoxins particularly aflatoxins, from the chain. Preharvest strategies are aimed to prevent fungal infection of the host plant or to impair the ability of the fungal pathogen to grow or synthesize mycotoxins on the plant. Killing the organisms (fungi) may stop the production of mycotoxins but do not remove the mycotoxins already present in the feedstuff. Most of the mycotoxins are chemically stable and persist long after the concerned fungi have died. With reference to the post-harvest elimination strategies, specific measures are needed to identify the threat, quantify it and manage it.

Laboratory Tests

Rapid screening for identification of mycotoxin types and concentrations in the field prior to harvest, immediately post-harvest, at the purchase point or at the feed mill is helpful. Now commercial kits are available for aflatoxins, ochratoxin A, DON and other trichothecenes, zearalenone, fumonisins. The analysis of a sample to determine the concentration of aflatoxin involves extraction, purification of the extract and measurement of the toxin concentration using thin-layer chromatography (TLC) plates, high pressure liquid chromatography (HPLC), enzyme linked immunosorbent assays (ELISA).

Techniques to Lower the Risk of Mycotoxicoses

Once the mycotoxicosis is identified as the cause, the toxin-contaminated feed should immediately be withdrawn and a low fat, high quality protein ration should be offered. Increase the vitamins, minerals and amino acids, especially methionine by 30-40% and this nutrient density ration is suggested for the lowered feed intake (due to a mild contamination) suffered earlier.

If the contaminated feeds are to be utilized the alternative is to reduce the impact by modifying the diet. This includes physical segregation of the damaged or fungi infested kernels or seeds, if possible and/or diluting the contaminated feed with clean, uncontaminated feed, though this approach is risky sometimes or feed the suspected feed material exclusively to mature animals such as finishing swine, cattle, layer birds in case of poultry, since they are the least susceptible.

Managing the Mycotoxins

In order to salvage the mycotoxin-contaminated feeds the following approaches may also be tried.

1. Increase the content of methionine: In case of mild contamination, increased nutrient density, as mentioned earlier, is helpful to offset the lowered fed intake and depression in the performance. The absorbed mycotoxins enter the blood stream. It is then the task of the liver to detoxify the mycotoxins and the liver uses biological reduction-oxidation reactions based upon glutathione, a tripeptide comprising glutamic acid, cysteine and glycine. Methionine supplementation, 30-40% over NRC levels, helps to detoxify the aflatoxins faster and to overcome the depression in the performance of broilers, layers, etc.

2. Follow the decontamination techniques

Chemical treatments: Liquid extraction of mycotoxin using organic solvents or water based solutions of calcium chloride or sodium bicarbonate or heated salt water. This requires considerable handling time, equipment and labour. Ammonia (aqueous or gaseous) treatment is a promising method for commercial detoxification of mycotoxins to destroy aflatoxin.

Physical treatments: Heat treatment can destroy unstable agents such as ergot alkaloids and citrinin, which usually occur in temperate regions in wheat and rye. Heat has little effect on a range of other mycotoxins including zearalenone, vomitoxin and ochratoxin A. It was reported that sunlight could destroy about 50% of aflatoxin in groundnut cake. Autoclaving at 120°C with a pressure of 15 lb psi   resulted   in progressive detoxification of toxic groundnut meal and cottonseed with time.

Ultraviolet and ionizing radiation may be effective in destroying some mycotoxins, such as aflatoxins, but also are likely to destroy nutrients in the feedstuffs.

3. Addition of mould inhibitors, mycotoxin binding/inactivating agents   and antioxidants: Formic acid and propionic acid have been found to be efficient grain preservatives against fungal growth and toxin production. Mycotoxin binding agents include activated charcoal, yeast cell wall products, synthetic zeolites and mined mineral clays such as aluminosilicates, sodium bentonites and sepiolites. Effectiveness of these compounds depends on the adsorptive capacity of their molecular structure, their purity and the characteristics of the targeted mycotoxin. Vitamin E and vitamin C appear to be effective in lessening the adverse effects of ochratoxin contamination.

The binding agents are capable of adsorbing or trapping mycotoxin molecules. Adsorption refers to attachment of the mycotoxin molecule on to the surface of other, harmless molecules and/or absorption into their microscopic pores. The molecular surfaces of these compounds are saturated with water which attracts the polar functional atomic structure of aflatoxins. The dipole attitude of water (with both positively and negatively charged areas) attracts the aflatoxin molecule and traps it against its surface. Thus adsorption isolates the aflatoxin from absorption or digestion by the animals preventing it from entering the animal's circulatory system. However, these binding agents alone have no effect on other harmful mycotoxins like zearalenone and trichothecenes.

Examples:

(i) Alfalfa fibre can have protective effects against zearalenone and T-2 toxin.

(ii) Hydrated sodium calcium aluminosilicate (HSCAS) has been shown to have potential to reduce aflatoxicosis.

(iii) Bentonite has been shown be effective against T-2 toxin, but only at levels that are not practical in animal feeds.

(iv) Glucomannan mycotoxin adsorbents (GMA): Mycosorb (Mannan oligosaccharides), developed by esterifying yeast cell wall, can specifically adsorb certain toxin molecules (aflatoxins, ochratoxin, fusariotoxins [zearalenone, T-2 toxin]). It is used at lower inclusion rates; about 50g is as effective as 4kg of clay.

(v) In case of trichothecenes, acutely exposed animals can be treated with oral adsorbents (e.g., highly activated charcoal, bentonite) in order to minimize absorption of the toxin from the GI tract and to short-circuit the enterohepatic recirculation of the toxins and/or their metabolites. Pretreatment with antioxidants such as vitamin C, vitamin E and ethoxyquin have proven effective in decreasing lethality of T-2 toxin in experimental animals. However, antioxidants are of no benefit after T-2 toxin exposure.

4. Enzymes: One of the recent techniques for mycotoxin decontamination is the use of enzymes to decompose the toxins. These enzymes lack the polar functional atomic groups of aflatoxins. Enzymes are available to inactivate zearalenone, all trichothecenes (T-2, HT-2, DON, DAS, etc.). The enzymes degrade the toxin by breaking the molecule apart to form harmless metabolites e.g. esterase and epoxidase. The enzyme esterase breaks the lactone ring of zearalenone, while the enzyme epoxidase degrades the 12, 13-epoxy group in the trichothecenes. Removal of the 12, 13-epoxide ring of trichothecenes using de-epoxidase enzyme entails a signficant reduction in its toxicity. The challenge to this approach is to identify enzymes non-specific enough to detoxify combinations of mycotoxins that might produce toxicological synergies, but also specific enough not to cause structural damage to the digestive tract or to interfere with digestive function. Thermal stability of enzymes in pelleted or extruded feeds is also a concern.

5. Microbial detoxification: Eubacterium strain (identified originally in bovine rumen contents), known as BBSH 797, exhibits de-epoxidation, ester hydrolysation and deacetylation activity, all of which are useful in detoxifying common feed mycotoxins. The bacterium was shown to be effective against DON in piglet feeding trials. *Clostridium sporogenes* and *Lactobacillus vitulinus* are able to cleave ochratoxin-A into non-toxic metabolites. A strain of yeast (Trichosporan) appears to destroy zearalenone's oestrogenic effects.

Flavobactrium multivorum and *Aspergillus repens* are potential aflatoxin (B_1 and G_1) degrading organisms.

A Word of Caution on Mycotoxin Binders

Many mycotoxin binders are available in the market. One is inclined to have a reasonable doubt that a mycotoxin binder or sequestering agent can be so selective that it only traps toxic substances without impairing the absorption of valuable nutrients, medications, etc.

The different mycotoxins have extremely diverse molecular structures and they are simlar to the vitamins. So it would seem reasonable to suppose that, until data to the contrary is presented, any material capable of sequestering multiple mycotoxins is also to trap one or more of the 40 or so vitamins, minerals, essential amino acids, medications, etc., that are present in feeds and are of value of the bird or animal.

TABLE 2. Maximum Permissible Levels of Aflatoxin as Stated by Different Agencies.

Food/Feed	Maximum level	
US FDA		
Human food (except milk)	20	ppb
Milk	0.5	ppb
Dairy feed, feed for immature animals	20	ppb
Feed for breeding cattle, swine or		
mature poultry	100	ppb
Feed for finishing swine	200	ppb
Feed for feedlot beef cattle	300	ppb
BIS		
Feeds for poultry	20	ppb
Feeds for ducks	3	ppb
CARI, Izatnagar		
Feeds for chicks	150	ppb
Feeds for broilers	400	ppb
Feeds for layers	900	ppb
Feeds for breeding stock	300	ppb
Europe		
Infant Milk	10 ng kg^{-1} aflatoxin M$_1$	
Dairy cattle feed	10 µg kg^{-1} aflatoxin B$_1$	
	2 µg kg^{-1} infant milk	

Storage and Preservation of Food Grain

There are two important reasons for storing food grain over varying periods.

1. If the ruling prices are low, farmers have to store grains till the market is favourable.
2. Food grains are stored for one year for household consumption. This improves cooking quality. For example, new rice will cook to a mass whereas stored rice absorbing more water gives discrete, puffed up grains.

But unless stored properly, food grains are lost in storage. It is estimated that nearly 9.3% of food grains produced are lost during storage. The post-harvest loss is mainly due to insect pests, rodents, birds and degradation by moisture.

The department of Food, Government of India, has taken several steps to propagate scientific techniques of foodgrains storage and preservation at different levels.

1. To educate farmers on the need to minimise the losses of foodgrain during storage, the department has launched the 'Save Grain Campaign' (S.G.C), as a pilot project in 1965-66 which became a regular scheme since 1969-70. The scheme was implemented through a network of 17 central teams, located in different states in collaboration with the respective state governments.
2. For conducting applied research on grain storage and for carrying out related developmental work, the department established the Indian Grain Storage Institute (IGSI) at Hapur (U.P.) with field stations at Ludhiana, Hyderabad, Jabalpur, Udaipur and Jorhat. The results of this research are being used in the campaign for minimising losses.

Buffer food grain stocks are to be build up to have food security to meet the public distribution system and guard against natural calamities such as floods and droughts. Food Corporation of India (FCI), Central Warehousing Corporation (CWC) and State Warehousing Corporation (SWC) are the agencies engaged in building large-scale godowns for storage.

The cover and plinth (CAP) system of storage which was susceptible to damage on account of rain, cyclones and other natural factors is on its way out. Concerted efforts are being made to bring down the loss of foodgrains as less as possible. However nearly 75% of the foodgrains is handled at the trade and farm levels. So here losses are to be minimized.

Control Measures

I.   Prophylactic spraying with insecticides like malathione over empty gunny bags, godowns. Malathione 50% of 10 ml per litre water; 3L for 100 sq m.

II. Fumigation of storage structure and rat burrows: Fumigation with e.d.b. (ethylene dibromide) ampoules gives adequate protection against insect attack. The storage place is sealed for 7 days after fumigation.

Ecofume is a newly developed biologically safer product for the management of stored product insects. It is a colourless gas with a garlic odour. Ecofume fumigant gas is a non-flammable pre-mixed cylinderised mixture of phosphine (2% by weight) and carbon dioxide (98% by weight), which provides highly effective fumigation in both sealed and unsealed storage facilities such as empty godowns, transport facilities, food processing facilities, etc. Carbon dioxide is an excellent carrier for phosphine and diluting phosphine to this concentration ensures that ecofume is nonflammable. It acts as a viable alternative for methyl bromide, which is an ozone depletory substance. It comes in ready-to-use cylinders and can be dispensed directly into sealed storages or sturctures from the outside.

III. Rodent control measures: Brown or Norwegian rat invariably follow wall and the edge of buildings. Black rat (seen in warmer countries) are more likely seen along the rafters of the roof or making use of pipes and wires. Rodent control includes construction of godowns with rodent proof measures, traping and hunting, use of cats and dogs, rodent repellents and rodenticides.

a. Anti-coagulant rodenticide: relatively slow-acting, needing 4-5 days to kill the animal by internal bleeding after a lethal dose has been ingested. Multiple feeding is essential, with the bait continuously available until control is achieved. Suppliers say this may take about 15 days from the start of the programme. These don't cause bait shyness. They may be ineffective due to resistance. e.g. warfarin, comarin (0.05%).

b. Alternatives: Acute poison, zinc phosphide acts much more quickly and death occurs within a few hours through paralysis and asphyxia. Other examples include calcium cyanide and aluminium phosphide (0.5%).

These acute poisons cause a phenomenon known as bait shyness. This means the poisoned rat suspects the bait eaten for its sudden illness and therefore is deterred from eating more of the substance even though this is highly palatable. So the aim must be to make sure the rodent eats a lethal dose at its first visit. That depends on denying it access to other food sources around the baiting area.

c. Other examples: 1. Cholecalciferol: It produces death from an excess of calcium in the blood. 2. Bromethalin: Affects CNS. Both are marketed as single-dose rodenticides that apparently do not lead to bait shyness.

Newer forms of anti-coagulants: (Second generation anti-coagulants): e.g. brodifacoum, bromadiolone. These are more potent so that fewer feedings are needed to give a lethal dose.

Brand Products

1. Prolin® has warfarin + Sulfaquinoxaline (Sulfaquinoxaline inhibits the growth of intestinal bacteria producing vitamin K).
2. EPIBLOC® contains Alpha-chlorhydrin. It is raticide and rodenticide. It is unique that sublethal doses produce sterility in male rats without affecting the sex drive. It is a biodegradable rodenticide, and is destroyed by the rat eating the chemical.

IV. Controlling the Growth of Moulds in Stored Feed/Food

Prevention programme include control of moisture, inspection of incoming grain, good housekeeping and use of chemical preservatives.

a. *Moisture level* should be about 10% at the time of storage. Because grains are hygroscopic in nature, grains improperly dried initially later pick up moisture from seepage, leakage and contact from air of high humidity.

b. *Evaluation of incoming grains* should include visual observation for insect infestation, mould growth and physical damage.

c. *Good housekeeping practices* should include such procedure as:
  1. Cleaning out feed bins after emptying and before refilling.
  2. Keeping trucks, feed mill equipment in good working order and clean.
  3. Constructing storage facilities so that insects and rodents do not have ready access.
  4. Eliminating trash and sources of dampness around grains and grain storage facilities.

d. *Chemical preservatives (mould inhibitors):* Most commonly used are acid-type inhibitors. These include acetic, propionic, sorbic and benzoic acids accompanied by their various salts. Propionic acid and acetic acid are added at 0.1 to 1% concentration to high moisture feeds to reduce moulds effectively. Propionates and sorbates are routinely used today in preservation of foods such as bread and cheese.

e. *Botanical preservatives:* Neem leaves and neem seed powder, custard apple leaves and seed powder, crushed garlic cloves are useful.

Modern Approaches in Combating Grain Pests

1. Low temperature warehouses have been installed in Japan for storing rice.
2. A technology of controlled atmospheric storage using CO_2 was established for grain storage as alternative measures to both, methyl bromide and phosphine fumigation.
3. Subsequently, a high pressure CO_2 system was developed to not only destroy the insect pests quickly, but also allow continuous operation.
4. More recently, a modern rational strategy, integrated pest management (IPM) is being proposed, comprising conventional disinfestation measures, pheromone traps, packaging materials, etc.

Nutritive quality of stored foodgrain: It depends upon its chemical composition. The chemical composition of the grains control their storage life as the fat, acidity and non-reducing sugar contents may increase or decrease with the longevity of storage under specific temperature and moisture levels.

Grains are living entity and they respire continuously during storage if aeration is allowed in godown. Carbohydrates decompose during respiration by grains converting into CO_2 and water. However, crude protein remains unchanged in wheat stored for 8 years under long-term commercial storage conditions. Germ damage has been reported in moist wheat storage under anaerobic conditions.

Fat content of grains may result in increased free fatty acids due to hydrolytic actions while oxidation of fats will give typical rancid odours. Among the vitamins, there is negligible loss in thiamin content; considerable loss of carotenoid pigments and tocopherols is reported with increased storage period.

Equilibrium moisture content and grain quality

The moisture level that is dependent on ambient temperature and relative humidity and that varies between types and grades of cereal grain is called the 'equilibrium moisture content'.

TABLE 3   Equilibrium moisture (%) for cereal grains at temperature of 25 °C

Cereal grain	Relative humidity (%) and Equilibrium moisture (%)		
	50	70	90
Barley	10.8	13.5	19.5
Yellow maize	11.2	14.0	19.6
Oats	10.3	13.0	18.5
Rice, whole grain	12.2	14.1	19.1
Sorghum	11.0	13.8	18.8
Wheat	10.9	13.8	19.7

Source: Feed International September, 2005, pp 12-17.

Although grain spoilage is both physical and chemical in nature, the direct cause is biological. High moisture content is the culprit for the growth and feeding activities of mould fungi and bacteria. At relative humidity of 70%, the equilibrium moisture contents for most types of grain fall in the range of 13-14%. Beyond this level in temperate countries (where the ambient temperature is around 25°C), commodity feedstuffs begin to deteriorate primarily due to mould activity; in case of tropical countries the optimum moisture for safe storage is not more than 11%. If relative humidity is 90% (which occurs over time in the tropics), then the equilibrium moisture level of grain shoots up to around 18-20%, and mould growth is rampant.

When feed grains (mostly maize) are imported from temperate zones to countries in Southeast Asia, the consequences are well-known: Physical degradation of grain due to mould and bacterial activity; chemical deterioration of grain and loss of nutritional quality; threat of mycotoxin contamination and further damage from stored product - insect pests such as maize weevil and lesser grain borer, encouraged by 'hot spots' or localized rises in temperature in the grain store caused by microbial activity and grain spoilage.

Organic acid treatment with propionic acid (3 kg per metric ton) is safe alternative to preservation of grain in shipment and storage. The pure acid is corrosive and emits penetrating pungent, acrid and irritating odour, while calcium or sodium propionate is slower acting but more 'user-friendly' and safer for workers.

Chapter 19

Conservation of Fodders-Silage and Hay Making

Silage Making

When green fodders are in plenty, they are conserved as either silage or hay to meet the demand of good quality fodder during lean season. The awns (spear grass) and thorns in some species may be rendered quite innocuous through ensiling. Weed seeds die off in the silo. Silage can be defined as a green material produced by controlled anaerobic fermentation of green fodder crop retaining its moisture content. Silage is the green succulent roughage preserved more or less in its original condition, with a minimum deterioration and minimum loss in respect of various nutritive constituents of fodders. The process of conserving green fodder is called as ensilage. Silo is the receptacle in which silage is made. The best silages are moist to the touch, soft but not slimy and fragrant in their own characteristic way.

Green, fruity silage is the most palatable and nutritious type. This can be produced only under careful management from crops that are cut at the right stage with a dry matter of 35%. A dark-brown colour indicates excessive heating.

Crops Suitable for Silage Making

1. Kind of crop
   (a) Crops rich in soluble sugars/carbohydrates are most suitable for ensiling, e.g. maize, sorghum, bajra.
   (b) Cultivated and natural grasses can be ensiled with addition of molasses at 3 to 3.5%.
   (c) Mixture of grasses/cereal fodders and legumes such as berseem, lucerne, etc. in a ratio of 3:1.
   (d) Unwilted leguminous leafy fodders and dry forage in the ratio of 4:1.
2. Stage of harvesting: Crop should be harvested between flowering and milk stage. In general, crops with thick stems are conserved in the form of silage while thin stemmed crops are conserved as hay.

Preparation of Silage

There are different types of ensiling. Apart from making silage under farm conditions, the same can be done under laboratory conditions.

Laboratory Method of Silage Making:

Under laboratory conditions silage can be prepared using Polythene bag silos.

Steps in ensiling:
1. A 45 X 60cm polythene bag is taken for the experiment.
2. The crop chosen for ensiling is chaffed to 2-4cm in length and wilted to 35% DM.
3. The crop is thoroughly mixed. Molasses can be added to ensure the availability of soluble carbohydrate for efficient bacterial fermentation to an extent of 3 to 3.5%. Salt and urea are added at 0.5 and 1% respectively, to improve palatability and nitrogen ontent of silage.
4. The material is then packed tightly into the bags.
5. The open end is sealed perfectly and kept in an identical bag and placed in a metal can/cement tub after sealing.
6. The remaining space is filled with sand before closing the lid, thus minimizing the possibility of the air, permeating the polythene film.
7. The silo is then stored in a room and opened for sampling after 4-6 weeks.

Preparation of Silage Under Field Conditions: Silo

A silo is an air tight structure designed for the storage and preservation of high moisture feed as silage. Pit silos are more common in India. The pits are dug 2.4 to 3.0 m deep, with variable sizes. One cubic metre of space is required for 400 kg fodder.

Requisites of a Silo

1. The walls should be impermeable so that water can't gain entry into silo pit. Walls may be made of cement or brick and mortar.
2. Silo should be sufficiently deep. It should not be shallow. The depth depends on the water table in the locality.
3. Silo must be located on an elevated ground.
4. The size of the silo should be calculated on the basis of the number of animals to be fed, the length of feeding period.

Method of Preparing Silage

1. Select the crop that is to be ensiled when it has 30-35% dry matter. In case the crop has less than 30% dry matter, allow it to dry for 3-4

hours so that the dry matter content would increase to 30-35%.

2. Generally the crops are harvested and ensiled when the ears start coming.

3. Select the days of the week when the weather is fair and not rainy.

4. Silo can be filled with long fodder as well as with chopped fodder. It is always better to chop the fodder first since packing is better. Thus loss of nutrients is minimized with chaffed fodder. Further, filling and removal of silage is easier.

5. After chaffing and ensuring that dry matter is around 35% the silo is filled with fodder.

6. The fodder should be evenly distributed throughout the pit. Trampling should be done properly either with men or tractor or bullocks depending upon the size of the pit. At the top of The silo the fodder should be packed 3-4 feet above the ground level.

7. From all the sides it should be covered with long paddy straw or poor quality grasses and then covered with wet mud and dung to seal the material preventing the entry of air and water. The layer of straw/grasses (over the green fodder) may be about 4 to 5". The silage would be ready in two months after covering.

8. Salt at 0.5% and urea at 1% are added to cereals and grasses to improve the palatabiliry and nitrogen content. In grass silages, molasses is added at 3 to 3.5% to improve the sugar content and thus quality of silage. In a more mature crop higher level of molasses (5%) may be added.

Changes During Fermentation

Carbohydrates

When green crops are cut up and packed in air-tight silo pits or towers, fermentation occurs to convert it into silage. Plant respiration continues for a short time after the material is packed in the silo pit. Enzymes, aerobic bacteria, yeast and moulds become active until all the oxygen in the packed material is used up. The respiration also uses up some of the carbohydrates in the plant material, giving off CO_2 and water. There is also a production of energy which contributes to the heat with a rise of temperature to about 27 to 38°C, particularly in the early stages of the fermentation process (aerobic phase).

The remaining carbohydrates are then broken down to their monomers glucose and fructose, which are water soluble and are the major carbohydrate sources for microbial purposes.

Proteins

Proteases are important enzymes responsible for undesirable changes in plant proteins during the first 5-7 days of ensilage. A proportion of the protein is degraded to nonprotein nitrogen compounds, mainly free amino acids, ammonia, amides and amines. The free amino acids may be metabolized further. Aspartate is thus degraded to α-alanine and glutamate to α-amino butyrate. These two reactions are particularly important, since the two amino acids are limiting factors for the growth and development of lactic acid bacteria. The activity of plant proteases is influenced by factors such as the pH and dry matter content. The optimum pH for proteolysis is around 6 for most silage crops, with activity declining linearly between pH 6 and 4 because proteases are acid labile and cease to function 5-7 days after ensilage when the acidic condition is established.

Other plant enzymes such as polyphenol oxidases may contribute to changes in the protein value of silage. Under improper ensilage conditions and in the presence of oxygen, the enzyme causes formation of quinones which combine with proteins and eventually leads to the formation of brown colour by the Maillard reaction process. While proteases convert proteins to soluble compounds of some value, the polyphenol oxidases and the Maillard reaction sequence make proteins biologically unavailable to the animal.

Types of Fermentation

Two main types of fermentations occur: Lactic acid type and Butyric acid type. When the fodder contains 65 to 75% moisture and sufficient sugar in the plant juices, anaerobic lactic acid bacteria become active, to produce eventually a good, clean-smelling silage of high quality. If the acidity rises to about 1% at the start itself, the silage will be of good quality, as the lactic acid checks the activity of undesirable organisms (pH around 4.0). Harmful bacteria, for example, those producing butyric acid are inhibited. It is thus essential that the forage used should contain a high percentage of carbohydrates.

Two fermentation types of lactic acid bacteria are involved: homofermentative type and heterofermentative type. In case of homofermentative type, 2 moles of lactic acid are formed per mole of glucose or fructose under anaerobic conditions; heterofermentative type forms anaerobically 1 mole of lactic acid, 1 mole of ethanol, and 1 mole of carbon dioxide per mole of glucose and mannitol, acetic acid and less lactic acid per mole of fructose. Heterofermentative type is less efficient than the homofermentative one in terms of lactic acid production. The homofermentative lactic acid bacteria remain active only in the first few days (10-14) of ensilage, during which time they account for 85% of the total bacterial population. As fermentation of silage proceeds, the heterofermentative bacteria become dominant because the homofermentative bacteria are less tolerant to acidity than the heterofermentative types. In well-made silages, the overall amount of lactic acid should be 60% of the total acids by the end of ensilage so that homofermentation of silage is encouraged.

If the forage is too rich in proteinaceous substances, the butyric acid type of fermentation will predominate. Butyric acid has a sharp, disagreeable odour and the silage is not relished by the animals. Clostridia are the principal anaerobic microorganisms which are detrimental to silage quality. They are classified into saccharolytic and proteolytic groups, both of which require wet conditions for an active growth. The result of the saccharolytic clostridial fermentation is mainly butyric acid, with some byproducts such as carbon dioxide and hydrogen. Proteolytic fermentation results in a variety of products such as ammonia and volatile amines. The presence of ammonia in silage may contribute to the high silage pH and often leads to a reduced intake of silage by ruminant animals. Hence optimum moisture content of the fodder ensiled is important.

Under optimal conditions, lactic acid forms rapidly and lowers the pH to 4.0 or below, where it remains constant. This normally inhibits clostridial growth but, with excessive moisture, clostridial growth can occur at a pH as low as 4.0. Clostridia attack already formed lactic acid and residual soluble carbohydrates and thereby raises the pH and set the stage for putrefactive organisms to operate. Clostridia also act on the amino acids normally resulting from proteolysis in the silage to produce amines, ammonia and fatty acids and CO_2.

A rapid fall in pH inhibits such degradation of amino acids and its effect on the quality of the silage.

Some of the Reactions in the Ensiling Process: Homofermentative Lactic Acid Bacteria:

1 Glucose + 2 ADP $\rightarrow$ 2 lactic acid + 2 ATP
1 Fructose + 2 ADP $\rightarrow$ 2 lactic acid + 2 ATP
1 Pentose + 2 ADP $\rightarrow$ 1 lactic acid + 1 acetic acid + 2 ATP

Heterofermentative lactic acid bacteria

1 Glucose + ADP $\rightarrow$ 1 lactic acid + 1 ethanal + 1 CO_2 + ATP
3 Fructose + 2 ADP $\rightarrow$ 1 lactic acid + 2 mannitol + 1 acetic acid + 1 CO_2 + 1 H_2O + 2ATP
1 Pentose + 2 ADP $\rightarrow$ 1 lactic acid + 1 acetic acid + 2 ATP

Clostridia

1 Alanine + 2 glycine $\rightarrow$ 3 acetic acid + 3 NH_3 + 1 CO_2
3 Alanine $\rightarrow$ 2 Propionic acid + 1 acetic acid + 3 NH_3 + 1 CO_2
Arginine $\rightarrow$ Putrescine

Histidine	$\rightarrow$	Histamine
1 Leucine	$\rightarrow$	1 Isovaleric acid + 1 NH_3 + 1 CO_2
Lysine	$\rightarrow$	Cadaverine
Phenylalanine	$\rightarrow$	Phenylethylamine
Tyrosine	$\rightarrow$	Tyramine
Tryptophan	$\rightarrow$	Tryptamine

Grasses, legumes are more difficult to ensile. Grasses are low in soluble carbohydrates. Legumes have higher moisture levels, higher proteins and minerals which raise the buffering capacity of plants and thereby their ability to resist pH change and these must be overcome to make satisfactory silage.

Buffering Capacity of Plants

The buffering capacity of plants or their ability to resist pH change is an important factor in ensilage. Most of the buffering properties of herbage can be attributed to the anions (organic acid salts, orthophosphates, sulphates, nitrates and chlorides) with only about 10-20% resulting from the action of plant proteins. Legumes usually contain higher amounts of organic acids than grasses. The level of organic acids is about 60-80 g/kg DM in legumes compared to 20-60 g/kg DM in grasses. Malate and citrate are the major acids, and they are metabolized by plant enzymes to varying degrees to succinic acid and lactic and acetic acids, respectively. Other acids include malic, quinic, fumeric, shikimic. Because of the buffering power of these products, there are often difficulties in ensiling legumes successfully.

Preservatives: Sodium metabisulphite causes partial sterilization. Dose is 4 to 8 kg per 1000 kg of forage. It checks bacterial growth, and reduces the final acidity.

Bacterial cultures and other microorganisms: Mixed culture of lactic acid producing bacteria.

Bioactive forage legumes as a strategy to improve silage quality and minimize nitrogenous losses

The use of forage legumes as a source of protein for ruminants is a sustainable strategy to reduce the use of inorganic-nitrogen fertilizer. Further, some legumes species contain naturally bioactive secondary compounds, such as condensed tannins or polyphenol oxidase, which could improve silage quality. Study revealed that all silages that contained bioactive legumes were better conserved than the pure grass silo (Ginane et al., 2014). In addition, bioactive legumes were able to preserve protein from degradation during the silage process.

Important Conditions for Success in Silage Making:

1. Storing the plant material at a moisture content of 65
2. Excluding air
3. Encouraging a rise of temperature to 30 to 38°C. When it is not possible to secure these optimum conditions, it is helpful to add some preservatives or 'silage conditioners'. Molasses, salt, cereal grains, citrus pulp act as preservatives and enhance feeding value. Sodium metabisulphite modify fermentation process and reduce the smell.

Why is Exclusion of Air from the Silo Needed?

1. To minimise the loss of nutrients due to respiration
2. To initiate the growth of lactic acid producing bacteria rapidly
3. To prevent the development of undesirable aerobic organisms which produce a lot of heat at the expense of nutrients which they oxidise
4. Aeration promotes the activity of mould, which spoil the silage and make it unpalatable.

Colour of the Silage

When the temperature in the silo is moderate the silage tends to be yellowish or brownish green and sometimes even golden in colour. This is due to the action of the organic acids on the chlorophyll, and converts chlorophyll into the brown magnesium-free pigment, phaeophytin. Silage is dark brown or black, when temperature in the silo is high.

A.I.V. Method of Silage Making

Silage was popularised in America in 1917, when lucerne was successfully ensiled. The method of making silage by using acid additives was developed principally by Professor A.I. Virtanen in 1925 in Finland, and the process has come to be known as A.I.V. method of silage making. He recommended the addition of equal quantities of dilute (2N) H_2SO_4 and HC1 to the green fodder when ensiling clover and clover-grass mixtures. Later it was recognised that the addition of other materials rich in carbohydrates kept the silage good for longer periods. The use of germinated maize and molasses improved the quality further.

Nutrient Content of Silage in Comparison to the Green Fodder

The ash, ether extract, crude fibre, crude protein, and NFE contents of silage can be very similar to the crop from which the silage was made. Proper amounts of moisture and fermentable carbohydrates and proper storage influence the ensiling process and the nutritive value of the silage.

Silage can greatly influence the loss of oxidizable vitamins. Carotene is fairly easily oxidized. Vitamin C or ascorbic acid is easily decomposed under the conditions prevailing even in the best-made silage. When oxidation and temperature are controlled a large proportion of carotene is conserved in silage. In a good quality silage (pH 4-4.5) β-carotene appears to be relatively stable and thus losses are likely to be low. A part of the minerals may be leached out and lost, but a large proportion will remain unchanged or simply take part in some new combination.

With crops cut and ensiled within 24 hours, losses of DM of no more than 1 or 2% may be expected. DM losses as high as 6 to 10% after 5 to 8 days of wilting have been reported. Under optimum conditions, the soluble carbohydrate fraction is almost entirely converted to organic acids, principally lactic acid and smaller amounts of the volatile acids, and the protein is converted to amino acids. Oxidation losses due to the oxygen trapped within the plant tissues during filling the silo pit is negligible (may be about 1%), since silo is rapidly filled and sealed. In lactic acid type of fermentation overall DM losses are less than 5%, while in clostridial and enterobacterial fermentations nutrient losses will be much higher. In most silos, free, drainage occurs and the liquid or effluent carries with it soluble nutrients. Effluent losses vary with initial moisture content, and little effluent is produced with optimum moisture level when ensiled.

Silage Quality

Shephered *et al.* (1948) have classified the silage into the following categories.

1. **Very good silage:** Silage having acidic taste and odour, being free from butyric acid, moulds, sliminess, showing a pH range of 3.5-4.2, and with ammoniacal nitrogen less than 10% of the total nitrogen. Lactic acid content is 1-2%.

2. **Good silage:** Silage possessing acidic taste and odour, traces of butyric acid (less than 0.2%), pH 4.2-4.5 and ammoniacal nitrogen 10-15% of the total nitrogen.

3. **Fair silage:** Ensiled material with some butyric acid, a slight proteolysis, some moulds, pH 4.8 and above and ammoniacal nitrogen 20% of the total nitrogen.

During the early stage of ensilage, the predominant microorganisms are coliform bacteria. These belong to the family *enterobacteriaceae* which are facultative anaerobic acting mainly on the breakdown of carbohydrates. They are undesirable because they compete with lactic acid bacteria for fermentable sugars.

Yeast and mould may either be found naturally on a crop or generated from spores which have survived the ensilage. They are most often linked with silage aerobic deterioration when the silo pit is not closed properly.

Flieg Index

Flieg index is a commonly used method for evaluation of silage quality. The index is calculated by determining the relative amounts of lactic, acetic, and butyric acids, expressed as % of the total acids in the silage. Scores are given to each value of these acids, and the higher the total score the better quality of fermentation. The Flieg index is also correlated positively to the feeding value of silage according to the following equation:

$$Y = 55.95 + 0.07\,X$$

Y = TDN expressed as % of dry matter

X = Flieg score

Flieg index takes into account butyric acid, the main product of saccharolytic clostridia and it makes no reference to the ammonia produced by the proteolytic species.

TABLE 1. The Flieg Index.

Lactic acid Relative		Acetic acid Relative		Butyric acid Relative	
% acid in total silage	Flieg index	% acid in total silage	Flieg index	% acid in total silage	Flieg index
0-20.0	–	0-15	20	0-1.5	50
20.1-25	0	15.1-20	18	1.6-3	30
25.1-30	2	20.1-24	16	3.1-4	20
30.1-34	4	24.1-28	13	4.1-6	15
34.1-38	6	28.1-32	10	6.1-8	10
38.1-42	8	32.1-36	7	8.1-10	9
42.1-46	10	36.1-40	4	10.1-12	8
46.1-50	12	40.1-45	2	12.1-14	7
50.1-54	14	45.1-50	0	14.1-16	6
54.1-58	16	50.1-55	0	16.1-18	4
58.1-62	18	55.1-60	0	18.1-20	2
62.1-66	20			20.1-25	0
66.1-70	24			25.1-30	0
70.1-75	28			30.1-40	– 5
>75	30			> 40	– 10

Haylage

When grasses and legumes generally meant for hay are ensiled, the term 'haylage' is used. Material wilted to 40-45% dry matter before ensiling is often referred to haylage. The dry straws are improved by the addition of suitable additives namely urea, mineral mixture and water. The straws are chaffed into fine pieces (2-3 cm). One kg of urea and 1.5 kg of mineral mixture are dissolved in 20 kg of water and mixed with 97.5 kg of the chaffed material. This is stored in silo pits like silage and is allowed to ferment under anaerobic conditions. The soluble carbohydrates present in the dry straws act as a source of energy for the bacteria to grow well. After about 2 months the pits are opened, and fed to livestock. It is termed as "haylage". It is supplemented with 2 kg of green fodder per day per animal to take care of the requirement of vitamin A.

Wastelage

Silage containing animal organic waste (poultry droppings, poultry litter, swine excreta, and bovine dung) is called wastelage. Wastelage is anaerobically fermented animal waste containing other feed ingredients with the help of lactic acid producing bacteria.

Example: Ensiling of paddy straw/sorghum or maize stover with animal waste

Poultry droppings/dung	40 kg
Molasses	10 kg
Mineral mixture	1 kg
Salt	0.5 kg

The above are mixed in about 22 litres of water and is sprayed on straw.

Straw (chaffed)	48 kg

Ensile for 6 weeks

Nitrate in Silage

Spoelstra (1985) reviewed the effect of nitrate content on ensilability of grasses and other related things. High rates of N fertilizer diminish the ensilability of grass by lowering the concentration of fermentable carbohydrates and increasing the protein concentration and buffering capacity. The nitrate content of the grass is also increased by N fertilizer. All or part of the nitrate present in the fresh crop is broken down during silage fermentation. Degradation is complete in poor quality silages. It is reported that high pH values, high ratios of NH_3-N to total N and low ratings in Flieg's evaluation system correlate with nitrate reduction.

Within few hours after ensiling nitrate reduction starts and nitrite (NO_2^-) and nitric oxide (NO) are temporarily accumulated to disappear again within 1 or 2 weeks. Further end products of nitrate in silage are ammonia (NH_3) and nitrous oxide (N_2O). The formation of nitrous oxide gas started 2 days after ensiling and continued for about a week. Enterobacteria appear to be mainly responsible for the degradation of nitrate in silage.

In well-preserved silages volatile nitrosamines are absent or present in very low amounts. Higher amounts have been found in badly preserved silages and in silages that have been exposed to air.

Silo-filler's Disease

Silo-filler's disease is an illness of farm workers that is caused by inhalation of oxides of nitrogen (NO_x) during ensiling or after entering a silo after filling. In the anaerobic environment of silage, nitric oxide (NO) is the predominant nitrogenous gas formed. Minor amounts of nitrogen dioxide (NO_2) and nitrous oxide (N_2O) may also be present. Nitric oxide is a colourless gas. Upon contact with oxygen it is oxidized to a mixture of NO_2 (red), N_2O_3 (brown) and N_2O_4 (yellow). This mixture is responsible for the frequently reported brownish fumes in and near silos. High amounts of NO can be expected when nitrate-rich, rapidly fermenting material is ensiled. Upon inhalation, NO_x gases are oxidized in the lung to mixture of nitrous and nitric acids. These strongly oxidizing acids damage lung tissue and can cause chemical pneumonia. In addition, reactions with haemoglobin (nitrosylhaemoglobin and methaemoglobin) occur, causing impaired oxygen transfer. Animals are also affected.

Hay Making

The forage, crop is cut before it is fully ripe and dried for storage as hay. Hay is more nutritious and palatable than straw. It is leafy, pliable, green and free from mould, and has a pleasant characteristic smell and aroma. The hay should not have more than 12-14% of moisture so that it can be safely stored without risk of fermentation and combustion.

Hay is the product obtained by cutting and curing the entire herbage of fine stemmed grasses or legumes so that the moisture content of the product is not more than 12-14%.

Crops Suitable for Hay Making

All thin-stemmed grasses and legumes can be conveniently and quickly dried unlike thick-stemmed fodders, which take more time for drying, e.g. grasses (Cyanodon, Cenchrus, Marvel, etc.), M.P. chari (*Sorghum bicolor*), oats, legumes (Stylosanthes, siratro, sunhemp, cowpea, berseem, lucerne, horse gram, pillipesara). In case of spear grass, the sharp pointed 'spears' or awns on the inflorescences make the hay unpalatable. Thin napier grass, sudan grass and Johnson grass can make fairly good quality hay only if they are cut at early flowering stage, before the heads set seed.

However, if the thick-stemmed fodders are required to be dried quickly they should necessarily be chopped into small pieces or crushed by passing the material in between rollers.

Stage of Harvesting the Crop for Hay Making

The nutritive value of the fodder goes down as the plant matures. At a very early stage the protein and energy contents of the fodder are very high but the dry matter yield of the fodder per unit area is very low. At the later stage when the crop is in full bloom the protein value goes down and the digestibility of nutrients is also reduced. The best time for cutting a crop for hay making is when it is $\frac{1}{3}$ to $\frac{1}{2}$ in blossom; in case of cereals the grain is in the milk stage while in legumes tender pod formation stage is optimum.

Kinds of Hay

1. Legume hay

Good legume hay has many characteristics that make it of special value in feeding of animals. It has got a higher percentage of digestible nutrients. It has got more of digestible protein because of the high protein content. Further more, the protein of legumes is of superior quality as compared to that from other plants. Well cured legume hays are higher in vitamin content. They are particularly rich in carotene and may contain vitamin D. They are also rich source of vitamin E. The legume hays are particularly rich in calcium and are generally palatable.

2. Non-legume hay

Non-legume hays are made from grasses and cereals. They are, as a rule, less palatable and contain less protein, minerals and vitamins than the legume hays but rich in carbohydrates. Non-legume hays have the advantage over legume hays because their outturn per hectare is more than that of legume hays and the former can be grown easily. Hays made from crops like oats, barley, etc. compare very favourably with the other grass hays.

3. Mixed hay

Hay prepared from mixed crops of legumes and non-legumes is known as mixed hay. The chemical composition of such a kind of hay will depend on the proportion of the different species grown as a mixed crop. Such a crop is generally cut earlier because of the variation in the seeding time of the mixed crops. If harvested early, the cereals are generally richer in proteins.

Different Methods of Hay Making

There are three methods of hay making. They are field curing, barn drying, and artificial drying.

1. Field curing

As the name indicates, cut plants are cured in the field itself to make hay. The various steps in this process are:

(i)   Cutting the crop: Any type of power or hand cutting may be used. It is highly desirable to cut in the same direction. The crop is left there itself in the swath to dry partially.

(ii) Swath curing: Hay is dried much more rapidly in the swath than in the windrow. Therefore maximum advantage of swath curing may be taken to speed up the operations. But after a certain degree of curing, there will be shattering and bleaching of leaves reducing the nutritive value of hay considerably. The forage should be left to cure in the swath until it is wilted sufficiently but before there is danger of shattering and loss of carotene due to bleaching action of sun. No definite time can be assigned to swath curing but at this time the moisture is roughly 40%.

(iii) Raking: After wilting forage to about 40% moisture in the swath, it is rolled into small loose fluffy cylindrical bundles known as windrow. It is better to do raking in the morning as dew makes the hay a little more tough and prevent shattering.

(iv) Cocking: This is the process of making bigger heaps after hay has been cured partially in windrows. Cocks are even protected with hay caps where ram is expected. If there is labour shortage this step may be discarded. Under such circumstances hay is completely cured in the windrow. However, cocking is advisable as it will give better hay with more carotene content.

(v)   Baling and storing: Pick-up baling directly from windrow is the most automated system where the baler attached to tractor picks up hay in the form of windrows and bale it. Where such machines are not available hay may be stored as loose bundles in hay stacks.

2. Mow curing (barn drying)

This refers to the practice of curing partially dried hay inside the barns in mows. Heated or unheated air is blown on to the mows until the moisture is reduced to 20-25%. Swath curing is completed in the field itself and when the moisture is 35-40%, it is taken into the barns and placed on the mows. It takes 7-14 days on the mows with unheated air to cure the hay fully. With heated air it takes less time. Generally the hay produced in this manner will be greener and leafier and of a higher quality than field cured hay.

3. Dehydration or artificial drying

This is the process of chopping freshly cut or wilted fodder and drying it in artificial driers. This is limited to large commercial operations where alfalfa meal or alfalfa leaf meal for use chiefly as a vitamin supplement for poultry and swine are produced. Such hay is consistently of superior quality.

Losses of Nutrients in Hay Making

The losses in nutritive value in hay making are:
1. Losses of leaves by shattering
2. Losses of vitamins due to bleaching and fermentation
3. Losses of soluble nutrients by leaching in heavy rain.

1. Losses by shattering

The loss due to shattering of leaves and finer parts in hay making is of importance, especially in the case of legumes. The leaves are much richer in digestible nutrients than the stem and hence losses by shattering decrease the nutritive value of hay. To avoid these losses, hay should never be overdried or handled during warm periods of the day. Handling of hay, while field curing, is preferably done in the morning hours of the day.

2. Losses of vitamins due to oxidation

In the process of drying, much of the green colouring matter containing carotene (provitamin A) is bleached. Exposure of the green plants to Sun rays decreases vitamin A content of the hay. Sun cured hays are rich in vitamin D_2 (ergocalciferol).

3. Losses due to fermentation

After the crop is harvested the plant enzymes act on the soluble carbohydrates forming thereby CO_2 and water. Therefore, in a normal hay making process some of the nutrients are lost. This loss results in the higher crude fibre content of dry matter of hay as compared to the green fodder. In addition to carbohydrates, protein is affected. Proteins are hydrolysed to amino acids which will be lost if there is rain on the hay due to leaching. In normal curing there is a loss, about 5-9% of dry matter.

4. Losses due to leaching

If hay is almost cured and is exposed to heavy and prolonged rains, especially when it is in the field, severe losses may occur through leaching. Unless the rain is so heavy as to soak the material, losses by leaching will not occur and the losses will be much less even in heavy rains if the hay is in good sized windrows. Leaching causes loss of protein, soluble carbohydrates and other soluble nutrients.

Total losses in hay making

Loss of dry matter	20-30% in legumes
	10-15% in grasses
Loss of protein	28%
Loss of carotene	90%
Loss of energy	25%

Brown Hay

The optimum moisture level for safe storage of hay is 12-14% under tropical Indian conditions. If hay is stored with moisture more than this fermentation takes place and the hay may become very hot and turn brown. Such hay is often quite unpalatable and less nutritious. Starches are broken down to sugars and alcohol and a type of hay called 'Mow-burnt hay' is obtained. Sometimes hay stacks may catch fire spontaneously due to excess fermentation and heat. Therefore a moisture level of 12-14% is important before stacking.

Chapter 20

Harmful Natural Constituents Present in Livestock Feedstuffs

Antinutritional Factors and their Classification

Antinutritional factors (ANFs) may be defined as those substances present in the diet which by themselves or their metabolic products arising in the system interfere with the feed utilization, reduce production or affects the health of the animal. These anti-nutritive substances are often referred to as "toxic factors' because of the deleterious effects they produce when eaten by animals. Toxic substances of natural origin can be classified based on their chemical properties and on the basis of their effect on utilization of nutrients.

A. According to their Chemical Properties

Group I	:	Proteins	1.	Protease inhibitor
			2.	Haemagglutinins (Lectins)
Group II	:	Glycosides	1.	Saponins
			2.	Cyanogens
			3.	Glucosinolates (Goitrogens) or Thioglucosides
Group III	:	Phenols	1.	Gossypol
			2.	Tannins
Group IV	:	Miscellaneous	1.	Antimetals
			2.	Antivitamins

B. On the Basis of Nutrients they Affect Directly or Indirectly

1. Substances depressing digestion or metabolic utilization of proteins.
   a. Protease inhibitor (Trypsin and Chymotrypsin inhibitor)
   b. Haemagglutinins (Lectins)
   c. Saponins
   d. Polyphenolic components

2. Substances reducing solubility or interfering with the utilization of minerals.

    a. Phytic acid
    b. Oxalic acid
    c. Glucosinolates (Thioglucosides)
    d. Gossypol

3. Substances increasing the requirements of certain vitamins.
    a. Anti-vitamin A, D, E, K.
    b. Anti-vitamin B_1, B_6, B_{12} and nicotinic acid.

4. Substances with a negative effect on the digestion of carbohydrates
    a. Amylase inhibitors
    b. Phenolic compounds
    c. Flatulence factors

α-Amylase inhibitors: It has been reported that α-amylase inhibitor is responsible for the impaired digestion of starch from kidney beans.

Flatulence factors: Flatulence factors are related to oligosaccharides which are fermented by intestinal bacteria in the large intestine. These oligosaccharides are not broken down in the small intestine because of a lack of appropriate enzyme, and subsequently enter the large intestine and broken down by bacterial α-1, 6-galactosidase. The monomers of these sugars are converted into VFA, carbon dioxide, hydrogen, methane, resulting in flatulence, diarrhoea, nausea, cramps and discomfort.

5. Substances that stimulate the immune system (antigenic proteins): Antigenic proteins in feed or raw materials are macromolecular proteins or glycoproteins capable of inducing a humoral immune response when fed to animals. In this case humoral immune response means the synthesis of specific polyclonal antibodies secreted in body fluids, such as blood, for eliminating the antigenic protein. The humoral immune response, together with the cellular immune response, forms the specific immune system, which is one of the defence mechanisms of man and animals to keep the integrity of the body. As a result of the specific immune response man and animals can become immune to the antigen.

    When the antigen is an infectious microbial agent immunity is a desired effect. In the case of a feed antigen it is questionable whether an immune response attractive. In case of feed antigens, man and animals are continuously exposed. This continuous exposure increases the chance that the immune response develops into an acute hypersensitivity reaction (causing tissue damage) or into a chronic hypersensitivity reaction. Chronic hypersensitivity is common in case of feed antigens. Antigenic globulins of soybean are glycinin and β-conglycinin.

Effect of Feed Antigens
1. Increased endogenous protein secretion.

2. Lowered apparent protein digestibility.
3. Increased maintenance requirement due to activation of the immune system.
4. Decreased utilization of feed proteins because part of the protein is absorbed as intact macromolecular proteins instead of amino acids and small peptides.

Inactivation of feed antigens: Heat is not appropriate; chemical or enzymatic treatments are preferred; a hot aqueous ethanol extraction may also be used. In preruminant calves ethanol extraction may develop low levels of soya-specific antibodies. Hydrolysis of proteins by means of acid or proteases results in products apparently free of antigenic proteins.

Brief Description of Antinutritional or Toxic Factors
Group - I Proteins

1. Protease inhibitors

Substances that have the ability to inhibit the proteolytic activity of certain digestive enzymes. e.g. Legume seeds: Soybean, kidney bean, mung bean. Protease inhibitors are concentrated in the outer part of the cotyledon mass. Protease inhibitors are two types: a. Kunitz inhibitor (inhibits only trypsin) and b. Bowman - birk inhibitor (inhibits trypsin and chymotrypsin).

The inhibitory substances are mostly heat labile and thus proper heat treatment inactivates the protease inhibitors. Since overheating can damage some nutrients such as amino acids and vitamins, quality control tests have been developed to assess the adequacy of heat treatment. These include trypsin inhibitor and urease assays.

Trypsin inhibitor of soybean interferes with the availability of methionine from the raw soybean. Young chicken fed raw soybean developed hypertrophy of the pancreas. Pancreatic hypertrophy and hyperplasia are not observed in large animal species such as pigs, dog and calves.

The important factors controlling trypsin inhibitor destruction are: 1. temperature 2. duration of heating 3. particle size and 4. moisture level. The trypsin inhibitor activity of solvent extracted SBM was destroyed by exposure to steam for 60 minutes, or by autoclving under the following conditions. 5 psi for 45 min, 10 psi for 30 min and 15 psi for 20 min. duration.

2. Haemagglutinins (Lectins)

Soybean, Castor bean (ricin) and other legume seeds contain haemagglutinins. These are found in both plant and animal tissue. These toxic substances are able to combine with the carbohydrate moieties of cell membranes. Soybean lectin strongly binds to mannose of red blood cells (RBC) and causes agglutination of the cells.

Ricin is extremely toxic. It causes severe inflammatory changes in the intestines, kidney, thyroid gland, etc. Lectins are resistant to digesion by pancreatic juice. Although resistant to destruction by dry heat, lectins are destroyed by the same conditions as those used to inactivate protease inhibitors i.e. by steam.

Group - II Glycosides

1. Saponins: These are glycosides characterised by bitter taste, foaming in aqueous solution and haemolyse RBC. They are able to form complexes with sterols, including those associated with the plasma membranes of animal cells. Generally, saponins are less important because their levels are low in most common feed ingredients for monogastric animals. Their toxicity is related to their activity in lowering surface tension in ruminants.

The important common forages which cause saponin poisoning of livestock are lucerne, soyabean, etc. Average saponin content of the leaves are twice as much as those of the stems and that the saponin content declines as the plant becomes older.

Poultry are more sensitive than pigs. 0.4-0.5% saponin in the feed depress feed consumption in birds. Egg production and body weights are also depressed. Feeding lucerne meal beyond 5-7% in poultry mash show decreased weight gain and egg production. The effect can partly be reversed by feeding of cholesterol and cottonseed oil in the diet with which saponins get binded.

Saponins are degraded by rumen microbes and hence no growth depression is noticed. However, upon excess feeding of green lucerne, etc. legume forages saponins lower the surface tension of ruminal contents leading to accumulation of gas in the digesta. This condition is known as "bloat". This is also known as tympany/tympanitis. It is characterised by the distension of the rumen due to accumulation of gas (CO_2 and CH_4). The presence of saponins has been cited as one of the factors responsible for formation of foam in the rumen and thereby gas is trapped in the rumen contents with the result of which animals can not eliminate it by belching. The rumen distension impedes the blood flow and anorexia develops which is responsible for respiratory failure. Turpentine and paraffin oil are helpful in reducing bloat. For ruminants 1 to 2 kg dry fodder should be fed before letting the animals for legume pastures or before excessive feeding of green legume fodders as a preventive measure.

The negative effect of saponins might be because of their well-known effect as a surface-active component on the biological membrane by which the permeability of the intestinal mucosal cells is increased and the active nutrient transport hindered.

2. Cyanogens: Cyanide in trace amounts is present in the plant kingdom. It occurs mainly in the form of cyanogenetic glycoside. In plants the glycoside is non-toxic in the intact tissues. These glycosides can be hydrolysed to prussic acid or hydrocyanic acid (HCN) by the enzyme usually present in the same plant or as they are being digested by animals. This reaction can take place in the rumen by microbial activity. The HCN is rapidly absorbed and some is eliminated through the lungs, but the greater part is rapidly detoxified in the liver by conversion to thiocyanate. Excess cyanide ion can quickly produce anoxia of the central nervous system inactivating the cytochrome oxidase system and death can result within a few seconds. There are three distinct glycosides.

Glycoside		Plant source
1. Amygdalin	–	Bitter Almonds
2. Dhurrin	–	*Sorghum vulgare* and other immature grasses
3. Linamarin or phaseolunatin	–	Linseed, cassava, Java beans (*Phaseolus lunatus*)

Ruminants are more susceptible to HCN poisoning than are horses and pigs, because the enzyme required for the release of HCN is destroyed in horses and pigs by the gastri HCl. Cattle are most susceptible than sheep. It usually causes reduced growth, poor feed efficiency and result in death if consumed in increased amounts. Clinical symptoms are characterised by mental confusion, generalised muscle peresis and respiratory distress, abdominal pain and vomiting. Sorghum and sudan fodder, linseed may develop toxic levels of HCN in the new growth that follows either a period of drought, or a period of heavy trampling or physical damage by frost, etc. Heavy nitrate fertilisation followed by an abundant irrigation or rainfall may increase the potential of HCN poisoning of these crops.

Feeding of immature jowar green fodder should be avoided to prevent HCN poisoning. Animals which have not shown much evidence of toxicity may be injected intravenously with 3 g sodium nitrate and 15 g sodium thiosulphate in 200 ml H_2O for cattle; for sheep 1 g sodium nitrate and 2.5 g sodium thiosulphate in 50 ml H_2O.

In the UK, linseed cake or meal must, by law, contain less than 350 mg of hydrocyanic acid per kg of food with a moisture content of 12%.

3. Glucosinolates: Most plants of crucifera family (cabbage, turnips, rutabaga, rapeseed and mustard green) contain these substances. These glucosinolates are responsible for the pungent flavours found in plants belonging to the genus *Brassica*. Their main biological effect is to depress the synthesis of the thyroid hormone (Thyroxine, T_4) and Triiodothyronine (T_3), thus producing goitre, although the latter is not caused by the glucosinolates *per se* but by their products of hydrolysis.

The glucosinolates occur in the root, stem, leaf and seed and are always accompanied by the enzyme myrosinase (thioglucosidase), which is capable of hydrolysing them to thiocyanates, glucose and acid sulphate and isothiocyanates or nitriles depending on pH. These volatile isothiocyanates undergo cyclization in the presence of myrosinase to vinyloxazolidinethione which is potently goitrogenic. These cause depressed iodine uptake with an enlargement of the thyroid gland and liver damage. Growth depression and enlargement of liver and kidneys are also observed in chicks and pigs. Ruminants appear to be less susceptible to the toxic effect of glucosinolates compared to pigs and poultry. This is probably the result of the glucosinolates being relatively unhydrolysed in the rumen.

Myrosinase is present not only in the plant and in the seed but also intestinal bacteria have appropriate enzyme systems for glucosinolate hydrolysis. Because of the presence of myrosinase in the intestine, inactivation of myrosinase in the seed is not an appropriate way to eliminate the antinutritional effects of glucosinolates. High-or-low-glucosinolate cultivars of rapeseed are available. Double-zero cultivars were developed in Canada. (p. 256)

Group-III Phenols

1. Gossypol: In genus Gossypium, gossypol is present in pigment glands of leaves, stems, roots and seeds. These pigments can exist either in a free form or as a gossypol-protein in complex. It is highly toxic to monogastric animals. Pigs and rabbits are more sensitive than poultry. Horses are resistant. Ruminants are more resistant due to the formation of stable complexes with soluble protein in rumen which are resistant to enzymatic breakdown. Gossypol form complex with metals like iron and the toxic effect can be overcome by supplementing iron as ferrous sulphate. Whole cotton seed contain a total of 1.09 to 1.53%, of which free form is 0.19%.

The physiological effects of free gossypol are reduced appetite, loss of body weight, accumulation of fluid in the body cavities, cardiac irregularity, reduced oxygen carrying capacity of the blood (reduced haemoglobin content) and an adverse effect on certain liver enzymes. Decreased egg size and decreased egg hatchability are also observed. Free gossypol content of 0.06% depresses growth in chicks while 0.1% causes severe effect. In laying hens, 0.15% free gossypol reduced egg production.

Egg yolk will have an olive green colour. Further higher levels cause yellow, brown pigments in liver and spleen due to destructive effect on red blood cells. In case of pigs a dietary level of 0.01% reduced growth rate while 0.015% showed toxic symptoms. Now new varieties of cotton seed with less than 0.01% total gossypol (0.002% in the free form) are available.

Although heat treatment as in the commercial production of cottonseed meal decreases the content of free gossypol, the availability of lysine is reduced because of the interaction of the aldehyde groups of gossypol with the amino group of lysine.

2. *Tannin:* It is polyphenolic substance with molecular weight greater than 500. The term tannin was coined by Seguin in 1796. Tannins are of two types.

A. *Hydrolysable tannins:* These can be readily hydrolysed by water, acids, bases or enzymes and yield gallotannins and ellagitannins.

B. *Condensed tannins:* These are Flavonoids-polymers of flavonol. Both hydrolysable and condensed tannins are widely distributed in nature. Tannin content of certain feedstuffs are presented here. Chlorogenine is a polyphenolic compound present in sunflower seed meal. See Table 1 also (page No. 550).

Sorghum	2.0 to 10%
Salseed meal	9.0 to 12%
Mangoseed kernel	5.0 to 7%
Mustard oil cake	2.5 to 3.5%
Lucerne meal	0.1 to 3.0%

Tannins are astringent in nature leading to poor palatability. They cause a dry or puckery sensation in the mouth, probably by reducing the lubricant action of the glycoproteins in the saliva. They bind the proteins and are thus inhibitors of proteolytic enzymes. High tannin content also depresses cellulase activity and thus affects digestion of crude fibre. So tannins reduce the digestibility of protein and dry matter. Sorghum contains high levels of condensed tannins. Most of the tannins are located in seed coats. Decortication of seeds will reduce the tannin content. Germination of legumes also result in a decrease in the tannin content.

Tannins found in some tree leaves form complexes with plant proteins which decrease their rate of digestion in the rumen, thereby decreasing rumen ammonia concentrations and increasing the amount of plant protein bypassing the rumen. When the tannin-protein complexes are dissociated in the low pH of the abomasum, an additional source of protein is made available for absorption by the animal. But in some cases, the tannins protect the proteins from digestion even in the small intestine. Tannins may, therefore, have a beneficial effect (increasing bypass protein

TABLE 1. Polyphenolic Compounds of Certain Tree Leaves*.

Tree leaves/ Constituents	Total phenolics[1]	Non-tannin phenolics[1]	Total tannin phenolics[1]	Condensed tannins[2]
Acacia auriculiformis	13.44–14.68	0.48–0.51	12.96–14.17	12.29–13.62
Cashew	20.31–22.26	0.86–0.90	19.45–21.36	16.43–16.84
Gliricidia	5.63	0.35	5.28	3.44
Guava**	17.02	0.84	16.18	14.00
Jack	15.63	0.94	14.69	13.23
Sesbania grandiflora	9.38	0.74	8.64	5.71
Subabul	11.25	0.48	10.78	7.28
Yellow gold mohur	12.50	0.53	11.98	11.03

[1]as tannic acid equivalent, [2]as leucocyanidine equivalent.
*D.V. Reddy and N. Elanchezhian 2008, Livestock Research for Rural Development, 20, 5, 8 pages; **N. Elanchezhian, personal communication.

or decreasing ammonia loss) or a detrimental effect (depressing palatability, decreasing rumen ammonia, decreasing post-ruminal protein absorption) on protein availability.

It is clear that the interpretation of the nutritional value of protein in fodder tree leaves requires information on the nature and action of tannins. The protein in the leaves of species which do not have tannins will be rapidly degraded in the rumen, providing high levels of rumen ammonia, much of which will ultimately be wasted by excretion as urinary urea. Species which contain some tannin will, therefore, provide both degradable and undegraded rumen N and will be more effective sources of supplemental N for ruminants.

Condensed tannins (CT; procyanidins or proanthocyanidins) form complexes containing proteins which protect the latter from rumen digestion and augment the bypass protein available for absorption in the small intestine. This seems to apply to species such as *Sesbania grandiflora*, *Leucaena leucocephala*, *Gliricidia sepium* which often contain moderate levels of condensed tannins (Table 1) exhibit moderate protein degradability. On the other hand, high levels of CT are inimicable to intake and protein complexes may be protected from digestion even in the small intestine.

Further, tannins suppress methanogenesis by reducing methanogenic populations in the rumen either directly or by reducing the protozoal population, thereby reducing methanogens symbiotically associated with the protozoal population. Tannin sources containing both hydrolysable tannins and condensed tannins are more potent in suppressing methanogenesis than those containing only hydrolysable tannins.

Detannification of Feedstuffs

Methods of detannification: The methods available for removal/ inactivation of tannins can be divided into two main categories:

1. **Physical treatments:** Soaking and cooking decrease the tannin content. However, these treatments, cause a substantial loss of dry matter between 20 to 70%. Anaerobic storage of moist sorghum grains for two and nine days resulted in 40% and 92% reduction in tannins, respectively.

2. **Chemical treatments:** Addition of tannin complexing agents like polyethylene glycol (PEG) and polyvinylpyrrolidone (PVP) prevent formation of complexes between tannin and protein as well as break the already formed complex thus liberating protein. Alkalies, formaldehyde, organic solvents like acetone, acids, oxidizing agents (KMnO$_4$, Potassium dichromate, alkaline H$_2$O$_2$), ferrous sulphate reduce the tannin content.

3. Simple methods based on post-harvest technology, treatment with low-cost chemicals, biological treatments, and supplementation with tannin-complexing agents are developed to enhance the feeding value of tannin-containing feeds.

4. H.P.S. Makkar did series of experiments on chemistry and estimation of tannins and on several detannification methods. Oak leaves are rich in tannins and young oak leaves cause toxicity. Although consumption of mature oak leaves does not normally lead to the death of animals, their consumption impairs production. The detoxification (by inactivation or removal of tannins) methods employed in case of oak leaves may also be followed to any feed resource rich in tannins.

1. Wood ash: Wood ash is a good source of alkali. A 10% of solution of oak wood ash decreased the content of total phenols, condensed tannins and protein precipitation capacity by 66, 80 and 75% in oak leaves.

2. Chopping and storage: The 'chopping of leaves and then storage' has been found practical application at the farmer's level. Instead of feeding the leaves on the same day as they are lopped, they need only be chopped and stored for about 5-10 days before feeding. The higher extent of inactivation of tannins by chopping of leaves could be due to oxidation of tannins by phenol oxidases present in leaves, as chopping is expected to increase the availability of tannins to the enzyme. In addition, inactivation of tannins during storage was due to their polymerization to higher 'inert' polymers.

3. Drying: Drying of mature oak leaves under different conditions (60° C for 48h, 90°C for 24h, shade drying for 1 day, 2 days and 3 days and sun drying for 24h, 48h) had no effect on the levels of total phenols, condensed tannins, protein precipitation capacity, degree of polymerization, specific activity of tannins and bound condensed tannins. On the other hand, drying conditions (90°C for 24h) decreased tannin content in cassava and leucaena leaves. One of the reasons for this difference was found to be different level of moisture in these leaves. Cassava and leucaena leaves had about 65% moisture whereas oak leaves had 40%. Increase of moisture of oak leaves followed by the heat treatment decreased tannin levels.

4. Solid state fermentation: Biodegradation of tannins using white-rot fungi (*Sporotricum pulverulentum, Ceriporiopsis subvermispora* and *Cyathus steroreus*) is a promising approach.

5. Tannin complexing agents: Polyethylene glycol, a non-nutritive synthetic polymer having high affinity for condensed tannins, makes them inert by forming PEG-tannin complex. Polyvinylpyrrolidone (PVP) is also used as tannin-complexing agent. These tannin-complexing agents are also considered to break 'the already formed tannin-protein complexes' since their affinity for tannins is higher than for proteins. The affinity of PVPs for tannins was lower than of PEG. The PEG 6000 may be preferred for inactivation of tannins in feedstuffs as its binding to tannins was highest at near neutral pH values.

Makkar (2003) advocated use of PEG both by farmers (give to animals through water, feed or spraying on tannin-rich feedstuffs) as well as by industry (incorporate PEG in a pelleted diet). The incorporation of PEG had beneficial effects for feedstuffs such as *Zizyphus nummularia* (Kumar and Vaithiyanathan, 1990) which are rich in tannins (condensed tannin content: 5-10%). On the otherhand, for *L. corniculatus*, the condensed tannin content of which varied from 2 to 4 %, addition of PEG decreased wool growth, weight gain, reproduction and milk yield. From these observations, it is clear that incorporation of PEG in diets containing high levels of condensed tannins is beneficial for ruminants.

Group-IV

1. Antimetals: Substances depressing the utilization of minerals.

Phytic acid: Phytic acid is an ester formed by combination of the 6 alcoholic groups of inositol with 6 molecules of hexaphosphoric acid. Hence its name inositol hexaphosphoric acid.

Inositol   Phytic acid

Because of the presence of the large number of phosphoric acid radicals it can form simple salts or mixed salts as well as metabolic or protein complexes. Sodium and potassium salts are soluble. Calcium, iron, magnesium, copper, zinc and lead salts (phytates) are insoluble even at pH 3-4. Phytate phosphorus is a poor source of phosphorus. Seeds of cereals, dried legumes, oilseeds and nuts are rich in phytic acid. Phytic acid concentration is more in the rind (pericarp + aleurone layer) and the embryo than the core (endosperm).

Ingredient		Phytic acid content (mg%)
Wheat	-	170-280
Maize	-	157-240
Rice	-	70-300
Soybean	-	402
Linseed	-	741
Cotton seed	-	366
Castor beans	-	500

About 67% or more of the phosphorus in cereal grains is in the form of phytin phosphorus. The availability of phosphorus from plant feeds to nonruminants may be safely assumed as no more than 33%. By contrast, phosphorus from inorganic mineral supplements and of animal origin are usually available at the rate of more than 80%. Phytin phosphorus is less effectively utilized than the inorganic form in poultry, pigs and horses since phytin is incompletely broken down in their digestive tract. Horses utilize it less efficiently than ruminants but more efficiently than pigs. Both dietary phytase and microbial phytase are concerned in the extent of this breakdown. Addition of the enzyme phytase to the ingredients of vegetable origin can increase phosphorus digestibility considerably. Phytase produced by rumen microorganisms makes phytin phosphorus available to ruminants. Phytic acid depresses the utilization of several mineral elements such as Ca, Mg, Fe, Zn, etc. It forms insoluble compounds which are eliminated in the faeces.

Oxalic acid: Plant foodstuffs have much oxalic acid. Foodstuffs of animal origin have relatively little oxalic acid. Oxalic acid is present as free and in salt form. It is a dicarboxylic acid $(COOH)_2$. The greater part of oxalic acid in plants is present in the form of soluble oxalates (potassium, sodium and ammonium oxalates) and only 10-20% appears as insoluble calcium and magnesium oxalate especially within the cells. The leaves are richer than other parts. In general young leaves contain smaller quantities than mature leaves. Ageing as well as over ripening of vegetables is accompanied by an increase in the proportion of calcium oxalate.

Pigs and poultry are affected. Growth is depressed and blood calcium is decreased. Animal response to oxalate poisoning varies with species of animal and species of plant (kind of oxalate differs in different plant species) consumed. Thus cattle, sheep and horses differ in their responses to oxalate. Cattle fed on paddy straw or other grasses (napier, bajra, etc.) containing 2% oxalate develop a negative calcium balance but sheep do not develop at this level. Rumen microflora (Pseudomonas, Streptomyces, etc.) decompose much of soluble oxalic acid and to a less extent its calcium salts.

When the dietary amount exceeds certain level, normal degradation (by microbes) is interrupted and the excess oxalates combine with feed calcium to form insoluble calcium oxalate and thus calcium becomes unavailable for absorption or the excess oxalate (20-30 mg per cent) may be absorbed from the rumen into the blood stream where it can combine with calcium to produce hypocalcaemia. The insoluble calcium oxalate may then crystalise in various tissues, specially kidneys and rumen wall.

Oxalate poisoning in livestock results principally from ingesting oxalate-producing plants, which are highly palatable to livestock. Oxalate poisoning in cattle and sheep are characterised by rapid and laboured respiration, depression, weakness, coma and death.

2. Antivitamins: These are organic compounds which either destroy certain vitamins or combine and form unabsorbable complexes or interfere with digestive and/or metabolic functions.

a. Antivitamin A: Raw soybean contains enzyme lipoxygenase which can be destroyed by heating 5 min with steam at atmospheric pressure. Lipoxygenase catalyses oxidation of carotene, the precursor of vitamin A.

b. Antivitamin E: Lipoxygenase destroys vitamin E also. Present in kidney bean. Diets with raw kidney beans produced muscular dystrophy in chicks and lambs by reducing plasma vitamin E. Autoclaving destroys the factor.

c. Antivitamin K: Eating mould infected sweet clover cause fatal haemorrhagic condition in cattle. This is known as "Sweet clover disease". Dicoumarol present in sweet clover is responsible for this. Dicoumarol reduce prothrombin levels in blood and affects blood clotting (see p. 147 also).

d. Antivitamin D: Rachitogenic activity of isolated soya protein (unheated) has been found with chicks and pigs. Autoclaving eliminates this rachitogenic activity.

e. Anti-pyridoxine: An antagonist of pyridoxine from linseed has been identified as 1-amino-D-proline. It occurs naturally in combination with glutamic acid as a peptide and it is called linatine. Nutritive value of linseed meal for chicks can be considerably improved after water treatment and autoclaving.

f. Antiniacin: An antagonist of niacin, niacytin is found in maize, wheat bran, etc. which cause perosis and growth depression.

g. Antithiamine: The enzyme thiaminase present in bracken fern (*Pteridium aquilinum*) acts as antithiamine factor by destroying it.

Nitrate Poisoning

Nitrate *per se* is not toxic. Nitrate poisoning or 'Oat hay poisoning' in cattle is due to the consumption of nitrates present in some grasses and other crops; examples include sorghum, sudan grass, maize, lucerne, wheat, barley, soybean. The nitrates are reduced to nitrites in the rumen. (See below). When high levels of nitrites accumulate in the GI tract, they are absorbed into the bloodstream. Nitrites oxidize the ferrous iron of haemoglobin to the ferric iron of methaemoglobin which does not transport oxygen. In severe cases, the blood becomes almost chocolate brown and there is a brownish discolouration of nonpigmented areas of the skin and mucous membranes.

The pulse is rapid and breathing is laboured. Death may result because of anoxia. Nonruminants can tolerate nitrate but ruminants don't (See the Figure) because the bacteria in the rumen convert nitrate to nitrite.

Sources of nitrate/nitrite: Water contaminated with animal or industrial wastes (page no. 86), feeds containing high levels of nitrate. Cornstalks and oat hay were two of the feeds first reported to occasionally contain high level of nitrate. Hay or straw containing more than 2.2% potassium nitrate is toxic.

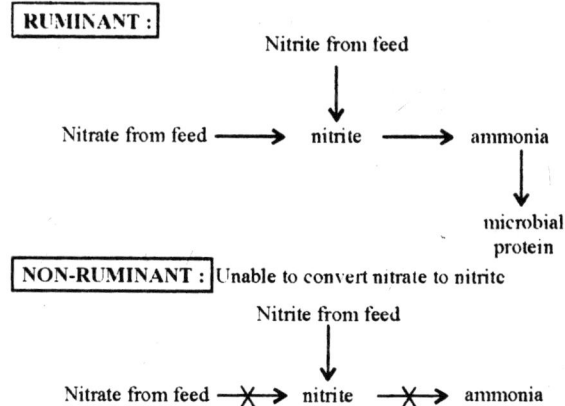

Nitrite poisoning

There is considerable variation between species in their susceptibility to nitrite poisoning. Pigs are the most susceptible, then, in order, cattle, sheep and horses. Non-ruminants, such as horses and pigs, have no mechanism for converting nitrate to nitrite (see figure on page no. 555) in their digestive tract, so they are not susceptible to nitrite poisoning from excessive intake of nitrates. However, they are highly susceptible to poisoning from nitrite intake (for instance in mouldy hay) because they cannot convert the nitrite to ammonia. Sheep are more efficient at converting nitrite to ammonia; that is why probably, they are less susceptible to nitrite poisoning than cattle.

Hasan H.Oruc et al (2010; Journal of Equine Veterinary Science, 30: 159-162) reported nitrate poisoning in thoroughbred mares from Turkey. High nitrate concentrations were found in their grass and lucerne feed samples. The clinical symptoms, postmortem findings together with the nitrate levels supported the nitrate and nitrite poisoning as the cause of deaths.

Treatment

Treatment involves conversion of methaemoglobin into oxyhaemoglobin by administration of suitable reducing agents such as methylene blue, thionin or ascorbic acid. Acute nitrate toxicity is treated with intravenous administration of methylene blue solution. Methylene blue apparently accepts electrons for NADPH reductase in the blood and acclerates the reconversion of methaemoglobin to functional haemogobin. The recommended dosage of methylene blue is 2 to 4 mg/kg to 15 mg/kg body weight (in severe methaemoglobinemia), intravenously in a one percent solution. The dosage should be repeated if clinical signs recur. Oral doses of mineral oil (one litre for adult cattle) or saline cathartics (sodium sulphate 500 g per adult cattle) are recommended as supportive treatment, which help in removing toxic materials from gastrointestinal tract.

To be at safer side, the fodder cut in the early part of regrowth may be fed mixed with other dry roughages to neutralize the nitrate concentration.

Mimosine Toxicity

Subabul green forage contain a toxic amino acid, mimosine at 2-5% in the leaves on DMB. When fresh leaves are masticated and mostly on rumen microbial degradation, a goitrogen 3-hydroxy - 4 (1H) - pyridone (3, 4DHP) is autocatalytically formed from the mimosine. The DHP is toxic and symptoms of toxicity include alopecia, excessive salivation, enlarged thyroid glands, low serum thyroxine (T_4), low serum triiodothyronine (T_3), oesophageal lesions, poor appetite, weight loss and death. Abortion of pregnant animals, death of calves are also reported. Some animals developed cataract.

It is reported that ruminants in Hawaii and Indonesia possess rumen bacteria (*Synergistes jonesii*) which can rapidly degrade DHP and thus are not susceptible to leucaena toxicity. The DHP is eventually excreted in the urine in a simple or a conjugated form as non-toxic compounds. Mimosine toxicity is observed in ruminants if subabul constitutes more than about 30% of the total diet dry matter intake and 5 to 7% in pigs and rabbits.

Subabul is toxic to poultry and other monogastric animals. The maximum quantity of subabul leaf meal acceptable to layers was 2.5% and 5% to broilers.

Sundrying has been reported to reduce the mimosine content to the extent of 10%. Drying at high temperature, ensiling and addition of ferrous sulphate reduce the mimosine content of subabul. Ferrous sulphate binds mimosine, hinders in its absorption and promotes its excretion through faeces; this is more useful for monogastric species.

Secondary Plant Compounds (SPC)

Plants contain lignin, cutin, suberin, biogenic silica and a far more diverse and active chemical defence arsenal of secondary plant compounds. They physically impede digestive enzymes or microorganisms and their effects can range from feeding deterrence to toxicity. They have been labeled "secondary" because few have primary metabolic functions within the plant and at one time they were viewed as end products of other metabolic systems.

Secondary Plant Compounds are antiherbivory chemicals. Although SPC are invariably viewed as antinutrients, some may have beneficial roles in animal nutrition. The three most prevalent groups of SPC are soluble phenolics, alkaloids and terpenoids. Soluble plant phenolics include flavonoids, isoflavonoids (phytoestrogens) and hydrolysable and condensed tannins.

Chapter 21

Quality Control of Feedstuffs

Quality control of feedstuffs can play a vital role in the development of feed manufacturing industry and also for maximum exploitation of the production efficiency. It is essential at all stages in the production of compound feed so that animals could get wholesome balanced and nutritious feed.

Organisations and Acts

The quality control of feed is regulated by the legislation laid down by the Bureau of Indian Standards (BIS), New Delhi. BIS is a statutory institution established under the BIS Act, 1986 to promote harmonious development of the activities of standardization, marketing and quality certification of goods and attending to connected matters in the country. It has set up Animal Feeds Sectional Committee and the members of this Committee are drawn from ICAR Institutes, State Agricultural Universities, Feed Industry and Government departments having specialization in Animal Nutrition and Feed Technology and concerned with Animal Husbandry Activities.

Objectives of the Animal Feeds Sectional Committee
1. To describe the feeds accurately
2. To lay down standards on feed ingredients
3. To lay down standards for compounded feed formulations and mineral mixtures for cattle, poultry, pigs, laboratory animals, etc.

In the United States, two organizations publish manuals which contain methods approved for analysis of food and feeds. They are the Association of Analytical Communities (AOAC) and the American Oil Chemist's Society (AOCS). In India, BIS methods are also available for analysis of some nutrients and antinutritional factors.

The Agricultural produce (Grading and Marketing) Act empowers the Government of India to fix quality standards, known as 'Agmark' standards and prescribe terms and conditions for using the seal.

The objective of quality control of feedstuffs is to ensure that a consumer obtains feeds that are unadulterated, true to their nature and give desired results. A good system of quality control may therefore, be defined as the maintenance of quality at levels and tolerances acceptable to the buyer while minimising the cost of processing.

Monitoring the quality of livestock/poultry/fish feeds

There is a need to regulate the quality of animal feed vis-à-vis the BIS standards. BIS specifications for certain concentrate ingredients (See page No. 412) and BIS specifications for mineral mixtures and cattle feeds (Tables 11 and 12, page 72 and 73 of Applied Nutrition 3rd edition) are furnished for follow up. "Cattle fodder, including oilcakes and other concentrates" are the deleted items from the Essential Commodities Act, 1955. Hence it is not possible to regulate the quality of feed under the said act. An advisory had been issued on 24th January 2013 (by the dept of Animal Husbandry, Dairying and Fisheries, Government of India) on using the provisions under the 'Consumer Protection Act, 1986' and 'The Bureau of Indian Standards Act, 1986' to regulate the quality of feed sold in the market.

Quality Control of Raw Materials

Quality control of raw materials i.e., feed ingredients is the first step to be done to ensure that they meet the minimum contract specifications, that they are suitable for inclusion in the compounded feeds and also to indicate the maximum proportions in which they can be included.

1. Preliminary Inspection of Raw Materials

A thorough 'physical inspection' for the following is to be done when they are received at the mill.

1. Colour, odour, texture, density of the material
2. Evidence of wetting
3. Presence of adulterants such as stones, dirt or other foreign materials.
4. Storage pests
5. Evidence of damaged or broken kernels, etc.
6. Evidence of presence of rat faecal pellets or hair, etc.
7. Moisture should not be more than 10% (Determine moisture of the feed rapidly).

Automatic control of moisture content in feed: Though the maximum moisture content of feed is prescribed by law, their actual moisture values are often substantially lower. This is primarily due to the fact that the fine-tuning of the moisture content is an extremely complex matter and hence, animal feed producers prefer to observe a safety margin in order to avoid exceeding the maximum legal value. On the other hand, a higher (within the legal limit) and constant moisture content would ensure a consistently high product quality, reduce the raw material requirement, and therefore boost a feed manufacturer's profit.

Now it is possible with the 'advances in automation technology'. It helps the online testing and adjustment of the moisture content of animal feed in the ongoing process by using NIR measurement probe (Buhler Multi-Online NIR System). This NIR probe offers feed manufacturers great potential for cutting costs and increasing margins.

2. Chemical Tests

Draw a representative sample for laboratory analysis very carefully:

Analyse for proximate principles. This indicates possible constraints on usage due to the presence of excessive content of crude fibre, fat or total ash.

Additional tests should be carried out on materials with high ash content, to determine acid insoluble ash. The amount of acid insoluble ash is a good guide to the amount of sand or other dirt which may be present.

It is also desirable to determine the free fatty acid content of oily materials as this will affect palatability due to rancidity.

3. Toxicological Tests

Some ingredients contain 'endogenous' toxic substances which may at low concentration adversely affect feed conversion and palatability and at higher concentration, even result in the death of animals.
e.g. Gossypol in cotton seed (cotton seed cake is to be treated with ferrous sulphate to overcome toxicity in nonruminants)

Glucosinolates in rape seed
Cyanogenic glycosides in linseed and cassava
Mycotoxins, primarily aflatoxins in maize, groundnut cake, etc.

Ultra violet screening is used whereby a greenish yellow fluorescence is observed (when the sample is exposed to ultra violet light to detect mycotoxins), if the sample contains aflatoxin.

Obviously it will not be practicable to assess the toxicity on routine basis. One should get from the best source of supply and one should have some idea of normal levels of toxicity which may be expected.

Fish meal, meat meal and bone meal should be free from pathogenic bacteria like Salmonella which may cause diseases in animals to which they are fed.

Rapid Methods of Feed Quality Control (D. Narahari, Feed Tech 6, 6, 2002, pp. 23)

A combination of field and laboratory tests will aid in better quality control. The field methods are mainly based on organoleptic evaluation, using the senses of touch, taste, vision, smell and hearing. Simple field tests can also be carried out as well. Certain laboratory tests may be carried out.

By touching the grains moisture level, coarseness, fat level in rice polish can be felt. By biting and tasting oil cakes, one can define the freshness, rancidity, mould and mustiness and adulteration if any. During storage, the oil or fat in it will undergo rancidity, leading to an undesirable burning taste due to presence of free fatty acids. Visual evaluation helps to examine the feedstuffs for natural colours, consistency and presence of foreign materials, mould growth, cake and clump formation, weevil attack and any other abnormalities. Smelling the feed reveals rancidity and musty odours. Musty odour is an indication of mould growth. Rancid feedstuffs in feeds lead to destruction of fat-soluble vitamins. Well-dried grains and fish on shaking in the hands will give a dry metallic sound whereas high moisture grains and fish will give soft dull sound.

Commercially available soybean meal is roasted solvent extracted meal. It can be tested by a rapid field method for its proper processing to destory the trypsin inhibitor with the help of a mixture containing cresol red + urea + thymol blue + glycerol. Proper heat processing reveals developing a red colour, that too slowly, only in 10% of soybean meal sample.

Finished Feed Quality

Finished feed assays are necessary because they provide the mill with a final report on how well the quality was controlled. One sample of each formula per week or per batch has to be analysed.

Test for Soybean Meal (Popular in-plant test)

While purchasing soybean meal it is tested for the absence of trypsin inhibitors, haemagglutinins and urease enzyme. The former two antinutritional factors depress the utilization of proteins while urease presents no practical problem to monogastric animals but of concern to ruminant feeds. The urease activity of the feed is an indication of the level of cooking or processing applied during the preparation of soybean meal. The urease enzyme is denatured at approximately the same rate as that of the trypsin inhibitors and it is easier to assay for urease enzyme than for trypsin inhibitors. Hence urease analysis is accepted by the feed industry world wide for use in monitoring the soybean meal quality.

No (urease) activity at all hints overheating and possible denaturation of protein (overheating of soybean meal reduces the availability of essential amino acids, especially lysine and arginine). Excessive activity indicates a lack of proper heat treatment at the processing plant. The former condition could mean reduced protein availability while the latter can cause palatability problems since the urease of such meal reacts with urea (in ruminant feeds consisting urea) and release ammonia. Excessive urease activity also indicates presence of trypsin inhibitors.

Visual Examination of Soybean Meal when Treated with Urea-phenol Red Solution*

	Urease Activity	Approximate range of urease	Assessment
No visible red colour	Inactive	0.00	over cooked
Few scattered red particles	Slightly active	0.05 - 0.10	properly cooked
Approximately 25% or red particles	Moderately active	0.20	properly cooked
Approximately 50% or more red particles	Very active	Above 0.20	under cooked

*Urea - phenol red solution is made as follows. Dissolve 0.14g of phenol red in 7 ml 0.1N NaOH and 35 ml distilled water. Dissolve 21g of urea in 300 ml distilled water. Mix these two solutions together and titrate to amber colour with 0.1N H_2SO_4.

Common Adulterants in Feeds and Fodders

Adulteration is defined as the intentional admixture of a pure substance with some cheaper and low quality substances to make money. Costly feed ingredients like oil cakes and feed products from animal origin like fish meal are adulterated. However, sometimes brans, molasses are also adulterated (Table 1).

Adulteration can be checked in the laboratory by the following methods.

1. Chemical analysis
2. Bioassay assessment: But bioassay technique is less common for detecting adulteration
3. Feed microscopy

TABLE 1. Common Adulterants of Different Feed Ingredients.

Feed ingredient	Adulterant
Groundnut cake	Groundnut husk, urea, non-edible oil cakes
Mustard cake	*Argimona maxicana* seeds, fibrous feed ingredients urea
Soybean meal	Urea, hulls
Deoiled rice bran, wheat bran	Ground rice hulls, saw dust
Fish meal	Common salt, urea
Mineral mixture	Common salt, marble powder, sand, lime stone
Molasses	Water
Meat and bone meal	Leather meal, blood meal, sand
DCP	Calcite powder, rock phosphate

Chemical Analysis

Proximate analysis of the feed in question gives some idea about the adulteration.

1. Lower CP and higher fibre content of an oilseed cake than its specifications indicate about the presence of some fibrous feed such as hulls.

2. If the fibre remains higher than the specified limits but CP within normal range, it may be inferred that the cake is adulterated with urea and/or some inferior quality oil cake, like mahua cake, castor cake, karanj cake, etc.

The presence of these oil cakes may be visualised by their abnoxious flavour or specific taste. Moreover, these could be determined chemically.

1. Presence of **mahua cake** in compound feed or in raw oil cake	Water extract of the test feed + conc. H_2SO_4: **Violet or pink colour** indicates the presence of mahua cake
2. Presence of **argimona seeds** in mustard cake	Water extract of test feed + conc. HNO_3: **Brown-reddish** colour indicates the presence of argimona seeds
3. Presence of **urea**	1 part of test feed + 3 parts of water and mix: Supernatant + few drops of DMAB reagent (2 g dimethylamino benzaldehyde dissolved in 90 ml methyl alcohol + 10 ml HCl): **Deepening of yellow colour** indicates the presence of urea.

Spot tests:

Identification of adulterants by use of certain reagents: These tests are best applied by placing about *two drops of the reagent* in a clear or white spot plate or filter paper and *sprinkling* a small portion of the *feed.* They may also be used to identify single particles.

Reagent	Reaction	Compound indicated
HCl 0.5 N	Effervescence	Carbonates/bicarbonates
Ammonium molybdate	No precipitate	Calcium carbonate or absence of phosphorus
Ammonium molybdate	Yellow precipitate	Bone meal, Dicalcium phosphate (presence of phosphorus)
Silver nitrate 0.1 N	White precipitate	Salt (in min. mixture, etc.)
Distilled water	White solution	Milk products
Concentrated H_2SO_4	Effervescence	Carbonates or NaCl
	Blue colour	Chloretetracycline
	Light red	Oxytetracyline
	Red purple	Tetracycline
	Orange brown	Riboflavin

Feed Microscopy: It is commonly used for confirming the adulteration and identifying the adulterants. Official procedures for basic feed microscopy are given by AOAC (1970).

Under low magnification (8 to 50X) the material examined are identified by their outward physical characteristics like shape, colour, particle size, softness, texture, etc. It needs very little sample preparation.

Under high magnification (100 to 500X) the plant cells and structural features of the material are taken into consideration which are not lost during grinding or even after powdering.

A Microscopist must be familiar with all types of feed ingredients and adulterants. He must have a collection of

a. pure feed ingredients
b. adulterants
c. contaminants

These must be studied under low and high magnification for familiarisation with their distinguishing features whether coarsely or finely ground.

Floatation technique: Separatory funnel is used to separate mineral (inorganic) from organic matter by using carbon tetrachloride or chloroform as solvent.

In this technique the sample is soaked in the solvent then stirred and allowed to settle until the two fractions have been clearly separated. The top layer is of organic and the bottom layer is of inorganic material. Each fraction is removed in petri dishes and allowed to dry at room temperature. The use of carbon tetrachloride or chloroform not only causes separation of organic and inorganic material, but also removes fat from the sample, which does help for a more clear examination. The floatation technique is very useful in microscopy work particularly in estimating the amount of adulterant of major ingredients in the mixture. In feed mills with laboratory facilities, microscopic inspection can support chemical findings.

Mad Cow Disease - Feeding of Rendered Products

Feed manufacturers and animal nutritionists have to protect the animals from various forms of zoonotic prion diseases. These prion (an acronym derived from 'Proteinaceous infectious particle') diseases include bovine spongiform encephalopathy (BSE) or mad cow disease in cattle, sheep scrapie and other strains of BSE-like transmissible spongiform encephalopathies (TSE) in human beings, cats, mink, hamsters, ostrichs. Normal transmission of prion - associated diseases is through feed intake. Hence prevention of BSE in food animals and companion animals is easy by avoiding the feeding of animal byproducts to the animals. However animal byproducts such as meat and bone meal (MBM) is a valuable animal protein supplement in feeding of ruminants as well as monogastric animals and poultry.

Proliferation of BSE in the British cattle (in 1986) thought to have emerged originally from initial interspecies transmission of the scrapie agent into cattle by the feeding of scrapie - infected sheep and goat meal, plus bone meal products to cattle. This led to an EU - wide MBM ban for ruminant feeding while some other countries, most notably the UK, have a complete MBM ban for all animal feed. If animal proteins are not allowed to be used in feed not only feed cost would be increased but also cost of disposal of dead animals and byproducts from slaughter houses would increase.

Life - threatening salmonellosis and BSE epidemic had brought about a drastic overhaul of rendering technology and procedures within the EU. The new regulations required that mammalian material with a maximum particle size of 50 mm be processed at 133°C at 3 atmospheres pressure for a minimum of 20 minutes. In case of MBM processed according to these conditions, it was considered safe for use in animal feeds, except for ruminants.

In USA these processing conditions are not mandatory. However many American renderers follow pressurised processes. Moreover, the US

FDA implemented its own ban on feeding any rendered products containing ruminant proteins to ruminants since 1997.

Consequent upon recent reports of clinical diseases caused by TSE group of agents occurring in different countries, Government of India instructed all state governments to take appropriate measures to strengthen the TSE surveillance and monitoring system through its order dated 21-6-1999. "Though there is no prevalent practice of using meat meal, bone meal, and blood meal in ruminant feeds, it is considered necessary as a matter of abundant precaution, to reiterate the prohibition on the use of these animal meals in the manufacture of ruminant feeds". It also cautions the state governments to enhance the surveillance to prevent cross contamination of feeds.

The new FDA regulations of 2009 prohibit specified high-risk materials (bovine offals such as brain, spinal cord, eyes and connective nerves, thymus, spleen, tonsils) from all animal feeds, including petfoods. The FDA's "enhanced feed ban" will likely affect the availability of some ingredients for use in petfoods. FDA considers this ban as prudent to further protect public and human health. The removal of high-risk materials from all animal feed will protect against inadvertent transmission of the agent thought to cause BSE, which could occur through cross-contamination of ruminant feed, with non-ruminant feed or feed ingredients during manufacture and transport or through misfeeding of non-ruminant feed to ruminants on the farm. FDA expects all parties to practice due diligence in excluding "cattle materials prohibited in animal feed (CMPAF)" from their respective products.

Quality Control of Feed

Animal byproducts such as meat meal, blood meal, meat and bone meal, fish meal, etc. have a high content of good quality protein and a high energy value. They are rich sources of lysine and the sulphur containing amino acids and biologically available sources of minerals. In view of the ban of meat and bone meal in ruminant feeds, there is a potential to adulterate fish meal with these banned terrestrial animal products. Analytical methods are available to detect the presence of ruminant animal protein, other protein meals in animal feeds.

Methods for detection

Rapid identification of bovine and other animal materials in animal feedstuffs is essential for effective control of a potential source of BSE. Several methods for the detection and identification of animal materials in feed have been developed ever since BSE was recognized. Species identification of animal products is possible by three major methods.

1. **Enzyme-linked immunosorbent assay (ELISA):** ELISA is simple and convenient, but not sensitive enough to detect heat-treated proteins produced during the rendering process.
2. **Feed microscopy:** It is based on microscopic structure identification. It is tissue-specific and mostly unaffected by heat treatment of the samples. But feed microscopy is reliable only when the operator is expert.
3. **DNA analysis:** It is said that the PCR finds a needle in the haystack and then produces a stack of needles. In DNA analysis, use of the polymerase chain reaction (PCR) has improved feed analysis for traceability of foods of animal origin because of its simplicity, species specificity and sensitivity for detecting feed components. With species-specific primers and analysis of restriction fragment length polymorphism, material from cattle, sheep, goats, pigs and chickens can be detected and identified.

Similarly, tests are available to detect the presence of very small amount of GM material in the feed by DNA-based PCR and the protein-based ELISA; PCR takes 2-10 days while ELISA is an on-site test that takes 2 hours; a faster and simpler dipstick test that provides a "yes - no" result takes 5-10 minutes.

DIOXIN CONTAMINATION OF FEED

The occurrence of dioxin contamination in feed and food in Belgium in May 1999 scared the consumers of the animal products and shaked the consumers faith on the regulatory systems of food safety.

What are dioxins?

Dioxins and dioxin - like compounds are created by the manufacture of chlorine and such chlorinated compouds as chlorinated phenols, polychlorinated bipnenyls. (PCBs), phenoxy herbicides, chlorinated benzenes, chlorinated aliphatic compounds, chlorinated catalysts, and halogenated dipheny 1 ethers. The most toxic compound is 2, 3, 7, 8 - tetrachlorodibenzo-p-dioxin or TCDD. The toxicity of other dioxins- and chemicals like PCBs that act like dioxins - is measured in relation to TCDD.

Dioxin is a toxic heterocyclic hydrocarbon. Dioxins are widely distributed in the environment. Dioxin is produced as an unintentional byproduct of many industrial processes involving chlorine, importantly combustion and incineration, chemical manufacturing and processing, paper making, garbage incineration and pesticide prodution. Forest fires also release dioxins and are deposited onto the leaves of trees. Eventually dioxins find their way into rivers, lakes and seas and can thus be found in fish, concentrated in the fat. Dioxins tend to concentrate in the milk of the dairy cow.

Health risks associated with dioxins: Dioxins are highly toxic and present a real hazard to health. Even minute amounts of dioxin have been shown to cause damage to the nervous system and liver, apart from causing cancer. They can cause birth defects as well as mimic hormones that disrupt reproduction and human develoment. Dioxins released into the environment reach the food chain and get accumulated in fat. By far the greatest exposure to dioxin (over 90%) is from food.

Dioxin contamination: Dioxin contamination is global. In 1994, a U.S. Environmental Protection Agency (EPA) report claimed that the averge North American got approximately 32% of dioxin contamination from beef ingestion, 35% from milk and dairy products, 11% from chicken, 10% from pork, 7% from fish and 3% from eggs, as well as a small amount from soil, water and inhalation. Inhalation may be of greater significance near emission sources, such as incinerators.

Dioxin contaminated feed sources: These include fish meal, fish oil, recovered vegetable oil, grease and many byproducts from the food industry, bleaching earths and kaolinitic clays, milk products. When these are included in animal rations dioxins get concentrated in animal products.

It all happened when 90 tons of contaminated fat had gone into 1700 tons of feeds (5.3%) distributed to over 1500 farms in Belgium. The problem apparently began with a leakage of coolant from electrical transformers in January 1999. The news was not announced until May.

Since the results of a test for dioxin in animal products take several weeks to complete, more rapid testing was brought in based on the indicator substance polychlorinated biphenyl (PCB).

Codex Alimentarius Commission (CAC) and food safety

The Food and Agriculture Organisation (FAO) and the World Health Organisation (WHO) created the Codex Alimentarius (meaning food law or code in Latin) in 1963. The CAC is an international body with 172 member countries. The CAC aims at developing global food standards, guidelines and related texts such as codes of practice under the food standards programme of FAO and WHO, the bodies under the aegis of United Nations Organization (UNO).

In the open market scenario, India is facing challenges of global competitiveness. India is a signatory to World Trade Organisation (WTO) agreement on Technical Barriers to Trade (TBT). The only way to sustain in the global market is to harmonize Indian Standards as far as possible with International Standards. Harmonization is aligning the National Standards with International Standards and BIS had been doing this.

Hazard Analysis and Critical Control Point (HACCP) is a process control system designed to identify and prevent microbial and other hazards in food production. HACCP can be applied throughout the food chain from primary producer to final consumer.

CAC, which has been responsible for setting standards of food safety largely ignored the role of feed in the food chain. In 2004 during its 27th general session, it was formally approved after more than five years of intense negotiations involving government-level bodies. The Codex code of practice (COP) makes practical sense as a feed safety system for food-producing animals. **Now feed is part of the food industry.** The COP had risen in response to a spate of feed-related problems in Europe, from BSE and dioxin contamination to accusations over the inclusion of sewage sludge in feeds for some animals. **Melamine-tainted pet food brands** and melamine-tainted baby milk powder, in 2008, are recent happenings.

Office International des Epizooties (OIE) or World Organization for Animal Health has a permanent working group on Animal Production and Food Safety. This group has developed a synthesis between the Codex Alimentarius and the OIE on Food Safety throughout the food chain.

Tracking and tracing of feeds to recall

Tracking and tracing are magic words in modern feed/food production. Tracking involves the follow-up from the raw material/batch to the semi-finished or finished product that is supplied to the customer. Tracing means starting from the semi-finished or finished product and going back to the original raw materials / batches.

Following the BSE epidemic in Europe, safety of livestock-derived foods is high on research and regulatory agendas. DNA techniques are already in use for **tracking** of sources of *Salmonella enterica* and *Escherichia coli* outbreaks, as well as for **traceability** of product in the food chain. Recall of the pet foods in March 2007 due to contamination with melamine is a recent happening in the US. **Melamine** scrap was added to plant ingredients (wheat gluten) in China to enhance the protein content cheaply and the melamine can cause kidney failure and deaths. Melamine-tainted pet food from China was blamed for the deaths of large number of cats and dogs.

Health hazards associated with animal feed

Food safety hazards associated with animal feed can be biological, chemical, or physical. Hazards in feed may be inherent to feed ingredients as well as introduced during feed production, processing, handling, storage, transportation, and use (FAO, 2015). Hazards may also result from accidental or deliberate (e.g. fraud or bioterrorism) human intervention.

The chemical hazards include persistent organic pollutants such as dioxins and related things; veterinary drug residues; organochlorine and other pesticides; potentially toxic elements like arsenic, cadmium, lead, mercury; mycotoxins; and plant toxins like genotoxic pyrrolizidine alkaloids anti-nutritionals such as glucosinolates as well as other potential and emerging chemical hazards.

The biological hazards include primarily bacteria (Salmonella, Mycobacterium, Brucella, Clostridium spp, enterohaemorrhagic E.coli and Listeria) but also parasites (from pasture and forage), viruses and prions (e.g. the causative agent of bovine spongiform encephalopathy).

The physical hazards include radionuclides, residues of nanomaterials, micro- and nano-plastics and other relevant materials. Physical hazards (except nanomaterials and radionuclides) do not transfer to animal tissues and as such were not considered in terms of food safety.

Appendix I

1. Some Feedstuffs along with their Scientific Names

A. Cereal Grains   Synonym, if any
1. Oats (*Avena sativa*)   -
2. Barley (*Hordeum sativum*)   -
3. Rice (*Oryza sativa*)   -
4. Wheat (*Triticum aestivum*)   -
5. Maize (*Zea mays*)   -
6. Bajra (*Pennisetum typhoides*)   Pearl millet; Bulrush millet
   P. americanum
7. Ragi (*Eleusine coracana*)   Finger millet; Birdsfoot millet
8. Sorghum (*Sorghum bicolor*)   Great millet
9. Korra (*Setaria italica*)   Foxtail or Italian or German millet
10. Kodo millet   Ditch millet
    (*Paspalum scorbiculatum*)
11. Samulu (*Panicum miliare*)   Little millet
12. Variga (*Panicum miliaceum*)   Proso or Broomcorn or Hog millet
13. Rye (*Secale cereale*)   -
14. Triticale (Hybrid cereal)   -

B. Roots and Tubers
1. Tapioca   Manioc or Cassava
   (*Manihot esculenta syn. utillissima*)
2. Carrots
   (*Daucus carota*)
3. Sweet potatoes
   (*Ipomoea batatas*)
4. Turnips
5. Beet-Root
6. Potatoes (*Solanum tuberosum*)

C. **Legumes and others**
1. Pea (*Pisum sativum*)
2. Chick pea (*Cicer arietinum*) Gram
3. Groundnut (*Arachis hypogaea*)
4. Cottonseed (*Gossypium hirsutum, G. arboreum*)
5. Soybean (*Glycine max*)
6. Linnseed/Flax seed (*Linum usitatissimum*)
7. Sunflower (*Helianthus annus*)
8. Gingelly, Sesame, Til (*Sesamum indicum*)
9. Mustard (*Brassica juncea*)
10. Rapeseed, Brown sarson, (*brassica campestris var. brown sarson*)
11. Rapeseed, Gobhi sarson (*Brassica napus*)
12. Rapeseed, Toria (*B. campestris var. toria*)
13. Rapeseed, Yellow sarson (*B. campestris var. yellow sarson*)
14. Safflower (*Carthamus tinctorius*)
15. Coconut (*Cocos nucifera*)
16. Castor (*Ricinus cummunis*)
17. Oil palm (*Elaeis quineensis*)
18. Salseed (*Shorea robusta*)
19. Tamarind seed (*Tamarindus indica*)
20. Mango seed (*Mangifera indica*)
21. Sugarcane (*Saccharum officinarum*)
22. Khesari (*Lathyrus setivus*)
23. Lentil, Masoor (*Lens esculenta*)
24. Silk Cotton or Kapok (Ceiba pentandra)
25. Red Silk cotton or Indian Kapok tree (Bombax malabaricum)

2. **Fodder crops - popular varieties**
   I. **Cereal Fodders**
      1. Maize   - African tall variety, Ganga - 1, Ganga - 5
      2. Sorghum   - M.P. Chari, Sweet Sudan Grass (SSG)- 59-3
      3. Oats   - Kent, Fleming gold
      4. Teosinte   - a wild relative of maize (*Euchlaena mexicana*)
      5. Bajra   - Giant bajra, Rajko

   II. **Leguminous fodders**
      1. Berseem or Egyptian clover   -   Pusa giant, Mescawi, Khadrawi
         (*Trifolium alexandrium*)
      2. Lucerne or Alfalfa   -   Sirsa - 9
         (*Medicago sativa*)

3. Sunnhemp (*Crotalaria juncea*)
4. Horse gram (*Dolichos biflorus*)
5. Pillipesara (*Phaseolus trilobus*)
6. Field bean (*Lablab purpureus var. lingnosus; var. typicus*)
7. Cowpea (*Vigna sinensis*)   -   Russian giant variety
    (*Vigna unguiculata*)
8. Perennial redgram (*Pigeon pea*) (*Cajanus cajan*)
9. Kudzu vine (*Pueraria thunbergiana*)
10. Cluster beans (*Cyamopsis tetragonaloba*) Guar in Hindi
11. Hedge lucerne (*Desmanthes virgatus*)
12. Rice bean (*Phaseolus calcartus*) K-1 variety.

III. Perennial cultivated grasses

1. Napier grass (*Pennisetum purpureum*)
2. Hybrid napier/Pusa giant napier grass:
    (Napier x Bajra cross)
    NB-21, Co - 4 variety
3. Guinea grass (*Panicum maximum*) - Hamil variety
4. Para grass (*Brachiaria mutica*) Buffalo or water grass
5. Signal grass (*Brachiaria decumbens, B. brizantha*)
6. Rhodes grass (*Chloris gayana*)
7. Thin napier grass (*Pennisetum polystachyon*)
8. Blue panic grass (*Panicum antidotale*)
9. Dinanath grass (*Pennisetum pedicellatum*)
    (*Deenabandhu grass*)

IV. Indigenous grasses

1. Kolukkattai (*Tamil*) grass (*Cenchrus ciliaris*) Kusa gaddi
    (Telugu), Anjan (Hindi)
    C. setigeres (*Black Kolukkattai*)
2. Hariali grass (*Cynodon dactylon*), garika (*Telugu*),
    Doob grass
3. Giant star grass (*Cynodon plectostachyus*)
4. Marvel grass (*Dichanthium annulatum*), Molava gaddi -
    Telugu, Apang - Hindi
5. Spear grass (*Heteropogon contortus*), Pandumullu
    gaddi (Telugu)
6. Chengali gaddi (*Iseilema anthephoroides*)
7. Yerra chengali gaddi (*Iseilema laxum*)
8. Nendra gaddi (*Sehima nervosum*), Pavan grass
9. Johnson grass (*Sorghum halepense*)
10. *Desmostachya bipinnata* (Dharbha, Kusa darbha - Telugu)

V. Important pasture grasses

Cenchrus ciliaris, C. setigerus, Sehima nervosum, Pennisetum pedicellatum

VI. Important pasture legumes

Stylosanthes hamata, S. scabro, S. humilis, S. gracilis, Siratra (Macroptilium atropurpureum), Butterfly pea (Clitorea ternatea), Centrosema pubescens.

VII. Fodder trees / shrubs

1. Subabul (*Leucaena leucocephala*) - Peru, K-8 varieties
2. *Gliricidia maculata*
3. Agathi/Avisa (*Sesbania grandiflora*), Sesbania sesban, Shevri (*Sesbania aegyptica*)
4. The rain tree (*Samanea saman*), *Nidraganneru* - Telugu
5. *Acacia arabica, A. nilotica (Babul tree)*
6. Banyan tree (*Ficus bengalensis*)
7. Peepal tree (*Ficus religiosa*)
8. Water hyacinth (*Eichhornia cressipes*)
9. Khejri tree (*Prosopis spicigera*) - Sanjeevani of the desert
10. *Prosopis juliflora*
11. *Pongamia glabra (Kanuga* - Telugu)
12. *Butea frondosa, Dhak* (Hindi), *Moduga* (Telugu).

3. Acid - binding capacity (ABC) of foodstuffs

The standard test involves finding how much hydrochloric acid is needed per kilo foodstuff to reach pH 3.0 after one hour at 37°C. The greater the quantity in meq/kg, the more that foodstuff will be able to neutralise the digestive acid secreted by the gastric mucosa. Grains such as maize, wheat and barley have a rather low ABC value around 200 meq/ kg. Ingredients such as soybean meal, skimmed milk powder and fish meal have values of 1200 or more. Minerals have ABC values around 20,000.

The digestibility of a diet is affected adversely by ingredients which bind acid. Acid – binding capacity of 750 meg/kg or more can favour the development of *E. coli* in the piglets gut, increasing the risk of bacterial diarrhoea. Acidification can promote better growth and improved feed conversion ratio in addition to avoiding a diarrhoea in early weaned (3 weeks of age) piglets. Danish standards recommend a maximum ABC of 720 meq/kg for the finished feed in pigs.

Appendix II

1. Pathways for pyruvate utilization
2. Conversion factors
3. Table: Example of conversion of nitrogen and crude protein of feeds from as fed basis to dry matter basis (DMB)
4. Common functional groups and linkages in molecules

1. Pyruvate that is Produced in Glycolysis Can Take one of the Following Directions:

1. It can enter the mitochondria and thereby go through the TCA cycle. This is the most frequent pathway.
2. It can be reversibly reduced to form lactic acid.
3. It can be converted back to carbohydrate by glycogenesis (reverse glycolysis).
4. It can be oxidized to oxaloacetate for the TCA cycle.
5. It can be converted to the amino acid alanine by transamination.
6. It can be reduced to malate (malic acid) and enter TCA cycle.
7. It can be oxidatively decarboxilated to acetyl Co A in mitochondria and follow lipid synthesis pathway after reaching cytosol.

2. Conversion Factors

1 mg retinol is 3333 IU vitamin A.

1 mg cholecalciferol is 40000 IU vitamin D_3.

1 mg DL α- tocopherol acetate is 1 IU vitamin E.

One IU of vitamin C is the activity contained in 0.05 mg of the vitamin. Thus, 1 mg of vitamin C is the same as 20 IU of vitamin C.

3. Table: Example of Conversion of Nitrogen and Crude Protein of Feeds From as Fed Basis to Dry Matter Basis (DMB)

Tree leaf	Moisture	On as fed basis		On DM Basis	
	%	Nitrogen, %	Crude protein, %	Nitrogen, %	Crude Protein, %
Acacia auriculiformis	62.51	0.93	5.84	2.48	15.50
Cashew	65.45	0.52	3.26	1.51	9.41
Gliricidia	79.99	0.78	4.87	3.90	24.38
Jack	67.60	0.67	4.26	2.07	12.94
Sesbania grandiflora	79.40	1.15	7.18	5.58	34.88
Subabul	63.11	1.30	8.13	3.52	22.00
Yellow gold mohur	67.11	0.64	3.94	1.95	12.16

4. TABLE   Common functional groups and linkages in molecules

Compound Name	Structure ^{a}	Functional Group or Linkage
Amine ^{b}	RNH_2 or $R\overset{+}{N}H_3$ R_2NH or $R_2\overset{+}{N}H_2$ R_3N or $R_3\overset{+}{N}H$	$-N\langle$ or $\overset{+}{-}\overset{\vert}{\underset{\vert}{N}}-$ (amino group)
Alcohol	ROH	— OH (hydroxyl group)
Thiol	RSH	— SH (sulfhydryl group)
Ether	ROR	— O — (ether linkage)
Aldehyde	$R-\overset{O}{\overset{\|}{C}}-H$	$-\overset{O}{\overset{\|}{C}}-$ (carbonyl group)
Ketone	$R-\overset{O}{\overset{\|}{C}}-R$	$-\overset{O}{\overset{\|}{C}}-$ (carbonyl group)
Carboxylic acid ^{b}	$R-\overset{O}{\overset{\|}{C}}-OH$ or $R-\overset{O}{\overset{\|}{C}}-O^-$	$-\overset{O}{\overset{\|}{C}}-OH$ (carboxyl group) or $-\overset{O}{\overset{\|}{C}}-O^-$ (carboxylate group)
Ester	$R-\overset{O}{\overset{\|}{C}}-OR$	$-\overset{O}{\overset{\|}{C}}-O-$ (ester linkage) $R-\overset{O}{\overset{\|}{C}}-$ (acyl group) ^{c}

Compound Name	Structure [a]	Functional Group or Linkage
Thioester	$$R-\overset{\displaystyle O}{\overset{\|}{C}}-SR$$	$-\overset{\displaystyle O}{\overset{\|}{C}}-S-$ (thioester linkage) $R-\overset{\displaystyle O}{\overset{\|}{C}}-$ (acyl group)[c]
Amide	$$R-\overset{\displaystyle O}{\overset{\|}{C}}-NH_2$$ $$R-\overset{\displaystyle O}{\overset{\|}{C}}-NHR$$ $$R-\overset{\displaystyle O}{\overset{\|}{C}}-NR_2$$	$-\overset{\displaystyle O}{\overset{\|}{C}}-N\big\langle$ (amido group) $R-\overset{\displaystyle O}{\overset{\|}{C}}-$ (acyl group)[c]
Imine (Schiff base)[b]	$R=NH$ or $R=\overset{+}{N}H_2$ $R=NH$ or $R=\overset{+}{N}HR$	$\big\rangle C=N-$ or $\big\rangle C=\overset{+}{N}\big\langle$ (imino group)
Disulfide	$R-S-S-R$	$-S-S-$ (disulfide linkage)
Phosphate ester [b]	$$R-O-\underset{\underset{\textstyle OH}{\|}}{\overset{\overset{\textstyle O}{\|}}{P}}-O^-$$	$-\underset{\underset{\textstyle OH}{\|}}{\overset{\overset{\textstyle O}{\|}}{P}}-O^-$ (phosphoryl group)
Diphosphate ester [b]	$$R-O-\underset{\underset{\textstyle O^-}{\|}}{\overset{\overset{\textstyle O}{\|}}{P}}-O-\underset{\underset{\textstyle OH}{\|}}{\overset{\overset{\textstyle O}{\|}}{P}}-O^-$$	$-\underset{\underset{\textstyle O^-}{\|}}{\overset{\overset{\textstyle O}{\|}}{P}}-O-\underset{\underset{\textstyle OH}{\|}}{\overset{\overset{\textstyle O}{\|}}{P}}-O^-$ (phosphoanhydride group)
Phosphate diester [b]	$$R-O-\underset{\underset{\textstyle O^-}{\|}}{\overset{\overset{\textstyle O}{\|}}{P}}-O-R$$	$-O-\underset{\underset{\textstyle O^-}{\|}}{\overset{\overset{\textstyle O}{\|}}{P}}-O-$ (phosphodiester linkage)

[a]**R** represents any carbon-containing group. In a molecule with more than one R group, the groups may be the same or different;

[b]Under physiological conditions, these groups are ionized and hence bear a positive or negative charge;

[c]If attached to an atom other than carbon.

Index